Osteopathy and Physical Medicine

Osteopathy and Physical Medicine

Edited by **Pete Edner**

SYRAWOOD
PUBLISHING HOUSE
New York

Published by Syrawood Publishing House,
750 Third Avenue, 9th Floor,
New York, NY 10017, USA
www.syrawoodpublishinghouse.com

Osteopathy and Physical Medicine
Edited by Pete Edner

International Standard Book Number: 978-1-68286-356-5 (Hardback)

Printed in China.

Contents

Preface

Osteopathy and physical medicine are both focused on the manipulation and restoration of the body's muscles. This book deals with the diagnostic practices and scope of treatment in these fields. It elucidates the various methods practiced across the globe and brings forth the most up-to-date researches revolving around them. This book is an essential guide for students and academicians in these fields. It will also prove beneficial to the professionals associated with these fields.

This book has been the outcome of endless efforts put in by authors and researchers on various issues and topics within the field. The book is a comprehensive collection of significant researches that are addressed in a variety of chapters. It will surely enhance the knowledge of the field among readers across the globe.

It gives us an immense pleasure to thank our researchers and authors for their efforts to submit their piece of writing before the deadlines. Finally in the end, I would like to thank my family and colleagues who have been a great source of inspiration and support.

Editor

Systematic review of clinical trials of cervical manipulation: control group procedures and pain outcomes

Howard Vernon*, Aaron Puhl, Christine Reinhart

Abstract

Objective: To characterize the types of control procedures used in controlled clinical trials of cervical spine manipulation and to evaluate the outcomes obtained by subjects in control groups so as to improve the quality of future clinical trials

Methods: A search of relevant clinical trials was performed in PubMed 1966-May 2010 with the following key words: "Chiropractic"[Mesh] OR "Manipulation, Spinal"[Mesh]) AND "Clinical Trial "[Publication Type]. Reference lists from these trials were searched for any additional trials. The reference lists of two prior studies, one review and one original study were also searched. Accepted reports were then rated for quality by 2 reviewers using the PEDro scale. Studies achieving a score of >50% were included for data extraction and analysis. Intra-group change scores on pain outcomes were obtained. For determining clinically important outcomes, a threshold of 20% improvement was used where continuous data were available; otherwise, an effect size of 0.30 was employed

Results: The PubMed search yielded 753 citations of which 13 were selected. Eight (8) other studies were identified by reviewing two systematic reviews and through reference searches. All studies scored >50% on the PEDro scale. There were 9 multi-session studies and 12 single-session studies. The most commonly used control procedure was "manual contact/no thrust". Four (4) studies used a placebo-control (patient blinded). For two of these studies with VAS data, the average change reported was 4.5 mm. For the other control procedures, variable results were obtained. No clinically important changes were reported in 57% of the paired comparisons, while, in 43% of these, changes which would be considered clinically important were obtained in the control groups. Only 15% of trials reported on post-intervention group registration.

Conclusions: Most control procedures in cervical manipulation trials result in small clinical changes, although larger changes are observed in 47% of paired comparisons. The vast majority of studies do not result in subject blinding; the effect of unmasking of control subjects in these studies makes the interpretation of the existing clinical trials challenging. The greatest majority of trials do not report on post-intervention blinding. A small number of candidate procedures for effective control interventions exist. Much more research is required to improve this important aspect of clinical trial methodology in cervical manipulation studies.

Introduction

Clinical trials of spinal manipulation for neck pain have been published since the early 1980's. Numerous reviews of these trials have been published in the ensuing years [1-3]. The lack of a valid control group has been a consistent criticism of this body of studies [1-5]. In 2005, Vernon et al. [6] reported on a candidate manoeuvre for a cervical sham manipulation (sham cervical thrust using a "drop" headpiece). In a small group of neck pain patients, 60% mis-registered the sham manoeuvre as a "real treatment". In these subjects, no clinically important changes were obtained post-intervention in paraspinal pressure pain thresholds (R-PPT decreased by an average of 1.2%; L-PPT decreased by an average of 6%) as well as in cervical ranges of motion.

* Correspondence: hvernon@cmcc.ca
Canadian Memorial Chiropractic College 6100 Leslie St., Toronto, Ontario, M2H 3J1, Canada

In that report, the literature on studies of manipulation with sham/placebo manoeuvres was briefly reviewed. Of note were the studies of Hawk and her colleagues [7-9] who identified numerous issues attendant with the development and use of sham manipulations. Their work was focused on the lumbar spine and low back pain patients. The review by Ernst and Harkness [4] was also mentioned as one of the works critical of the extant clinical trials in manipulation for neck pain.

Vernon et al. [10] conducted a systematic review of the outcome of control groups used in clinical trials of conservative treatments for chronic neck pain. These trials included primarily laser and acupuncture studies; no study of manual therapy was included. In this review, the mean [95% CI] effect size of change in pain ratings in the no-treatment control studies at outcome points up to 10 weeks was 0.18 [-0.05, 0.41] and for outcomes from 12-52 weeks it was 0.4 [0.12, 0.68]. In the placebo control groups it was 0.50 [0.10, 0.90] at up to 10 weeks and 0.33. [-1.97, 2.66] at 12-24 weeks. None of the comparisons between the no-treatment and placebo groups were statistically significant. It was concluded that changes in pain scores in subjects with chronic neck pain not due to whiplash who are enrolled in no-treatment and placebo control groups were similarly small and not significantly different. As well, they do not appear to increase over longer-term follow-up. The placebo and no-treatment control procedures in these trials appeared to be successful in inducing relatively little therapeutic benefit.

There has been no similar review of the control procedures and control group outcomes of trials of manipulation in the cervical spine for neck pain and headaches, although a review of control group outcomes in lumbar spine trials has recently been published [11]. Such a review would assist clinicians and researchers in determining the validity of the existing evidence base as well as the applicability and generalizability of the control procedures which have been employed to date. It would also identify issues for consideration by future clinical trial groups.

Methods

Search Strategy

A search for randomized controlled clinical trials was performed in PubMed 1966-May 2010 with the following key words: "Chiropractic"[Mesh] OR "Manipulation, Spinal"[Mesh]) AND "Clinical Trial "[Publication Type]. Reference lists from these selected trials were searched for any additional trials. The reference lists of two prior studies, one review [4] and one original study [6] were also reviewed. Finally, after reviewing the retrieval lists from these searches, the authors identified some additional trials from the general literature.

Inclusion Criteria

Studies were included into the quality review round if they fulfilled the following criteria:

a) randomized clinical trial
b) cervical spinal manipulation was the index treatment (studies of thoracic manipulation were excluded)
c) a control group was used in any of the following forms
   a. placebo treatment
   b. non-blinded control treatment
   c. no-treatment or waiting list control
d) the clinical complaint was neck pain, neck and arm pain or headaches
e) data from a pain-related outcome was provided for each group at relevant times
e) English language

Study Selection

The inclusion criteria were applied by the senior author to the titles and abstracts of the studies identified in the searches.

Quality reviewing

Studies included in the review were then subjected to quality rating by two independent raters (not the senior author). Ratings were derived using the PEDro Scale [12] for a score out of 11. Scores were converted into a percentage figure. Each rater conducted a separate rating. After this, ratings were compared. When exact agreement was not achieved, a consensus method was used to resolve any disagreements in ratings. This method involved the two raters working together first. If any disagreements could not be resolved between them, the senior author joined the discussion and forced a consensus rating. Studies scoring higher than 50% were included in the review.

Categorization of the included studies

Studies were separated into two categories: 1) single and 2) multiple intervention session trials.

Data extraction and analyses

Data were extracted by a single author. The following data was extracted: complaint type, number of subjects in the control group, control intervention type, type of primary outcome measure, whether blinding was checked post-intervention, primary pain-related outcome data for the control group(s) (typically a VAS: means, variance measures, effect sizes). For determining clinically important changes, several criteria were employed. Where continuous data were available, a threshold of 20% improvement was used; otherwise, an effect size of 0.30 was employed [similar to Vernon et al. [10,13,14]. Data were not formally pooled, although, when possible, means (sd) of the outcomes of selected groups of trials were computed. Data from the index treatment group was not analyzed.

Results

The PubMed search yielded 753 citations of which 13 were selected [15-26]. The manual search of Ernst and Harkness' study [4] identified no additional studies. The search of Vernon et al. [6] identified 3 additional studies [27-29]. The senior author identified 5 additional studies [30-34] for a total of 21 studies. There were four exceptions to the inclusion rules as follows: the trial by Bakris et al [33] was accepted for its unique approach to creating a control procedure; the trials by Buchman et al. [17], Tuttle et al. [23] and Dunning and Rushton [24] were accepted as manual control studies, even though the outcome measure was not pain-related.

The types of control interventions are described in Table 1. The quality scores and data extraction for these 21 studies are depicted in Table 2. All studies scored above 50% and were included in the review. The mean quality score for all these studies was 77.8 (11.7) %. There were 9 multiple session studies [15,16,27-29,31,33,34] whose average quality score was 82.5% (9.2). Of these, 6 were for headaches [15,28,29,31,34,35], 2 were for neck pain [16,27] and 1 was for another complaint (hypertension [33]). There were 12 single session studies whose average quality score was 74.2% (11.9). Of these, 10 were for neck pain and 2 were for other complaints in the upper limb. There was a statistically significant difference in the quality scores favouring the multi-session studies ($t = 2.49$, $p = 0.01$). Both groups of studies had an average of 24 subjects per group (range for multi-session = 9-40; range for single session = 8-54).

Pain outcomes

Ten (10) trials [15,16,18,26-30,32,34] employed a pain visual analogue scale (VAS) to record neck pain or headache intensity; one [Haas 10] used an 11-point numerical rating scale. Six (6) trials [19-22,25,26], all single-session, employed a pressure threshold algometer to measure pressure pain thresholds over the neck, upper back or upper limb.

Pain outcomes by control group type

Four trials employed some form of placebo control. Sloop et al.'s trial for neck pain [27] employed anamnestic valium in both groups with the control group receiving no actual manipulations. Outcomes were obtained at an average of two weeks post-treatments. Most patients received only one treatment, while some received two. The mean change in VAS scores in the control group was -5 mm; however, the standard deviation for this value was quite large at 32 mm. Vernon et al.'s [31] trial for tension-type headache employed a factorial design whereby three of four groups received at least one placebo/sham version of the therapies (amitryptiline and spinal manipulation) with one of these groups receiving both placebo treatments. This was the only trial to employ a sham cervical manipulation treatment; however, there was no report of the outcomes for each group separately, so no data were available for this review on the outcome of the double placebo group.

Two trials used de-tuned therapy devices as the control treatment. Tuchin et al.s' [15] multi-session trial for migraine headaches employed de-tuned interferential therapy and reported an average headache intensity reduction in the control group of 17 mm with an effect size of 1.17. Pikula's single session study [32] employed two control groups, one of which received du-tuned ultrasound. The immediate pain reduction averaged 4 mm with an effect size of 0.18.

Using the Sloop et al. and Pikula trials for estimating pain reduction on a VAS in the placebo control groups provides an average of 4.5 mm reduction, which is well below the level most often adopted for minimal clinically important difference and is in accord with the

Table 1 Types of control interventions

Intervention type	Multiple session studies	Single session studies
Placebo: drug only	1	0
Placebo: non-manual therapy	1	1
Placebo: drug + sham manual therapy	1	0
Manual thrust at alternate site (randomly different [30], contralateral [32], ineffective site [33])	1	2
Manual contact: no thrust	2	10
Low level manual therapy	1	0
Low level non-manual therapy only	0	0
Low level manual + non-manual therapy	1	0
Waiting list	1	0

Figures add up to 22 due to use of 2 control groups in [Pikula].

Table 2 Review of studies of manipulation and control or placebo comparison

STUDY (First author name)	PEDro	REGION/COMPLAINT	"PLACEBO" MANEUVER	N (CONTROL GROUP)	BLINDING CHECKED?	PRIMARY OUTCOME MEASURE	PRIMARY OUTCOME FOR CONTROL GROUP
Multi-session							
Sloop, 1982 [27]	**8/11**	Neck pain	Diazepam (anamnestic) with no treatment	18	Yes	For neck pain: - VAS - NVS	VAS change @ 3 wks = 5 mm (±32 mm) NVS = 28% subjects reported treatment helped
Nilsson et al., 1997 [28]	**9/11**	Cervical: headache	Low power laser light and deep friction massage	25	NR	- headache hrs - headache intensity - analgesic use	Avg HA (hrs/day ± inter4tile range) pre = 4.0; post = 2.4; Δ = -1.6 ± 2.5 Avg HA intensity (mm ± inter4tile range) Pre = 41; post = 36; Δ = -4.2 ± 26 Avg analgesics/day ± inter4tile range Pre = 1.0; post = 0.7; Δ = -0.3 ± 1
Bove and Nilsson, 1998 [29]	**9/11**	Cervical spine: Headache	Low power laser light and deep friction massage (described as both an "active control" and as the "placebo" group)	37	NR	pre = 2 wks post = 7 wks follow-up = 19 wks -headache hrs -headache intensity (VAS) -analgesic use	Avg HA hrs/day (95% CI) Pre = 3.4 (2.4-4.4) post = 1.9 (0.9-2.9); Δ = -1.5 follow-up = 2.2 (1.2-3.2); Δ = -1.2 Avg HA intensity (95% CI) Pre = 37 mm (33-41) post = 34 mm (26-38); Δ = -3 follow-up = 26 mm (20-32); Δ = -11 * Avg analgesics/day (95% CI) Pre = 0.82 (0.5-1.14) post = 0.59 (0-1.49); Δ = -0.23 follow-up = 0.56 (0.22-0.9); Δ = -0.26
Tuchin et al., 2000 [15]	**7/11**	Cervical spine - migraines	De-tuned interferential therapy	40	NR	Headaches per month Headache intensity (VAS) Headache duration (hrs) analgesics/month	Avg HA/month (SD) Pre = 7.3 (6.53) post = 6.9 (6.6); ES = 0.06 Avg HA intensity VAS (SD) Pre = 7.89 (1.2) post = 6.2 (1.7); ES = 1.17 * Avg HA duration in hrs/episode (SD) Pre = 22.6 (27.4) post = 19.8 (17.7); ES = 0.12 Avg analgesics/month (SD) Pre = 20.1 (28.4) post = 16.2 (12.4); ES = 0.19

Table 2 Review of studies of manipulation and control or placebo comparison *(Continued)*

Alison et al., 2002 [16]	**8/11**	Neck and arm pain	Waiting list	10	N/A	-SF-MPQ - NPQ - VAS	Median SF-MPQ (inter4ile range) Pre = 10.0 (9.0) Post = 7.5 (4.0); Δ = -2.5 * median NPQ (inter4tile range) Pre = 12.5 (4.0) Post = 11.5 (6.0); Δ = -1.0 median VAS (inter4tile range) Pre = 3.3 (3.5) Post = 3.8 (3.9); Δ = 0.5
Bakris et al., 2007 [33]	**9/11**	Cervical spine - hypertension	Manual contact, Inappropriate direction of thrust	25	NR	BP & pulse	Systolic BP: Pre = 145.3; post = 142.1; Δ = -3.2 Diastolic BP: Pre = 91.0; post = 89.2; Δ = -1.8 Pulse rate Pre = 73.3; post = 73.8, Δ = -0.5
Vernon et al., 2009 [31]	**9/11**	Cervical spine: headache	Sham manipulation with head thrust, but no segmental thrust + placebo meds	9	Yes[##]	Reduction of headache days	Outcome not reported for sham manipulation only
Borusiak et al., 2009 [34]	**8/11**	Cervical spine: pediatric headache	Light touch/no thrust	28	Yes	- % of days with HA - Duration of HA - Intensity of HA	% of days with HA (SD) Pre = 41.2 (28.5) Post = 31.8 (28.3); ES = 0.33 * Duration of HA in hours (SD) Pre = 113.8 (115.1) Post = 107.2 (121.1); ES = 0.06 Intensity of HA VAS (SD) Pre = 4.9 (1.8) Post = 5.0 (1.8); ES = 0.06
Haas et al., 2010 [35]	**11/11**	Cervical spine/ cervicogenic headache	Heat + light massage:		NR	Numerical rating scales for: A - Headache intensity	
			Group 1- 8 sessions	20			Percentage score - Group 1: Pre = 56.8 (15.8) 12 wk = 42.0 (20.6); ES = 0.81 * 24 wk = 41.5 (18.2); ES = 0.90 *
			Group 2- 16 sessions	20		B - Neck pain	Percentage score - Group 2: Pre = 58.7 (17.1) 12 wk = 49.4 (19.0); ES = 0.52 * 24 wk = 48.6 (21.4); ES = 0.52 * Percentage score - Group 1: Pre = 60.5 (21.4) 12 wk = 47.1 (24.2); ES = 0.59 * 24 wk = 47.2 (21.8); ES = 0.58 * Percentage score - Group 2: Pre = 48.5 (23.6) 12 wk = 42.8 (21.6); ES = 0.25 24 wk = 48.4 (23.1); ES = 0.004

Table 2 Review of studies of manipulation and control or placebo comparison *(Continued)*

Single session							
Pikula, 1999 [32]	**6/11**	Neck pain	1. SMT- contralateral 2. Detuned US	1-12 2-12	NR	VAS neck pain	1. Contralateral manip VAS (SD) Pre = 44.1 (27.5) post = 41.4 (28.4) ES = 0.10 2. Placebo UltraSound VAS (SD) Pre = 50.4 (22.5) post = 46.5 (21.8) ES = 0.18
Haas et al 2003 [30]	**11/11**	Neck pain	Alternate site manipulation	52	NR	Pain (VAS) Measured immediately after and later that evening (~ 6 hours)	Pain VAS (SD) Pre = 40.4 (20.9) post = 24.7 (19.5); ES = 0.78 * follow-up = 28.7 (19.6); ES = 0.58 *
Buchmann et al., 2005 [17]	**6/11**	Cervical spine	Manual contact, no rotation, no thrust	8	NR	Dysfunctional motion segments	Pre contact = 13 dysfunctional segments Post contact = 13 dysfunctional segments
Martinez-Segura et al., 2006 [18]	**8/11**	Cervical spine - Neck pain	Manual contact, cervical rotation, no thrust	37	NR	Resting neck pain (VAS)	Resting neck pain VAS (SD) Pre = 5.5 (1.7) post = 5.1 (1.9) ES = 0.22
Fernandez De Las Penas et al., 2007 [19]	**7/11**	Cervical spine - healthy subjects	Manual contact, cervical rotation, no thrust	15	NR	PPT at elbow both ipsi and contral.	Ipsi elbow PPT Pre = 2.3(0.4); post = 2.3 (0.5); ES = 0 Contra elbow PPT Pre = 2.3(0.5); post = 2.3 (0.6); ES = 0
Ruiz-Saez et al., 2007 [20]	**8/11**	Cervical spine - trapezius MTrP's	Manual contact, cervical rotation, no thrust	36	NR	PPT at trapezius trigger points	Pre = 1.34 (0.4) Post = 1.27 (0.4); ES = -0.18 Post 5 min = 1.15 (0.4); ES = 0.48 * Post 10 min = 1.1 (0.5); ES = 0.53 *
Fernandez-Carnero et al., 2008 [21]	**8/11**	Cervical spine - tennis elbow	Manual contact, cervical rotation, no thrust	10	NR	- PPT	Affected elbow PPT Pre = 314.4 (11.6); post = 327.7 (18.6) ES = 0.88 * Contralateral elbow PPT Pre = 475.2 (78.5); post = 481.2 (84.6) ES = 0.07
						- Thermal pain threshold (TPT)	Affected elbow TPT (°C) Pre = 41.1 (3.4); post = 41.8 (1.3) ES = 0.3 Contralateral elbow TPT (°C) Pre = 44.3 (1.5); post = 43.4 (0.9) ES = 0.75
						- Pain free grip strength (PFG)	PFG (KG) affected side Pre = 14.7 (6.0); post = 13.6 (6.2) ES = 0.18

Table 2 Review of studies of manipulation and control or placebo comparison *(Continued)*

Fernandez De Las Penas et al., 2008 [22]	**8/11**	Cervical spine- healthy subjects	Manual contact, cervical rotation, no thrust	10	NR	C5-C6 Z-joint tenderness (PPT)	Left Z-joint PPT Pre = 316.4 (30.5); post = 311.8 (32.8) ES = 0.15 Right Z-joint PPT Pre = 315.0 (43.8); post = 312.3 (47.7) ES = 0.06
Tuttle et al., 2008 [23]	**7/10[1]**	Cervical spine - neck pain	Mobilization applied to non-symptomatic level	20	NR	AROM stiffness	NS decrease in flex/ext AROM NS increase in lat flex and rotation NS decrease in stiffness (data not reported; only graphic data)
Dunning and Rushton, 2009 [24]	**6/10[1]**	Cervical spine - EMG of biceps muscle	Manual contact, cervical rotation, no thrust	54	NR	Biceps resting EMG	21.12% (±5%) increase in resting EMG of right bicep after sham 17.15% (±7%) increase in resting EMG of left bicep after sham
Mansila-Ferragut et al., 2009 [25]	**8/11**	Upper cervical spine - neck pain	Manual contact, cervical rotation, no thrust	19	NR	- PPT at the sphenoid - Active mouth opening	PPT (95% CI) Pre = 0.8 (0.7 - 0.9) Post = 0.7 (0.5 - 0.9); Δ = -0.1 Active mouth opening in mm (95% CI) Pre = 36.2 (34.3 - 38.2) Post = 35.9 (33.7 - 38.0); Δ = -0.3
Sterling et al., 2010 [26]	**8/11**	Neck pain findings	Manual contact	17	NR	- PPT at C6 - Nociceptive Flexion Reflex (NFR) threshold - VAS pain from NFR	PPT at C6 (SD) Pre = 216.1 (103.2) Post = 253.4 (114.2); ES = 0.34 * NFR threshold (SD) Pre = 8.0 (5) Post = 7.9 (5.4); ES = -0.02 VAS pain from NFR (SD) Pre = 4.5 (3.8) Post = 3.6 (2.8); ES = 0.27

VAS = visual analogue scale; NVS = numerical verbal scale; HA = headache; avg = average; inter4tile = interquartile; US = ultrasound; NR = not reported; SF-MPQ = Short-form McGill Pain Questionnaire; NPQ = Neck Pain Questionnaire; PPT = pressure pain threshold; ipsi = ipsilateral; contra = contralateral; MTrP's = myofascial trigger points; BP = blood pressure; z-joint = zygapophyseal joint; AROM = active range of motion; EMG = electromyogram.

Reported on double placebo registration (not just for sham manipulation).

* Clinically important change.

[1]In these two studies, subjects received all treatments; intention-to-treat was not applicable: PEDro score out of 10.

values of placebo control group outcomes reported by Vernon et al. [10] in non-manual therapy trials.

Three trials employed, as the control treatment, cervical manipulation at an "alternate" site. Bakris et al. [33] employed recoil manipulation at what they defined as an ineffective site. As their study investigated the effect of manipulation on blood pressure, no pain-related outcomes were available. They did report virtually no difference in systolic and diastolic blood pressure pre-post intervention in this control group. Pikula [32] employed manipulation to the contralateral side in his single-session control group. He reported an average of 3 mm reduction on a pain VAS (effect size = 0.10). Haas et al. [30] employed a cervical manipulation at an alternate site from the target pain site. This site was determined randomly and compared to sites which had been determined by manual palpation. They reported an average VAS reduction of 16 mm (effect size = 0.78) which is considered a clinically important change.

Data on pain outcomes was available from fourteen (14) trials with non-placebo control groups (5 multi-session; 9 single session). In the five multi-session trials, control groups received either low-level manual contact with no thrust [28,29,34,35] or a waiting list [16]. In three of these studies [16,28,29], the average pain reduction on a VAS was 3 mm. Bove and Nilsson [29] also reported a 7-week follow-up of an average 11 mm reduction in their tension-type headache patient's headache intensity. Haas et al. reported relatively small percentage reductions in headache pain (14.8% for the 8-treatment group, 9.3% for the 16-treatment group at 12 weeks, 15.3% and 9.9% respectively at 24 weeks); however, the effect sizes for these changes were above our threshold (0.90 and 0.52 for 12 weeks; 0.52 and 0.52 for 16 weeks). The fifth trial [34] reported virtually no change in their pediatric headache control group.

Of the nine (9) single-session studies [18-20,22, 23,25,26,30,32], two [30,32] employed a contra-lateral or alternate site thrusting manipulation; the other 7 studies used a "manual contact/no thrust" procedure. The mean [95% CI] effect size for VAS reduction of neck pain (five groups [Pikula x2 [32], Haas et al. [30], Martinez-Segura et al. [18], Sterling et al. [26]) was 0.31 [-0.02,0.64]. The mean [95% CI] effect size for neck, trapezius and elbow PPT reduction in 6 groups [19-22,25,26] was 0.34 [0,0.68]. These mean ES just exceeded our threshold for minimally important clinical difference.

Three single-session studies which used manual contact/no thrust controls did not report pain-related outcomes. Their results were as follows: in Buchman et al. [17], the control procedure appeared to have no effect on the presence of palpable cervical segmental dysfunctions; in Tuttle et al. [23], there was no significant change in active ranges of motion; in Dunning and Rushton's trial [24], resting EMG of the biceps muscle increased by an average of 21% on the ipsilateral side and 17% on the opposite side. The first two of these studies provided some support for the proposition that non-thrust procedures do not result in changes in the mobility of the cervical spine.

With regard to clinically important changes, the 21 reviewed studies provided 35 comparisons of baseline to post-treatment pain scores (some trials had no pain-related outcomes; some trials had 2 or 3 comparison times for a pain-related outcome (Haas et al. [35] had 8 such comparisons). In 15 (43%) of these comparisons (8 trials), the control group outcomes exceeded the minimum threshold of 20% reduction of pain/tenderness or effect size greater than 0.30 (See Table 2 for *). In these 8 trials, 5 employed manual contact/no thrust controls [20,21,26,30,35], 1 employed a waiting list [16], 1 employed low level laser and deep massage [29] and 1 employed detuned ultrasound [15]. This latter trial is notable as it was the only one of these 8 trials to use a single-blind placebo treatment; the control group effect size for average headache intensity reduction was 1.17.

The nine (9) multi-session studies merit additional analysis. Seven of these trials [15,16,27-29,34,35] provided pain-related outcome comparisons; however, five of them were for headache and only two [16,27] were for neck pain. Within these trials, the control procedures which did not result in a mean reduction of pain that reached the clinically important threshold included anamnestic valium, low power laser + deep frictions, light touch/no thrust.

With respect to the issue of confirming the success of the blinding or the subject's identification of their group assignment, only 3 trials (15%) reported performing this check [27,31,34], all of which used placebo controls. These studies reported that the blinding was generally successful. Two studies which did use a placebo control [32,33] did not report post-intervention registration. None of the studies which used non-placebo control groups reported on the degree to which subjects in each of their study groups could identify their group registration.

Discussion

The primary objective of this review was to characterize the types of control procedures used in controlled clinical trials of cervical spinal manipulation and the outcomes obtained by subjects in these groups. The goal of this analysis was to identify areas for improvement in future controlled clinical trials. Twenty-one (21) trials were identified, 9 multi-session trials and 12 single-session trials. The most commonly employed control group procedure was "manual contact/no thrust" (12 groups). The clinical outcomes obtained in these control groups are varied, as discussed below.

Clinical trial theory posits that the ideal control treatment should account for all of the non-specific effects of the index treatment but carry none of the direct therapeutic benefits [5-11]. Machado et al. [11] used the following terms to describe these attributes: a placebo treatment that has no known or substantiated therapeutic mechanism is termed "inert"; an inert placebo which mimics the index treatment in all aspects, including the replication of any common side effects is termed "indistinguishable"; when placebos cannot be made indistinguishable, researchers should strive to create "structural equivalence". This term refers to the degree to which the control procedures are as similar in nature and delivery as possible to the index treatment.

Any difference between the index and control treatments that is obtained in the trial ("the trial effect size") should, theoretically, result from the therapeutic mechanism purported to exist in the index therapy. Any deviation from this ideal circumstance has important effects on the potential success of a clinical trial by, for example, increasing the therapeutic effect of the control treatment, thus reducing the trial effect size (Type II error) or by increasing the therapeutic effect of the index treatment (Type I error).

Hawk and colleagues [7-9] and Hancock et al. [5] have noted that the development of placebo manipulation procedures by researchers in manipulative therapy has been challenging. They identified two important objectives of placebo manipulation procedures: 1) the equalization of the non-specific effect of physical touch between groups of subjects, and 2) the blinding of the subject as to the nature of the treatment. Hawk et al. identified the essence of such a placebo manoeuvre in that it "increase(es) the believability of the intervention, thus equalizing the effect of expectation of improvement between groups" [7].

Strong placebogenic effects of manipulation [4-9,36] have been hypothesized. Key factors in this regard include the encouragement of patient relaxation in order to facilitate the procedure, the generic or non-specific effects of manual contact, including fulfillment of patients' expectations regarding manual contact on subjectively felt problem sites and the effect of the thrust and cavitation in fulfilling patient expectations that "something important has just happened". This latter point is often reinforced or amplified by positive feedback statement or behavior from the clinician [36].

Sham cervical manipulation procedures should account for the following issues: tactile contact with the skin, head and neck motions involved in the procedure, mechanical loads applied to the tissues and the sounds associated with them. Differences between a sham and an actual procedure for any one or more of these characteristics might be responsible for cuing the patient as to the nature of the procedure applied. These criteria can be applied to an evaluation of the control procedures described above.

Aside from the control procedure used in Vernon et al., [6,31], which did not involve an actual thrusting manipulation, all other control procedures identified in this review do not provide for the following important elements: a) simulated manual thrust, b) distracting noise to create ambiguity on the issue of cavitation and, c) proven lack of therapeutic effectiveness *a priori*. This combination creates the maximum level of "indistinguishability" possible in manual therapy research. However, with Vernon et al.'s clinical trial [31], the results of the sham manipulation as a control procedure cannot be confirmed separately from the placebo medication, as both were used in the true control group (see below).

The few studies that did employ a single thrusting manipulation control procedure did so on the basis of applying it to sites designated by the investigators as alternative to the "clinically important manipulation site". Whether this was at an alternate segment in the cervical spine [30,32] or at a supposedly non-effective site at the same segment (Bakris et al. [33] who also used a supposedly ineffective thrust direction), by actually providing a "real" manipulation (but at a supposedly inert site), these procedures did not accomplish the goals of simulating thrust and cavitation sounds (they actually produced them). Furthermore, these procedures were not tested previously for their inertness; in other words, there may have been some element of "indistinguishability", but the level of inertness was not established *a priori*.

In the case of Haas et al. [30], the alternate site procedure produced clinically important changes that were roughly equivalent to the index procedure; thus invalidating this procedure as a useful control manipulation (although the intention of these authors was not to establish the alternate site approach as a "control" procedure). In the case of both Pikula [32] and Bakris et al. [33], their control groups' results were only confirmed posteriorly. Pikula's small study provides very limited support for the idea that a real manipulation at a site designated as clinically less important may work as a control procedure in a single session. In the case of Bakris et al., it appears that their control procedure is highly dependent on the model of manipulation and the skill of the chiropractor involved and may not be generalizable to other circumstances.

Distinguishing control procedures which do and don't employ thrusts becomes important for two reasons. These will be discussed with respect to manual-type procedures and then non-manual type procedures. With respect to manual-type procedures, the first issue pertains to the control group subjects who receive non-thrust procedures, particularly those that involve manual contact without thrust (the predominant category in this review). While the strategy of "manual contact without thrust" does account for some similarities with real manipulation in patient positioning and in initial manual contact, such subjects do come to know after-the-fact that they have not received a thrusting procedure (because there is no simulation of thrust and cavitation noise). This may become incongruent with their expectations, especially in multi-session trials, and create a psychological factor superimposed on the more direct treatment-related outcome (which should, theoretically, be minimal). This could even rise to the status of a "nocebo" effect if the subject's posterior knowledge and resultant unmet expectations (especially over several sessions) combine to result in a negative attitude to the circumstances and in a poorer response on clinical outcome measures.

On the other hand, from Table 3 it can be seen that, in single session studies using manual contact/no thrust procedures, most often the control groups reported no significant or clinically important changes in pain, tenderness or other singular physical findings. Despite the issues raised above on lack of equivalence and the effects of unmasking, this type of procedure may be satisfactory for single session studies of the immediate effects of cervical manipulation. Given the fact that, in a small number of studies, clinically important changes in pain or tenderness were reported, it is advisable that researchers conduct a pre-test of this procedure in their hands to insure that it is generally inert before using it in a larger randomized trial.

The second issue applies to those subjects who receive the "real manipulation" in studies where other groups of subjects do not. By experiencing thrusting manipulations (with resultant audible cavitations (i.e., clicking sounds), subjects in these groups automatically receive indications which they would interpret to mean that they did receive the "index" treatment. This may result in an effect opposite to the one described above, where their treatment expectations are strongly confirmed. This may result in a non-specific effect which adds to that of the direct effects of the therapy, leading to a positive augmentation of the clinical outcomes (especially those that require subjective responses, and especially those related to satisfaction ratings). In passing, it should be remarked that in virtually all prior clinical trials of manipulation for neck pain and headaches, this is the situation that prevails in the groups receiving spinal manipulation.

With regard to non-manual control procedures, these do more readily lend themselves to the creation of placebo versions by, for example, de-tuning the equipment or applying very low doses of therapy. However, these procedures account for none of the manipulation-specific issues discussed above, making comparisons between these groups problematic, especially when issues of "mechanism of action" become important for the investigation. On strictly pragmatic grounds, non-manual placebo control procedures (such as those reviewed in Vernon et al. [10]) may be satisfactory for manipulation trials as they clearly result in clinical outcomes below the threshold of minimal clinically important difference.

With the exception of Vernon et al. [31], all studies have employed a single control procedure. Even if a single procedure is somewhat successful at masking subjects, it must do so entirely on its own. The "double placebo technique" [37-41] uses two procedures (either in a factorial design or in a simpler 2 or 3-group design) to increase the effectiveness of masking. While there is some evidence from the trial by Vernon et al. that this strategy was successful, more studies on this approach are needed.

It is difficult to summarize the clinical outcomes of the control groups analysed in this review on account of the highly variable methods and results. In 43% of the pain-related comparisons used in approximately one-third of the trials (8/21), the control procedure resulted in mean changes (reductions) that would be deemed clinically important. On the other hand, in some

Table 3 Summary of single-session studies using manual contact/no thrust control procedure

Buchman et al. [17]	Single session	No change in fixations
Martinez-Segura et al. [18]	Single session	No change in neck pain
Fernandez De Las Penas et al. [19]	Single session	No change in elbow PPT
Ruis-Saez et al. [20]	Single session	Moderate change trapezius TP at 5 and 10 minutes follow-up
Fernandez-Carnero et al. [21]	Single session	No change in elbow PPT
Fernandez De Las Penas et al. [22]	Single session	No change in neck PPT
Tuttle [23]	Single session	No change in ROM
Dunning and Rushton [24]	Single session	Moderate change in biceps EMG
Mansila-Ferragut et al. [25]	Single session	No change in TMJ PPT
Sterling et al. [26]	Single session	Moderate change in Neck PPT

proportion of each of the categories of control procedures, these procedures resulted in mean changes which were below the minimal clinically important threshold.

With regard to the multi-session studies, where three trials did report mean changes in the control groups that did not exceed the minimal clinically important threshold, several caveats are offered. In the case of Sloop et al. [27], while the control group receiving anamnestic valium + no manipulation reported very little improvement, most of the subjects in that study received only one treatment session and the outcome was obtained two weeks following treatment. In the case of Borusiak et al. [34], it should be noted that this trial, which employed a light touch/no thrust control procedure, included only children as subjects; this finding makes it difficult to justify the use of this control procedure in multi-session clinical trials with adults.

Beyond the issues of indistinguishability, equivalence and clinical effect, a very serious issue is the lack of determination of the level of blinding in the vast majority of these studies. In many cases, a result in favor of the manipulation group (especially in single-session studies) has been superficially interpreted to mean that a beneficial effect exists for manipulation, when, in fact, the investigators have no idea as to the degree to which subjects in the control group(s) may have become unblinded and how that may have affected their responses. There is a strong possibility of a Type I error which is then ignored. This problem is not confined to spinal manipulation as a therapy nor is it confined to treatments for the neck alone. Machado et al. [11] and Puhl et al. [42] have shown that the same problem exists for other pharmacologic and non-pharmacologic treatments for low back pain.

Finally, for single-session studies of clinical efficacy, every attempt should be made to report on randomization concealment and intention-to-treat, as this would make for more complete reporting and easier quality scoring.

This review has limitations. The entry-level search strategy was more broadly defined in order to identify the largest range of potential studies. While a search strategy with a more highly specified algorithm might have been employed, we are confident that our strategy is ultimately replicable by other investigators.

We did not specify the results of each item of the PEDro scale for each study, as all studies achieved a score above our threshold for acceptability. In this review, we felt that such an analysis, typically found in other systematic reviews, was not necessary, as the primary objective was not a methodological review of the studies themselves, but of the control group procedures used.

As noted in the Methods, pooling of outcomes data was not conducted. This was due to several factors. First, contrary to other systematic reviews, it was not our intention to derive a pooled estimate of the effect of a specific treatment on specific clinical entities; rather, we sought to characterize the various control group procedures used in a broad range of studies whose primary objective was the determination of the treatment effect of the index treatment, i.e., spinal manipulation. This lead to our review including a wide variety of studies with considerable heterogeneity on issues of clinical condition, subjects selected, outcomes measures and end points used, etc.

This heterogeneity made the reporting of outcomes more difficult, and less conventional, leading to our narrative account of the results.

Conclusion

The most commonly used control group procedure in clinical trials of cervical manipulation is manual contact/no thrust. Most control procedures in cervical manipulation trials do not result in subject blinding. Clinical outcomes of these groups were varied with about one third of groups demonstrating a clinically important change. The greatest majority of trials do not report on post-intervention blinding. The effect of unmasking of control subjects makes the interpretation of the existing clinical trials challenging. At the very least, future clinical trial reports should include an indication of the post-intervention registration of group allocation by subjects. A small number of candidate procedures exists for effective control interventions which create optimum combinations of inertness and practical equivalence with real manipulative therapies. Much more research is required to improve this important aspect of clinical trial methodology in cervical manipulation studies.

Acknowledgements
This study was supported by: NIH NCCAM grant R21 AT004396-01A1 to HV.

Authors' contributions
HV was responsible for following: the design of the study, selection of the studies, data collection and analysis, preparation of the manuscript.
AP was responsible for: scoring all studies, data extraction and preparation of the manuscript.
CR was responsible for: scoring all studies, data extraction and assistance with the preparation of the manuscript.
All authors read and approved the final manuscript.

Competing interests
The authors declare that they have no competing interests.

References

1. Vernon H, Humphreys BK: **Manual therapy for neck pain: an overview of randomized clinical trials and systematic reviews.** *Eura Medicophys* 2007, **43**:91-118.
2. Miller J, Gross A, D'Sylva J, Burnie SJ, Goldsmith CH, Graham N, Haines T, Brønfort G, Hoving JL: **Manual therapy and exercise for neck pain: a systematic review.** *Man Ther* 2010, **15(4)**:334-54.

3. D'Sylva J, Miller J, Gross A, Burnie SJ, Goldsmith CH, Graham N, Haines T, Brønfort G, Hoving JL, the Cervical Overview Group: **Manual therapy with or without physical medicine modalities for neck pain: a systematic review.** *Man Ther* 2010, **15(5)**:415-433.
4. Ernst E, Harkness E: **Spinal manipulation: A systematic review of sham-controlled, double-blind, randomized clinical trials.** *J Pain Sympt Manage* 2001, **22**:879-889.
5. Hancock MJ, Maher CG, Latimer J, McCauley JH: **Selecting an appropriate placebo for a trial of spinal manipulative therapy.** *Aust J Physiother* 2006, **52**:135-138.
6. Vernon H, MacAdam K, Marshall V, Pion M, Sadowska M: **Validation of a sham manipulative procedure fro the cervical spine for use in clinical trials.** *J Manipulative Physiol Ther* 2005, **28**:662-666.
7. Hawk C, Long C: **Use of a pilot to refine the design of a study to develop a manual placebo treatment.** *J Neuromusculoskel Sys* 2000, **8**:39-48.
8. Hawk C, Azad A, Phongphua C, Long C: **Preliminary study of the effects of a placebo chiropractic treatment with sham adjustments.** *J Manip Physiol Therap* 1999, **22**:436-443.
9. Hawk C, Long C, Reiter R, Davis C, Cambron J, Evans R: **Issues in planning a placebo-controlled trial of manual methods: results of a pilot study.** *J Altern Complement Med* 2002, **8(1)**:21-32.
10. Vernon H, Humphreys BK, Hagino C: **The outcome of control groups in clinical trials of conservative treatments for chronic neck pain: a systematic review.** *BMC Musculoskel Dis* 2006, **7**:58.
11. Machado LAC, Kamper SJ, Herbert RD, Maher CG, McAuley JH: **Imperfect placebos are common in low back pain trials: a systematic review of the literature.** *Eur J Spine* 2008, **17**:889-904.
12. Maher CG, Sherrington C, Herbert R, Moseley A, Elkins M: **Reliability of the PEDro scale for rating quality of randomized controlled trials.** *Phys Ther* 2003, **83**:713-721.
13. Cohen J: **Statistical Power Analysis for the Behavioral Sciences.** New York, NY: Academic Press;, 2 1988.
14. Ottenbacher KJ, Barrett K: **Measures of effect size in the reporting of rehabilitation research.** *Amer J Phys Med* 1989, **68(2)**:52-58.
15. Tuchin PJ, Pollard H, Bonello R: **A randomized controlled trial of chiropractic spinal manipulative therapy for migraine.** *J Manipulative Physiol Ther* 2000, **23(2)**:91-5.
16. Allison GT, Nagy BM, Hall T: **A randomized clinical trial of manual therapy for cervico-brachial pain syndrome - a pilot study.** *Man Ther* 2002, **7(2)**:95-102.
17. Buchman J, Wende K, Kundt G, Haessler F: **Manual treatment effects to the upper cervical apophysial joints before, during, and after endotracheal anesthesia.** *Am J Phys Med Rehabil* 2005, **84(4)**:251-7.
18. Martinez-Segura R, Fernandez-de-las-Penas C, Ruiz-Saez M, Lopez-Jimenez C, Rodriguez-Blanco C: **Immediate effects on neck pain and active range of motion after a single cervical high-velocity low-amplitude manipulative in subjects presenting with mechanical neck pain: a randomized controlled trial.** *J Manipulative Physiol Ther* 2006, **29**:511-17.
19. Fernandez-de-las-Penas C, Alonso-Blanco C, Cleland JA, Rodriguez-Blanco C, Alburquerque-Sendin F: **Changes in pressure pain thresholds over C5-C6 zygapophysial joint after a cervicothoracic junction manipulation in healthy subjects.** *J Manipulative Physiol Ther* 2008, **31**:332-7.
20. Ruiz-Saez M, Fernandez-de-las-Penas C, Rodriguez-Blanco C, Martinez-Segura R, Garcia-Leon R: **Changes in pressure pain sensitivity in latent myofascial trigger points in the upper trapezius muscle after a cervical spine manipulation in pain-free subjects.** *J Manipulative Physiol Ther* 2007, **30**:578-83.
21. Fernandez-Carnero J, Fernandez-de-las-Penas C, Cleland JA: **Immediate hypoalgesic and motor effects after a single cervical spine manipulation in subjects with lateral epicondylalgia.** *J Manipulative Physiol Ther* 2008, **31**:675-81.
22. Fernandez-de-las-Penas C, Perez-de-Heredia M, Brea-Rivero M, Miangolarra-Page JC: **Immediate effects on pressure pain threshold following a single cervical spine manipulation in healthy subjects.** *J Orthop Sports Phys Ther* 2007, **37(6)**:325-9.
23. Tuttle N, Barrett R, Laakso L: **Relation between changes in posteroanterior stiffness and active range of movement of the cervical spine following manual therapy treatment.** *Spine* 2008, **33**:E673-9.
24. Dunning J, Rushton A: **The effects of cervical high-velocity low-amplitude thrust manipulation on resting electromyographic activity of the biceps brachii muscle.** *Man Ther* 2009, **14**:508-13.
25. Mansila-Ferragut P, Fernandez-de-las-Penas C, Alburquerque-Sendin F, Cleland JA, Bosca-Gandia JJ: **Immediate effects of atlanto-occipital joint manipulation on active mouth opening and pressure pain sensitivity in women with mechanical neck pain.** *J Manipulative Physiol Ther* 2009, **32**:101-6.
26. Sterling M, Pedler A, Chan C, Puglisi M, Vuvan V, Vicenzino B: **Cervical lateral glide increases nociceptive flexion reflex threshold but not pressure or thermal pain thresholds in chronic whiplash associated disorders: a pilot randomized controlled trial.** *Man Ther* 2010, **15**:149-53.
27. Sloop PR, Smith DS, Goldenberg E, Dore C: **Manipulation for chronic neck pain: a double-blind controlled study.** *Spine* 1982, **7(6)**:532-5.
28. Nilsson N, Christensen HW, Hartvigsen J: **The effect of spinal manipulation in the treatment of cervicogenic headache.** *J Manipulative Physiol Ther* 1997, **20(5)**:326-30.
29. Bove G, Nilsson N: **Spinal manipulation in the treatment of episodic tension-type headache: a randomized controlled trial.** *JAMA* 1998, **280(18)**:1576-9.
30. Haas M, Groupp E, Panzer D, Partna L, Lumsden S, Aickin M: **Efficacy of cervical endplay assessment as an indicator for spinal manipulation.** *Spine* 2003, **28**:1091-6.
31. Vernon H, Jansz G, Goldsmith CH, McDermaid C: **A randomized, placebo-controlled clinical trial of chiropractic and medical prophylactic treatment of adults with tension-type headache: results from a stopped trial.** *J Manipulative Physiol Ther* 2009, **32**:344-51.
32. Pikula JR: **The effect of spinal manipulative therapy (SMT) on pain reduction and range of motion in patients with acute unilateral neck pain: a pilot study.** *J Can Chiropr Assoc* 1999, **43(2)**:111-9.
33. Bakris G, Dickholtz M Sr, Meyer PM, Kravitz G, Avery E, Miller M, Brown J, Woodfield C, Bell B: **Atlas vertebra realignment and achievement of arterial pressure goal in hypertensive patients: a pilot study.** *J Hum Hypertens* 2007, **21**:347-52.
34. Borusiak P, Biedermann H, BoBerhoff S, Opp J: **Lack of efficacy of manual therapy in children and adolescents with suspected cervicogenic headache: results of a prospective, randomized, placebo-controlled, and blinded trial.** *Headache* 2010, **50(2)**:224-30.
35. Haas M, Spegman A, Peterson D, Aickin M, Vavrek D: **Dose response and efficacy of spinal manipulation for chronic cervicogenic headache: a pilot randomized controlled trial.** *Spine J* 2010, **10**:117-128.
36. Coulehan JL: **Chiropractic and the clinical art.** *Soc Sci Med* 1985, **21(4)**:383-90.
37. Boutron I, Estallat C, Ravaud P: **A review of blinding in randomized controlled clinical trials found results inconsistent and questionable.** *J Clin Epidemiol* 2005, **58**:1220-6.
38. Boutron I, Tulbach F, Giraudeau B, Ravaud P: **Blinding was judged more difficult to achieve and maintain in nonpharmacologic than pharmacologic trials.** *J Clin Epidemiol* 2004, **57**:543-50.
39. Hrobjartsson A: **What are the main methodological problems in the estimation of placebo effects?** *J Clin Epidemiol* 2002, **55**:43-435.
40. Day SJ, Altman DG: **Blinding in clinical trials and other studies.** *Br Med J* 2000, **321**:504.
41. Morin CM, Colecchi C, Brink D, Astruc M, Mercer J, Remsberg S: **How "blind" are double-blind placebo-controlled trials of benzodiazepine hypnotics?** *Sleep* 1995, **18**:240-245.
42. Puhl Aaron A, Reinhart CJ, Rok ER, Injeyan HS: **An Examination of the Observed Placebo Effect Associated with the Treatment of Low Back Pain - A Systematic Review.** *Pain Res Manage* 2011.

2

The effect of spinal manipulative therapy on spinal range of motion: a systematic literature review

Mario Millan[1,2,3*], Charlotte Leboeuf-Yde[1,2,3,4], Brian Budgell[5], Martin Descarreaux[6] and Michel-Ange Amorim[1,7]

Abstract

Background: Spinal manipulative therapy (SMT) has been shown to have an effect on spine-related pain, both clinically and in experimentally induced pain. However, it is unclear if it has an immediate noticeable biomechanical effect on spinal motion that can be measured in terms of an increased range of motion (ROM).

Objective: To assess the quality of the literature and to determine whether or not SMT is associated with an immediate increase in ROM.

Design: A systematic critical literature review.

Method: Systematic searches were performed in Pubmed, the Cochrane Library and EMBASE using terms relating to manipulation, movement and the spine. Selection of articles was made according to specific criteria by two independent reviewers. Two checklists were created based on the needs of the present review. Articles were independently reviewed by two reviewers. Articles were given quality scores and the data synthesized for each region treated in the literature. Findings were summarized in tables and reported in a narrative fashion.

Results: Fifteen articles were retained reporting on experiments on the neck, lumbar spine, hip and jaw. The mean quality score was 71/100 (ranges 33/100 - 92/100). A positive effect of SMT was reported in both studies where mouth opening was assessed after cervical manipulation. In five of the nine studies on cervical ROM a positive effect was reported, whereas the remaining four studies did not show improvement. None of the three studies of the lumbar spine showed an effect of SMT on lumbar ROMs and one study of sacroiliac manipulation reported no effect on the ROM of the hip joint.
In relation to the quality score, the seven highest ranked studies, showed significant positive effects of SMT on ROM. Continuing down the list, the other studies reported no significant differences in the outcomes between groups.

Conclusion: SMT seems sometimes to have a small effect on ROM, at least in the cervical spine. Further research should concentrate on areas of the spine that have the potential of actually improving to such a degree that a change can be easily uncovered.

* Correspondence: mariomillan@live.fr
[1]EA 4532 CIAMS, UFR STAPS, Univ Paris-Sud, Orsay, France
[2]The Research Department, The Spine Centre of Southern Denmark, Hospital Lillebælt, Odense, Denmark
Full list of author information is available at the end of the article

Introduction

It is well known that back pain is highly prevalent in the general population, with serious economic consequences both on an individual and societal level. One of the treatments frequently used for back pain is spinal manipulative therapy (SMT). Although it has been shown that SMT is a reasonable treatment option for some people and some conditions [1], the mechanisms by which SMT achieves its effects remain unclear.

A manipulation is said to occur when a joint is brought to the extreme of its passive range and thereafter submitted to a rapid but shallow thrust, a so-called high velocity low amplitude (HVLA) manipulation [2]. The manipulation has, indeed, been shown to be a mechanical event as it causes slight momentary deformations of the spine and surrounding soft tissues [3-5]. It has also been confirmed that SMT carries the vertebrae beyond their normal physiological range of motion (ROM) without exceeding the boundaries of anatomic integrity [5,6]. Vertebral rotations and facet joint capsule strain magnitudes during SMT have been shown to be within the ranges that occur during physiological movements [6]. This maneuver is often accompanied by a crack [7].

SMT is usually differentiated from mobilization, which is described as more of a slow, long-lasting stretch of an articulation at the extreme of its passive range [8,9] and usually without causing a crack. Many clinicians make a strict distinction between SMT and mobilization[10] but some clinical studies have shown the effects to be similar for the two [11], indicating that such a distinction may not be relevant, at least not from a clinical point of view. Furthermore, the literature reports that, in clinical practice, the external forces applied during HVLA treatments vary considerably depending upon the treatment site, clinician and the technique used [7,12].

To better understand the true role of SMT in health care, more information is needed regarding the effects of SMT on the articular and peri-articular structures, and joint function; i.e. movement. Theoretically, SMT could have an effect on a number of structures and tissues within and surrounding the spinal articulation. These structures include muscles, aponeuroses, peri-articular receptors, tendons, discs, and ligaments, which all, singly or in combination, would have the capacity to cause dysfunction and pain as they are all potential starting points of proprioceptive and nociceptive pathways. For SMT to have a positive effect on vertebral movement, it must modulate the function of some or all of these structures/tissues. SMT has, in fact, been shown to modify spinal reflex excitability [13], paraspinal cutaneous temperature [14], visceral activity (e.g. cardiovascular function)[15], and electromyographic activity of paraspinal muscles [16,17]. It has also been hypothesized to alter motoneuron excitability [18], increase muscle strength [19,20], alter sensorimotor integration [21], and affect pain regulation in the dorsal horn of the spinal cord [22] and the periaqueductal grey area [23-25]. However, it is unclear as to what this brings in terms of a biomechanical effect, such as an increased range of movement (ROM). It has already been shown that SMT has a pain reducing effect [26,27]. It seems logical that if pain is reduced after SMT, ROM might increase, independently of any effect that it may have on pain. However, ROM might well increase after SMT, regardless of whether the treated segment was painful or not. Therefore, it is important to consider the effect that SMT may have on ROM, specifically. Because the literature is unclear on this topic, this systematic critical literature review was performed to assess the quality of the available literature and to determine whether or not SMT is associated with an immediate increase in ROM.

Methods

Design: systematic critical literature review.

Searches were conducted in PubMed, the Cochrane library and EMBASE without any date limitations and using the following combinations of search terms:

"spinal" + "manipulation" + "range" + "motion"
"chiropractic" + "manipulation" + "range" + "motion"
"spinal" + "manipulation" + "stiffness"
"spinal" + "mobilization" + "range" + "motion"
"spinal" + "mobilization" + "stiffness"

Thereafter, two of the authors (MM and CLY) independently applied specific inclusion criteria to select the potentially relevant articles from the titles, abstracts, and keywords of the references retrieved in the literature search. These inclusion criteria were:

- Languages: English, French, Spanish, Danish, Swedish and Norwegian.
- Spinal Manipulative Therapy (SMT), anywhere in the spine.
- Humans or animals.
- Experimental studies with at least one control group. Thus, studies without a random allocation procedure were accepted.
- ROM had to be one of the outcome variables.
- Immediate effect was reported. (This review did not examine long term effects at, for example, weeks or months following SMT, due to the risk of contamination from factors other than the manipulative procedure.)

The following studies were excluded:

- Studies of subjects with specific pathologies, such as inflammatory diseases, tumors or severe spinal degeneration, because these might influence the spinal structures in such a way as to limit ROM permanently and therefore confuse the results.
- Studies of combined/concomitant therapies (drugs, physiotherapy), as it would not be possible to know if the results were obtained from SMT or the other therapies.
- Literature reviews

Data extraction

Two authors (MM and CLY) extracted data from each article, independently of each other, into two check-lists, one descriptive and one qualitative. Data were later compared in order to minimize reading errors. The other authors were designated as judges in case of disagreement between the first two reviewers.

Descriptive check-list

The descriptive checklist for the selected articles (see Table 1) contained the following items:

- ID n°; author and year of publication;
- Study design;
- Type of study sample;
- Number of study subjects;
- Numbers of males and females;
- Age range and mean/median age of final study sample;
- Type and area of symptoms (if any);
- Duration of symptoms (if any);
- Description of the SMT/mobilization group and the type(s) of control group (sham treatment, another treatment or no treatment at all).
- Number of experiments performed on each study subject;
- Time when ROM was measured (immediately after the SMT or later);
- Whether SMT was performed at the level of a spinal complaint;
- Type of measurement (distance or angle) ;
- Method of measurement;
- Approval from ethics committee (yes/no)

Quality checklist

A number of issues related to quality of study were identified by consensus among the authors and used to develop a quality checklist (see Table 2). We designed this checklist based on concepts presented in the PRISMA statement [28], the CONSORT statement [29] and Cochrane guidelines [30] bearing in mind that there can be no general recipe for such work, as review procedures have to be topic specific. The risk of bias was assessed following the criteria suggested by the method guidelines for systematic reviews of trials of treatments for neck and back pain by Furlan et al. [30]. Additional items were mainly adapted from PRISMA [28]. Thus, the items selected for our review were:

Study population

1. Ideally, study subjects should be naïve or at least disinterested, meaning that they should not have any preconceived ideas about SMT that could affect their reactions to the experiment. This would exclude, for example, studies of chiropractic students. Patients referred for physiotherapy treatment and thereafter included in a study were considered suitable for inclusion because they did not actively select participation in the study.
2. If the study samples contained people older than 45, the age distribution should be similar among the treatment groups, as an uneven number of older people could influence the degree of spinal degeneration and so response to treatment as degeneration has been shown to modify the effect of SMT [31,32].

Procedure

3. The study subjects should have been randomly allocated to study groups.
4. Sham treatments, if any, should be credible, to reduce the risk of negative expectations from study subjects.
5. Physical conditions, such as room temperature, time of day, time of warm-ups, should be similar for all treatment groups, and also constant before/after SMT because such conditions might have an effect on spinal movement [33].
6. The manipulative maneuver should be well described to make it possible to ascertain whether it was actually a manipulation, but also to make it possible to reproduce the study.
7. The manipulative maneuver should be performed by an experienced person, to ensure that it was correctly carried out.
8. The person assessing the ROM should be blinded to treatment group to ensure absence of expectation bias.
9. The pre/post treatment ROM-test should be performed by the same person to optimize the reliability of the test procedure.
10. The ROM should be assessed by a method previously shown to be highly reliable or the study

Table 1 Descriptive check-list of selected articles in the literature review of the action of SMT on ROM

Author year and references	Design	Type of study sample	n° of subjects	n° males	n° females	Ages	Type and area of symptoms (if any)
Cassidy 1992 [36]	RCT	Patients	100	?	?	34.5 SD13.0	Unilateral neck pain with radiation to trapezius
Pollard 1997 [48]	RCT	Chiropractic students	34	?	?	21-33	None
Goodsell 2000 [45]	Cross-over	Patients	26	13	13	(16–69) 39.5	Low back pain
Whittingham 2001 [40]	Cross-over	Volunteers obtained through adverts	105	42	63	Group=39.4 Group2=41.9	Cervicogenic headache occipital region
Martinez Segura 2006 [37]	RCT	Patients referred to physiotherapy to osteopathic clinic	70	25	45	(20–55) 37	Neck pain
Konstantinou 2007 [46]	Cross-over	Patients referred for physiotherapy suitable for SMT	26	15	11	>18 38.3 SD11.7	Low back pain +/– Leg pain
Tuttle 2008 [41]	Cross-over	Volunteer staff and students from university	20	10	10	(19–55) 31	Neck pain that limited movement
Krauss 2008 [42]	RCT	Patients referred for physical therapy	32	6	26	(19–50) 34.2	Neck pain
Kanlayanaphotporn 2009 [43]	RCT	Patients	60	24	36	Goup1 39.7 Goup2 44.8	Neck pain
Mansilla-Ferragut 2009 [34]	RCT	Volunteers obtained through advert	37	-	37	(21–50) 35+/–8	Neck pain < 40 mm mouth opening
Mc Clatchie 2009 [38]	Cross-over	Orthopedic patients	21	7	14	49.8 (+/–9.8)	Shoulder pain No neck pain last year
Passemore 2010 [39]	RCT	Volunteer chiropractic students with C1-C2 fixation	15	?	?	21-42	N/A
Kanlayana-photporn 2010 [44]	RCT	Patients	60	18	42	42.2 (23–68)	Neck pain
Oliveira Campello 2010 [35]	RCT	Volunteer students	122	31	91	18-30	N/A
Stamospapastomous 2011 [47]	Cross-over study	Volunteer students	32	16	16	25.5 SD4.5	N/A

Table 1 Descriptive check-list of selected articles in the literature review of the action of SMT on ROM *(Continued)*

Duration of symptoms	Treatment and control activity (sham, other or nothing)	N° experiments	When was ROM measured?	Was SMT performed at level of problem?	What was measured?	How was ROM measured?	Approval from ethics committee?
<1week n=16 1w - 6m=34 >6 months n=50	- SMT (cervical, clinically determined) (n=52) - Mobilization (cervical) (n=48)	1	Before and 5′ after	Yes	Cervical ROM, 3 planes	Goniometer 3 D	Yes
N/A	- Sacroiliac manipulation (n=18) - Sham=Mastoid pressure (n=16)	1	Before and 30″ after	N/A	Straight leg raise on SMT side	Digital goniometer	Yes
0.5 – 60 months	- Clinically determined lumbar mobilization - Nothing (lying down)	2	Before and after	Yes	Lumbar motion (extension/flexion)	Fingertips-to-floor Inclinometer	?
> 6 months	- SMT upper cervical - Sham (deactivated instrument)	3	Before and after weeks 3, 6, 9	Yes	Lateral flexion, rotation	Strap-on head goniometer	Yes
>1Month	- SMT (C3-C5) - Sham neck mobilization	1	Before and 3′ after	Yes	Cervical ROM, 3 planes	Goniometer	Yes
>3 months	- PA mobilization - Nothing	2	Before and 5′ after	Yes	Lumbar flexion/ extension	Double inclinometer	Yes
>2 weeks	- PA cervical mobilization at symptom level - Placebo (PA mobilization but asymptomatic side) - Nothing (lying down) - general MT but no high velocity thrust	4	Before and after	Yes	Cervical ROM 3 planes	Post/ant assessment device and head sensor	Yes
?	- Thoracic SMT - Nothing	2	Before and after	No (thoracic adjustment)	Active ROM - Left/right rotation	Inclinometer compass system	Yes
Mean Goup1 804d Goup2 999d	-Clinically determined mobilization - Random mobilization	1	Before and 5′ after	Yes	Cervical ROM, 3 planes	Magnetic neck brace + 3 inclinometers	Yes
>6 months	- SMT atlanto-occipital - Sham (cervical manual contact)	1	Before and after	Yes (atlanto-occipital)	Mouth opening	Universal caliper	Yes
>6 weeks	- Mobilization (C5- C7) - Sham (same mobilization position but without external force)	2	Before and after	Yes	Cervical ROM, 3 planes	Goniometer	Yes
N/A	- SMT(C1-C2) - Nothing (wait 5′)	1	Before and 5′ after	N/A	Cervical ROM, 3 planes	Goniometer	Yes
Mean Group1 1575d Group2 1811d	- Post/ant (PA) cervical mobilization - random mobilization (PA, right or left)	1	Before and after	Yes	Cervical ROM 3 planes	Magnetic neck brace + 3 inclinometers	Yes
N/A	- SMT atlanto-occipital - Soft occipital tissue treatment - Nothing	1	Before and 2′ after	N/A	Mouth opening	Universal caliper	Yes
N/A	- SMT(lumbar) - Mobilization (lumbar)	2	Before and after	N/A	Bending stiffness and ROM lumbar extension/flexion	Electromagnetic tracking device	Yes

Table 2 Quality check-list of articles reviewed

Author and references	Random allocation		Study subjects naïve*/disinterested		Was there a credible sham treatment?		Was SMT well described?		Was SMT performed by experienced person?		Was the ROM assessor blinded?		Were pre/post treatment ROM-test performed by the same person?	
Oliveira Campello [35]	Yes	1	Yes	1	Yes	1	Yes	1	Yes	1	Yes	1	Yes	1
Kanlayanaphotporn [43]	Yes	1	No	0	Yes	1	Yes	1	Yes	1	Yes	1	Yes	1
Konstantinou [46]	Yes	1	Yes	1	No	0	Yes	1	Yes	1	Yes	1	Yes	1
Whittingham [40]	Yes	1	Yes	1	Yes	1	Yes	1	?	0	Yes	1	Yes	1
Stamospapastomous [47]	Yes	1	Yes	1	Yes	1	Yes	1	Yes	1	No	0	Yes	1
Krauss [42]	Yes	1	Yes	1	No	0	Yes	1	Yes	1	Yes	1	Yes	1
Martinez Segura [37]	Yes	1	Yes	1	Yes	1	Yes	1	Yes	1	Yes	1	Yes	1
Goodsell [45]	Yes	1	Yes	1	No	0	Yes	1	Yes	1	Yes	1	Yes	1
Mc Clatchie [38]	Yes	1	Yes	1	Yes	1	Yes	1	?	0	Yes	1	Yes	1
Mansilla-Ferragut [34]	Yes	1	?	0	Yes	1	Yes	1	Yes	1	Yes	1	Yes	1
Cassidy [36]	Yes	1	Yes	1	Yes	1	Yes	1	Yes	1	Yes	1	?	0
Tuttle [41]	Yes	1	?	0	Yes	1	No	0	Yes	1	Yes	1	Yes	1
Kanlayanaphotporn [44]	Yes	1	No	0	Yes	1	Yes	1	Yes	1	Yes	1	No	0
Passmore [39]	Yes	1	No	0	No	0	Yes	1	Yes	1	Yes	1	?	0
Pollard [48]	Yes	1	No	0	No	0	Yes	1	?	0	?	0	?	0

Table 2 Quality check-list of articles reviewed *(Continued)*

Was ROM assessed by a valid method or own inter/intra validation?		Were losses reported?		Were results reported and estimates shown in tables/graphs?		Were results tested for statistical significance?		Physical conditions controlled for all treatment groups		If study samples contained people older than 45, was the age distribution shown in treatment groups to be similar?		Total score	Score /100
Yes	1	Yes	1	Yes	1	Yes	1	?	0	N/A	-	11 /12	**92**
Yes	1	Yes	1	Yes	1	Yes	1	?	0	No, but compared base line variable for both	-	10 /12	**83**
Yes	1	Yes	1	Yes	1	Yes	1	?	0	Upper level age is known, but N/A because cross-over	-	10 /12	**83**
Yes	1	Yes	1	Yes	1	Yes	1	?	0	Age range are known, but N/A because cross-over	-	10 /12	**83**
Yes	1	Yes	1	Yes	1	Yes	1	?	0	N/A	-	10 /12	**83**
Yes	1	Yes	1	Yes	1	Yes	1	?	0	No (19 – 50)	0	10 /13	**77**
Yes	1	No	0	Yes	1	Yes	1	?	0	No (20 – 55)	0	10 /13	**77**
Yes	1	No	0	Yes	1	Yes	1	?	0	Yes	1	9 /13	**69**
Yes	1	No	0	Yes	1	Yes	1	?	0	No (>16)	0	9 /13	**69**
Yes	1	No	0	Yes	1	Yes	1	?	0	No (21–50)	0	9 /13	**69**
Yes	1	No	0	Yes	1	Yes	1	?	0	Age not known	0	9 /13	**69**
Yes	1	No	0	Yes	1	Yes	1	?	0	Age range known, but N/A because cross-over	-	8 /12	**67**
Yes	1	No	0	Yes	1	Yes	1	?	0	No, but compared base line variable for both	-	8 /12	**67**
?	0	No	0	Yes	1	Yes	1	?	0	N/A	-	6 /12	**50**
?	0	No	0	Yes	1	Yes	1	?	0	N/A	-	4 /12	**33**

should contain a satisfactory report of own inter/intra reliability evaluation.

Data reporting

11. Losses and exclusions should be reported to minimize the risk of selective removal of data.
12. Estimates should be reported as exact values or shown in tables/graphs and not only as significance levels.
13. If there were any differences between groups, these should be tested for statistical significance.

Classifying articles by their quality

For the selected articles, all descriptive and quality items were checked independently by the first two reviewers and a summary quality score was assigned. One point was awarded for each fulfilled quality item.

If the quality item was not satisfied ("no") or if the article did not mention this condition ("?"), no point was given. However, if the item was not applicable ("N/A"), this was not counted in the denominator. Thus the maximum total score could be different from one article to the next. Finally, the total score was normalized to a 100 point scale in order to compare quality across studies.

Although a summary quality score was calculated, no cutoff-point was defined for acceptable or unacceptable level of quality. This allowed us (and the readers) to use the quality scores and the information on each individual quality item as a guide to determine whether articles would be considered more or less credible. In other words, the quality assessment was meant to be informative rather than proscriptive. Because we decided not to use a scoring system to establish levels of quality, we have not defined any discrete levels of evidence, e.g. high, moderate or low.

Data synthesis

Four data tables were constructed according to the area of the spine where treatment was provided and ROM assessed: 1. cervical treatment and ROM, 2. lumbar treatment and ROM, 3. cervical treatment and range of mouth opening, and 4. sacroiliac treatment and hip ROM. The tables were scrutinized, one by one, to obtain answers to our research question. Results were thereafter interpreted and reported in a narrative fashion.

Results

Study selection

Figure 1 shows a flow diagram of the study selection process. A total of 242 articles were identified from the systematic search of MEDLINE, 51 from EMBASE, and 3 from the Cochrane library. Nine other articles were added from an additional hand search of reference lists. After duplicates were removed, 247 articles remained to be assessed for inclusion. Of these, 67 were retrieved in full and examined against our inclusion criteria. In all, 15 studies fulfilled all inclusion criteria and are reviewed herein (see Figure 1).

Description of data

Table 1 provides a full description of the key characteristics of each study. Articles have been listed chronologically based on the date of publication.

Of the 15 selected studies, two measured the effects of SMT on mouth opening, nine studied effects about the three cervical axes of movement, one measured only the range of cervical rotation, three studied flexion/extension in the lumbar spine, and one investigated the ROM of the hip. There were nine randomized controlled trials and six cross-over studies. All of them measured the ROM before and immediately after treatment. No papers on the thoracic spine satisfied the inclusion criteria.

ROM was measured differently depending upon the spinal region under study. Mouth opening ([34] and [35]) was measured with a universal caliper. Cervical ROM was assessed with a three- dimensional goniometer ([36], [37], [38] and [39]), a strap-on head goniometer ([40]), a postero-anterior assessment device with a head sensor ([41]), an inclinometer with a compass system ([42]), and a magnetic neck brace with three separate inclinometers ([43] and [44]). Lumbar ROMs were measured with a fingertip-to-floor inclinometer[45], a double inclinometer [46] and an electromagnetic tracking device [47]. Hip ROM was measured with a digital goniometer ([48]).

Some researchers (n=11) performed their experiments on people with symptoms, either patients (n=8) or volunteers with symptoms recruited by advertisements (n=3), whereas the remaining four studies dealt with healthy students.

Eight authors performed only one experiment, five reported two experiments, and two studies reported on three and four experiments, respectively.

Only one article did not report whether approval had been received from an ethics committee.

Quality

Table 2 presents a description of the quality items. The quality scores ranged from 33/100 to 92/100, with a mean score of 71.4 (SD 10.4) and a median of 69. Articles are listed in the order of decreasing quality score. There were no disagreements between the reviewers in relation to the quality items.

All articles fulfilled the following four quality criteria: "Random allocation", "SMT well described", "Estimates reported and shown in tables/graphs" and "Results tested

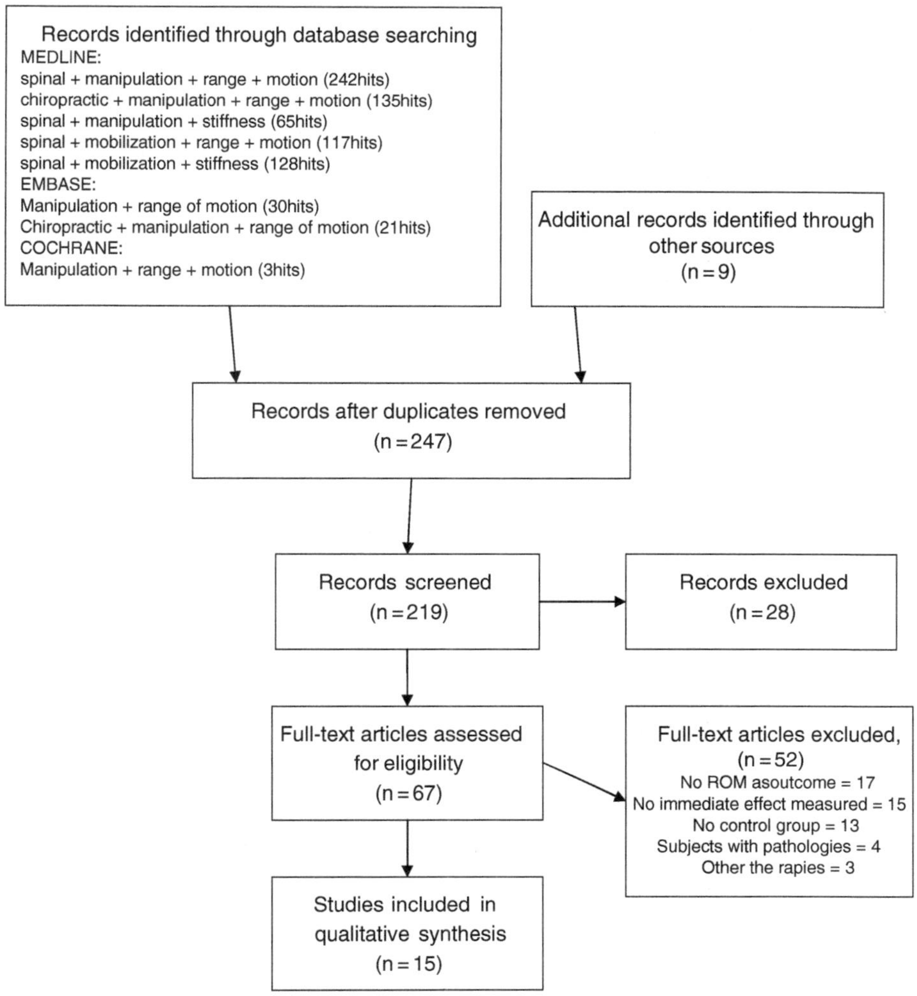

Figure 1 Flowchart describing the process for a systematic critical review of the literature on the effect of SMT on spinal range of motion (from The PRISMA Statement [56]).

for statistical significance". The item "Age distribution similar in studies with study sample consisting of people older than 45" was applicable to six studies ([36], [45], [37], [42], [34], and [38]) of which only [45] fulfilled the criterion.

Nine articles dealt with "disinterested/naïve study samples". Ten studies included what we considered a credible sham treatment in comparison to the spinal manipulation. However, some studies investigated differences in outcome in relation to different types of manipulation (such as manipulating in different planes), i.e. not comparing manipulation to a sham treatment making this issue superfluous. Eleven authors specified that SMT was performed by an experienced person (all except [36,39,44,48]), and twelve assured that pre/post assessment was made by the same person (all except [36,39,48]).

Outcome assessments were blinded in thirteen studies, and thirteen assessed ROMs with a validated method. In two of the studies, ([48] and [39]), the validity of the assessment method was not described.

In none of the studies were the experimental conditions stated to have been equal for treatment and control groups or before and after the manipulation. Only six studies reported if there were any exclusions or losses during the study.

Outcomes reported

The results for mouth opening, cervical ROM, lumbar ROM and hip ROM are shown in Tables 3, 4, 5 and 6 and are described below.

Outcomes were reported as either degrees or millimeters and there were generally no large improvements in ROM. In fact, although a statistically significant effect of SMT was seen in several studies, the differences between pre and post treatment, when clearly reported, were, for the best results, in the order of 3.5mm for mouth opening ([34]) and 10° ([37]) for unilateral cervical rotation.

Table 3 Effects of SMT on mouth opening

Author	Quality score /100	Treatment and control activity (sham, other or nothing)	Preintervention in mm	Postintervention in mm	Change of score in mm	Summarized results given by authors	Were the differences in outcome tested between groups and were they significant?
Oliveira Campello [35]	**92**	- SMT atlanto-occipital (n=41) - Soft occipital tissue treatment (n=41) - Nothing (n=40)	46.4 ± 6.8 (44.4, 48.4) 47.2 ± 6.2 (45.2, 49.3) 46.8 ± 6.8 (44.8, 48.9)	47.9 ± 6.8 (45.9, 49.9) 47.7 ± 6.1 (45.6, 49.7) 46.8 ± 6.7 (44.8, 48.9)	**1.5** ± 1.5 (1.0, 1.9) **0.5** ± 1.7 (0.0, 1.0) **0.0** ± 1.1 (−0.4, 0.3)	SMT increases maximum active mouth opening, but need of further studies to elucidate the clinical relevance of that.	Yes and yes
Mansilla-Ferragut [34]	**69**	- SMT atlanto-occipital (n=18) - Sham (cervical manual contact) (n=19)	35.4 (95% CI, 33.3-37.4) 36.2 (95% CI, 34.3- 38.2)	38.8 (95% CI, 36.6-41.1) 35.9 (95% CI, 33.7-38.0)	**3.5** (95% CI, 2.4, 4.6) **−0.3** (95% CI, -0.4, 1.2)	SMT increases maximum active mouth opening.	Yes and yes

A positive effect of SMT was reported in both of the studies where mouth opening was assessed after cervical manipulation (+3.5mm ([34]) and 1.5mm ± 1.5 [35]). In five of the nine studies on cervical ROM ([40], [37], [42], [43], and [39]) a positive effect was reported, whereas the remaining four studies ([36], [41], [38], and [44]) did not show improvement. See Table 4 for examples of increased ROM in the studies with significant results.

None of the three studies of the lumbar spine (Table 5) showed an effect of SMT on lumbar ROMs ([46], [47], and [45]) and one study ([48]) of sacroiliac manipulation (Table 6) reported no effect on the ROM of the hip joint.

The lack of homogeneity in the various reports made a meta-analysis impractical. For example, different areas of the spine were studied, all of which have different movement patterns. Concerning the cervical region, study [42] measured only rotation and not all three planes; study [40] showed only the baseline values and not the post-manipulative values. Study [41] did not report exact measures but showed the results in a graph. Finally, study [39] reported only exact numerical values for the significant findings but provided no estimates for those with non-significant differences. Also the study populations differed between papers, some including patients with back problems and others using healthy people. Only two studies, ([41] and [35]), compared the outcome of SMT in three groups: treatment, sham procedure and a control group which did not receive any type of treatment. The first of these two studies, which examined cervical ROM, did not find an effect, whereas the second, which examined mouth opening, did.

Nine studies compared the action of SMT to only a sham procedure ([36], [48], [40], [37], [43], [34], [38], [44], and [47]). Five of them ([40], [37], [43], [34], and [47]) found the outcome of SMT to be statistically significant but four ([36], [48], [38], and [44]) did not.

Four authors compared the action of SMT to the outcome in a control group which did not receive any treatment ([45], [46], [42], and [39]). The first of these studies ([45]) did not find any difference between the outcomes after SMT and the control process, whereas the three others did ([46], [42], and [39]).

Finally, if articles are listed by total quality score, the seven highest ranked studies ([35], [43], [46], [40], [47], [42], and [37]), with scores ranging from 92 to 77, showed significant positive effects of SMT on ROM. Continuing down the list from scores of 69 to 33, studies [45], [38], [36], [41], [44], and [48] reported no significant differences in the outcomes between groups, while studies [34] and [39] did report significant effects of SMT.

Discussion

Summary of results

This appears to be the first systematic critical literature review of the immediate effect of SMT on ROM. The fifteen articles that met our inclusion criteria for review did not provide a coherent picture; some studies found a small effect, others none. The differences in results between studies were related to the quality of studies, with the better studies reporting significant findings. Interestingly, it did not matter if SMT was compared with a sham treatment or if it was compared with some type of control procedure, suggesting that results were unaffected by expectation or observation bias. The only studies showing a positive effect in the spine were those performed in the cervical spine, while no effect was discerned after pelvic or lumbar treatment. When positive findings were present, they were generally modest.

Heterogeneous methods make meta-analysis unsuitable

Many different tools are used in research and in clinical practice to measure ROM: single/double/triple inclinometers, goniometers, a rangiometer, tape measures, visual estimation, spine motion analyzer, etc. It was not the purpose of this review to describe and compare these methods, but we refer to the literature concerning their reliability and validity [33,49-52]. The main point is that there are quite a number of studies on the topic but that the measurement tools used often differed from one study to another, making it difficult to compare results between studies. In addition, this multitude of outcome variables plus other differences such as choice of study population and area of manipulation make it impossible to combine results in a meaningful meta-analysis.

Why such small effects- if any?

The small improvement in ROM, when an improvement was seen at all, may come as a surprise to those who have clinical experience with SMT. However, perhaps in clinical practice, the biomechanical effect of SMT is influenced by a reduction in pain. In this review, we did not take into account changes in level of pain, but rather focused on ROM, which is a less common outcome variable in randomized clinical trials on SMT and back pain [11,46]. The choice of researchers to avoid measures of ROMs as outcome variables might well be because SMT does not generally produce substantial changes in ROMs.

Another possibility for this discrepancy between the clinical experience and the results of this review is that ROMs may improve gradually as treatment progresses over days or weeks. Our review dealt only with the immediate effects of SMT, in order not to confuse the effects of SMT with those of other factors that could come into play over a period of time. Other possible

Table 4 Effects of SMT on cervical range of motion

Author	Quality score /100	Treatment and control activity (sham, other or nothing)	Δ ROM pre/post treatment in degrees: flexion	Δ ROM pre/post treatment in degrees: extension	Δ ROM pre/post treatment in degrees: right lateral flexion
Kanlayanaphotporn [43]	**83**	- Clinically determined mobilization - Random mobilization	1.9 ± 4.1 −0.7 ± 4.5	1.8 ± 6.3 0.8 ± 4.6	- 0.3 ± 6.3 1.2 ± 4.9
Whittingham [40]	**83**	- SMT upper cervical - Sham (deactivated instrument)	-	-	Gr. 1=39° ± 1.1 Gr. 2=38° ± 1.4
Krauss [42]	**77**	- Thoracic SMT - Nothing	-	-	-
Martinez Segura [37]	**77**	- SMT (C3-C5) - Sham neck mobilization	7 (Cohen's d=5) 1.5 (Cohen's d=2.5)	8 (Cohen's d=7) 1.4 (Cohen's d=3.3)	5 (Cohen's d=4) 0.8 (Cohen's d=1.6)
Mc Clatchie [38]	**69**	- Mobilization (cervical) - Sham (same mobilization position but without external force)	−1.2 ± 6.5 −1.4 ± 5.3	0.8 ± 5.5 −0.5 ± 5.5	−0.7 ± 5.2 −0.1 ± 5.3
Cassidy [36]	**69**	- SMT(cervical) (n=52) - Mobilization (cervical) (n=48)	5.1 (SD 8.3) 3.9 (SD 9.4)	3.1 (SD 7.8) 1.3 (SD 7.5)	3.4 (SD 7.5) 2.0 (SD 5.2)
Kanlayanaphotporn [44]	**67**	- Post/ant (PA) cervical mobilization - random mobilization (PA, right or left)	1.4 (SD 5.2) −0.4 (SD 7.6)	1.8 (SD 5.4) −0.4 (SD 5.9)	−0.2 (SD 4.0) 0.6 (SD 4.1)
Tuttle [41]	**67**	- PA cervical mobilization at symptomatic level - Placebo (PA mobilization but asymptomatic side)			
- Nothing (lying down)	* initial values flexion/ extension ROM =119° (SD-17)	* initial values flexion/ extension ROM=119° (SD-17)	* initial values lateral flexion ROM=93° (SD-12)	* initial values lateral flexion ROM=93° (SD-12)	* initial values rotation ROM=93° (SD-12)
Passmore [39]	**50**	- SMT(C1-C2) - Nothing (wait 5')	No difference No difference	No difference No difference	No difference No difference

Table 4 Effects of SMT on cervical range of motion *(Continued)*

Δ ROM pre/post treatment in degrees: left lateral flexion	Δ ROM pre/post treatment in degrees: right rotation	Δ ROM pre/post treatment in degrees: left rotation	Summarized results given by authors	Comments	Were the differences in outcome tested between groups and were they significant?
0.8 ± 4.8 1.3 ± 4.1	0.5 ± 5.5 0.6 ± 6.9	1.1 ± 4.2 0.8 ± 6.0	The preferred mobilization group showed an increased flexion/extension compared to random mobilization group.		Yes and yes
Gr. 1=38° ± 1.3 Gr. 2=36° ± 1.2	Gr. 1=56° ± 1.4 Gr. 2=57° ± 1.5	Gr. 1=54° ± 1.6 Gr. 2=54° ± 1.6	SMT increase significantly ROM	Those are given baseline values. ROM values immediately after treatment. Effect is observed on weeks 3, 6, 9 and 12.	Yes and yes
-	8.23 (SD=7.41) −0.1 (SD=2.33)	7.09 (SD=5.83) −0.6 (SD=3.66)	Cervical rotation ROM is improved following SMT		Yes and yes
5 (Cohen's d=4) 0.8 (Cohen's d=1.5)	10 (Cohen's d=5) 0.4 (Cohen's d=1.5)	9 (Cohen's d=5) 0.3 (Cohen's d=0.8)	SMT was more effective than control mobilization on ROM. Large effect sizes.		Yes and yes
−0.4 ± 4.1 0.3 ± 4.4	1.1 ± 4.4 −0.4 ± 5.9	1.3 ± 6.6 - 0.3 ± 4.9	No significant difference		Not tested
4.3 (SD 7.0) 3.0 (SD 4.7)	5.0 (SD 9.0) 4.2 (SD 9.0)	3.6 (SD 7.0) 2.4 (SD 6.4)	Both treatments increase ROM to similar degree.		Yes and no
0.9 (SD 4.2) 1.5 (SD 7.8)	1.2 (SD 5.9) 1.2 (SD 6.1)	2.7 (SD 5.3) 2.0 (SD 5.8)	No significant effect on ROM		Yes and no
* initial values rotation ROM=93° (SD-12)	No significant ROM increase	* No differences. pre/post treatment values are given but only shown in a graph.	Not tested		
No difference No difference	3.75 No difference	-	SMT increases cervical active ROM		Not tested

Table 5 Effects of SMT on lumbar range of motion

Author	Quality score /100	Treatment and control activity (sham, other or nothing)	Mean ROM measures in degrees pre-treatment (SD) Flexion	Mean ROM measures in degrees pre-treatment (SD) Extension	Mean ROM measures in degrees post-treatment (SD) Flexion	Mean ROM measures in degrees post-treatment (SD) Extension	Differences pre –post treatment in degrees Flexion	Differences pre –post treatment in degrees Extension	Comments	Were the differences in outcome tested between groups and were they significant?
Konstantinou [46]	83	- Mobilization (n=26) - Lying down (n=26)	69.5 (19.0)	21.9 (10.2)	76.7 (22.4) 69.7 (21.5)	24.0 (11.0) 21.2 (11.1)	7.2 0.2	2.1 −0.7	Values pre-treatment are baseline for both groups. Small changes.	Yes and no
Stamospapastomous [47]	83	- SMT(lumbar) (n=32) - Mobilization (n=32)	54.22 (12.76) 54.11 (11.13)	27.02 (14.42) 22.8 (10.0)	56.07 (12.22) 54.81 (11.36)	28.56 (14.23) 23.66 (11.39)	1.85 0.7	1.54 0.86	No significant effect for the whole group, but some individual effects reported by author.	Not tested
Goodsell [45]	69	- PA mobilization - Nothing	A=105 (11) B=95 (22)	A=52 (8) B=46 (14)	A=106 (13) B=97(21) A=108 (12) B=95 (24)	A=52 (11) B=47 (14) A=52 (9) B=47 (14)	0.9 1.4	0.9 1.4	No effect on ROM.	Yes and no

Table 6 Effects of SMT on hip flexion range of motion

Author	Quality score /100	Treatment and control activity (sham, other or nothing)	Pre-test ROM in degrees relative to vertical plane	Post-test ROM in degrees relative to vertical plane	Changes in %	Summarized results given by authors	Were the differences in outcome tested between groups and were they significant?
Pollard [48]	33	- Sacroiliac manipulation (n=18) - Sham=mastoid pressure (n=16)	62.22 (2.40) 67.06 (3.23)	60.06 (2.22) 66.37 (3.21)	3.47 1.03	A single manipulation of the sacroiliac joint did not significantly affect hip ROM.	Yes and no

explanations are that SMT might produce changes in kinematics (i.e. how the spine moves) rather than changes in the total ROM. It is also possible that changes in one manipulated joint among several in a spinal region would not contribute greatly to changes in regional movement.

Significant effects only in the cervical spine

In this review, SMT only showed discernible effects in the cervical spine. There may be several explanations for this. First, gross ranges of motion are largest in the cervical spine and so there is the potential for treatment in that area to cause a larger, hence measureable, effect. Secondly, more than 50% of the total rotation of the cervical spine is attributed to movement at a single level, the atlanto-axial joint [53]. Hence, SMT targeting the atlanto-axial joint could potentially lead to a substantial overall increase in the rotation of the entire cervical spine. In the lumbar and thoracic spine no single segmental level is responsible for a substantial proportion of movement of the entire region. Therefore, an increase in movement at a single level below the neck is less likely to result in a large change in regional ROM, as shown in this review.

Post hoc analysis

In order to investigate this matter further, all articles that tested the effect of SMT specifically in the upper cervical spine were re-analyzed, in relation to the size of the effect. Two studies [39,40] treated C1-C2, with different results: the first one [39], showed a difference pre/post treatment (3.75 degrees) only for right neck rotation. The other [40], showed that SMT significantly increased neck flexion and rotation (see Table 4). Studies [37,41] treated at the C3-C6 level and they also had different results: [37] showed that SMT was more effective than control mobilization, whereas [41] showed no significant effect on ROM. One study [42] was conducted at the thoracic level and showed improved cervical ROM. Finally four studies [36,38,43,44] treated a clinically determined area and only one [36] showed improved cervical ROM with SMT. These results, therefore, do not corroborate the theory that upper cervical SMT has a particularly obvious effect on cervical rotation. Further study is obviously needed on this aspect of spinal ROM.

Technical challenges in measuring ROM

There are also some technical issues that have to be taken into account in interpreting the results presented herein. For example, measurements of ROM face the problem of where to start and stop; i.e. how to identify the neutral or starting position. Therefore, measurements are probably more accurate when the full ROM is reported. Although most studies in our review did measure the full range, for some reason they reported on each individual movement component (e.g. left rotation and right rotation).

It is also possible that ROM does increase immediately following treatment but that the methods used in the reviewed studies did not capture this effect. In this regard, most of authors either claimed to be using a previously tested and acceptable instrument in relation to reliability, or they presented their own reliability study with acceptable results.

Interestingly, many studies of cervical ROM seem to concentrate on the reliability of measurement tools, but construct validity and what has been referred to as 'responsiveness' - the ability to capture change - are studied less often [54]. Whether a particular device is capable of accurately measuring ROM with appropriate precision is of utmost importance. However, it has been pointed out [33] that certain methodological procedures, rather than the device itself, are problematic, at least for cervical ROMs. Such items are wide variations in study designs, the characteristics of the observers and study populations, whether warm-ups were allowed, whether the movements were active or passive, and the time intervals between repeated measurements. Furthermore, it is difficult to assess ROMs, and outcomes may not be reliable if there is pain in the examined area [55]. These were all items that we examined in our critical review of articles, and it was apparent that a number of studies did not take these concerns into consideration.

Methodological considerations of this review

As with all systematic literature reviews, it is likely that not all relevant articles were found, and the review process itself has a subjective element even with the systematic approach of using checklists. Other researchers may prefer to scrutinize other methodological items and may judge the contents differently. However, as there were no disagreements between the two primary reviewers, the protocol appears to have been appropriate and clearly defined.

Research findings are of course dependent on the study methodology; it is often seen that the weakest studies have the "best" results. However, in this review, the methodological score was, generally, associated with study outcome in the opposite way, i.e. studies with better quality scores were more likely to show statistically significant differences, suggesting that the effects of SMT on ROM are robust, albeit not very large. Nevertheless, the fact that there was no set cut-point for methodological acceptability and because the evidence tables report on both descriptive and quality items, the reader is able to make his/her own additional analysis of the data, should this be relevant.

Implications of findings for future research

It has been shown that it is difficult to evaluate ROM if there is pain [55]. On the other hand, it does not seem relevant to manipulate non-painful articulations in order to study the effect on movement, as these likely already have a full ROM. Therefore, it is difficult to know whether clinical improvements following SMT in patients with neck pain [11] or patients with low-back pain [1] are due mainly to improved biomechanical status, a direct reduction of pain, or a combination of the two. A previous review concluded that there is a direct action of SMT on experimentally induced pain [26] but the present review cannot isolate a general direct effect of SMT on ROM. Consequently, other information seems to be necessary to better understand the relationship between pain and motion in relation to SMT.

Implications of findings for clinical practice

The results do not support the concept that SMT has an immediate, strong and obvious effect on ROM in the human spine. In clinical practice, it is possible that measurements of ROM should be clearly separated from the experience of pain in relation to movements.

Conclusion

Based on the studies reviewed herein, SMT sometimes seems to have a small effect on ROM, at least in the cervical spine. The studies reviewed did not reveal an effect of SMT on temporomandibular, lumbar or hip ROMs. Future studies into ROM should take into account various stages of degeneration, should standardize the experimental situation, and should include both pain and ROM as outcome variables. It would also be useful to include study subjects who actually have a decreased ROM, in order to have the potential for improvement. Also, it seems obvious that the measured movement should have the potential to improve with the treatment. Therefore, the effect of SMT on the upper cervical spine should be tested in relation to rotation and treatment to the lower cervical spine in relation to lateral bending, flexion and extension. The full ROM should be measured with validated instruments and all estimates should be clearly reported, including full statistical analysis.

Competing interests

Authors declare there are no conflicts of interest.

Authors' contributions

All authors instigated this review. MM and CLY designed the check-lists. MM and BB searched in the databases. MM and CLY reviewed the literature and wrote the first draft. BB, MDC and MAA provided expertise on the topic, assisted with the literature review and provided critical comments to the first draft. All authors reviewed the final manuscript and approved the final version.

Author details

[1]EA 4532 CIAMS, UFR STAPS, Univ Paris-Sud, Orsay, France. [2]The Research Department, The Spine Centre of Southern Denmark, Hospital Lillebælt, Odense, Denmark. [3]Institut Franco-Européen de Chiropratique, Paris, France. [4]Institute of Regional Health Services Research, Faculty of Health Sciences, University of Southern Denmark, Odense, Denmark. [5]Canadian Memorial Chiropractic College, Toronto, ON, Canada. [6]Département de Chiropratique, Université du Québec à Trois-Rivières, Trois-Rivières, QC, Canada. [7]Institut Universitaire de France, Paris, France.

References

1. Rubinstein S, Van Middelkoop M, Assendelft W, De Boer M, Van Tulder M: **Spinal manipulative therapy for chronic low-back pain: an update of a cochrane review.** *Spine* 2011, **36**(13):E825–E846.
2. Leach RA: ***The chiropractic theories***. Fourthth edition. Baltimore: Lippincott Williams & Wilkins; 2004:131–197–235–246.
3. Walter H: **The biomechanics of spinal manipulation.** *J Bodyw Mov Ther* 2010, **14**(3):280–286.
4. Maigne J-Y, Vautravers P: **Mechanism of action of spinal manipulative therapy.** *Joint Bone Spine* 2003, **70**(5):336–341.
5. Vernon H, Mrozek J: **A revised definition of manipulation.** *J Manipulative Physiol Ther* 2005, **28**(1):68–72.
6. Ianuzzi A, Khalsa P: **Comparison of human lumbar facet joint capsule strains during simulated high-velocity, low-amplitude spinal manipulation versus physiological motions.** *Spine J* 2005, **5**:277–290.
7. Herzog W: **The biomechanics of spinal manipulation.** *J Bodyw Mov Ther* 2010, **14**(3):280–286.
8. Sung P, Kang Y-M, Pickar J: **Effect of spinal manipulation duration on low threshold mechanoreceptors in lumbar paraspinal muscles: a preliminary report.** *Spine* 2005, **30**(1):115–122.
9. Stoddard A: **Osteopathic techniques of manipulation.** *Physiotherapy* 1970, **56**(1):29–30.
10. Snodgrass SJ, Rivett DA, Robertson VJ, Stojanovski E: **Forces applied to the cervical spine during posteroanterior mobilization.** *J Manipulative Physiol Ther* 2009, **32**(1):72–83.
11. Gross A, Miller J, D'Sylva J, Burnie SJ, Goldsmith CH, Graham N, Haines T, Brønfort G, Hoving JL: **Manipulation or mobilisation for neck pain: a Cochrane review.** *Man Ther* 2010, **15**(4):315–333.
12. Forand D, Drover J, Suleman Z, Symons B, Herzog W: **The forces applied by female and male chiropractors during thoracic spinal manipulation.** *J Manipulative Physiol Ther* 2004, **27**(1):49–56.

13. Dishman JD, Burke J: **Spinal reflex excitability changes after cervical and lumbar spinal manipulation: a comparative study.** *Spine J* 2003, **3**(3):204–212.
14. Roy RA, Boucher JP, Comtois AS: **Paraspinal cutaneous temperature modification after spinal manipulation at L5.** *J Manipulative Physiol Ther* 2010, **33**(4):308–314.
15. Bolton PS, Budgell B: **Visceral responses to spinal manipulation.** *J Electromyogr Kinesiol*, http://www.sciencedirect.com/science/article/pii/S1050641112000478.
16. DeVocht JW, Pickar JG, Wilder DG: **Spinal manipulation alters electromyographic activity of paraspinal muscles: a descriptive study.** *J Manipulative Physiol Ther* 2005, **28**(7):465–471.
17. Lehman G: **Kinesiological research: the use of surface electromyography for assessing the effects of spinal manipulation.** *J Electromyogr Kinesiol* 0, http://www.sciencedirect.com/science/article/pii/S1050641112000417.
18. Pickar JG: **Neurophysiological effects of spinal manipulation.** *Spine J* 2002, **2**(5):357–371.
19. Botelho MB, Andrade BB: **Effect of cervical spine manipulative therapy on judo athletes' grip strength.** *J Manipulative Physiol Ther* 2012, **35** (1):38–44.
20. Grindstaff TL, Hertel J, Beazell JR, Magrum EM, Ingersoll CD: **Effects of lumbopelvic joint manipulation on quadriceps activation and strength in healthy individuals.** *Man Ther* 2009, **14**(4):415–420.
21. Taylor HH, Murphy B: **Altered sensorimotor integration with cervical spine manipulation.** *J Manipulative Physiol Ther* 2008, **31**(2):115–126.
22. Bialosky JE, Bishop MD, Robinson ME, Zeppieri G Jr, George SZ: **Spinal manipulative therapy has an immediate effect on thermal pain sensitivity in people with low back pain: a randomized controlled trial.** *Phys Ther* 2009, **89**(12):1292–1303.
23. Fernández-Carnero J, Fernández-de-las-Peñas C, Cleland J: **Immediate hypoalgesic and motor effects after a single cervical spine manipulation in subjects with lateral epicondylalgia.** *J Manipulative Physiol Ther* 2008, **31**(9):675–681.
24. Ruiz-Sáez M, Fernández-de-las-Peñas C, Blanco C, Martínez-Segura R, García-León R: **Changes in pressure pain sensitivity in latent myofascial trigger points in the upper trapezius muscle after a cervical spine manipulation in pain-free subjects.** *J Manipulative Physiol Ther* 2007, **30**(8):578–583.
25. Sterling M, Jull G, Wright A: **Cervical mobilisation: concurrent effects on pain, sympathetic nervous system activity and motor activity.** *Man Ther* 2001, **6**(2):72–81.
26. Coronado RA, Gay CW, Bialosky JE, Carnaby GD, Bishop MD, George SZ: **Changes in pain sensitivity following spinal manipulation: A systematic review and meta-analysis.** *J Electromyogr Kinesiol* 2012, http://www.sciencedirect.com/science/article/pii/S1050641112000065.
27. Millan M, Leboeuf-Yde C, Budgell B, Amorim M-A: *The effect of spinal manipulative therapy on experimentally induced pain: a systematic literature review.* Accepted for publication in Chiropractic Manual Therapies.
28. Liberati A, Altman D, Tetzlaff J, Mulrow C, Gøtzsche P, Ioannidis J, Clarke M, Devereaux P, Kleijnen J, Moher D: **The PRISMA statement for reporting systematic reviews and meta-analyses of studies that evaluate health care interventions: explanation and elaboration.** *J Clin Epidemiol* 2009, **62**(10):e1–e34.
29. Moher D, Hopewell S, Schulz K, Montori V, Gøtzsche P, Devereaux P, Elbourne D, Egger M, Altman D: **CONSORT 2010 explanation and elaboration: updated guidelines for reporting parallel group randomised trials.** *Int J Surg* 2011, **1**:27–54.
30. Furlan A, Pennick V, Bombardier C, Van Tulder M: **2009 updated method guidelines for systematic reviews in the Cochrane back review group.** *Spine* 2009, **34**(18):1929–1941.
31. Colloca CJ, Keller TS, Moore RJ, Gunzburg R, Harrison DE: **Effects of disc degeneration on neurophysiological responses during dorsoventral mechanical excitation of the ovine lumbar spine.** *J Electromyogr Kinesiol* 2008, **18**(5):829–837.
32. Colloca C: **Intervertebral disc degeneration reduces vertebral motion responses.** *Spine* 2007, **32**(19):E544–E550.
33. Jordan K: **Assessment of published reliability studies for cervical spine range-of-motion measurement tools.** *J Manipulative Physiol Ther* 2000, **23**(3):180–195.
34. Mansilla-Ferragut P, Fernández-de-las Peñas C, Alburquerque-Sendín F, Cleland JA, Boscá-Gandía JJ: **Immediate effects of atlanto-occipital joint manipulation on active mouth opening and pressure pain sensitivity in women with mechanical neck pain.** *J Manipulative Physiol Ther* 2009, **32**(2):101–106.
35. Oliveira-Campelo N, Rubens-Rebelatto J, Marti N, Vallejo F, Alburquerque-Sendi N, Fernandez-de-Las-Penas C: **The immediate effects of atlanto-occipital joint manipulation and suboccipital muscle inhibition technique on active mouth opening and pressure pain sensitivity over latent myofascial trigger points in the masticatory muscles.** *J Orthop Sports Phys Ther* 2010, **40**(5):310–317.
36. Cassidy JD: **The immediate effect of manipulation versus mobilization on pain and range of motion in the cervical spine: a randomized controlled trial.** *J Manipulative Physiol Ther* 1992, **15**(9):570–575.
37. Martínez-Segura R, Fernández-de-las-Peñas C, Ruiz-Sáez M, López-Jiménez C, Rodríguez-Blanco C: **Immediate effects on neck pain and active range of motion after a single cervical high-velocity low-amplitude manipulation in subjects presenting with mechanical neck pain: a randomized controlled trial.** *J Manipulative Physiol Ther* 2006, **29**(7):511–517.
38. McClatchie L, Laprade J, Martin S, Jaglal SB, Richardson D, Agur A: **Mobilizations of the asymptomatic cervical spine can reduce signs of shoulder dysfunction in adults.** *Man Ther* 2009, **14**(4):369–374.
39. Passmore SR, Burke JR, Good C, Lyons JL, Dunn AS: **Spinal manipulation impacts cervical spine movement and Fitts' task performance: a single-blind randomized before-after trial.** *J Manipulative Physiol Ther* 2010, **33**(3):189–192.
40. Whittingham W, Nilsson N: **Active range of motion in the cervical spine increases after spinal manipulation (toggle recoil).** *J Manipulative Physiol Ther* 2001, **24**(9):552–555.
41. Tuttle N, Barrett R, Laakso L: **Relation between changes in posteroanterior stiffness and active range of movement of the cervical spine following manual therapy treatment.** *Spine* 2008, **33**(19):E673–E679.
42. Krauss J, Creighton D, Ely JD, Podlewska-Ely J: **The immediate effects of upper thoracic translatoric spinal manipulation on cervical pain and range of motion: a randomized clinical trial.** *Journal of Manual & Manipulative Therapy (Journal of Manual & Manipulative Therapy)* 2008, **16**(2):93–99.
43. Kanlayanaphotporn R, Chiradejnant A, Vachalathiti R: **The immediate effects of mobilization technique on pain and range of motion in patients presenting with unilateral neck pain: a randomized controlled trial.** *Arch Phys Med Rehabil* 2009, **90**(2):187–192.
44. Kanlayanaphotporn R, Chiradejnant A, Vachalathiti R: **Immediate effects of the central posteroanterior mobilization technique on pain and range of motion in patients with mechanical neck pain.** *Disabil Rehabil* 2010, **32**(8):622–628.
45. Goodsell M, Lee M, Latimer J: **Short-term effects of lumbar posteroanterior mobilization in individuals with low-back pain.** *J Manipulative Physiol Ther* 2000, **23**(5):332–342.
46. Konstantinou K, Foster N, Rushton A, Baxter D, Wright C, Breen A: **Flexion mobilizations with movement techniques: the immediate effects on range of movement and pain in subjects with low back pain.** *J Manipulative Physiol Ther* 2007, **30**(3):178–185.
47. Stamos-Papastamos N, Petty NJ, Williams JM: **Changes in bending stiffness and lumbar spine range of movement following lumbar mobilization and manipulation.** *J Manipulative Physiol Ther* 2011, **34**(1):46–53.
48. Pollard H, Ward G: **The effect of sacroiliac manipulation on hip flexion range of motion.** *Australasian Chiropractic & Osteopathy* 1997, **6**(3):80–84.
49. Prushansky T, Deryi O, Jabarreen B: **Reproducibility and validity of digital inclinometry for measuring cervical range of motion in normal subjects.** *Physiother Res Int* 2010, **15**(1):42–48.
50. O'Sullivan K, O'Sullivan L, Campbell A, O'Sullivan P, Dankaerts W: **Towards monitoring lumbo-pelvic posture in real-life situations: Concurrent validity of a novel posture monitor and a traditional laboratory-based motion analysis system.** *Man Ther* 2012, **17**(1):77–83.
51. Gelalis I, DeFrate L, Stafilas K, Pakos E, Kang J, Gilbertson L: **Three-dimensional analysis of cervical spine motion: reliability of a computer assisted magnetic tracking device compared to inclinometer.** *Eur Spine J* 2009, **18**(2):276–281.
52. Assink N, Bergman GJD, Knoester B, Winters JC, Dijkstra PU: **Assessment of the cervical range of motion over time, differences between results of the Flock of Birds and the EDI-320: A comparison between an electromagnetic tracking system and an electronic inclinometer.** *Man Ther* 2008, **13**(5):450–455.

53. Bogduk N, Mercer S: **Biomechanics of the cervical spine. I: Normal kinematics.** *Clin Biomech* 2000, **15**:633–648.
54. de Koning C, van den Heuvel S, Staal J, Smits-Engelsman B, Hendriks E: **Clinimetric evaluation of active range of motion measures in patients with non-specific neck pain: a systematic review.** *Eur Spine J* 2008, **17**(7):905–921.
55. Lehman GJ: **Biomechanical assessments of lumbar spinal function. How low back pain sufferers differ from normals. Implications for outcome measures research. Part I: kinematic assessments of lumbar function.** *J Manipulative Physiol Ther* 2004, **27**(1):57–62.
56. *Preferred Reporting Items for Systematic Reviews and Meta-Analyses: The PRISMA Statement*; www.prisma-statement.org.

3

A replication of the study 'Adverse effects of spinal manipulation: a systematic review'

Peter Tuchin*

Abstract

Objective: To assess the significance of adverse events after spinal manipulation therapy (SMT) by replicating and critically reviewing a paper commonly cited when reviewing adverse events of SMT as reported by Ernst (J Roy Soc Med 100:330–338, 2007).

Method: Replication of a 2007 Ernst paper to compare the details recorded in this paper to the original source material. Specific items that were assessed included the time lapse between treatment and the adverse event, and the recording of other significant risk factors such as diabetes, hyperhomocysteinemia, use of oral contraceptive pill, any history of hypertension, atherosclerosis and migraine.

Results: The review of the 32 papers discussed by Ernst found numerous errors or inconsistencies from the original case reports and case series. These errors included alteration of the age or sex of the patient, and omission or misrepresentation of the long term response of the patient to the adverse event. Other errors included incorrectly assigning spinal manipulation therapy (SMT) as chiropractic treatment when it had been reported in the original paper as delivered by a non-chiropractic provider (e.g. Physician).
The original case reports often omitted to record the time lapse between treatment and the adverse event, and other significant clinical or risk factors. The country of origin of the original paper was also overlooked, which is significant as chiropractic is not legislated in many countries. In 21 of the cases reported by Ernst to be chiropractic treatment, 11 were from countries where chiropractic is not legislated.

Conclusion: The number of errors or omissions in the 2007 Ernst paper, reduce the validity of the study and the reported conclusions. The omissions of potential risk factors and the timeline between the adverse event and SMT could be significant confounding factors. Greater care is also needed to distinguish between chiropractors and other health practitioners when reviewing the application of SMT and related adverse effects.

Keywords: MeSH, Chiropractic, Spinal manipulative therapy, Adverse effects

Introduction

The use of a treatment by health care providers requires examination of the evidence of effectiveness and assessment of the evidence for risks or adverse events (AE) caused by the treatment [1]. Spinal manipulation therapy (SMT) has strong evidence for treatment of low back pain, neck pain, headache and migraine [2-6]. This is supported by numerous systematic reviews of a large number of randomized controlled trials [7-10].

Adverse events following SMT are common but usually result in minor, short term problems [11-14]. The most commonly expressed area of concern regarding these adverse effects of spinal manipulation includes conditions such as vertebral artery dissection (VAD) or carotid artery dissection (CAD), which results in cerebrovascular accidents (CVA) [15]. These serious AE can occur immediately following SMT but are reported as rare and unpredictable consequence of all neck movements [16]. However, there appears to be conflict over the frequency or severity of serious events which may follow SMT. A paper written by Ernst "Adverse effects of spinal manipulation: a systematic review" was published in the Journal of the Royal Society of Medicine in July 2007 [17]. In the paper, 28 articles reporting a total of 32 case reports were identified with 22 cases involving chiropractors. The

Correspondence: peter.tuchin@mq.edu.au
Macquarie University, Bld E5A Rm 355, Waterloo Rd, North Ryde, Sydney, NSW 2109, Australia

majority of cases involved complications from cervical manipulation, the most notable problem being VAD. According to the 2007 Ernst paper, "the symptoms were frequently life-threatening", and in the majority of cases "spinal manipulation was deemed to be the probable cause of the adverse effect" [17]. In addition, SMT applied by chiropractors was specified by a separation of the papers noting chiropractic as the cause of the AE.

It is important that all the clinical features for these AE are clearly identified and recorded, with any potential predisposing risk factors described [14]. As the 2007 Ernst paper is commonly cited when assessing any risk with cervical spine SMT, it may be regarded as a significant paper [18]. This paper is a replication of the 2007 Ernst paper, and a critical review of the initial results reported in the 2007 paper.

Methods

The case reports in the reference list from the 2007 Ernst paper were retrieved and reviewed in detail. The clinical details of each case were then cross-checked with Ernst's paper for accuracy and relevance towards assessing adverse events. Particular interest was paid towards papers that involved chiropractic SMT and its subsequent effects.

Each paper was reviewed to assess significant risk factors for CVA that had been identified in the literature [18,19]. These include factors such as use of oral contraceptive pill (OCP), any history of hypertension, atherosclerosis, family history of cardiac conditions, smoking, previous headaches or migraine, and genetic factors [19-24]. Also, each paper was reviewed to assess the likelihood that the provider that rendered the treatment was a qualified chiropractor. This was determined by a review of the details provided describing the SMT procedure, and by reviewing the country of origin for the case report. Any description of the SMT was assessed to determine if this was a commonly performed chiropractic procedure or if it described SMT commonly performed by other practitioners.

In addition, other items that were assessed included the description of the presenting symptom(s), the time lapse between treatment and the type of adverse event. This included examining any diagnosis of the presenting symptom to the SMT practitioner, the onset of symptoms relating to the adverse event, and assessing any other events that could be a confounding factor for assessment of the relationship between SMT and the adverse event.

Papers from the 2007 Ernst study were excluded if the abstract or full text could not be obtained.

Results

In the 2007 Ernst paper, 28 articles reporting a total of 32 case reports were identified with 22 cases involving chiropractors. Case reports where the paper was not published in English often had only an abstract which could be reviewed. The outcome of these papers is presented as separate issues.

The review of the original case reports and case series papers described by Ernst found numerous errors or inconsistencies (See Table 1- Errors Or Inconsistencies In The 2007 Ernst Paper). These errors included alteration of the age or sex of the patient, and omission or misrepresentation of the long term response of the patient to the adverse event.

More serious concerns involved the interpretation of clinical features for each case and the subsequent conclusions regarding the safety of chiropractic SMT. For example, Table 1 in the 2007 Ernst paper summarizes case reports of AE after SMT administered by chiropractors. However, two case reports clearly state the SMT was administered by non-chiropractors. Morandi reported a 49 year old female that developed caudal spinal cord ischaemia after a lumbar SMT [25]. The paper state's "*Three weeks into the episode, a physician performed lumbar vertebral manipulation*". Also, Chen reported a 72 year old male that developed a haematoma in the ligamentum flavum [26]. The paper states "*.... following traditional massage therapy*".

Nine cases originated from countries where there is no legislation governing chiropractic, which therefore allows non-qualified people to administer SMT, and this may be incorrectly termed "chiropractic" [27-35]. In four of these cases only the abstract was available in English, so a less detailed review could be performed for these papers. However, in the seven cases with full English papers, a detailed review is discussed later in this paper.

Therefore, in 11 cases of the 21 (one paper has been withdrawn from circulation) that Ernst reported as SMT administered by chiropractors, it is unlikely that the person was a qualified chiropractor. Whilst most cases did not describe the SMT procedure, the three cases which did, describe SMT procedures not commonly used by chiropractors [25,28,30]. For example, facet joint infiltration after the SMT and SMT with axial traction, which was initially described by Cyriax (a medical practitioner) [36]. This supports the theory that these 11 cases had SMT from a non-chiropractor, which has previously been reported [37]. (See Table 2: Countries With Legislation For Chiropractic).

Importantly, in five of the seven cases (with full English versions available) complete resolution of the AE was reported after appropriate treatment. Also, three of the seven cases describe the time interval following SMT to the onset of symptoms as greater than 24 hours (i.e. 24 – 96 hours). Given that many VAD occur spontaneously or due to simple everyday activities, a time interval of greater than 24 hours is not appropriate.

Table 1 Errors or Omissions to 2007 Ernst paper

Author	Presenting symptoms	Outcome	Comments	Error or omission
Chiropractic				
Jeret	Not noted	Complete resolution	Dural tear vs IH inconsistency	
Siegel	HA- several weeks, no IHS categories noted;	Permanent	Letter to the editor	
Parwar	Shoulder strain	Horner's syndrome; no further neurologic abnormalities developed	9 previous, uneventful treatments	noted as male; outcome "not reported"
Schram	Neck pain and stiffness after sleeping on sofa	Shortness of breath on exertion and breathing in the supine position	NB ref 12 notes stretch trauma;	Residual dyspnea
Stevinson	Unknown	Complete resolution after surgery	Subdural haematoma; Recall cases over 12mths	
Jeret	Neck pain, OCP	Complete resolution		
	Unknown	Flow re-established after recanulization		Outcome "not mentioned"
	Unknown	Horner's syndrome (opposite side) after 2 weeks hospital	new Horner's syndrome	"significant recovery after surgery"
Jay	4 day HA, fever, cough, sinusitis, antibiotics	Complete resolution	Polycysytic ovarian disease	Outcome "not mentioned"
Nadgir	Neck cramping	Minimal residual hemianasthesia and dysethesiae	B/L ICA & VAD	"residual hemianasthesia and dysethesiae"
Non chiropractic				
Se'dat	Chronic headaches, anti-inflam and pain medication	Positive outcome after 3 weeks	Genetic variation	"mild" removed from outcome statement
Beck	Unknown	Complete resolution confirmed by MRI	IH but reported as Wallenberg's syndrome,	"no information provided"; not Wallenberg's syndrome
Oehler	Unknown, past HA	Resolution	10yrs chiro and HA	Outcome "not mentioned"
Morandi	CLBP, aggravated by heavy lifting	Permanent neuro loss	CLBP with acute episode	Noted as 44 yo,
Saxler		Complete resolution	no translation	
Chen	Neck pain- relieved by chiropractor		Haematoma after massage	Massage therapy
Suh	Chronic neck and shoulder pain)	Complete resolution	IH	Reported as 36 yo female
Abstract only				
Yokota	Unknown	Dejerine syndrome	no translation	
Izquierdo-Casas	Unknown		no translation	
Menendez-Gonzalez	Unknown	Wallenberg's syndrome,	no translation	
Tome	Unknown	Multiple cervical disc lesions	no translation	
Wojcik		Publication withdrawn		

In the remaining 10 cases it is more likely that the person was a qualified chiropractor [38-44]. However, as most of these cases (n = six) did not describe the SMT procedure, it cannot be determined if the SMT procedure was a type commonly used by chiropractors. In addition, there is the possibility of poor execution of the SMT procedure or inappropriate use of the procedure (i.e. professional negligence).

Many of these 10 cases also had a plausible alternative explanation as to why the AE may have occurred (See Table 3: Features And Outcomes Of Cases). For example, Jeret described a case of a 51-year-old man who presented to the hospital five days after rotatory chiropractic manipulation of his neck [38]. For 2–3 days prior to admission, the patient was reported to have had intermittent slurred speech, left facial droop, and mild left hand weakness. The case had no description of the presenting symptom and no description of any risk factors for CVA. Interestingly, the initial symptoms were all related to a left side infarct and 2 weeks after admission to hospital the patient had a right side infarct. It is plausible this man had CVA due to risk factors other than chiropractic SMT.

Table 2 Reference papers and their country of origin and relevant legislation for chiropractic licensing

Reference	Country	Legislation regulating chiropractic
[25]	France	No
[26]	China/Taiwan	No
[27]	France	No
[28]	German (English translation)	No
[29]	German (in german)	No
[30]	German	No
[31]	Korea	No
[32]	Japan (in japanese)	No
[33]	Spain (in spanish)	No
[34]	Spain (in spanish)	No
[35]	Spain (in spanish)	No
[38]	USA	Yes
[39]	USA	Yes
[40]	USA	Yes
[41]	USA	Yes
[42]	Unknown –survey of UK neurologists	Yes
[43]	USA	Yes
[44]	USA	Yes
[45]	USA	Yes
[46]	USA USA	Yes Yes

Parwar (2001) reported a case of a 44-year-old woman who presented to an emergency room with severe headache, right-sided neck pain, ptosis, and miosis [40]. It was reported that this happened several days after her ninth chiropractic session for her presenting symptom of "a strained right shoulder muscle". The patient was diagnosed with Horner's Syndrome due to a right internal carotid artery dissection. None of the risk factors for CVA were reported, for example, migraine, which has been reported to cause Horner's Syndrome [19]. The case report also stated that no further neurological abnormalities occurred, which Ernst reported as "not reported".

Schram reported a case of a 41-year-old male who sought chiropractic care for pain and stiffness in his neck and shoulders [41]. The pain developed after the patient had slept on a sofa while on vacation, one week previous to the treatment. The case report stated the "chiropractor did a number of manipulations that the patient described as forcing his shoulders downward and turning his head laterally" (not a common chiropractic technique). There was no record that the patient experienced increased neck pain or any alteration in breathing pattern. He returned to his chiropractor the next day with this complaint, and was subsequently transferred to an emergency department for evaluation of his orthopnea.

Stevinson (2001) described a case of a 46 year old male that was reported to suffer a subdural haematoma after a chiropractic treatment [42]. The case was obtained from a survey to UK neurologists, who were asked to recall patients that had a neurological complication within a 12 month period. The entire case history is reproduced below:

> *A man aged 46 was diagnosed with acute subdural haematoma occurring immediately after chiropractic treatment. A burrhole was required. There was no neurological deficit at one month or six month follow up.*

Apart from the obvious weakness of recall bias with the survey, the case details could at best only be described as scant. It is more likely this is a case of negligence, with the chiropractor failing to adequately investigate any previous trauma that would have caused the subdural haematoma. This would then become a contra-indication for SMT and require immediate referral for emergency medical treatment.

Jeret reported a case of a 34 year old male who had a whiplash injury in a motor vehicle accident (MVA), for which chiropractic treatment gave some relief [43]. One month after the MVA, the chiropractor performed a SMT and approximately 36 hours after this the patient reported a severe, throbbing, positional headache. The clinical diagnosis was intracranial hypotension, which is commonly reported as spontaneous.

Jay et al (2003) described a case of bilateral occipital-parietal hemorrhagic infarctions following chiropractic cervical manipulation [44]. A 26-year-old woman presented to a chiropractor with mild headache, cough, and low-grade fever for four days (for which she had been prescribed antibiotics). The patient had received over 20 chiropractic manipulations over the previous two years without event. CT scan and MRI were reported to show bilateral, symmetric occipital-parietal hemorrhagic infarctions. The patient was taking the OCP (for polycystic ovarian disease), however, other risk factors for stroke were not recorded. In addition, the time between onset of visual changes and SMT was over 36 hours. It is plausible this woman had CVA due to risk factors other than chiropractic SMT. The patient also made a full recovery.

Discussion

The general quality of the original case information used by Ernst was poor, which should have called into question the conclusions published in the 2007 Ernst paper. The lack of clinical detail in the original cases does not

Table 3 Features And Outcomes Of Cases

Author	Patient	Presenting symptoms	SMT Procedure	Time after SMT for onset of symptoms	Additional information
Jeret	34 yo male	Not noted	Not noted	36 hrs after	Recent MVA
Siegel	33 yo female	HA- several weeks, no IHS categories noted;	HVLA	immediate	
Parwar	44yo female	Shoulder strain	Not noted	Several days	9 previous CSMT without incident
Schram	47yo male	Neck pain and stiffness after sleeping on sofa	Shoulders forced down and turning head laterally	Later at night; initial relief by SMT	Neck position whilst sleeping
Stevinson	46yo male	Unknown	Unknown	immediate	Subdural haematoma from previous unreported trauma
Jeret	31yo female	Neck pain,	Rapid rotation	immediate	Complication from OCP
	64 yo male	Unknown	Gentle SMT (daughter DC)	4 days	Age related CVA
	51 yo male	Unknown	rotation	2-3 days	
Jay	26 yo female	4 day HA, fever, cough, sinusitis, antibiotics	20 previous DC treatments-not described	36hrs	Complication from inflammatory response
Nadgir	34 yo male	Neck cramping	Several previous sessions, not described	Immediate, but symptoms not described	Neck cramping a symptom of impending CVA
Non chiropractic					
Se'dat	42 yo female	Chronic headaches, anti-inflammatory and pain medications	Gentle SMT	immediate	Complication from inflammatory response, Un-registered practitioner
Beck	40 yo female	Unknown	Axial tension and rotation-(Cyriax manoeuver)	24 hrs	Not chiropractic SMT
Oehler	31 yo female	Unknown, past HA	Unknown, previous regular chiropractic	Minimum of 24 hrs	Un-registered practitioner
Morandi	49 yo female	CLBP, aggravated by heavy lifting	Physician	Few hours	Not chiropractic SMT
Saxler	27 yo female		C5/6 SMT, facet joint infiltration	10 min	Not chiropractic SMT
Chen	72 yo male	Neck pain- relieved by chiropractor	Massage therapy	1 week, symptoms began after hospital treatment	Not chiropractic SMT
Suh	37 yo female	Chronic neck and shoulder pain)	Cyriax treatment (reported as "chiropractic manoeuver")	5 days	Not chiropractic SMT
Abstract only			**probably not chiropractic**		
Yokota	38 yo male	Unknown	Unknown	Unknown	Un-registered practitioner
Izquierdo-Casas	37 yo female	Unknown	Unknown	Unknown	Un-registered practitioner
Menendez-Gonzalez	Not noted	Unknown	Not noted	A few hours	Un-registered practitioner
Tome	Not noted	Unknown	"non qualified personnel"	Unknown	Un-registered practitioner

Key: *IH* = intracranial hypotension; *HVLA* = high velocity, low amplitude; *OCP* = oral contraceptive pill; *HA* = headache; *IHS* = international headache society; *B/L* = bilateral; *CVA* = internal carotid artery; *VAD* = vertebral artery dissection; *CLBP* = chronic low back pain; *SMT* = spinal manipulative therapy.

allow adequate conclusions to be drawn from these cases. For example, the vast majority of the original cases did not contain information about well-established confounding variables for these types of cases. Subsequently, no conclusions can be correctly derived about the impact of SMT on the development of VAD. The author of the 2007 paper should have concluded previous cases material was inadequate for any relationship between SMT and VAD to be assessed.

The terms chiropractic treatment, chiropractic manipulation, chirotherapy and/or chiropractic procedure were used repeatedly, without identification of the practitioners' qualifications. A study by Terrett found that "the words chiropractic and chiropractor have been incorrectly used in numerous publications dealing with SMT injury by medical authors, respected medical journals and medical organisations. In many cases, this is not accidental; the authors had access to original reports that identified the practitioner involved as a non-chiropractor" [36]. Wenban also suggests that the words 'chiropractor' and 'chiropractic manipulation' are used inappropriately by European biomedical researchers

[45]. This appears to be continuing with the Ernst's paper giving the impression that most AE after SMT are due to chiropractic procedures "....(SMT) is the hallmark treatment of chiropractors".

Another weakness in many of the original case studies involved poor information on the time period between the onset of the AE and the administration of the SMT. Few cases described any events which may have occurred after the SMT that could have had a direct bearing on the subsequent AE occurrence. For example, one person drove home after her treatment and whilst she was reversing the car, the AE occurred. The sustained neck rotation could have had more impact than the SMT.

There were also further examples were plausible alternative processes may have led to the development of a VAD, which was independent to the SMT. For example, Ernst failed to acknowledge the anatomical variance in the patient's vertebral arteries causing them to originate below the level of the foramen magnum which the author acknowledges to have played a vital role in the patient's complications following spinal manipulative therapy [27].

There was also no discussion on the relevance of time lapse between SMT and the AE, where, in some cases, periods of greater than 24 hours occurred. This combined with many cases not describing the presenting symptom, creates significant weaknesses in establishing a link of the AE to SMT.

Conclusion

It is unwise to make conclusions regarding causality from any case study or multiple case studies. The number of errors or omissions in the 2007 Ernst paper significantly limit any reported conclusions. Standard risk factors for VAD and the timeline between the VAD and SMT could be significant confounding factors. Whilst SMT may coincide with development of VAD, the quality of the 2007 paper does not add to the understanding of whether there is any link of SMT to VAD. A much more thorough peer review needs to occur regarding papers such as Ernst 2007. Further research is required to assess the relationship between SMT and VAD.

Competing interests

The author declare that they have no competing interests.

Authors' information

Peter Tuchin: Senior Lecturer.

References

1. Harlan WR Jr: **Research on complementary and alternative medicine using randomized controlled trials.** *J Altern Complement Med* 2001, **7**(Suppl 1):S45–S52.
2. UK BEAM Trial Team: **United Kingdom back pain exercise and manipulation (UK BEAM) randomised trial: cost effectiveness of physical treatments for back pain in primary care.** *BMJ* 2004, **329**: doi:10.1136/bmj.38282.607859.AE.
3. Meade TW, Dyer S, Browne W, *et al*: **Randomized comparison of chiropractic and hospital outpatient management for low back pain: Results from an extended follow up.** *Br Med J* 1995, **311**:349–351.
4. Bronfort G, Evans R, Anderson AV, Svendsen MS, Bracha Y, Grimm RH: **Spinal Manipulation, Medication, or Home Exercise With Advice for Acute and Subacute Neck Pain: A Randomized Trial.** *Ann Intern Med* 2012, **156**:1–10.
5. Jull G, Trott P, Potter H, Zito G, Niere K, Shirley D, *et al*: **A randomized controlled trial of exercise and manipulative therapy for cervicogenic headache.** *Spine* 2002, **27**:1835–1843.
6. Tuchin PJ, Pollard H, Bonello R: **A RCT of Chiropractic SMT and migraine.** *J Manipulative Physiol Ther* 2000, **23**:91–95.
7. Chou R, Qaseem A, Snow V, *et al*: **Diagnosis and treatment of low back pain: a joint clinical practice guideline from the American College of Physicians and the American Pain Society.** *Ann Intern Med* 2007, **147**:478–491.
8. Bronfort G, Haas M, Evans R, Triano J: **Effectiveness of manual therapies: the UK evidence report.** *Chiropr Osteopat* 2010, **18**:3–36.
9. Airaksinen O, Brox JI, Cedraschi C, *et al*: **Chapter 4. European guidelines for the management of chronic nonspecific low back pain.** *Eur Spine J* 2006, **15**(Suppl 2):S192–S300.
10. Chaibi A, Tuchin PJ, Russell M: **Manual Therapies for Migraine A Systematic Review of the Literature.** *J Headache* 2011. doi:10.1007/s10194-011-0296-6.
11. Thiel HW, Bolton JE, Docherty S, Portlock JC: **Safety of Chiropractic Manipulation of the Cervical Spine. A Prospective National Survey.** *Spine* 2007, **32**:2375–2378.
12. Hurwitz EL, Morgenstern H, Harber P, *et al*: **A Randomized Trial of Chiropractic Manipulation and Mobilization for Patients with Neck Pain: Clinical Outcomes from the UCLA Neck-Pain Study.** *Am J Publ Health* 2002, **92**:100.
13. Rubinstein SM, *et al*: **The benefits outweigh the risks for patients undergoing chiropractic care for neck pain: a prospective, multicenter, cohort study.** *J Manipulative Physiol Ther* 2007, **30**(6):408–418.
14. Cagnie B, Vinck E, Beernaert A, Cambier D: **How common are side effects of spinal manipulation and can these side effects be predicted?** *Man Ther* 2004, **9**:151–156.
15. Ernst E: **Vascular accidents after neck manipulation: cause or coincidence?** *Int J Clin Pract* 2010, **64**:673–677.
16. Haldeman S, Kohlbeck FJ, McGregor M: **Unpredictability of cerebrovascular ischaemia associated with cervical spine manipulation therapy.** *Spine* 2002, **27**:49–55.
17. Ernst E: **Adverse effects of spinal manipulation: a systematic review.** *J Roy Soc Med* 2007, **100**:330–338.
18. Debette S, Leys D: **Cervical-artery dissections: predisposing factors, diagnosis, and outcome.** *Lancet Neurol* 2009, **8**:668–678.
19. Chatzikonstantinou A, Wolf ME, Hennerici MG: **Ischemic stroke in young adults: classification and risk factors.** *J Neurol*, doi:10.1007/s00415-011-6234-3.
20. Chandra A, Suliman A, Angle N: **Spontaneous dissection of the carotid and vertebral arteries: the 10-year UCSD experience.** *Ann Vasc Surg* 2007, **21**:178–185.
21. Gallai V, Caso V, Paciaroni M, *et al*: **Mild hyperhomocystaeinemia: a possible risk factor for cervical artery dissection.** *Stroke* 2001, **32**:714–718.
22. Grau AJ, Brandt T, Buggle F, *et al*: **Association of cervical artery dissection with recent infection.** *Arch Neurol* 1999, **56**:851–856.
23. Brandt T, Orberk E, Weber R, *et al*: **Pathogenesis of cervical artery dissections: association with connective tissue abnormalities.** *Neurology* 2001, **57**:24–30.
24. Campos CR, Evaristo EF, Yamamoto FI, *et al*: **Spontaneous cervical carotid and vertebral arteries dissection: study of 48 patients.** *Arq Neuropsiquiatr* 2004, **62**:492–498.
25. Morandi X, *et al*: **Caudal spinal cord ischemia after lumbar vertebral manipulation.** *Joint Bone Spine* 2004, **71**:334–337.
26. Chen H-C, Hsu P-W, Lin C-Y, Tzaan W-C: **Symptomatic hematoma of cervical ligamentum flavum.** *Spine* 2005, **30**:E489–E491.

27. Se'dat J, Dib M, Mahagne MH, Lonjon M, Paquis P: **Stroke after chiropractic manipulation as a result of extracranial postero-inferior cerebellar artery dissection.** *J Manipulative Physiol Ther* 2002, **25:**588–590.
28. Beck J, Raabe A, Seifert V: **Intracranial hypotension after chiropractic manipulation of the cervical spine.** *J Neurol Neurosurg Psychiatry* 2003, **74:**820–826.
29. Oehler J, *et al*: **Vertebralisdissektion nach chiropraktischer behandlung.** *Der Orthopade* 2003, **32:**911–913.
30. Saxler G, Barden B: **Extensive spinal epidural haematoma – an uncommon entity following cervical chiropractic manipulation.** *Z Orthop Grenzgeb* 2004, **142:**79–84.
31. Suh S-I, Koh S-B, Choi E-J, *et al*: **Intracranial hypotension induced by cervical spine chiropractic manipulation.** *Spine* 2005, **30:**E340–E342.
32. Yokota J, Amakusa Y, Tomita Y, Takahashi S: **The medial medullary infarction (Dejerine syndrome) following chiropractic neck manipulation.** *No To Shinkei* 2003, **55:**121–125.
33. Izquierdo-Casas J, *et al*: **Diseccion vertebral como causa del syndrome de enclaustramiento y opciones terapeuticas con fibrinolisis intraarterial durante la fase aguda.** *Rev Neurol* 2004, **38:**1139–1141.
34. Menendez-Gonzalez M, *et al*: **Sindrome do Wallemberg secundario a diseccion de la arteria vertegral por manipulacion quiropractica.** *Rev Neurol* 2003, **37:**837–839.
35. Tome F, Barriga A, Espejo L: **Herniacion discal multiple tras manipulacion quiropractica cervical.** *Revista de Medicina de la Universidad de Navarra* 2004, **48:**39–41.
36. Terrett AGJ: **Misuse of the literature by medical authors in discussing spinal manipulative therapy injury.** *J Manipulative Physiol Ther* 1995, **18:**203–210.
37. Cyriax J: *Textbook of Orthopaedic Medicine. Volume one: Diagnosis of Soft Tissue Lesions.* 8th edition. London: Baillière Tindall; 1982. ISBN 0 7020 0935.
38. Jeret JS: **More complications of spinal manipulation.** *Stroke* 2001, **32:**1136–1137.
39. Siegel D, Neiders T: **Vertebral artery dissection and pontine infarction after chiropractic manipulation.** *Am J Emerg Med* 2001, **19:**172–173.
40. Parwar BL, Fawzi AA, Arnold AC, Schwartz SD: **Horner's syndrome and dissection of the internal carotid artery after chiropractic manipulation of the neck.** *Am J Ophthalmol* 2001, **131:**523–524.
41. Schram DJ, Vosik W: **Diaphragmatic paralysis following cervical chiropractic manipulation: case report and review.** *Complementary/ Alternative Medicine for Asthma* 2001, **119:**638–640.
42. Stevinson C, Honan W, Cooke B, Ernst E: **Neurological complications of cervical spine manipulation.** *J Roy Soc Med* 2001, **94:**107–110.
43. Jeret JS, Bluth M: **Stroke following chiropractic manipulation. Report of three cases and review of the literature.** *Cerebrovasc Dis* 2002, **13:**210–213.
44. Jay WM, Shah MI, Schneck MJ: **Bilateral occipital-parietal hemorrhagic infarctions following chiropractic cervical manipulation.** *Semin Ophthalmol* 2003, **18:**205–209.
45. Nadgir RN, Loevner LA, Ahmed T, Chalela J, Slawek K, Imbesi S: **Simultaneous bilateral internal carotid and vertebral artery dissection following chiropractic manipulation: case report and review of the literature.** *Neuroradiol* 2003, **45:**311–314.
46. Wenban AB: **Inappropriate use of the title chiropractor and the term chiropractic manipulation in the peer-reviewed biomedical literature.** *Chiropr Osteopat* 2006, **14:**1–7.

Self-reported recognition of undiagnosed life threatening conditions in chiropractic practice: a random survey

Dwain M Daniel[1*], Harrison Ndetan[2], Ronald L Rupert[2] and Daniel Martinez[2]

Abstract

Background: The purpose of this study was to identify the type and frequency of previously undiagnosed life threatening conditions (LTC), based on self-reports of chiropractic physicians, which were first recognized by the chiropractic physician. Additionally this information may have a preliminary role in determining whether chiropractic education provides the knowledge necessary to recognize these events.

Methods: The study design was a postal, cross-sectional, epidemiological self-administered survey. Two thousand Doctors of Chiropractic in the US were randomly selected from a list of 57878. The survey asked respondents to state the number of cases from the list where they were the first physician to recognize the condition over the course of their practice careers. Space was provided for unlisted conditions.

Results: The response rate was 29.9%. Respondents represented 11442 years in practice and included 3861 patients with a reported undiagnosed LTC. The most commonly presenting conditions were in rank order: carcinoma, abdominal aneurysm, deep vein thrombosis, stroke, myocardial infarction, subdural hematoma and a large group of other diagnoses. The occurrence of a previously undiagnosed LTC can be expected to present to the chiropractic physician every 2.5 years based on the responding doctors reports.

Conclusion: Based on this survey chiropractic physicians report encountering undiagnosed LTC's in the normal course of practice. The findings of this study are of importance to the chiropractic profession and chiropractic education. Increased awareness and emphasis on recognition of LTC is a critical part of the education process and practice life.

Keywords: Chiropractic, Education, Professional role, Primary care, Diagnosis, Life threatening

Background

There are several different definitions of what constitutes a primary care physician [1,2]. Most of these definitions incorporate the concept of "assumption of longitudinal responsibility for the patient regardless of the presence or absence of disease" [3]. Based on this definition a physician, at a minimum, has the moral and legal responsibility to be able to identify and refer, when necessary, conditions which if left unrecognized and untreated may result in serious and even deadly consequences to the patient.

There is an ongoing controversy within the healthcare community regarding role of the chiropractic physician as well as debates on this issue within the chiropractic profession itself. There are three basic positions argued; primary care, neuromusculoskeletal care and subluxation based care. The Council on Chiropractic Education mandates that chiropractic educational institutions "train a competent doctor of chiropractic who will provide quality patient care and serve as a primary care physician" [4]. Duenas et al. found 94% of chiropractic colleges utilize the term "primary care provider" or similar variants when describing the product of their educational programs [1]. In spite of primary care training some argue the proper role of the chiropractor is as a neuromusculoskeletal or musculoskeletal specialist [5,6]. This position is supported at least in part by the profile of the typical chiropractic patient. According to The National Board of Chiropractic Examiners, 82.9% of presenting complaints in the typical chiropractor's office consist of back pain, extremity pain,

* Correspondence: ddaniel@txchiro.edu
[1]Texas Chiropractic College, Pasadena, TX, USA
Full list of author information is available at the end of the article

neck pain and headache. Less than 10% of patients present with non-neuromusculoskeletal complaints [7]. A third position argues chiropractic is a separate and distinct health care specialty that should limit itself to detecting and correcting subluxations [8].

The training students receive in chiropractic college is broad based and similar to medical training [9]. A 2005 study tested 4th year chiropractic students and 4th year medical students on their knowledge of primary care activities. Overall chiropractic students scored slightly lower than medical students in all areas but musculoskeletal diagnosis [10]. Considering the differences on emphasis relating to primary care between the disciplines the outcomes are not surprising, except possibly that the chiropractic student did so well compared to their medical counterpart. Additionally, a 1995 survey of 753 chiropractors reported 78.5% of respondents considered their training as primary care providers as "adequate" [11].

It has been suggested chiropractic training is deficient to medical training for primary care due to the lack of patient contact [12]. The chiropractic student usually encounters patients with musculoskeletal conditions or asymptomatic patients presenting for wellness care during their internship [13]. Although a medical doctor can be granted a license to practice with as little as 1 year in a post graduate residency [14], most have a minimum of 2 to 3 years in a residency program. This additional exposure provides patient contact with a wide variety of conditions. Essentially the chiropractic physician is limited to knowledge gained in the classroom and limited patient contact. Whether this difference produces a physician that is insufficiently trained to recognize undiagnosed life threatening conditions (LTC) has not been determined.

A review of the Job *Analysis of Chiropractic* reveals that chiropractors have contact with patients with a wide variety of serious conditions and often co-manage these patients with a medical provider [7]. What is not included in the analysis is whether the chiropractor was the first to recognize these conditions in an undiagnosed patient.

There is relatively little information in the scientific literature relating to the chiropractic physician's ability to recognize LTC. The purpose of this paper is to begin the process to determine whether chiropractic training equips the chiropractic physician to recognize conditions which were previously undiagnosed, may be fatal if left untreated and usually fall outside the scope of chiropractic practice. Thus, the specific purpose was to identify the type and frequency of self-reported cases of undiagnosed life threatening conditions which doctors of chiropractic claim have presented in their offices during their careers. If these conditions were commonly reported, it was also of interest to explore any potential associations between college of graduation, years in practice, type of practice or prior medical training and the rate of recognition.

Methods

The study was a self-administered, epidemiological survey involving randomly selected doctors of chiropractic (DC) practicing in the United States. The survey instrument was a self-administered one paged questionnaire that asked DCs to state the number of cases (patients), based on their recall over the course of their careers, which presented in their offices with LTC which had not been previously diagnosed or recognized. Included in the survey was a list of the following conditions: carcinoma, abdominal aneurysm, deep vein thrombosis, stroke, myocardial infarction, subdural hematoma and other. This list was developed from an earlier unpublished study of chiropractors which did not include a list of conditions. The operational definition of "life threatening" provided to the doctor was "an illness or injury that, if it remains unrecognized and untreated, could result in the death on the individual within 24 months." The initial and follow up survey included a request to complete the survey even if the doctor had never encountered a LTC in their practice. Based on the responses given it is possible some doctors did not read or ignored the definition of "life threatening condition" the authors provided. There was evidence this occurred in some responses. In reviewing the surveys the authors attempted to correct for these errors. The authors recognize their exclusions were not systematic. Since this is a survey and by nature biased, the authors did not feel it necessary to develop a system to rule out specific responses. The authors used their training as physicians to eliminate those responses that were, in their opinion, not life threatening or excessive reporting. Data were reviewed prior to statistical analysis and data points that were determined to be invalid were excluded.

The survey also solicited demographic information such as gender, college of graduation of the doctor and whether or not they have had any prior health care experience. They were also asked to provide information on some practice characteristics such as number of years in practice, type of practice (solely subluxation-based or not), and practice settings (rural, suburban, urban, solo, multi-DC, or multi-discipline practice) as well as whether or not they were employed by the Veteran Administration (VA) or the military. In early November 2010, 2000 doctors were randomly selected by computer program from a mailing list of 57878 chiropractors provided by MPA Media. Two mailings to each doctor were performed over a two month period. The study was approved by both the research committee and the institutional review board of the institution where this research was conducted.

Statistical method

All survey responses were entered into a PASW statistics 18 spread sheet (SPSS Inc., Chicago, IL) for analysis. For the purpose of analysis, a response variable 'rate of occurrence' (the number of undiagnosed LTC (count) per year in practice) was defined as the ratio of the number of cases identified to the number of years in practice for each respondent. This variable was defined for each of the 6 specific conditions listed as being most common on the current survey (carcinoma, myocardial infarction, stroke, subdural hematoma, abdominal aneurism, and deep vein thrombosis), all other cases seen combined, and for the total number of cases seen in general. The colleges of graduation were grouped into three categories based on the cultures of the colleges as 'liberal, mixed or conservative' based on information provided in a report developed by the Institute for Alternative Futures [15]. Years of experience was also categorized into three levels: "education dominant" (less than 5 years in practice), "education and experience equal" (above 5 to 15 years in practice), and "experience dominant" (above 15 years in practice). Poisson regression models were used in generating mean 'rate of occurrence' for each of the conditions and the total occurrences. In order to identify factors that would predict 'rate of occurrence' a Poisson regression model was constructed with 'rate of occurrence' for the total number of cases seen in general as the response and all the demographic and practice characteristics as predictors. Statistical significance was assessed at the 5% level. The actual effect estimates generated by the Poisson regression models were mean rates of occurrence (the number of undiagnosed LTC per years in practice) but for the sake of easy comprehension we have reported the reciprocals of these estimates which give the number of years in practice per presentation of an undiagnosed LTC (years-per-case).

Results

A total of 588 completed surveys were received (a 29.9% response rate) and 35 uncompleted surveys were returned as undeliverable (31), doctor was deceased (2), or retired (2). Of the completed surveys 12 (2%) were eliminatedfrom the analysis due invalid responses. Thirty seven responses were removed from the list of reported LTC which in the opinion of the authors did not qualify as life threatening. Additionally the responses of 12 doctors who reported between 171 to 500 encounters were also excluded as being excessive.

Most of the respondents were male DCs (79.4%) and had been in practice for over 15 years (60.7%). The mean number of years in practice reported was 20.0 +/− 10.5. Most of the DCs reported practicing in a suburban setting (46.3%) and in solo practice (52.3%). No doctor reported working with the Veteran Administration or military. Graduates from Palmer Chiropractic College in Davenport represented the highest percentage of respondents (23.2%). Based on the culture of the colleges of graduation, 61.6% were mixed, 23.7% liberal and 14.8% conservative. The complete list of demographic and practice characteristics of the respondents are shown in Table 1.

A total of 470 (81.6%) respondents reported having been the first to identify at least one LTC during their practice career. The maximum number of cases for all conditions in general identified by a single doctor was 71 and a total of 3861 cases were noted by all the respondents combined. Based on the total number of years in practice (11442 years) reported by these respondents, this amounted to an average of 2.5 years-per-case. The conditions reported most (percentage of doctors who reported) were carcinoma (58.9%), abdominal aneurism (43.4%), deep vein thrombosis (29.9%), stroke (27.4%), and myocardial infarction (25.0%). Other conditions commonly reported (21.7%) included severe hypertension, diabetes, meningitis, cervical fracture and appendicitis. Details on the maximum number of cases reported by a single doctor, total number of reported cases by all the doctors, and the mean number of years in practice per case for each of these conditions as well as for other reported conditions are outlined in Table 2. Factors that may be predictive of occurrence, based on self-reports, of a condition presenting in their office include gender of doctor, years in practice, and practice characteristics such as whether or not a doctor practiced traditional chiropractic, practiced in a rural setting or group (multi-DC) setting (Table3).

Discussions

The purpose of this study was not to establish whether chiropractic training prepares the chiropractor to be a primary care physician, neuromusculoskeletal specialist or subluxation based provider. The role of the chiropractor in healthcare has been eloquently debated in several articles [1,2,5,16-18]. Our interest was to provide preliminary data in the process of determining if chiropractic training provides the chiropractor the ability to recognize undiagnosed LTC which is a fundamental requirement of all physicians. The 576 surveys validated for our study represent 11442 years in practice and a reported 3861 patients with an undiagnosed LTC. Based on this data the typical chiropractor could expect to have 1 patient with an undiagnosed LTC to present in their office every 2.5 practice years using Poisson Regression analysis. Respondents identified over 50 different conditions that fit the operational definition of "life threatening". Considering the total number and wide variety of diagnoses reported the authors feel there is preliminary evidence to support the position that chiropractic training provides an educational base to the chiropractor to be able to recognize undiagnosed LTC when they present in their office.

The concern relating to missed or delayed diagnosis is common throughout the healthcare professions. Between 2007 and 2009 the NCMIC Insurance Company reported 7.5% of claims made against their insured chiropractors were related to missed diagnosis or delayed referral based on personal communications with Keith P.

Table 1 Demographics and practice characteristics for DC's who responded to the survey on identifying life threatening conditions in their offices [N = 576 (98%)]

	N(%)
Gender	
Male	452 (79.4)
Female	117 (20.6)
Years In practice	
Education dominant	27(4.7)
Education/Experience mixed	198 (34.6)
Experience dominant	348 (60.7)
Traditional Chiro	221 (39.7)
Rural setting	128 (22.3)
Suburban	266 (46.3)
Urban	142 (24.7)
Multi-Discipline	59 (10.3)
Veterans	0 (0)
Solo	300 (52.3)
Multi DC	121 (21.0)
Other Healthcare Experience	63 (11.0)
College of Graduation	
Palmer CC Davenport (M)	126 (23.2)
National University (L)	53 (9.8)
Life University (C)	51 (9.4)
Logan (M)	47 (8.7)
New York CC (M)	39 (7.2)
Northwestern HS Univ. (M)	33 (6.1)
Parker CC (M)	32 (5.9)
Southern California Univ. of HS (L)	31 (5.8)
Cleveland CC KS (M)	26 (4.8)
University of Western States CC (L)	21 (3.9)
Texas CC (L)	20 (3.7)
Palmer CC WEST (M)	18 (3.3)
Sherman CC (C)	18 (3.3)
Cleveland LA (M)	11 (2.0)
Life CC WEST (C)	11 (2.0)
University of Bridgeport (L)	3 (.6)
Canadian Memorial CC	1 (.2)
Palmer CC Florida (M)	1 (.2)
Type of College of Graduation (grouped)	
Liberal	128 (23.7)
Mixed	333 (61.6)
Conservative	80 (14.8)

* Top 3 states with at least 30 respondents (DCs) were California (12.1%), New York (5.9%), and Texas (5.4%).
(M) Mixed educational culture, (C) Conservative educational culture, (L) Liberal educational culture.

Table 2 Number of doctors reporting conditions, maximum number of cases per doctor, total number of cases by all reporting doctors and the ratio of total year in practice to total cases of life threatening conditions identified in chiropractic offices (N = 576)

Conditions	N (%)	Max # of cases	Total # of cases	Mean (S.D.)	Year to Case Ratio%	Year to case ratio#
Total (in all)	470 (81.6)	71	3861	6.7 (10.3)	3.0	2.5
Carcinoma	339 (58.9)	38	1226	2.1 (3.6)	9.3	7.8
Abdominal aneurism	250(43.4)	30	856	1.5 (3.3)	13.4	11.8
Deep vein thrombosis	172 (29.9)	40	628	1.1 (3.1)	18.2	15.0
Stroke	158 (27.4)	12	340	0.6 (1.4)	33.7	33.3
Myocardial infarction	144 (25.0)	21	375	0.7 (1.8)	30.5	27.0
Subdural hematoma	48 (8.3)	6	84	0.2 (0.6)	136.2	125.0
Others	125 (21.7)	30	352	0.6 (2.3)	32.5	27.8

*The maximum years in practice reported by all doctors combined was 60, minimum 1, mean 20.0+/−10.5, and total 11442.
% The ratio of sum of years in practice to sum of number of cases.
# Estimation from Poisson Regression analysis.

Henaman, Assistant Vice President of Claims. Within the medical community the most common malpractice lawsuits were related to missed diagnosis, failure to diagnose or delayed diagnosis [19] representing 34% of primary care cases according to Phillips et al. [20]. Interestingly the most common missed diagnoses in medical practice are similar to the most common presentations of LTC in chiropractor's offices. These include carcinoma, myocardial infarct, stroke and abdominal aneurysm [20-22]. This is not to suggest chiropractors are diagnosing conditions missed in the medical doctor's office but that these type conditions are common, easy to misdiagnose and can have deadly consequences. As one author noted the gold standard of diagnosis, the clinical autopsy, would not have been necessary in 12% of cases if the proper diagnosis had been made and the proper treatment given [23].

A very important component of our study was to identify the most common conditions chiropractors reported encountering. In rank order they include carcinoma, abdominal aneurysm, deep vein thrombosis, stroke, myocardial infarction and subdural hematoma. There was a large group of other conditions commonly reported which included severe hypertension, other cardiovascular disease, infection, diabetes, meningitis, cervical fracture and appendicitis. It is interesting to note that many of the most commonly reported presenting conditions often share one of two characteristics. The first is that many patients present with conditions that may manifest themselves as neuromusculoskeletal in origin thereby

Table 3 Factors that were predictive to number of cases of life threatening conditions a doctor is likely to identify for a given year in practice

Factors	Year-per-case	p-value
Gender		.047*
Male	2.9	
Female	3.4	
Years in Practice		
Education dominant	2.2	.718
Equal education/experience	1.9	<.0001
Experience dominant	3.4	Ref
Traditional chiropractic		.278
Yes	3.7	
No	2.6	
Rural setting		.007*
Yes	2.2	
No	3.3	
Suburban		.731
Yes	2.9	
No	3.0	
Multi-discipline		.462
Yes	3.2	
No	2.9	
Solo		.740
Yes	3.4	
No	2.6	
Multi-DC		.019*
Yes	2.0	
No	3.4	
Other healthcare experience		.668
Yes	2.4	
No	3.1	
Type of college of graduation		
Liberal	2.6	.112
Mixed	2.9	.181
Conservative	3.0	Ref

*Four factors were predictive of rate of occurrence of undiagnosed life threatening conditions in chiropractic practice: years in practice, gender, practicing in a group (multi-DC) and practicing in a rural setting.

causing them to choose a chiropractor as the physician of choice. These conditions could include myocardial infarction manifesting as thoracic tightness, carcinoma resulting in perceived muscle/bone pain, deep vein thrombosis resulting in leg pain and stroke or subdural hematoma resulting in headache or extremity weakness. Secondly many of the conditions reported could appear to be discovered incidental to radiographic examination such as abdominal aneurysm and carcinoma.

In addition to the number of LTC reported and the varied diagnoses, several findings of interest were discovered when analyzing relationships (Table 3). The reader is cautioned that the reasons for these differences may be due to the inherent bias of the survey instrument and should be interpreted as no more than points of interest requiring additional study.

1. Although the chiropractic profession continues to battle over philosophical questions, this study provided preliminary evidence that the reported ability to recognize LTC was equal among schools when divided into liberal, mixed and conservative categories. Additionally there was no significant differences in those doctors that categorized themselves as "subluxation based" compared to those that did not.
2. Rural practices appeared to experience an increase in reported recognition of patients with LTC compared to other practice environments.
3. A doctor in multi-DC practice reported recognizing more LTC than a doctor in solo practice.
4. Doctors with a blend of recent education and experience (6 to 15 year's experience) reported recognizing LTC at a greater rate than more recent graduates or those in practice over 15 years.
5. Male DC's reported recognizing LTC at a more frequent rate than female DC's.

This paper had several limitations which are common to survey instruments. Recall bias may have resulted in over reporting or under reporting of LTC.

The presence of LTC was determined by the survey takers themselves and did not require confirmation by any outside source. It is possible that what a responder thought was a LTC may have been misdiagnosed or not truly life threatening and as a result weakened our findings. It should be noted a total of 37 conditions were removed from data analysis because in the opinion of the authors they did not meet the operational definition of life threatening. Two examples of conditions removed included subluxation and mononucleosis. The response rate for this survey was lower than desired. The findings in a study by Russell et al. indicated that the response rates for postal surveys of chiropractors range from 7.0% to 91.4% with an a mean of 52.7% [24]. It should be noted many surveys reported in the Russell et al. study were of specific populations of chiropractors which generally provide higher response rates, while surveys which include all chiropractors generally have lower response rates [25-27].

Lastly this survey did not attempt to determine "missed" diagnoses on the part of the chiropractor as that was not the purpose of the paper. The authors acknowledge that diagnoses may have been missed which would have increased the frequency of these conditions.

Conclusions

The data from this study provides preliminary evidence that chiropractic education prepares the DC to recognize LTC when they present in their offices. Additionally this study provides preliminary identification and frequency of LTC which commonly present in the chiropractor's office. This information is important to chiropractic colleges, continuing education programs and the practicing DC. Heightened awareness and knowledge of these conditions should improve patient care by reducing the risk of missed or delayed diagnosis.

As stated previously this is a preliminary study. Additional prospective studies are required to develop more reliable and accurate information in this area of investigation.

Competing interests

The authors declare that they have no competing interests.

Author details

[1]Texas Chiropractic College, Pasadena, TX, USA. [2]Parker University, Dallas, TX, USA.

Authors' contributions

DD was primarily responsible for design, interpretation of data and drafting of the manuscript. HN was primarily responsible for statistical analysis. RR and DM provided substantial contribution to the design of the study, interpretation of data, revisions and editing of the manuscript. All authors read and approved the final manuscript.

References

1. Duenas R, Carucci GM, Funk MF, Gurney MW: **Chiropractic-primary care, neuromusculoskeletal care, or musculoskeletal care? Results of a survey of chiropractic college presidents, chiropractic organization leaders, and Connecticut-licensed doctors of chiropractic.** *J Manipulative Physiol Ther* 2003, **26:**510–523.
2. Gaumer G, Koren A, Gemmen E: **Barriers to expanding primary care roles for chiropractors: The role of chiropractic as primary care gatekeeper.** *J Manipulative Physiol Ther* 2002, **25:**427–449.
3. Bockenek WL, Currie DM: **Physical medicine and rehabilitation as a primary care specialty. Commentary.** *Am J Phys Med Rehabil* 1994, **73:**58–60.
4. *Standards for Doctor of Chiropractic Programs and Requirements for Institutional Status.* Greeley: CO, Council on Chiropractic Education; 2007. Ref Type: Report.
5. Horwitz AD, Hosek R, Boyle J, Cianciulli A, Glass J, Codario R: **A new gatekeeper for back pain.** *Am J Manag Care* 1998, **4:**576–579.
6. Nelson CF: **Chiropractic scope of practice.** *J Manipulative Physiol Ther* 1993, **16:**488–497.
7. Christiansen M, Kollasch M, Ward R, Webb K: *Job Analysis of Chiropractic, 2005.* Greeley: CO, National Board of Chiropractic Examiners; 2005. Ref Type: Report.
8. *Position Statement on Vertebral Subluxation as the Sole Rationale for Care. The World Chiropractic Alliance.*: The World Chiropractic Alliance; 2010. 11-2-2010. Ref Type: Electronic Citation.
9. Coulter I, Adams A, Coggan P, Wilkes M, Gonyea M: **A comparative study of chiropractic and medical education.** *Altern Ther Health Med* 1998, **4:**64–75.
10. Sandefur R, Febbo TA, Rupert RL: **Assessment of knowledge of primary care activities in a sample of medical and chiropractic students.** *J Manipulative Physiol Ther* 2005, **28:**336–344.
11. Hawk C, Dusio ME: **A survey of 492 U.S. chiropractors on primary care and prevention-related issues.** *J Manipulative Physiol Ther* 1995, **18:**57–64.
12. Morrison P: **Adjusting the role of chiropractors in the United States: why narrowing chiropractor scope of practice statutes will protect patients.** *Health Matrix Clevel* 2009, **19:**493–537.
13. Nyiendo J, Phillips RB, Meeker WC, Konsler G, Jansen R, Menon M: **A comparison of patients and patient complaints at six chiropractic college teaching clinics.** *J Manipulative Physiol Ther* 1989, **12:**79–85.
14. Robertson RG: **Health reform, primary care, and graduate medical education.** *N Engl J Med* 2010, **363:**2177.
15. *The Future of Chiropractic Revisited: 2005–2015. 1-1-2005.* Alexandria, Virginia: Institute for Alternative Futures; 2010. Ref Type: Report.
16. Cambron JA, Cramer GD, Winterstein J: **Patient perceptions of chiropractic treatment for primary care disorders.** *J Manipulative Physiol Ther* 2007, **30:**11–16.
17. Kremer RG, Duenas R, McGuckin B: **Defining primary care and the chiropractic physicians' role in the evolving health care system.** *J Chiropr Med* 2002, **1:**3–8.
18. Gaumer G, Gemmen E: **Chiropractic users and nonusers: differences in use, attitudes, and willingness to use nonmedical doctors for primary care.** *J Manipulative Physiol Ther* 2006, **29:**529–539.
19. McDonald C, Hernandez M, Gofman Y, Suchecki S, Schreier W: **The five most common misdiagnoses: a meta-analysis of autopsy and malpractice data.** *Internet J Fam Pract* 2009, **7.**
20. Phillips RL Jr, Bartholomew LA, Dovey SM, Fryer GE Jr, Miyoshi TJ, Green LA: **Learning from malpractice claims about negligent, adverse events in primary care in the United States.** *Qual Saf Health Care* 2004, **13:**121–126.
21. Gandhi TK, Kachalia A, Thomas EJ, Puopolo AL, Yoon C, Brennan TA, *et al*: **Missed and delayed diagnoses in the ambulatory setting: a study of closed malpractice claims.** *Ann Intern Med* 2006, **145:**488–496.
22. Schiff GD, Hasan O, Kim S, Abrams R, Cosby K, Lambert BL, *et al*: **Diagnostic error in medicine: analysis of 583 physician-reported errors.** *Arch Intern Med* 2009, **169:**1881–1887.
23. Croskerry P: **Diagnostic Failure: A Cognitive and Affective Approach.** In *Advances in Patient Safety: From Research to Implementation Volume 2: Concepts and Methodology.* Edited by Henriksen K, Battles JB, Marks ES. Rockville (MD): Agency for Healthcare Research and Quality (US); 2005:241–254.
24. Russell ML, Verhoef MJ, Injeyan HS, McMorland DG: **Response rates for surveys of chiropractors.** *J Manipulative Physiol Ther* 2004, **27:**43–48.
25. Hawk C, Byrd L, Jansen RD, Long CR: **Use of complementary healthcare practices among chiropractors in the United States: a survey.** *Altern Ther Health Med* 1999, **5:**56–62.
26. Stuber KJ, Grod JP, Smith DL, Powers P: **An online survey of chiropractors' opinions of Continuing Education.** *Chiropr Osteopat* 2005, **13:**22.
27. Smith DL, Spillman DM: **A survey of chiropractor's use of nutrition in private practice.** *J Chiro Hum* 2001, **10:**1–6.

5

Treatment preferences amongst physical therapists and chiropractors for the management of neck pain: results of an international survey

Lisa C Carlesso[1*], Joy C MacDermid[2,3], Anita R Gross[2], David M Walton[4] and P Lina Santaguida[5]

Abstract

Background: Clinical practice guidelines on the management of neck pain make recommendations to help practitioners optimize patient care. By examining the practice patterns of practitioners, adherence to CPGs or lack thereof, is demonstrated. Understanding utilization of various treatments by practitioners and comparing these patterns to that of recommended guidelines is important to identify gaps for knowledge translation and improve treatment regimens.

Aim: To describe the utilization of interventions in patients with neck pain by clinicians.

Methods: A cross-sectional international survey was conducted from February 2012 to March 2013 to determine physical medicine, complementary and alternative medicine utilization amongst 360 clinicians treating patients with neck pain.

Results: The survey was international (19 countries) with Canada having the largest response (38%). Results were analyzed by usage amongst physical therapists (38%) and chiropractors (31%) as they were the predominant respondents. Within these professions, respondents were male (41-66%) working in private practice (69-95%). Exercise and manual therapies were consistently (98-99%) used by both professions but tests of subgroup differences determined that physical therapists used exercise, orthoses and 'other' interventions more, while chiropractors used phototherapeutics more. However, phototherapeutics (65%), Orthoses/supportive devices (57%), mechanical traction (55%) and sonic therapies (54%) were *not* used by the majority of respondents. Thermal applications (73%) and acupuncture (46%) were the modalities used most commonly. Analysis of differences across the subtypes of neck pain indicated that respondents utilize treatments more often for chronic neck pain and whiplash conditions, followed by radiculopathy, acute neck pain and whiplash conditions, and facet joint dysfunction by diagnostic block. The higher rates of usage of some interventions were consistent with supporting evidence (e.g. manual therapy). However, there was moderate usage of a number of interventions that have limited support or conflicting evidence (e.g. ergonomics).

Conclusions: This survey indicates that exercise and manual therapy are core treatments provided by chiropractors and physical therapists. Future research should address gaps in evidence associated with variable practice patterns and knowledge translation to reduce usage of some interventions that have been shown to be ineffective.

Keywords: Survey, Neck pain, Treatment, Practice patterns, Complementary and alternative medicine

* Correspondence: lccarlesso@gmail.com
[1]Toronto Western Research Institute, University Health Network, 399 Bathurst Street - MP11-328, Toronto, Ontario M5T 2S8, Canada
Full list of author information is available at the end of the article

Background

Clinical practice guidelines (CPG) are developed to provide statements and recommendations with the intention of helping practitioners optimize patient care [1]. By examining the practice patterns of practitioners, adherence to CPGs or lack thereof, is demonstrated. Recommendations for practice can then be formed. Understanding existing practice patterns provides insight into how current evidence impacts on practice and can identify where greater efforts in knowledge translation are needed. Clinical practice will vary dependent on a number of factors such as location, resources available, patient population, and professional background. Several CPGs from varying professionals who treat patients with neck pain exist [2-5]. To our knowledge no examination of practice patterns across health care professionals who treat patients with neck pain has been published.

Neck pain is a common problem with an episodic course that affects a large proportion of the population. Estimates for the prevalence of neck pain vary from 0.4% to 86.8% (mean 23.1%) in the general population, whereas the range for the one year incidence is reported to be smaller (10.4% to 21.3%) [6]. Risk factors for new onset neck pain include being female, between the ages of 35 to 49 years and having a previous episode of neck pain [6-8]. Estimated expenditures on spine related care in the United States have almost doubled in the last decade [7,9]. The number of emergency room visits related to motor vehicle accidents (MVA) has been steadily increasing in the last three decades [10]. Direct healthcare costs may only be a small piece of this burden, while the indirect costs of work absenteeism and disability are much greater [6,11].

Over the past decade the evidence base guiding the choice of effective treatments for reducing symptoms and increasing function has evolved. The association between severity and disability of neck pain has been established by numerous studies [12-15]. There are numerous health care practitioners that treat patients with neck pain with a variety of interventions such as physical medicine, manual therapies, exercise, electrotherapeutic agents, and ergonomics [16]. Manual therapies in combination with exercise may provide optimal treatment effects [17]. Outcomes such as better pain reduction, better patient satisfaction, improved function, increased range of motion and increased strength in people with neck pain have been reported in patients who received manual therapy alone or in combination with other modalities [16,18-22]. While evidence exists for other interventions, the number of studies is few with conflicting results leading to less confidence in their effectiveness [16,23-25].

Our recent reviews of reviews [26,27] provide some guidance for practitioners. There is moderate evidence for specific modalities such as laser and acupuncture for pain reduction while there is evidence of no benefit for the use of collars, ergonomic or physical environment changes in the workplace. Ideally, providers make treatment choices based on their experience, the available evidence, and the clinical presentation of their patient.

In reality however, provider choices of care may be influenced by factors such as scope of practice, patient preferences, types of providers the patient chooses to see or insurance coverage, thereby influencing the types of treatments received and by their interaction with providers. Even within the same profession, providers' choices of care may vary depending upon the degree to which they are aware of current evidence on treatment effectiveness and the degree to which they choose to incorporate the evidence into their practice. For example, care provided by a physical therapist will differ, in some ways from care provided by a physician or from another physical therapist. Patient centered care and the shared decision making model have incorporated patient preferences into treatment planning. This denotes the importance of flexibility in the way that health professionals structure the decision-making process so that individual patient differences can be respected [28]. The incorporation of patient preferences has the potential to shift 'ideal' choices to more practical ones based on preferences of each individual. For example, a patient treated previously for a different problem and presenting with a new problem may have had a successful outcome using an evidence based intervention. However applying the same intervention to a different area may not be supported. Given the favourable outcome, the patient may request that the same intervention be used. The practitioner is therefore faced with making treatment decisions that incorporate patient expectation and it has been suggested that doing so may improve adherence and satisfaction with care [29]. The end result is more varied care and a modification of the 'ideal' treatment allowing incorporation of patient preferences and expectations but straying slightly from recommended guidelines.

There is little evidence in the literature about guideline adherence in patients with neck pain. A study by Oostendorp et al. (2013) used quality indicators of treatment based on guideline recommendations for patients with non specific neck pain [30]. The study by Oostendorp et al. used a sample of 38 physiotherapists and 96 patients in the Netherlands. Adherence to the identified treatment quality indicators ranged from weak (34%) to adequate (59%). These findings provide some initial insight into the potential variability in care that may exist for this patient population and practitioner group but does not provide details about the types of interventions or the frequency with which they were used.

The International Collaboration on Neck Pain (ICON) project is a collaborative project amongst internationally recognized experts in the field of neck pain. The goal of ICON is to establish clear, actionable messages in the areas of diagnosis, prognosis, interventions and outcomes measurement. To establish such data, ICON has implemented an international multidisciplinary survey of clinical practice patterns that will help shape evidence based recommendations.

The purposes of this study were 1. To describe the utilization of interventions in patients with neck pain by clinicians and 2. Where appropriate, to examine whether utilization varies by profession or subgroup of disorder.

Methods

A cross sectional survey to determine practice patterns of clinicians who provide care to patients with neck pain was conducted from February 2012 to March 2013. The survey was approved by the McMaster University Research Ethics Board (REB#11-025).

Survey development and validation

The survey was designed to acquire information in four principle content areas. These four areas included examination/diagnostic procedures, prognostic indicators, interventions (including adverse events), and outcome measures. Two additional content areas determined the demographic and caseload information of respondents.

The survey was developed using Streiner and Norman (2008) [31] methods in three distinct and iterative steps – item generation using literature review, consultation with clinicians which included clinical observation, and ICON content experts - before fielding the questionnaire. 1) The initial core set of items was generated from systematic reviews on conservative treatments for neck pain. 2) This set was then sent to expert clinicians identified within and external to ICON for review of usability, technical functionality of the electronic questionnaire and identification of issues/gaps. 3) The next set was tested using the ICON expert panel of interdisciplinary professionals; this included physicians, psychologists, physiotherapists, massage therapists, chiropractors, and other rehabilitative professions. Additional items created by these experts aimed to address areas missing from the initial item generation to ensure they were designed to be appropriate for administration across different health care professionals commonly treating people with neck pain.

This content area being sufficiently large was divided into the following two separate surveys: 1. Physical medicine or CAM interventions; and 2. Pharmacological and psychological interventions. Items in the physical medicine and CAM survey covered exercise, manual therapies, modalities, mechanical traction, orthoses/supportive devices, ergonomic and work related interventions. An 'other' response option was included where appropriate within each category and allowed respondents to add any interventions that may have been missed. Broadly, items asked about utilization of each treatment category (yes, no, outside scope of practice). The questions progressed in the following sequence. If a respondent indicated 'yes' to the initial utilization question, then inquiry of frequency of use (commonly, occasionally, never) followed. If respondents indicated 'common' or 'occasional' use of an intervention, then use of that intervention (commonly, occasionally, never, not applicable) among the following common subgroups of neck pain disorders was also inquired about:

1. Acute nonspecific neck pain,
2. Chronic nonspecific neck pain,
3. Facet joint dysfunction (as diagnosed by diagnostic block),
4. Acute whiplash associated disorder (WAD),
5. Chronic WAD and
6. Radiculopathy/WADIII.

For the modalities category, respondents were also asked about indications for use. Routing questions were sequentially designed to reduce respondent burden allowing avoidance of categories not relevant to respondents.

Face and content validity of the survey were addressed in an iterative process involving multiple revisions and content experts. In the first round, there was a focus on accuracy of item content and clarity in the wording of each item and response. In the second round, there was a focus on the organizational structure of the survey so as to have logical grouping, sequencing of items and routing questions. In the third round, responses were piloted within the electronic survey format to evaluate presentation and routing. Finally, the ICON working group (n = 38) that had representation from all the disciplines included in our target audience was used for field-testing. These experts reviewed the survey for accuracy, clarity, completeness and burden. After each round of revisions, editing occurred for clarity. This resulted in minor changes to items and a few additions. The finalized version was mounted using LimeSurvey[a], a software program for web-based survey administration.

Sampling frame

Our sampling frame was all health care professional groups identified as having a major role in the management of neck pain, relying on both our reviews and clinical experience to identify these groups. This included physicians (general practitioners, physiatrists, psychiatrists) physiotherapists, chiropractors, massage therapists, occupational therapists, psychologists and complementary medicine specialists. We wanted to include an international perspective. Given the number of national associations and a general lack of willingness for professional associations to burden their members with survey requests we relied on Snowball sampling strategies.

This method allowed clinician experts identified by ICON within each of the professions. Invitations were sent to the contact person identified for each association and requested they assist with sending out links to our survey to their professional links and colleagues. If the association responded and agreed to send out the link on our behalf, it was done so at their discretion. In total 37 groups were contacted, 19 of which did not respond. Survey invitations were distributed via e-mail blast to members, and electronic postings (e.g., e-newsletter, website, Facebook or Twitter pages) by national and international professional groups for chiropractors (Danish Chiropractors' Association; European Academy of Chiropractic; Netherlands Chiropractic Association; New Zealand Chiropractors' Association; Ontario Chiropractic Association); manual therapists (Canadian Academy of Manipulative Physical Therapy; Dutch Association for Manual Therapy; Finnish Association for Orthopedic Manual Therapy; German Manual Therapy Journal; International Federation of Orthopaedic Manipulative Physical Therapists); massage therapists (Massage Therapists' Association of British Columbia); physicians (North American Spine Society; University of British Columbia Department of Family Medicine); physiotherapists (American Physical Therapy Association – Orthopedic Section; Canadian Physiotherapy Association – Pain Sciences Division; Hong Kong Physiotherapy Association; Musculoskeletal Physiotherapy Australia; Physiopedia); and other health care professionals (Osteopathic Society of New Zealand). The method of recruitment meant we were unable to determine how many people received our requests for participation. We were unaware if the associations sent the survey link to all members or only those who agreed to receive it.

Survey administration

The survey was administered through the International Collaboration on Neck (ICON) group and was estimated to take 15-20 minutes to answer. An e-mail including information about the survey, and a registration link were provided. No incentives were offered. Public registration was required to participate in the survey and individuals who volunteered to receive the survey link were considered "registrants". Once respondents registered, an email containing the link to participate in this survey was sent out immediately. Respondents remained anonymous by storing the identification tokens (name and e-mail address) that provided access to the survey on a secure separate database. Registrants were notified that clicking the survey link indicated that they were electronically consenting to participate. Weekly reminders were sent to registrants until they completed the survey, opted out, or received a maximum of four reminders. Response rates amongst registrants were calculated based on the number of registrants who completed at least part of the survey.

Analysis

Data quality was assessed by randomly sampling 10% of the dataset to check for errors. Discrepant entries (< 1%) were resolved through this process. Descriptive statistics were used to summarize participants and their responses to each question. Chi-squared analyses were used to test for differences in the frequency of use of various treatment interventions based on profession. Rank order was used to assess frequency of use of interventions amongst subtypes of neck pain.

Results

There were 360 respondents (332 full and 28 partial) spanning 17 countries. Respondents were mainly physical therapists (38%) or chiropractors (31%) and largely male (41-66%). Due to lack of adequate representation from professions other than physical therapists and chiropractors, we focused the analyses on these two groups. Based on the relevant physiotherapy and chiropractic professional associations' membership information that we were able to ascertain, as many as 17773 individuals were invited to respond to our survey. This is likely a high estimate as more detailed information from a few organizations indicates that variation existed due to inactive emails, unsent links (one international body represents 22 countries) and membership number fluctuations throughout the year. Using this very conservative total, results in a response rate of approximately two percent. Table 1 provides the characteristics for the whole sample and physical therapists and chiropractors only. Within the two professions, there was an average of 15 years of clinical experience, and 34% had obtained a Master's degree. The majority (80%) worked in private practice, with reimbursement through private insurance (79%) in a fee for service private payment model (64%). Over half of the respondents indicated that patients with neck pain made up at least one quarter of their caseload. The largest subset of respondents was from Canada (38%). The gender distribution of this subset of respondents is representative of both professions (males 41% physical therapists; 66% chiropractors) [32,33].

Table 2 demonstrates the frequency of use ('Yes') of the various physical medicine and CAM treatment interventions along with their subtypes. Exercise prescription was used at least by 98% of respondents, as were manual therapies. Ergonomic advice (83%), work related interventions (73%) and thermal agents (73%) rounded out

Table 1 Demographics

Demographics	Respondents (n = 360)	Respondents (n = 251)	
		Chiropractor (n = 113)	Physical therapist (n = 138)
Years in practice since graduation (mean (sd))	16 (12)	16 (12)	16 (12)
Gender	44% female, 48% male	35% female, 66% male	59% female, 41% male
Profession			
Physical therapist (Manual therapist)	38% (13%)	-	55%
Chiropractor	31%	45%	-
Massage therapist	9%	-	-
Physician	5%	-	-
Other	14%	-	-
Country			
Canada	38%	56%	23%
United Kingdom	10%	3%	19%
United States of America	10%	1%	12%
Denmark	9%	26%	-
New Zealand	9%	1%	11%
Netherlands	6%	3%	9%
Other (Australia, Belgium, Brazil, Finland, Germany, Hong Kong, Italy, Norway, Portugal, South Africa, Sweden,)	18%	13%	25%
Practice setting			
Private clinic	72%	95%	69%
General hospital	7%	1%	14%
Teaching hospital	7%	3%	10%
Outpatient rehab facility	7%	6%	9%
Private consultant	6%	3%	7%
Other	9%	4%	12%
% of caseload with neck pain			
<5	3%	0%	3%
6-20	21%	14%	34%
21-50	47%	60%	49%
>50	24%	26%	15%
Health care reimbursement system			
Private insurance	72%	83%	75%
Public health insurance	45%	40%	51%
Workers compensation	36%	40%	36%
Salary reimbursement scheme			
Salary - Fixed	27%	17%	46%
Fee for service – Public	22%	27%	12%
Fee for service – Private	61%	75%	55%
Education - Highest level obtained			
Diploma	9%	4%	5%
Bachelor's degree	19%	6%	33%
Masters degree	29%	*	41%
Doctor of medicine	4%	3%	1%
Doctorate/PhD	16%	27%	15%
Other	14%	35% (Doctor of chiropractic)	4%

*This value for chiropractors is not reported as it overlaps with the 'Other' category.

Table 2 Provision of treatment interventions

Interventions	Yes %	Yes commonly %	Yes occasionally %	Yes never %	No %	Outside scope of practice
Exercise	98				2	0
Stretch neck/upper thorax		79	17	2		
Stretch other body part		47	43	8		
Strengthen neck/upper thorax		77	19	3		
Strengthen other body parts		51	41	7		
Local muscle endurance		63	26	9		
Postural control		84	13	2		
Exercises related to motor control		40	41	18		
Static/dynamic stabilization		55	32	12		
Cardiovascular retraining		25	51	23		
Other:		17	53	29		
Mechanical Traction	28				55	12
Modalities						
Electrotherapeutics	43				47	9
TENS		12	27	4		
EMG biofeedback		1	9	26		
Short wave diathermy		0	5	31		
Muscle stimulation		5	13	19		
Thermal agents	73				22	5
Heat or cold application		55	13	0		
Phototherapeutics	10				65	23
Laser therapy		5	4	1		
Sonic therapies	29				54	17
Ultrasound		11	13	0		
Shock wave		0	2	21		
Acupuncture	46				29	25
Traditional acupuncture		17	17	7		
Dry needling		18	11	12		
Manual therapies	99				1	0
Mobilization		90	8	1		
Manipulation		56	32	11		
Manual traction		55	37	7		
Massage/soft tissue work		79	19	1		
Orthoses/supportive devices	30				57	11
Collars		0	24	5		
Pillows		8	20	3		
Taping		4	16	10		
Adaptive equipment		0	5	25		
Other		0	1	28		
Ergonomic interventions	83				15	8
Work related interventions	73				22	9
Work hardening		8	35	29		
Work site modification		33	36	3		
Communication with employer		16	43	13		
Work site restrictions		19	47	7		
Other		7	23	42		
Other	13				70	6

the top 5 most frequently endorsed treatment approaches. Respondents indicated that they largely did not provide ('No') 'other' interventions (70%), phototherapeutics (65%), orthoses/supportive devices (57%), mechanical traction (55%), sonic therapies (54%) or electrotherapeutics (47%).

Different types of exercise were more *commonly* used such as those for postural control (84%), stretching of the neck/upper thorax (79%) and strengthening of the neck/upper thorax (77%). The exceptions were motor control (41%) and cardiovascular training (51%), which were used more *occasionally*. The most *commonly* used modalities included hot and cold applications (55%) and acupuncture (traditional 17%, dry needling 18%). A substantial number of respondents rarely or never used short wave diathermy (31%), biofeedback (26%), shock wave sonic therapy (21%) and muscle stimulation (19%). The majority of respondents *commonly* used manual therapies and this was most frequently mobilization (90%) compared to manipulation (56%). Work related interventions such as work hardening, site modification, communication with the employer and site restrictions were used *occasionally* (35-47%).

Table 3 highlights the use of modalities and their indications for use. The only two modalities that the majority of respondents indicated that they used were Thermal applications and TENS. Both were indicated for pain relief, 90% and 71% respectively. For the remaining modalities, for all but ultrasound and muscle stimulation (45% each), the majority of respondents indicated that they 'Do not use/outside scope of practice'.

Subgroup analysis

Provider

Looking across physical therapists and chiropractors, differences in their use of the various interventions were found. Table 4 shows that the two differ in their prescription of exercise, phototherapeutics, orthoses/supportive devices and the category of 'other' interventions. Both collars and taping are used more often by physical therapists than chiropractors ($p = 0.01$ and $p = 0.03$ respectively). Examples of 'other' interventions used more frequently by physical therapists include pain education, referral to other healthcare professionals, use of McKenzie methods [34], self-management strategies, breathing/relaxation strategies and prolotherapy. Figure 1 depicts the differences in exercise prescription between the two. Significant differences were found in the prescription of some types of exercise (greater by physical therapists $p \leq 0.01$) except stretching of other body parts, strengthening of neck/upper back and other body parts and cardiovascular training where there was no difference. Figure 2 shows the differences in use of modalities. Chiropractors use of laser ($p = 0.00$), and electrical muscular stimulation ($p = 0.01$) was significantly greater than physical therapists. Although there is no significant difference between the two in the overall use of manual therapies, there is a significant difference in the use of thrust manipulation ($p = 0.00$) with chiropractors performing it more often.

Disorder subgroup

Table 5 outlines the use of treatment interventions according to disorder subgroup. Respondents reported using exercises, manual therapy, and ergonomic interventions most frequently in patients with chronic nonspecific neck pain compared to the five other conditions. Differences between chronic nonspecific neck pain and chronic WAD were minimal. The use of orthoses/supportive devices was variable across the 6 subgroup disorders. Respondents indicated that collars were used most frequently for patients with acute WAD (24%), pillows for patients with chronic nonspecific neck (27%), while the use of taping (16%) was split across three subgroups and adaptive equipment (5%) in chronic non specific neck pain. Utilization of three of the four work related interventions was equal in patients with chronic non

Table 3 Indications for use of modalities

	Pain relief	Retrain or strengthen muscle	Enhance tissue healing	Alter tissue prior to MT	Do not use/outside scope of practice
TENS	71%	3%	5%	7%	26%
EMG biofeedback	2%	28%	1%	1%	66%
Short wave diathermy	5%	0%	4%	5%	83%
Muscle stimulation	16%	42%	11%	15%	45%
Heat or cold application	90%	1%	34%	42%	1%
Laser therapy	12%	1%	28%	3%	65%
Ultrasound	25%	1%	40%	18%	45%
Shock wave	1%	1%	8%	1%	86%
Traditional acupuncture	37%	5%	18%	12%	55%
Dry needling	34%	4%	15%	21%	55%

Table 4 Differences in provision of treatment interventions across professions

Interventions	Physical therapy versus chiropractic significance and direction
Exercise	p = 0.01, PT–138 CH–107
Electrotherapeutics	No difference
Thermal agents	No difference
Phototherapeutics	p = 0.00, CH–23 PT–10
Sonic therapeutics	No difference
Acupuncture	No difference
Manual therapies	No difference
Mechanical traction	No difference
Orthoses/support devices	p = 0.05, PT–53 CH–26
Ergonomic interventions	No difference
Work related interventions	No difference
Other	p = 0.00, PT–29 CH–4

PT = Physical therapist, *CH* = Chiropractor.

specific neck pain or chronic WAD (43 to 68%). Respondents indicated that they used mechanical traction most frequently for patients with radiculopathy or WAD III (27%). Rank ordering of interventions within the subgroups from most utilized to least utilized resulted in the following: 1. chronic nonspecific neck pain; 2. chronic WAD; 3. radiculopathy; 4. acute nonspecific neck pain; 5. acute WAD; and 6. facet joint dysfunction by diagnostic block. This would indicate that chronic conditions are being treated with the interventions we inquired about more frequently and that respondents are also utilizing a wider range of interventions.

Discussion

Summary of main findings

Our results from this survey demonstrate that the interventions most commonly used by physical therapists and chiropractors for the treatment of people with neck pain (exercise and manual therapy) are those that also have strong evidence for their effectiveness, [17,35-38] particularly when combined. It is these two interventions that are also recommended by clinical practice guidelines [2,4]. Other treatments do not reflect the best evidence for effective treatment. The results also indicate variable use of interventions with low or very low evidence. Some are being used to a larger degree (ergonomic and work related interventions) [39,40] while others are not being used (mechanical traction, orthoses/supportive devices and modalities) [23,24]. Other treatments may be used more as they address immediate or short term symptom relief but they lack sufficient focus on long-term functioning [17,27].

Exercise

A Cochrane review of exercise interventions for patients with neck pain highlighted that a combination of cervical and scapulothoracic stretching and strengthening improves pain and function and leads to greater patient satisfaction in people with chronic neck pain. Endurance exercises of the cervical and scapulothoracic regions are effective at reducing pain, improving function and global perceived effect for subacute/chronic cervicogenic headache, while neck strengthening is effective at reducing pain in acute cervical radiculopathy. Neither upper extremity stretching, strengthening or a general exercise program is recommended for chronic neck pain [35]. In this study, respondents' reported the greatest utilization

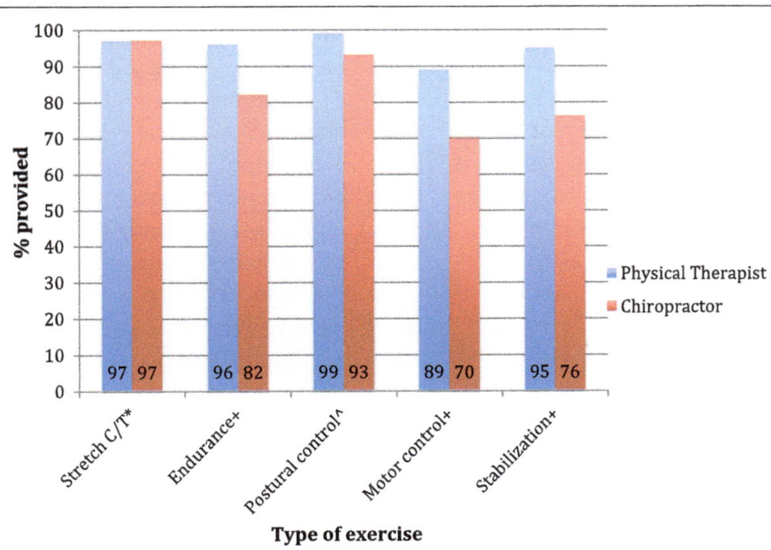

Figure 1 Significant differences between professions in exercise prescription.

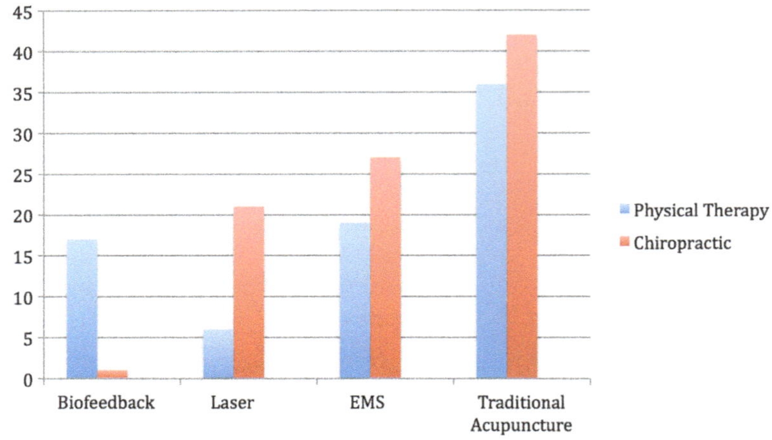

Figure 2 Significant differences between professions in modality use.

of exercise in chronic nonspecific neck pain and WAD conditions demonstrating that current practice patterns are in sync with evidence based recommendations. We did not have a specific category to capture cervicogenic headache so we cannot be certain of how this subgroup was considered. Our response options regarding exercise covered many general concepts ranging from stretching, strengthening, endurance, postural control, motor control and stabilization, but did not allow for details within these categories to be explored. Overall exercise prescription was reported most often in the two chronic neck pain conditions and radiculopathy, which is consistent with the findings of the systematic review.

Manual therapies

Manual therapies are a core skill for the majority of respondents so it is not surprising that they are used as frequently as exercise. Mobilization and massage therapy/soft tissue work were the two most commonly reported of the four techniques. Possible explanations for this lie in our sample representing physical therapists and chiropractors as well as in the evidence base. A Cochrane review has reported the benefit of using mobilization techniques and that no differential benefit for spinal manipulation as opposed to mobilization has been shown for the outcomes of pain, function and patient satisfaction [36]. Using the techniques alone compared to combining them with exercise is mainly of short term benefit on pain only [37]. Regarding the effectiveness of massage therapy/soft tissue techniques, findings of systematic reviews are concordant [41-43]. Evidence indicates some pain reduction and improvement in function for subacute and chronic neck pain immediately post massage therapy/soft tissue treatment but there is inconclusive evidence of any long-term benefit. Despite the lack of clear direction in the literature, the proportion of utilization of massage therapy/soft tissue techniques was similar between the physical therapists and chiropractors in this survey. Massage/soft tissue techniques may be selected for a variety of reasons including complementary or preparatory effects prior to vertebral mobilization/manipulations [43] and the fact that patients report it being very helpful for neck pain [44,45]. It is possible that there are differences in the type of soft tissue techniques performed by the two different professions, but the nature of survey work does not allow for these distinctions.

Ergonomics, work related interventions and Orthotics/ Supportive devices

The association between poor workstation design and awkward work postures with neck pain has been documented [46]. Recent systematic reviews reported limited evidence for decreased neck pain when physical ergonomic interventions were used compared to none at all [39,47]. The following interventions are reported to have no evidence of benefit: ergonomic education (for intervention), workplace physical environment changes (for intervention and primary prevention), and individual worker upper extremity stretching and endurance training program (for intervention, primary and secondary prevention) [26]. In the absence of strong evidence for ergonomic or work related interventions, and considering the difficulties and potential high costs of these interventions it may be that practitioners are less likely to select this treatment approach. Our survey does not allow us to determine why people select different interventions and thus whether it is perceived effectiveness, skills or resources that drive the lower utilization of ergonomic and workplace interventions. The lower rate of utilization of these interventions by respondents, particularly for complex patients like those with chronic WAD may reflect the challenge that practitioners face in addressing interventions for complex patients with limited evidence [48,49].

Table 5 Provision of treatment interventions by subgroups

	Acute non specific NP + %	Chronic non specific NP%	Facet joint dysfunction by diagnostic block %	Acute WAD%	Chronic WAD%	Radiculopathy (WAD III)%
Exercise						
Stretch neck/upper thorax	78	**97**	50	63	92	65
Stretch other body part	69	**86**	42*	63	83	65
Strengthen neck/upper thorax	69	**94**	51	62	92	75
Strengthen other body parts	61	**87**	47	57	86	65
Local muscle endurance	63	**87**	51	59	86	65
Postural control	84	**95**	57	81	92	85
Exercises related to motor control	56	**72**	40*	56	71	59
Static/dynamic stabilization	68	**84**	48	67	83	73
Cardiovascular retraining	29*	**57**	26*	31*	56	38
Manual therapies						
Mobilization (joint or neuromuscular)	95	**97**	61	86	95	89
Manipulation (thrust)	73	**82**	51	51	77	49
Manual traction	82	**83**	51	66	77	79
Massage/soft tissue work	93	**95**	58	85	92	84
Mechanical traction	17	25	15	12	24	**27**
Orthoses/supportive devices						
Collars	21	6*	6*	**24**	8*	20
Pillows	22	**27**	18	23	26	23
Taping	**16**	**16**	10	14	**16**	14
Adaptive equipment	3	**5**	2	3	4	4
Other	2	1	1	2	1	1
Ergonomic interventions	73	**83**	49	70	81	75
Work related interventions						
Work hardening	19*	**43**	21*	21*	**43**	27
Work site modification	56	**68**	37	57	**68**	63
Communication with employer	45	**55**	7*	50	**55**	52
Work site restrictions	59	55	31*	**61**	58	61
Other	21	**22**	13*	20	21	21
Other types of interventions	12	**15**	8*	11	14	12

+NP = Neck Pain.
* = percentage is ≤ to respondents indicating never use/not applicable.
Bolded = highest percentage amongst subgroups.

Overall, respondents provided little endorsement for the use of mechanical traction, and orthoses/supportive devices. However, responses suggest that there may be subgroups where clinicians feel these interventions could be beneficial. For example, mechanical traction was used most frequently in the radiculopathy/WAD III population compared to the other subgroups, despite inconclusive evidence for its use either intermittently or continuously [24]. This may suggest that practitioners expect that a force to unload pressure on the nerve is indicated in nerve root compression. Some evidence does exist for intermittent traction for generalized mechanical neck pain which may be influencing practitioner usage [50] and we have recently found evidence of moderate benefit for intermittent traction for chronic neck pain [27]. We did not ask about intermittent versus continuous application and therefore cannot be certain how this was interpreted.

Cervical pillows were used most commonly in chronic neck pain and WAD conditions while collar use was reported most often in acute non specific neck pain despite evidence of no benefit [51,52] or that collar use is detrimental to recovery [53]. In our concurrent review we found no evidence to support the effectiveness of soft collars in acute neck pain or WAD [26].

Modalities

We did not inquire about modality usage by disorder subgroup but by indications for use. When implemented, the rationale selected by respondents for specific modalities was consistent with their accepted indications. TENS, Heat/cold and acupuncture were used for pain relief and laser therapy for tissue healing. The existing literature base shows moderate evidence supporting the use of these modalities for neck pain [16,23,54] with the exception of heat/cold where little evidence is present. A survey of patients in one state in the USA seeking care for neck pain reported that heat and cold therapy were received by 57% and 48% respectively compared to prescribed exercise (53%), spinal manipulation (37%) or TENS (22%) [55]. A survey of chiropractors in two states in the USA also reported use of thermal and electrical modalities more than exercise [56]. There may be several reasons for these discrepancies between the practice patterns reported in these two American studies versus the current findings. This could include factors such as: patient preferences, time management in busy clinics, clinicians balancing observations of treatment efficacy with the published evidence or perhaps being unaware of the current recommendations for care.

Our concurrent review of reviews indicates that acupuncture (short term pain relief) and low-level laser (short and intermediate term pain relief and function improvement) both have moderate evidence of benefit for chronic neck pain. Evidence of no benefit was found for pulsed ultrasound, or continuous traction [27]. Our data shows that respondents are practicing in line with the evidence in their minimal use of ultrasound and traction and greater use of acupuncture, but deviates from the evidence in their minimal use of low level laser.

Disorder subgroups

Our data indicated some difference in treatment selection across different types of neck pain. Chronic neck pain conditions presented in our survey as non specific and WAD were more likely to be treated with physical medicine and CAM treatment interventions in comparison to radiculopathy/WAD III, (presented in our survey as acute neck conditions and facet joint dysfunction). Although it is tenuous to make assumptions about why respondents selected different interventions from this type of survey, it does appear that the pattern of utilization is consistent with variations in the complexity of the condition. Chronic neck pain conditions, particularly those arising following WAD [13,57] are often more complex, and associated with greater degrees of disability and impairment [57]. Our respondents indicated use of more varied interventions for chronic neck conditions compared to acute conditions, possibly in line with the complexity of the condition. Cervical nerve root pathology leading to upper extremity symptoms is often caused by space occupying lesions such as disc herniation, spondylosis, or osteophytosis that can be resistant to conservative treatment [58]. There is conflicting evidence around the efficacy of manual therapy, exercise, and other modalities for radiculopathy [3,58]. Acute neck pain and WAD if uncomplicated by high levels of pain severity, functional limitation or psychological distress will likely resolve within a reasonable timeframe. Our survey results seem to reflect this as these acute conditions had the lowest frequency of intervention utilization.

There is little published evidence on the effectiveness of conservative treatments for facet joint dysfunction confirmed by diagnostic block. The relative lack of evidence for treatment specific to this syndrome may be why respondents ranked it last of our listed disorders regarding overall frequency of utilization of interventions. Practitioners may suspect facet joint dysfunction after screening but it is likely that few are confirmed by diagnostic block thus making certainty of the diagnosis difficult.

Differences and similarities between professions

Our findings indicate that some differences exist in the utilization of interventions between physical therapists and chiropractors. Although the scope of practice of these two professions is similar, these findings are not unexpected, as differences based on education and clinical paradigms could be expected that may influence their approach to treatment. Practitioner's use of interventions can be shaped by factors other than their entry-level education such as courses taken post professionally, clinical environments, characteristics of the population treated, or use of evidence base medicine. The nature of the survey does not allow us to determine why differences existed between the professional groups. The higher utilization of exercise by physical therapists could reflect the fact that physical therapists have a strong focus on use of therapeutics exercise in their entry-level training or that there is a substantial body of therapeutic exercise evidence developed by physical therapists. We could anticipate that clinicians attend to research that is published within their own professional journals to a greater extent than literature from other disciplines [59-61]. Similarly, innovations in pain education have arisen in physical therapy literature and were cited in the 'other' category by physical therapists [62,63]. The higher use of manipulation by chiropractors (100%) is consistent with this intervention being at the core of chiropractic education. Explanations for the differences in the remaining categories were less dramatic and the reasons for them were less intuitive.

Similarities between the physical therapists and chiropractors were demonstrated in their utilization of electrotherapeutics, thermal agents, sonic agents, acupuncture, manual therapies, mechanical traction, ergonomic and work related interventions. Our review of the evidence has indicated that most of these categories have poor supporting evidence with the exception of manual therapies. The similarity in the use of manual therapies in general is not surprising since they are at the core of entry-level education for both professions. Reasons for their similarity in practice patterns with respect to the remaining interventions can only be speculated. It may be that a combination of factors is contributing to this practice pattern including caseload, patient expectations, infrastructure within the clinics, post-professional training, mentorship and others. For example, patients with neck pain may have a preference for heat applications and in busy private clinics supplementing the treatment sessions with heat may improve patient satisfaction and facilitate other aspects of the treatment program. Although workers compensation accounted for approximately one third of reimbursement in our respondents, it may be that practitioners are seeing patients who are having issues managing their neck pain at work even though the problem may not have directly resulted from a work injury. This along with practitioners implementing primary or secondary prevention strategies could explain the high use of ergonomic and work related interventions.

Overall the practice patterns demonstrated by this data suggest that chiropractors and physical therapists demonstrate strong utilization of interventions widely supported by the literature to manage neck pain. Interventions with limited or conflicting evidence have low to moderate use that is consistent with the uncertainty in the literature. The variability in use of interventions reflects the multimodal practice of practitioners that are commonly used to treat this population. Clinicians faced with applying the evidence-base must customize interventions to the presentation of the individual patient and we know that even within clinical trials response patterns vary across different patients. Therefore, some of the variability in practice patterns reflects this customization. There are multiple patient and practitioner preferences that affect the treatment choices made in clinician and patient interactions around managing neck pain. These can include previous experience, stage of healing, or practitioner type. However understanding the gaps between the evidence base and practice patterns is important for identifying areas needing targeted knowledge translation. Comparing current evidence with our survey results indicates that there are areas for education of chiropractors and physical therapists to increase utilization of interventions with supportive evidence. This includes low level laser and acupuncture therapy that were reported by only 13% and 45% respectively of our respondents. Our results also indicate an even greater need to educate practitioners about their use of interventions with weak supporting evidence such as work related and ergonomic interventions which were utilized by the majority of respondents. A greater understanding of explanatory factors of utilization may require further mixed methods research. As the evidence-based becomes clearer, it might be expected that practice patterns should become less variable.

To our knowledge our practice survey is the first to compare practice patterns of chiropractors and physical therapists for people with neck pain. Previous surveys pertaining to specific professions, reporting more broadly or on specific aspects of treatment have been published making comparison difficult. Within the physical therapy profession, surveys have focused on the utilization of manual therapies with greater attention to spinal (thrust) manipulation for neck pain. Internationally and in Canada, a decrease in manipulative procedures to the neck have been reported [64,65] and there is evidence of them generally being used less often in the neck compared to mobilization techniques [65-68]. Chiropractic surveys report much higher utilization of spinal (thrust) manipulative procedures [56,69,70], and this is not surprising since spinal manipulation is a core intervention within the paradigm of chiropractic practice. Chiropractors see a client base that consists mainly of people with back or neck pain [71] and are sought by the public for the treatment these problems [44,55]. In one population based survey, chiropractors and physical therapists were the second and third most utilized practitioners respectively for the treatment of chronic neck pain [55].

The effort to provide clear consistent messaging to relevant health professionals and the public regarding treatments with demonstrated effect as well as those without or even impeding recovery must continue and occur in multiple formats and mediums. This will help with the expenditure and appropriate allocation of healthcare dollars to minimize over-treatment with ineffective therapies or under-treatment of patients presenting with more complex conditions.

Limitations

This survey has limitations that should be considered when interpreting the results. Our survey was cross-sectional and therefore provides a one-time perspective of general treatment trends. The benefit of this is that it can be revisited over time and results compared to detect change. We are also aware that our sample was not proportional and over-represented Canadian clinicians compared to other countries. It also was largely representative of the chiropractic and physical therapy professions. Our snowball sampling technique was limited by the associations known within our network and likely resulted in the exclusion of several relevant associations, that had we been able to sample, their input could have altered our results. Also we cannot be certain of our response rate due to the limitations of the information that we were able to receive from the organizations that distributed the survey link. We are aware of the potential for significant variation in the numbers of people that actually received the link and therefore the response rate provided is likely a very conservative one, yet still quite low. Those who choose to participate in survey research may represent a systematically different type of practitioner than those who don't choose to participate. This survey was descriptive and to our knowledge the first of its kind. We did not conduct a Bonferroni correction to our results therefore allowing for the possibility that some reported differences in professions are due to chance. The results should not be considered generalizable but rather hypothesis generating to be further explored in future studies. Therefore, transferring the conclusions of this study to disciplines may not be appropriate.

Conclusions

Our survey respondents indicated that they widely use interventions with a strong evidence base for effectiveness and that they also use a variety of other interventions with limited support or conflicting evidence. This suggests there is a need for research to fill gaps in evidence that are associated with variable practice patterns and knowledge translation to reduce the usage of some interventions that have been shown to be ineffective. Examining the consistency or lack of it between available evidence and current treatment patterns can influence guideline dissemination as well as other interventions, such as payment reform, to improve the effectiveness of current care for neck pain.

Endnote

[a]LimeSurvey software, Survey Service & Consulting, Hamburg, Germany.

Competing interests

The authors declare that they have no competing interests.

Authors' contributions

LC provided input at all stages of survey development, conducted the analysis, drafted the manuscript and incorporated feedback from all co-authors. JCM, ARG, DM and PLS provided input at all stages of survey development and provided feedback on the analysis and on the draft of the manuscript. All have given final approval for publication.

Acknowledgements

ICON is a multi-disciplinary collaborative group that includes scientist-authors (listed below) and support staff (Margaret Lomotan) that conduct knowledge synthesis and translation aimed at reducing the burden of neck pain.
The ICON authors provided direction of the project; input into the survey questions and review of the findings/manuscript and includes (in alphabetical order): Gert Bronfort, Norm Buckley, Lisa Carlesso, Linda Carroll, Pierre Côté, Jeanette Ezzo, Paulo Ferreira, Tim Flynn, Charlie Goldsmith, Anita Gross, Ted Haines, Jan Hartvigsen, Wayne Hing, Gwendolen Jull, Faith Kaplan, Ron Kaplan, Helge Kasch, Justin Kenardy, Per Kjær, Janet Lowcock, Joy MacDermid, Jordan Miller, Margareta Nordin, Paul Peloso, Jan Pool, Duncan Reid, Sidney Rubinstein, P. Lina Santaguida, Anne Söderlund, Natalie Spearing, Michele Sterling, Grace Szeto, Robert Teasell, Arianne Verhagen, David M. Walton, Marc White.
Lisa Carlesso is supported by a Canadian Health Research Institute Fellowship.

ICON (International Collaboration on Neck)

- This work was supported by Canadian Institutes of Health Research (CIHR) grant(s) FRN: KRS-102084 and FRN: 114380.

Author details

[1]Toronto Western Research Institute, University Health Network, 399 Bathurst Street - MP11-328, Toronto, Ontario M5T 2S8, Canada. [2]School of Rehabilitation Sciences McMaster University, Hamilton, Ontario, Canada. [3]Clinical Research Lab, Hand and Upper Limb Centre, St. Joseph's Health Centre, London, Ontario, Canada. [4]School of Physical Therapy, Western University, London, Ontario, Canada. [5]Department of Clinical Epidemiology and Biostatistics, Hamilton, Ontario, Canada.

References

1. **About systematic evidence reviews and clinical practice guidelines.** In http://www.nhlbi.nih.gov/guidelines/about.htm.
2. Anderson-Peacock E, Blouin JS, Bryans R, Danis N, Furlan A, Marcoux H, Potter B, Ruegg R, Gross Stein J, White E: **Chiropractic clinical practice guideline: evidence-based treatment of adult neck pain not due to whiplash.** *JCCA J Can Chiropr Assoc* 2005, **49:**158–209.
3. Bono CM, Ghiselli G, Gilbert TJ, Kreiner DS, Reitman C, Summers JT, Baisden JL, Easa J, Fernand R, Lamer T, Matz PG, Mazanec DJ, Resnick DK, Shaffer WO, Sharma AK, Timmons RB, Toton JF, North American Spine S: **An evidence-based clinical guideline for the diagnosis and treatment of cervical radiculopathy from degenerative disorders.** *Spine J* 2011, **11:**64–72.
4. Childs JD, Cleland JA, Elliott JM, Teyhen DS, Wainner RS, Whitman JM, Sopky BJ, Godges JJ, Flynn TW, American Physical Therapy A: **Neck pain: clinical practice guidelines linked to the International Classification of Functioning, Disability, and Health from the Orthopedic Section of the American Physical Therapy Association.** *J Orthop Sports Phys Ther* 2008, **38:**A1–A34.
5. Chou R, Huffman LH, American Pain S, American College of P: **Nonpharmacologic therapies for acute and chronic low back pain: a review of the evidence for**

an American Pain Society/American College of Physicians clinical practice guideline. *Ann Intern Med* 2007, **147**:492–504.
6. Hoy DG, Protani M, De R, Buchbinder R: **The epidemiology of neck pain.** *Best Pract Res Clin Rheumatol* 2010, **24**:783–792.
7. Martin BI, Deyo RA, Mirza SK, Turner JA, Comstock BA, Hollingworth W, Sullivan SD: **Expenditures and health status among adults with back and neck problems.** *JAMA* 2008, **299**:656–664.
8. Croft PR, Lewis M, Papageorgiou AC, Thomas E, Jayson MI, Macfarlane GJ, Silman AJ: **Risk factors for neck pain: a longitudinal study in the general population.** *Pain* 2001, **93**:317–325.
9. Harkness EF, Macfarlane GJ, Silman AJ, McBeth J: **Is musculoskeletal pain more common now than 40 years ago?: two population-based cross-sectional studies.** *Rheumatology (Oxford)* 2005, **44**:890–895.
10. Haldeman S, Carroll L, Cassidy JD: **Findings from the bone and joint decade 2000 to 2010 task force on neck pain and its associated disorders.** *J Occup Environ Med* 2010, **52**:424–427.
11. Borghouts JA, Koes BW, Vondeling H, Bouter LM: **Cost-of-illness of neck pain in The Netherlands in 1996.** *Pain* 1999, **80**:629–636.
12. Sterling M, Kenardy J: **Physical and psychological aspects of whiplash: important considerations for primary care assessment.** *Man Ther* 2008, **13**:93–102.
13. Thompson DP, Urmston M, Oldham JA, Woby SR: **The association between cognitive factors, pain and disability in patients with idiopathic chronic neck pain.** *Disabil Rehabil* 2010, **32**:1758–1767.
14. Webb R, Brammah T, Lunt M, Urwin M, Allison T, Symmons D: **Prevalence and predictors of intense, chronic, and disabling neck and back pain in the UK general population.** *Spine (Phila Pa 1976)* 2003, **28**:1195–1202.
15. Lee KC, Chiu TT, Lam TH: **The role of fear-avoidance beliefs in patients with neck pain: relationships with current and future disability and work capacity.** *Clin Rehabil* 2007, **21**:812–821.
16. Gross A, Goldsmith C, Hoving J, Haines T, Peloso P, Aker P, Santaguida P, Myers C: **Conservative management of mechanical neck disorders: a systematic review.** *J Rheumatol* 2007, **34**:1083–1102.
17. Miller J, Gross A, D'Sylva J, Burnie SJ, Goldsmith CH, Graham N, Haines T, Bronfort G, Hoving JL: **Manual therapy and exercise for neck pain: a systematic review.** *Man Ther* 2010, **15**:334–354.
18. Gross AR, Hoving JL, Haines TA, Goldsmith CH, Kay T, Aker P, Bronfort G: **Manipulation and mobilisation for mechanical neck disorders.** *Cochrane Database Syst Rev* 2004, **1**:CD004249.
19. Gross AR, Hoving JL, Haines TA, Goldsmith CH, Kay T, Aker P, Bronfort G: **A Cochrane review of manipulation and mobilization for mechanical neck disorders.** *Spine* 2004, **29**:1541–1548.
20. Vernon HT, Humphreys BK, Hagino CA: **A systematic review of conservative treatments for acute neck pain not due to whiplash.** *J Manipulative Physiol Ther* 2005, **28**:443–448.
21. Vernon H, Humphreys BK: **Manual therapy for neck pain: an overview of randomized clinical trials and systematic reviews.** *Eura Medicophys* 2007, **43**:91–118.
22. Bronfort G, Haas M, Evans RL, Bouter LM: **Efficacy of spinal manipulation and mobilization for low back pain and neck pain: a systematic review and best evidence synthesis.** *Spine J* 2004, **4**:335–356.
23. Kroeling P, Gross A, Goldsmith CH, Burnie SJ, Haines T, Graham N, Brant A: **Electrotherapy for neck pain.** *Cochrane Database Syst Rev* 2009, **4**:CD004251.
24. Graham N, Gross A, Goldsmith CH, Klaber Moffett J, Haines T, Burnie SJ, Peloso PM: **Mechanical traction for neck pain with or without radiculopathy.** *Cochrane Database Syst Rev* 2008, **3**:CD006408.
25. Gross AR, Haines T, Goldsmith CH, Santaguida L, McLaughlin LM, Peloso P, Burnie S, Hoving J, Cervical Overview G: **Knowledge to action: a challenge for neck pain treatment.** *J Orthop Sports Phys Ther* 2009, **39**:351–363.
26. Gross AR, Kaplan F, Huang S, Khan M, Santaguida PL, Carlesso LC, Macdermid JC, Walton DM, Kenardy J, Soderlund A, Verhagen A, Hartvigsen J: **Psychological care, patient education, orthotics, ergonomics and prevention strategies for neck pain: an systematic overview update as part of the ICON project.** *Open Orthop J* 2013, **7**:530–561.
27. Graham N, Gross AR, Carlesso LC, Santaguida PL, Macdermid JC, Walton D, Ho E: **An ICON overview on physical modalities for neck pain and associated disorders.** *Open Orthop J* 2013, **7**:440–460.
28. Charles C, Gafni A, Whelan T: **Shared decision-making in the medical encounter: what does it mean? (or it takes at least two to tango).** *Soc Sci Med* 1997, **44**:681–692.
29. May SJ: **Patient satisfaction with management of back pain. Part 2 an explorative, qualitative study into patients' satisfaction with physiotherapy.** *Physiotherapy* 2001, **87**:10–20.
30. Oostendorp RA, Rutten GM, Dommerholt J, der Sanden MW N-v, Harting J: **Guideline-based development and practice test of quality indicators for physiotherapy care in patients with neck pain.** *J Eval Clin Pract* 2013, **19**(6):1044–1053.
31. Streiner DL, Norman GR: *Health measurement scales: a practical guide to their development and use.* 4th edition. New York: Oxford University Press; 2008.
32. **CCA membership demographics survey.** In http://www.chiropracticcanada.ca/en-us/members/practice-building/survey-highlights/demographics.aspx.
33. Canadian Physiotherapy Association: *Member Services.* 2013.
34. The MacKenzie Institute International: *The MacKenzie Method.* http://www.mckenziemdt.org/approach.cfm?section=int.
35. Kay TM, Gross A, Goldsmith CH, Rutherford S, Voth S, Hoving JL, Bronfort G, Santaguida PL: **Exercises for mechanical neck disorders.** *Cochrane Database Syst Rev* 2012, **8**, CD004250.
36. Gross A, Miller J, D'Sylva J, Burnie SJ, Goldsmith CH, Graham N, Haines T, Bronfort G, Hoving JL, COG: **Manipulation or mobilisation for neck pain: a cochrane review.** *Man Ther* 2010, **15**:315–333.
37. D'Sylva J, Miller J, Gross A, Burnie SJ, Goldsmith CH, Graham N, Haines T, Bronfort G, Hoving JL, for the Cervical Overview G: **Manual therapy with or without physical medicine modalities for neck pain: a systematic review.** *Man Ther* 2010, **15**:415–433.
38. Furlan AD, Yazdi F, Tsertsvadze A, Gross A, Van Tulder M, Santaguida L, Gagnier J, Ammendolia C, Dryden T, Doucette S, Skidmore B, Daniel R, Ostermann T, Tsouros S: **A systematic review and meta-analysis of efficacy, cost-effectiveness, and safety of selected complementary and alternative medicine for neck and low-back pain.** *Evid Based Complement Alternat Med* 2012, **2012**:953139.
39. Driessen MT, Proper KI, van Tulder MW, Anema JR, Bongers PM, van der Beek AJ: **The effectiveness of physical and organisational ergonomic interventions on low back pain and neck pain: a systematic review.** *Occup Environ Med* 2010, **67**:277–285.
40. Verhagen AP, Karels C, Bierma-Zeinstra SM, Feleus A, Dahaghin S, Burdorf A, De Vet HC, Koes BW: **Ergonomic and physiotherapeutic interventions for treating work-related complaints of the arm, neck or shoulder in adults. A Cochrane systematic review.** *Eura Medicophys* 2007, **43**:391–405.
41. Brosseau L, Wells GA, Tugwell P, Casimiro L, Novikov M, Loew L, Sredic D, Clement S, Gravelle A, Hua K, Kresic D, Lakic A, Menard G, Cote P, Leblanc G, Sonier M, Cloutier A, McEwan J, Poitras S, Furlan A, Gross A, Dryden T, Muckenheim R, Cote R, Pare V, Rouhani A, Leonard G, Finestone HM, Laferriere L, Dagenais S, *et al*: **Ottawa Panel evidence-based clinical practice guidelines on therapeutic massage for neck pain.** *J Bodyw Mov Ther* 2012, **16**:300–325.
42. Patel KC, Gross A, Graham N, Goldsmith CH, Ezzo J, Morien A, Peloso PM: **Massage for mechanical neck disorders.** *Cochrane Database Syst Rev* 2012, **9**, CD004871.
43. Bronfort G, Haas M, Evans R, Leininger B, Triano J: **Effectiveness of manual therapies: the UK evidence report.** *Chiropr Osteopathy* 2010, **18**:3.
44. Wolsko PM, Eisenberg DM, Davis RB, Kessler R, Phillips RS: **Patterns and perceptions of care for treatment of back and neck pain: results of a national survey.** *Spine (Phila Pa 1976)* 2003, **28**:292–297. discussion 298.
45. Sherman KJ, Cherkin DC, Connelly MT, Erro J, Savetsky JB, Davis RB, Eisenberg DM: **Complementary and alternative medical therapies for chronic low back pain: what treatments are patients willing to try?** *BMC Complement Altern Med* 2004, **4**:9.
46. Cote P, van der Velde G, Cassidy JD, Carroll LJ, Hogg-Johnson S, Holm LW, Carragee EJ, Haldeman S, Nordin M, Hurwitz EL, Guzman J, Peloso PM, Bone, Joint Decade -2010 Task Force on Neck P, Its Associated D: **The burden and determinants of neck pain in workers: results of the bone and joint decade 2000-2010 task force on neck pain and its associated disorders.** *Spine (Phila Pa 1976)* 2008, **33**:S60–S74.
47. Hoe VC, Urquhart DM, Kelsall HL, Sim MR: **Ergonomic design and training for preventing work-related musculoskeletal disorders of the upper limb and neck in adults.** *Cochrane Database Syst Rev* 2012, **8**, CD008570.
48. Walton DM, Macdermid JC, Giorgianni AA, Mascarenhas JC, West SC, Zammit CA: **Risk factors for persistent problems following acute whiplash injury: update of a systematic review and meta-analysis.** *J Orthop Sports Phys Ther* 2013, **43**:31–43.

49. Sterling M, Pedler A: **A neuropathic pain component is common in acute whiplash and associated with a more complex clinical presentation.** *Man Ther* 2009, **14**:173–179.
50. Graham N, Gross AR, Goldsmith C, Cervical Overview G: **Mechanical traction for mechanical neck disorders: a systematic review.** *J Rehabil Med* 2006, **38**:145–152.
51. Hurwitz EL, Carragee EJ, van der Velde G, Carroll LJ, Nordin M, Guzman J, Peloso PM, Holm LW, Cote P, Hogg-Johnson S, Cassidy JD, Haldeman S, Bone, Joint Decade - Task Force on Neck P, Its Associated D: **Treatment of neck pain: noninvasive interventions: results of the bone and joint decade 2000-2010 task force on neck pain and its associated disorders.** *Spine (Phila Pa 1976)* 2008, **33**:S123–S152.
52. Shields N, Capper J, Polak T, Taylor N: **Are cervical pillows effective in reducing neck pain?** *N Z J Physiother* 2006, **34**:3–9.
53. Teasell RW, McClure JA, Walton D, Pretty J, Salter K, Meyer M, Sequeira K, Death B: **A research synthesis of therapeutic interventions for whiplash-associated disorder (WAD): part 2 - interventions for acute WAD.** *Pain Res Manag* 2010, **15**:295–304.
54. Gross AR, Dziengo S, Boers O, Goldsmith CH, Graham N, Lilge L, Burnie S, White R: **Low Level Laser Therapy (LLLT) for Neck Pain: a systematic review and meta-regression.** *Open Orthop J* 2013, **7**:396–419.
55. Goode AP, Freburger J, Carey T: **Prevalence, practice patterns, and evidence for chronic neck pain.** *Arthritis Care Res (Hoboken)* 2010, **62**:1594–1601.
56. Mootz RD, Cherkin DC, Odegard CE, Eisenberg DM, Barassi JP, Deyo RA: **Characteristics of chiropractic practitioners, patients, and encounters in Massachusetts and Arizona.** *J Manipulative Physiol Ther* 2005, **28**:645–653.
57. Elliott JM, Noteboom JT, Flynn TW, Sterling M: **Characterization of acute and chronic whiplash-associated disorders.** *J Orthop Sports Phys Ther* 2009, **39**:312–323.
58. Boyles R, Toy P, Mellon J Jr, Hayes M, Hammer B: **Effectiveness of manual physical therapy in the treatment of cervical radiculopathy: a systematic review.** *J Manipulative Physiol Ther* 2011, **19**:135–142.
59. Falla D, Jull G, Russell T, Vicenzino B, Hodges P: **Effect of neck exercise on sitting posture in patients with chronic neck pain.** *Phys Ther* 2007, **87**:408–417.
60. Jull G, Falla D, Treleaven J, Hodges P, Vicenzino B: **Retraining cervical joint position sense: the effect of two exercise regimes.** *J Orthop Res* 2007, **25**:404–412.
61. Jull GA, Falla D, Vicenzino B, Hodges PW: **The effect of therapeutic exercise on activation of the deep cervical flexor muscles in people with chronic neck pain.** *Man Ther* 2009, **14**:696–701.
62. Louw A, Diener I, Butler DS, Puentedura EJ: **The effect of neuroscience education on pain, disability, anxiety, and stress in chronic musculoskeletal pain.** *Arch Phys Med Rehabil* 2011, **92**:2041–2056.
63. Moseley GL: **Widespread brain activity during an abdominal task markedly reduced after pain physiology education: fMRI evaluation of a single patient with chronic low back pain.** *Aust J Physiother* 2005, **51**:49–52.
64. Carlesso L, Bartlett D, Padfield B, Chesworth B: **Cervical manipulation and informed consent: Canadian manipulative physiotherapists opinions on communicating risk.** *Physiother Can* 2007, **59**:86–96.
65. Carlesso L, Rivett D: **Manipulative practice in the cervical spine: a survey of IFOMPT member countries.** *J Manipulative Physiol Ther* 2011, **19**:66–70.
66. Adams G, Sim J: **A survey of UK manual therapists' practice of and attitudes towards manipulation and its complications.** *Physiother Res Int* 1998, **3**:206–227.
67. Sweeney A, Doody C: **Manual therapy for the cervical spine and reported adverse effects: a survey of Irish manipulative physiotherapists.** *Man Ther* 2010, **15**:32–36.
68. Jull G: **Use of high and low velocity cervical manipulative therapy procedures by Australian manipulative physiotherapists.** *Aust J Physiother* 2002, **48**:189–193.
69. Gleberzon B, Stuber K: **Frequency of use of diagnostic and manual therapeutic procedures of the spine taught at the Canadian Memorial Chiropractic College: a preliminary survey of Ontario chiropractors. Part 1 - practice characteristics and demographic profiles.** *J Can Chiropr Assoc* 2013, **57**:32–41.
70. Rupert RL: **A survey of practice patterns and the health promotion and prevention attitudes of US chiropractors. Maintenance care: part I.** *J Manipulative Physiol Ther* 2000, **23**:1–9.
71. Cherkin DC, Deyo RA, Sherman KJ, Hart LG, Street JH, Hrbek A, Davis RB, Cramer E, Milliman B, Booker J, Mootz R, Barassi J, Kahn JR, Kaptchuk TJ, Eisenberg DM: **Characteristics of visits to licensed acupuncturists, chiropractors, massage therapists, and naturopathic physicians.** *J Am Board Fam Pract* 2002, **15**:463–472.

6

Commentary: we can tell where it hurts, but can we tell where the pain is coming from or where we should manipulate?

O'Dane Brady[1†] and Scott Haldeman[2,3*†]

Abstract

The shared decision making process has become increasingly important in the management of spinal disorders where there remains a variety of treatment options. Spinal manipulative therapy (SMT) is often recommended as a conservative option by evidence based clinical practice guidelines and a treatment modality frequently utilized by chiropractors and other clinicians who offer SMT to their patients. This article serves as a commentary to a review of the methods that are often used by chiropractors to determine the site for applying their manipulative intervention. Though it may be easy to criticize any review of this type of literature and point out shortcomings there are strong take away messages for the clinician interested in employing SMT as a part of their treatment protocol. Most notably, clinicians can be reassured that a history on the localization of pain, tissue palpation, provocative testing, range of motion testing and the demonstration by the patient of the locus and description of pain have reasonable consistency between observers. What this paper does not inform us on is the nature of the lesion causing the pain or where the manipulation should be applied to obtain the best outcome.

Keywords: Chiropractic, Spinal manipulative therapy, Spine palpation, Clinical decision making

Commentary

Clinicians faced with a patient with spinal pain must make a number of decisions prior to offering treatment options for the patient to consider in the shared decision making process [1]. This process is increasingly recommended before a treatment begins and is assumed to result in the most effective and patient preferred outcomes. Shared decision making is increasingly important in an era where there are over 200 treatment approaches for the management of spinal pain with very few of them having any real evidence of effectiveness [2].

The decisions that are part of this process are:

(1) Are there any red flags for serious pathology?
(2) Is there any evidence for neurological compromise?
(3) Where is the spinal pain and can the location of the pain be accurately determined?
(4) What structure or physiological process is causing the pain?
(5) What treatment is likely to improve the symptoms?

The first two components of this decision making process are incorporated in all guidelines on the management of spinal pain. However, despite being essential to the diagnostic process, there remains considerable concern about the reliability of many of the procedures used to rule out serious pathology and neurological deficits given the high false positive rates when these signs are used in isolation. What is clear, is that this process requires that every clinician who treats patients with spinal pain take a complete history and physical examination of the patient and correlate their findings with other clinical tests when necessary, before proceeding in the decision making process.

One of the few treatment approaches which have a reasonable level of research evidence of effectiveness and which is usually listed in widely recommended guidelines for the management of neck and back pain is manipulation [3,4]. Although spinal manipulation is offered by a number

* Correspondence: Haldemanmd@aol.com
†Equal contributors
[2]University of California, Irvine, USA
[3]University of California, Los Angeles, USA
Full list of author information is available at the end of the article

of professions chiropractors have been most closely identified as providers of spinal manipulative therapy (SMT) which has been considered the 'mainstay' of the profession for over 100 years [5]. The primary diagnostic tool that is stressed at chiropractic educational institutions and in most post graduate manipulation skills courses is the honing of exceptional palpation skills. Chiropractors spend entire semesters palpating each other and then use these skills when they begin treating patients in the clinical setting. Most of the procedures that are taught in the colleges have been an integral part of chiropractic and manual therapy throughout its history and includes the location of tender areas or provocation of pain on specific manoeuvres, static and motion palpation and range of motion testing. The generally accepted goal of palpation is to identify the source of pain, the so called subluxation or the level of spinal restriction and to determine where and what type of manipulative, adjustive, or manual therapy should be considered.

This process is complicated by the multiple undergraduate and post-graduate courses that promote very specific and complex diagnostic procedures to identify the site of manipulation. These procedures are often named after a particular method or system of spinal manipulation, not only in chiropractic but also in physical therapy and osteopathic courses. In addition there are a host of mostly controversial yet widely promoted and taught, instruments and diagnostic techniques used for detecting the site of the manipulative lesion. These methods include x-rays, skin temperature, complex muscle testing, skin conductance, and electrodiagnostic procedures that along with other diagnostic methods are often associated with some form of commercial or practice building incentive.

The article by Triano et al. in this issue of the journal [6] attempts to assess the current research that supports the methods that are used by chiropractors to determine the site for applying their manipulative intervention. They have done an intensive search of the literature to find research that has looked at this question and have adequately assessed the literature. It is easy to criticize any review of this type of literature and the shortcomings in this article are easily determined and mostly pointed out by the authors. These include the heterogeneity of the available literature, the fact that much of the evidence is conflicting or inconclusive and that most of the studies have been done on young healthy subjects rather than a wide spectrum of symptomatic patients. One should also consider the fact that almost all the recommendations are based on inter-observer reliability with little consideration as to whether the findings are meaningful or actually result in greater outcomes following treatment. Despite these criticisms it is possible to take a few important points away from this paper that can impact the daily practice of chiropractors and clinicians involved in spine care. The readers of this paper can take some reassurance that a history on the localization of pain, tissue palpation, provocative testing, and range of motion testing remain an integral part of the diagnostic process. Furthermore the authors have concluded that static and motion palpation and the demonstration by the patient of the locus and description of pain have reasonable consistency between observers. This therefore suggests that they may be an important part of chiropractic practice or for that matter the examination process by any clinician who is anticipating offering manual or manipulative treatment to a patient. However, further research remains necessary given the lack of strong evidence for palpation in localizing the site of care.

The authors of this review have also concluded that the literature does not provide convincing evidence for the use of x-rays or any diagnostic device in determining the site of care. It is therefore important for the clinician to keep in mind that, in the absence of a history to suggest serious pathology, x-rays to seek out postural or biomechanical changes within the spine are unlikely to change the course of the proposed treatment or add any additional information to the overall clinical picture and only serve to perpetuate the overutilization of diagnostic imaging procedures utilized for the assessment of spinal pain [7]. It is also evident from this paper that specific named systems of determining where to manipulate often taught by charismatic instructors including manual muscle testing or novel devices used for the same purpose or to generate income (e.g. surface EMG and thermography) have not been validated and are not worth considering.

The authors point out, that for some of the most widely used procedures such as simple palpation, there remain considerable weaknesses in the literature and this should be kept in mind when clinicians are interpreting their clinical findings. Of greater importance, however, is the fact that none of the studies that these authors quote have tested what the meaning of the diagnostic procedures are or how they should be interpreted. The fact that tenderness, range of motion or skin characteristics are reasonably reproducible between observers does not give us any information about what is actually being palpated, what lesion or tissue is causing the pain or anything about whether the proposed manipulation or adjustment actually changes the positive findings noted in the examination. It also does not tell us whether any change in these findings relate to patients symptoms or disability. Furthermore, in the absence of any gold standard there is no means of determining the sensitivity or specificity of the tests in assessing the patient's complaint.

These weaknesses, however, are not the sole problem of chiropractors. The same can be said for many of the diagnostic tests that are currently being used by family physicians, neurologists, orthopaedic or neurosurgeons, physical therapists, osteopathic physicians and the increasingly growing number of health care professionals that offer care to people with spinal pain. As the authors of this paper point out there is currently no gold standard for the assessment of spinal pain. The expensive and painful assessment procedures often used by medical specialists including pain provocation or blocking procedures such as discography, facet injections etc. have failed to convincingly isolate the painful lesion [8]. Furthermore the inter-observer reliability of some of the standard medical procedures including MRI have reliability estimates that are similar to those described for manual diagnostic procedures.

Given the shortcomings of diagnostic tests for non-specific spine pain there is a growing attempt on the part of some clinicians to seek alternative approaches to the assessment of patients. One tool that is gaining some attention in the management of spinal pain is the use of clinical prediction rules to identify patients most likely to respond to a specific treatment approach. These rules classify patients into sub-groups based on the clinical examination rather than a presumed identification of the painful lesion and have shown some promise [9] in identifying the patients likely to respond to specific treatment approaches. However, this approach still requires further refinement before it can be generally accepted.

The assumption in this article by Triano et al. is that the manipulation will be applied to the manipulable lesion identified in the testing. This question has to be considered by any clinician who may wish to apply SMT to an unrelated area of the spine (i.e. SMT to the thoracic spine for the management of neck pain or limiting SMT to the cervical spine irrespective of the presenting complaint and examination findings). It is clear that none of these studies can be considered to justify such an application.

Finally, these study findings should not be considered to be solely of interest and use by chiropractors. Any spine care provider who may be interested in employing SMT or referral of a patient with spinal pain to a chiropractor should consider using these examination tools. Educational institutions and examination boards should also be observant of the study findings and should make every effort to avoid teaching or examining chiropractors or any professional who is learning to apply SMT on those procedures that have no reasonable scientific support.

Competing interests

Both authors declared that they have no competing interests.

Authors' contributions

All authors critically appraised the review by Triano and colleagues. OB wrote the initial draft of the commentary. SH provided suggestions for changes to the draft which were then incorporated. The final draft was approved by all authors.

Author details

[1]World Spine Care, PO Box 49, Mahalapye, Botswana. [2]University of California, Irvine, USA. [3]University of California, Los Angeles, USA.

References

1. Dagenais S, Brady O, Haldeman S: **Shared decision making through informed consent in chiropractic management of low back pain.** *J Manipulative Physiol Ther* 2012, **35**:216–226.
2. Haldeman S, Dagenais S: **A supermarket approach to the evidence-informed management of chronic low back pain.** *Spine J* 2008, **8**:1–7.
3. Airaksinen O, Brox JI, Cedraschi C, Hildebrandt J, Klaber-Moffett J, Kovacs F, Mannion AF, Reis S, Staal JB, Ursin H, Zanoli G, COST B13 Working Group on Guidelines for Chronic Low Back Pain: **Chapter 4. European guidelines for the management of chronic nonspecific low back pain.** *Eur Spine J* 2006, **15**(Supp 2):S192–S300.
4. Chou R, Huffman LH: **Nonpharmacologic therapies for acute and chronic low back pain: a review of the evidence for an American Pain Society/ American College of Physicians clinical practice guideline.** *Ann Intern Med* 2007, **147**:492–504.
5. Coulter ID, Shekelle PG: **Chiropractic in North America: a descriptive analysis.** *J Manipulative Physiol Ther* 2005, **28**:83–89.
6. Triano JJ, Budgell B, Bagmulo A, Roffey B, Bergman T, Cooperstein R, Gleberzon B, Good C, Perro J, Tepe R: **Review of methods used by chiropractors to determine the site for applying manipulation.** *Chiropr Man Therap* 2013, **21**(36).
7. Chou R, Fu R, Carrino JA, Deyo RA: **Imaging strategies for low-back pain: systematic review and meta-analysis.** *Lancet* 2009, **373**:463–472.
8. Nordin M, Carragee EJ, Hogg-Johnson S, Weiner SS, Hurwitz EL, Peloso PM, Guzman J, van der Velde G, Carroll LJ, Holm LW, Cote P, Cassidy JD, Haldeman S, Bone and Joint Decade 2000–2010 Task Force on Neck Pain and Its Associated Disorders: **Assessment of neck pain and its associated disorders: results of the Bone and Joint Decade 2000–2010 Task Force on Neck Pain and Its Associated Disorders.** *Spine* 2008, **33**:S101–S122.
9. Fritz JM, Childs JD, Flynn TW: **Pragmatic application of a clinical prediction rule in primary care to identify patients with low back pain with a good prognosis following a brief spinal manipulation intervention.** *BMC Fam Pract* 2005, **6**:29.

7

Is manipulative therapy more effective than sham manipulation in adults?: a systematic review and meta-analysis

Gwendolijne GM Scholten-Peeters[1,2*], Erik Thoomes[1,2], Sophie Konings[3], Michelle Beijer[3], Karin Verkerk[2,3], Bart W Koes[2] and Arianne P Verhagen[1,2]

Abstract

Background: Manipulative therapy is widely used in the treatment of spinal disorders. Manipulative techniques are under debate because of the possibility of adverse events. To date, the efficacy of manipulations compared to sham manipulations is unclear. The purpose of the study is: to assess the efficacy of manipulative therapy compared to sham in adults with a variety of complaints.

Study design: Systematic review and meta-analysis.

Methods: Bibliographic databases (PubMed, EMBASE, CINAHL, PEDro, Central) along with a hand search of selected bibliographies were searched from inception up to April 2012.
Two reviewers independently selected randomized clinical trials (RCTs) that evaluated manipulative therapy compared to sham manipulative therapy in adults, assessed risk of bias and extracted data concerning participants, intervention, kind of sham, outcome measures, duration of follow-up, profession, data on efficacy and adverse events. Pooled (standardized) mean differences or risk differences were calculated were possible using a random effects model. The primary outcomes were pain, disability, and perceived recovery. The overall quality of the body of evidence was evaluated using GRADE.

Results: In total 965 references were screened for eligibility and 19 RCTs (n = 1080) met the selection criteria. Eight studies were considered of low risk of bias. There is moderate level of evidence that manipulative therapy has a significant effect in adults on pain relief immediately after treatment (standardized mean difference [SMD] - 0.68, 95% confidence interval (-1.06 to -0.31). There is low level of evidence that manipulative therapy has a significant effect in adults on pain relief (SMD - 0.37, -0.69 to -0.04) at short- term follow-up. In patients with musculoskeletal disorders, we found moderate level of evidence for pain relief (SMD - 0.73, -1.21 to -0.25) immediate after treatment and low level of evidence for pain relief (SMD - 0.52, -0.87 to -0.17) at short term-follow-up. We found very low level of evidence that manipulative therapy has no statistically significant effect on disability and perceived (asthma) recovery. Sensitivity analyses did not change the main findings. No serious adverse events were reported in the manipulative therapy or sham group.

Conclusions: Manipulative therapy has a clinical relevant effect on pain, but not on disability or perceived (asthma) recovery. Clinicians can refer patients for manipulative therapy to reduce pain.

Keywords: Spinal manipulation, Musculoskeletal manipulation, Manipulative therapy, Systematic review, Sham, Efficacy, Adverse effects

* Correspondence: ggm.scholten-peeters@avans.nl
[1]University of Applied Sciences AVANS, Research Group Diagnostics, PO Box 90116, Breda, RA 4800, The Netherlands
[2]Department of General Practice, Erasmus Medical Centre, University Medical Center, PO Box 2040, Rotterdam, CA 3000, The Netherlands
Full list of author information is available at the end of the article

Background

Manipulative therapy (MT) is widely used in the treatment of musculoskeletal and other kind of complaints. Its use has increased over the world in the past few decades [1]. Manipulative therapy consists of manipulations, which are passive, high velocity, low amplitude thrusts applied to a joint complex within its anatomical limit (active and passive motion occurs within the range of motion of the joint complex and not beyond the joint's anatomic limit). The intent of a manipulation is to create motion (including articular surface separation), function, and/or to reduce pain. It is often accompanied by a brief or repetitive popping noise within the affected joint [2]. The cracking sound is caused by cavitation of the joint, which is a term used to describe the formation and activity of bubbles within the fluid [3,4]. The mechanisms through which manipulations may alter musculoskeletal pain are unknown. Current evidence suggests an interaction between mechanical factors such as movement and forces and associated neurophysiological responses to these mechanical factors [5,6]. Various practitioners, including manipulative physical therapists, physicians, chiropractors or osteopaths use these interventions. However, the theoretic hypothesis, diagnostic tools and treatment methods between the professions differ considerably [7].

In the literature there have been reports published about an apparent association between cervical manipulation and serious complications such as arterial dissection and subsequent stroke, while others found no relation [8-13]. Minor adverse events such as aggravation of neck pain or headache, muscle soreness or stiffness are reported more often following manipulation [14]. Ideally to be justified, the risk-benefit ratio of (cervical) manipulations should be known. Manipulative therapy could be used if there is a substantial benefit that exceeds the risks (and costs). To provide insight into the active agent of manipulative therapy, research about the efficacy is needed. These trials will represent an attempt to differentiate between specific and non-specific therapeutic effects of manipulative therapy.

As far we know there are no systematic reviews published about the efficacy of manipulative therapy versus sham manipulative therapy in adults with a variety of complaints. Earlier systematic reviews evaluated manipulative therapy versus other conservative treatments, waiting list controls or sham in specific patient groups such as low back pain, asthma or dysmenorrhea [15-17]. Therefore, the aim of this systematic review was to evaluate the efficacy of manipulative therapy compared with 'sham manipulative therapy' in adults with a variety of complaints on pain, disability or perceived recovery immediate after treatment, at the short term and long term follow-up.

Methods

Selection criteria

We consider published randomised clinical trials (RCTs) studies eligible that stated to evaluate manipulative therapy, including manipulations (as defined by the original authors), compared to sham manipulative therapy in adult participants (18 years of age or older) with a diversity of complaints. Studies were selected that used at least one of our primary outcome measures namely, pain intensity, disability or perceived recovery. Functions (e.g. range of motion, endfeel, propriocepsis, pulmonary functions), adverse events, quality of life and return to work were considered as secondary outcomes.

Search strategy

We identified RCTs by electronically searching the following databases from inception until April 2012: MEDLINE, EMBASE, CENTRAL (The Cochrane Library April 2012), CINAHL and PEDro. The sensitive search strategy developed by the Cochrane Handbook for Systematic Review of Interventions was followed, using free text words and MeSH Headings (Medline), Thesaurus (EMBASE, CINAHL) [18]. Combinations were made based on a) intervention (manipulation, spinal manipulation, manipulative therapy, high velocity thrust, chiropractic manipulation, osteopathic manipulation, musculoskeletal manipulation), b) comparison (placebo, sham treatment, sham manipulation and c) design: randomised clinical trial or randomised controlled trial. The complete search strategy is available on request from the primary review author. References from the included studies as well as relevant systematic reviews were screened and experts approached in order to identify additional studies. One research librarian together with a review author (WS) performed the electronic searches. Two review authors (WSP, ET) independently selected the studies first by screening title and abstract, and secondly by screening the full text papers. No restrictions were applied to year of publication or language. Disagreements on inclusion were resolved by discussion or through arbitration by a third review author (AV).

Risk of bias assessment

Two review authors (WSP, ET) independently assessed the risk of bias (RoB) of the included RCTs using the 12 criteria recommended by the Cochrane Back Review Group [18]. The criteria were scored as "yes," "no," or "unclear" and reported in the *Risk of Bias* table. Disagreements were solved in a consensus meeting. When disagreement persisted, a third review author (AV or KV) was consulted. A study with a low RoB was defined as fulfilling six or more of the criteria items, which is supported by empirical evidence [19].

Data extraction

Two review authors (WSP, ET, SK and MB) independently extracted the data using a standardized form (including profession, participants, intervention, kind of sham, outcome measures, duration of follow-up, drop-outs, data on efficacy and adverse events). Follow-up time intervals were defined as immediate (within one day), short-term (≤ 3 months) and long-term (≥ 6 months). In cases of uncertainly about the data extracted, a third review author (AV) was consulted.

Data analysis

The inter-observer reliability of the risk of bias assessments was calculated using Kappa statistics and percentage agreement. We assessed the possibility of publication bias by creating funnel plots. For continuous data, we calculated weighted mean differences (WMD) with 95% confidence intervals (95% CI). Visual Analogue Scales (VAS) or Numerical Pain Rating Scales (NPRS) were converted to a 100-point scale, when necessary. In case different instruments were used to measure the same clinical outcome, we calculated standardized mean differences (SMD). For dichotomous outcomes, we calculated Risks Differences (RD) and 95% CI. All analyses were conducted in Review Manager 5.1, using a random-effects model. Prior to pooling, clinical heterogeneity sources were assessed such as participants, time-frame and outcomes. Statistical heterogeneity was considered using a cut-off point of 50%; then the results were thought to be too heterogeneous to pool. Stratified analyses were considered: 1) by time (immediate, short-term, long- term); 2) type of participants (musculoskeletal complaints versus non-musculoskeletal complaints); 3) profession (chiropractor, physical therapist, osteopath, physician). We planned sensitivity analyses a priori to explain possible sources of heterogeneity for RoB. Results are considered clinically relevant when the pooled SMD is at least ≥ 0.5 [20].

Strength of the evidence

The overall quality of the evidence and strength of recommendations were evaluated using GRADE (Grading of Recommendations Assessment, Development and Evaluation) [21]. The quality of the evidence was based on performance against five principal domains: (1) limitations in design (downgraded when more than 25% of the participants were from studies with a high RoB), (2) inconsistency of results (downgraded in the presence of significant statistical heterogeneity [$I^2 > 50\%$] or inconsistent findings (defined as ≤75% of the participants reporting findings in the same direction), (3) indirectness (e.g. generalizability of the findings; downgraded in those studies that used a specific subset of the population under investigation), (4) imprecision (downgraded when the total number of participants was less than 400 for continuous outcomes and 300 for dichotomous outcomes), and (5) other considerations, such as publication bias [21].

High quality evidence was defined as RCTs with low risk of bias that provided consistent, direct and precise results for the outcome. The quality of the evidence was downgraded when one of the factors described above was met [21]. Two independent review authors (WSP, ET) graded the quality of evidence. Single studies (N < 400 for continuous outcomes, N < 300 for dichotomous outcomes) were considered inconsistent and imprecise (i.e. sparse data) and provide "low quality evidence", which could be further downgraded to "very low quality evidence" if there were also limitations in design or indirectness [21]. The following grading of quality of the evidence was applied:

- High quality: further research is very unlikely to change our confidence in the estimate of efficacy;
- Moderate quality: further research is likely to have an important impact on our confidence in the estimate of efficacy and may change the estimate; one of the domains is not met;
- Low quality: further research is very likely to have an important impact on our confidence in the estimate of efficacy and is likely to change the estimate; two of the domains are not met;
- Very low quality: we are very uncertain about the estimate; three of the domains are not met.

Results

Results of the search

A total of 965 titles and abstracts were screened, of which 35 full text articles were selected (Figure 1). After screening the full text articles and searching bibliographies of included studies and systematic reviews, 19 papers were identified and included [22-40], and one study could not be assessed because of the language (Portuguese) [41]. Any differences between the two review authors were resolved by consensus.

Description of studies

Table 1 represents the characteristics of the 19 studies included in the review.

Interventions

In total, 11 of the 19 studies were identified which compared MT only versus sham [22-24,27-29,31-33,38,40]. Three studies combined MT with soft tissue therapy [39] or trigger point therapy [25,26] and compared this with sham MT and effleurage [25,26]. One study compared range of motion exercises with MT versus range of motion exercises with sham MT [36]. Three studies had three intervention groups [30,34,36], two of them included a no treatment group [30,34]. One study used

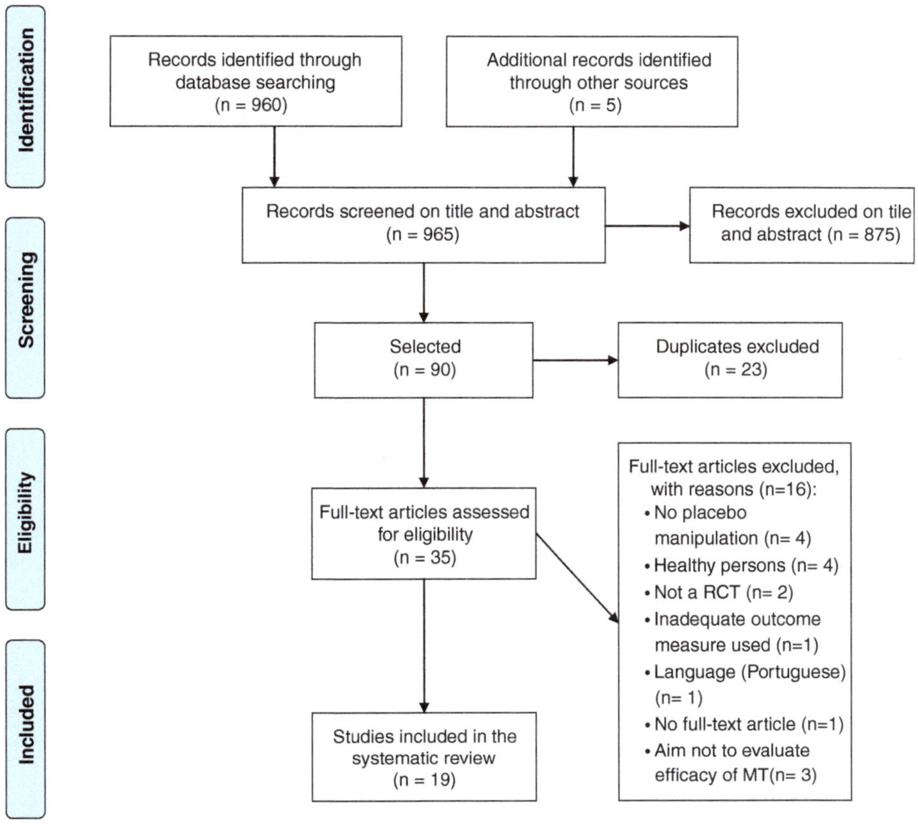

Figure 1 Flowchart of the inclusion and exclusion of RCTs.

four intervention groups and a double dummy design evaluating (sham) amitriptyline with (sham) MT [37].

Treatment was delivered by a chiropractor in 12 studies [22,25-28,32,34,35,37-40], a manipulative physical therapist in 4 studies [23,24,29,31], an osteopath in two studies [30,33], and a physician in one study [36].

Study population

In total, 1080 patients were included in this systematic review. Sample sizes per study group ranged from 4 to 69 patients. Thirteen studies included less than 25 patients in their smallest study group [22,23,25,28-34,37-39]. Patients were treated either for neck pain [23,31], osteoarthritis [22], chronic pelvic pain [25], chronic low back pain [24,26,29,30,36,38], primary dysmenorrhea [27,28], chronic asthma [32], obstructive pulmonary disease [33], acute low back pain [34], acute low back pain with sciatica [35], tension type headache [37], premenstrual syndrome [39], and cervicogenic headache [40].

Outcome measures

Fourteen studies examined pain [22-31,34-36,38], 13 of them used a VAS or NRS [22-30,34-36,38]. Six studies examined disability [22,24-26,30,36], and one study examined perceived (asthma) recovery [32]. Secondary outcomes ranged from quality of life [25,26,35,36], range of motion [22, 38 40], headache frequency [37], to pulmonary function tests [32,33]. Eight studies reported on adverse events [23,27,31-33,35-37]. No studies reported on return-to-work.

Follow-up measurement

Most studies examined short-term outcomes [22,24-26, 29,30,32,37-40], ranging from 1 week [29] to 3 months [25,30,37,39,40]. Five studies examined the immediate effects of MT [23,28,31,33,34]. Only three studies examined long-term outcomes [27,35,36], ranging from 4 months [27] to 10 months [36].

Risk of bias

Overall, high levels of agreement between review authors were achieved for risk of bias assessments with a Kappa of 0.84 (95% CI: 0.77 to 0.90) and a percentage of agreement of 89% (95% CI: 0.84 to 0.93). Kappa values ranged from 0.53 (for item 3 and 5) to 1.0 (for items 6, 7, and 12). The results of the RoB for the individual studies are summarized in Figure 2.

Eight studies scored low risk of bias [23,25-28,31,33,36]. Due to the nature of the interventions it was not possible for care providers to be blinded. Intention- to- treat analysis

Table 1 Study characteristics

Author (year) profession	Patient population	Intervention (n) follow-up	Sham specification	Outcome (instrument)	Results mean, sd (n) and WMD with 95% CI or n and RD with 95 CI	Author's conclusion
Brantingham et al (2003) [22]	Osteoarthritis of the hip (n = 8)	I1: hip manipulations (4)	Sham manipulation with deactivated Activator Instrument a spring loaded piston activated instrument to posterior superior iliac spine, iliac crest and greater trochanter	Pain (NRS)	*Final treatment*	MT may have noteworthy short term clinical benefit over sham.
		I2: sham manipulation of the hip (4)		Disability (WOMAC)	Pain: I1: 18.8 (4); I2: 48.8 (4)	
Chiropractic	Mean age:			Hip function (ROM)	Disability: I1: 7.3 (4); I2 37.5 (4)	
	I1: 60 ± 4; I2: 57 ±12	Six treatments over 3 weeks and a one month follow-up visit			ROM flexion: I1: 109.5 (4); I2: 94.3 (4)	
		Follow-up 7 weeks			ROM extension: I1: 10.0 (4); I2: 6.3 (4)	
					7 weeks follow-up	
					Pain: I1: 15.0 (4); I2: 36.6 (4)	
					Disability: I1: 7.4 (4); I2: 31.4 (4)	
Cleland et al (2005) [23]	Mechanical neck pain (n = 36)	I1: thoracic spine manipulation (19)	Participants in the exact same position as the MT group, deep inhalation and then exhale; no high-velocity low amplitude thrust .	Pain (VAS)	*Immediate*	A statistical significant improvement in pain in the MT group.
		I2: sham manipulation (17)			Pain: I1: 26.1 ± 17.2 (19); I2: 43.5 ± 19.5 (17); WMD: -17.4 (-29.8 to -5)	
Physical therapy	Mean age:					
	I1: 36 ± 8.5;	One intervention				
	I2: 35 ± 11.3	5 minutes post treatment				
Ghroubi et al (2007) [24]	Chronic low back pain (n = 64)	I1: spinal manipulation (32)	Sham manipulations under the same conditions as for I1 without the manipulative thrust	Pain (VAS)	*1 month follow-up*	Patients receiving the manipulations showed improvement in pain and disability.
		Four interventions		Disability	Pain: I1: 49.4 ± 16.8 (32); I2: 58.4 ± 28.8 (32); WMD: -9 (-20.8 to 2.8)	
Physical therapy	Mean age:	I2: sham manipulation (32)		(Oswestry)	*2 months follow-up*	
	I1: 39.1 ±11.1; I2: 37.4 ±7.5	One intervention			Pain: I1: 48.1 ± 22.8 (32); I2: 54.4 ± 25.8 (32); WMD: -6.3 (-18.5 to 5.9)	
		Follow-up at 1 and 2 months			Disability: I1: 12.3 ± 5.7 (32); I2: 12.1 ± 5.6 (32); WMD: 0.2 (-2.6 to 3)	
Hawk et al (2002) [25]	Chronic Pelvic Pain, (n = 39)	I1: lumbar spine flexion-distraction and trigger point therapy (20)	Sham manipulation with a hand-held adjusting instrument combined with light effleurage	Pain (VAS) Disability (PDI) Quality of life (SF-36)	Median change scores [range] (n)	Mean change scores were not consistent across sites so results were not combined and overall effect sizes were not estimated
Chiropractic	Mean age:	I2: sham manipulation and effleurage (19)			*6 weeks follow-up:*	
	I1: 34.7 ± 7.6; I2: 33.7 ± 7.6					

Table 1 Study characteristics *(Continued)*

		Six weeks of treatment with three visits a week for 2 weeks and twice a week for 4 weeks (total14 treatments at 3 different sites/practices) Follow-up 12 weeks			Pain: I1 site 1: 36 [0, 76] (9); I1 site 2: 20 [-16,50] (6); I1 site 3: -63 [-70, -3.0] (3); I2: site 1: 14 [-12,34] (7); I2 site 2: 11 [-5,60] (6); I2 site 3: 13 [-17,28] (5) Disability: I1 site 1: 9 [1,20] (9); I1 site 2: 7 [-5,21] (6); I1 site 3: 1 [-30,22] (3) I2: site 1: 4 [-18,32] (7); I2 site 2: 8 [2,15] (6); I2 site 3: 14 [1,28] (5) *12 weeks follow-up:* Pain: I1 site 1: 36 [-6, 76] (9); I1 site 2: 23 [-40,51] (6); I1 site 3: -23 [-49,2] (3) I2: site 1: 11 [-29,35] (7); I2 site 2: 4 (-14,38) (6); I2 site 3: 3 (-35,39) (5) Disability: I1 site 1: 9 [0,27] (9); I1 site 2: 9.5 [-14,16] (6); I1 site 3: 2 [-39,25] (3); I2: site 1: 7 [-10,46] (7); I2 site 2: 10.5 [0,19] (6); I2 site 3: 5 [1,20] (5)	
Hawk et al (2005) [26] Chiropractic	Subacute (4-12 weeks) or chronic low back pain (more than 12 weeks), (n = 111) Mean age: I1: 51 ± 14.2; I2: 53 ±15.2	I1: lumbar spine flexion-distraction and trigger point therapy (54) I2: sham manipulation and effleurage (57) Eight treatment over 3 weeks Follow-up 3 weeks	Sham manipulation with a hand-held adjusting instrument combined with light effleurage	Improvement of symptoms Disability (RMQ) Quality of life (SF-36)	Improvement symptoms I1: n = 29; I2: n = 20 RD: 0.19 (0.0 to 0.37) *3 weeks follow-up* Disability: I1: 1.6 ±3.2 (n = 54); I2: 2.1 ± 3.3 (n = 52) WMD: -0.5 (-1.8 to 0.8)	Patients in both groups improved on RMQ but there were no significant differences
Hondras et al (1999) [27] Chiropractic	Primary dysmenorrhea, (n = 138) Mean age:	I1: spinal manipulation (69) I2: low force mimic (69) Treatment took place on day 1of cycles 2, 3 and 4.	The low force mimic maneuver consisted of positioning the subject on one side with bilateral flexion of the hip and knee joints.	Pain (VAS)	*Mean pre- post change cycle 2* Pain: I1: 10.1 ± 14.8 (68); I2: 8.0 ± 16.6 (69) WMD: 2.1 (-3.2 to 7.4)	There are no statistically significant differences between the two interventions.

Table 1 Study characteristics *(Continued)*

	I1: 31.1; I1: 29.7	Follow-up after each of 4 menstrual cycles.				
Kokjohn et al (1992) [28]	Primary dysmenorrhea, (n = 45)	I1: spinal manipulation (24)	Positioning the subject on one side with bilateral flexion of the knee and hip joint; to minimize the mechanical effect	Pain (VAS)	Mean differences	MT is effective in relieving pain
		I2: sham manipulation (21)			Abdominal pain: I1: 20.91 ± 23.0 (23); I2: 8.1 ±15.0 (21); WMD: 12.8 (0.9 to 24.7)	
	Mean age: 30.3	One intervention, Post-treatment			Back pain: I1: 18.7 ±19.4 (23); I2: 7.8 ± 15.7 (21); WMD: 10.9 (0.09 to 21.7)	
Learman et al (2009) [29]	Chronic low back pain, (n = 33)	I1: first spinal manipulation second sham procedure(17)	Sham procedure was done in de manipulative position to simulate a manual technique	Pain (VAS) Trunk proprioception (Biodex system 3)	No data	MT had minimal immediate effect on trunk proprioception.
Physical therapy	Mean age:	Two interventions				
	I1: 37.4 ±9.21; I2: 37.25 ±8.65	I2: first sham procedure second spinal manipulation third sham (16)				
Crossover design		Three interventions				
		Intervention took place in a period of one week.				
		Post treatment and 1 week follow-up				
Licciardone et al (2003) [30]	Chronic low back pain, (n = 91)	I1: osteopathic manipulative treatment (48)	Subject receiving manipulation as a simulated osteopathic manipulative techniques	Pain (VAS) Disability (RMQ)	No data	Both groups scored better than the control group. No significant benefits were measured.
Osteopathic	Mean age:	Seven interventions				
	I1: 49 ±12; I2: 52 ±12; I3: 49 ±12	I2: sham manipulation (23)				
		Seven interventions				
		I3: no intervention (20)				
		Follow-up at 1, 3 months				
Mansilla-Ferragut et al (2009) [31]	Mechanical neck pain, (n = 37)	I1: spinal manipulation of the atlanto-occipital joint (18)	Manual contact intervention similar to cervical thrust manipulation. Head was rotated and maintained for 30 sec.	Pressure pain threshold (Mechanical pressure algometer, kg/cm^2)	Pressure pain threshold	MT group scored better on pressure pain and active mouth opening
	Mean age:	One intervention		Function: (Active mouth opening in mm)	I1: 0.9 ± 0.3 (18)	
Physical therapy	I1: 36 ±7; I2: 34 ± 8	I2: manual contact sham intervention (19)			I2: 0.7 ± 0.4 (19)	
		One intervention			WMD: 0.2 (-0.04 to 0.4)	
					Function	
					I1: 38.8 ± 4.5 (18)	
					I2: 35.9 ± 4.3 (19)	
		5 minutes post-treatment			MD: 2.9 (-0.1 to 5.9)	

Table 1 Study characteristics *(Continued)*

Nielsen et al (1995) [32]	Chronic asthma, (n = 31)	I1: Active chiropractic spinal manipulation followed by sham (16)	A drop table was used. Gentle pressure over the spinal contact point with one hand was applied, while the other hand trusted on the drop section with the purpose of releasing it.	Perceived recovery (VAS) Pulmonary functions (FEV1, FCV)	Mean change from baseline	No significant differences between MT and sham in perceived recovery and lung functions.
Chiropractic	Mean age: 28.6 ±7.2	I2: Sham chiropractic spinal manipulation followed by active spinal manipulation (15)			Recovery: I1: - 5.93 (16); I2: - 8.46 (15)	
Crossover study		Started with twice a week for a 4-week period. Two weeks cross over.			*FEV_1:* I1: 0.05 (16); I2: 0.09 (15)	
					FVC: I1: 0.13 (16); I2: 0.12 (15)	
Noll et al (2008) [33]	Elderly patients with obstructive pulmonary disease, (n = 35)	I1: seven osteopathic manipulative techniques 'commonly used for respiratory disorders' (18)	Light touch at the same anatomic regions in the same position as the manipulative group	Pulmonary functions (FEV1, FVC, RAW, residual volume)	*Post-treatment*	Overall worsing of air trapping immediate after manipulation compared to sham.
Osteopathic		I2: sham manipulative techniques (17)			FEV1: I1: 1.18 ±0.62 (18); I2: 1.28 ± 0.63 (17); WMD: -0.1 (-0.5 to 0.3)	
	Mean age:				FVC; I1: 2.36 ± 0.93 (18); I2: 2.66 ± 0.92 (17); WMD: -0.3 (-0.94 to 0.34)	
	I1: 69.6 ± 6.6; I2: 72.2 ± 7.1	One intervention.			FEF25-75 L/sec; I1: 0.43 ± 0.31 (18)	
		Post treatment and 1 day follow-up with a survey			I2: 0.55 ± 0.43 (17); WMD: 0.12 (-0.14 to 0.38)	
					RAW: I1: 6.15 ± 5.22 (18); I2: 7.71 ± 6.09 (17); WMD: -1.6 (-5.5 to 2.3)	
					Residual volume; I1: 5.02 ± 3.06 (18)	
					I2: 4.84 ± 1.84 (17); WMD: 0.18 (-1.6 to 2.0)	
Sanders et al (1990) [34]	Acute low back pain < 2 weeks, (n = 18)	I1: MT L4/L5-S1 region (6)	Light physical contact/touch at the L4/L5-S1 region of the spine	Pain (VAS)	No data	Significant reduction of pain in de manipulation group, not in the other groups. No between group analyses.
Chiropractic		I2: sham manipulation L4/L5-S1 (6)				
	Mean age:	I3: no treatment or physical contact (6)				
	Males 41 ± 13.9; Female 33 ± 8.6	One intervention. 5 and 30 minutes post treatment				
Santilli et al (2006) [35]	Acute low back pain and sciatica with disc protrusion	I1: soft tissue manipulations and rotational MT (53)	Soft muscle pressing similar to MT but not following any	Pain (number of patients pain-free) at	*180 days follow-up*	Active manipulations are more effective than sham on

Table 1 Study characteristics *(Continued)*

Chiropractic	on resonance imaging, (n = 102)	I2: soft muscle pressing (49)	specific patterns and not involving rapid thrusts	end of follow-up Quality of life (SF-36)	Pain: low back pain; I1: n = 15; I2: n = 3	percentage pain-free cases, not on SF-36 scores
	Mean age: 43.1	Maximum of 20 sessions, 5 days per week			RD: 0.22 (0.08 to 0.36)	
		Follow-up 15-30-45-90-180 days after first visit			Referred pain; I1: n = 29 (48); I2: n = 10 (48) RD: 0.34 (0.17 to 0.52)	
					Quality of life; I1: 53.8 ±16.8 (53)	
					I2: 57.5 ± 20 (49)	
					WMD: -3.7 (-10.9 to 3.5)	
Senna and Machaly (2011) [36]	Chronic nonspecific low back pain, (n = 93)	I1: maintained MT and ROM exercise (26)	Manually applied force of diminished magnitude, aimed purposely to avoid treatable areas of the spine.	Pain (VAS) Disability (Oswestry)	*1 month follow-up*	After 1 and 10 months the subjects receiving maintenance MT had lower pain and disability scores and higher quality of life scores compared to sham.
	Mean age:	I2: sham manipulation and ROM exercise (40)		Quality of life (SF-36)	Pain: I1: 29.4 ± 5.5 (25); I2: 33.2 ± 7.3 (37); I3: 29.5 ± 6.1 (26)	
Physician	I1: 41.6 ±11; I2: 42.4 ±9.7; I3: 40.3 ± 11.7	I3: non-maintained MT and ROM exercise (27)			WMD (I1 vs I2): -3.8 (-7.2 to -0.4)	
		I2 and I3 12 treatments of MT or sham MT over 1 month period in I2 and I3.			Disability: I1: 24.6 ± 8.0 (25); I2: 32.5 ± 12.8 (37); I3: 24.1 ± 9.2 (26)	
		I1 received the same treatments of MT as I3 and additional MT every two weeks for the next 9 months.			WMD (I1 vs I2): -7.9 (-13.7 to − 2.1)	
		Follow-up 1,4,7,10 months			Quality of life: I1: 32.1 ± 7.0 (25); I2: 27.1 ± 7.9 (37); I3: 31.6 ± 8.2 (26)	
					WMD (I1 v I2): 5.0 (1.1 to 8.9)	
					10 months Pain: I1: 23.5 ± 8.0 (25); I2: 38.3 ± 12.8 (37); I3: 38.5 ± 12.8 (26)	
					WMD (I1 vs I2): -14.8 (-20.6 to -9.0)	
					Disability: I1: 20.6 ± 7.5 (25); I2: 37.4 ± 13.4 (37); I3: 34.9 ± 12.2 (26)	
					WMD (I1 vs I2): -16.8 (-22.7 to -10.9)	

Table 1 Study characteristics *(Continued)*

					Quality of life: I1: 33.7 ± 7.0 (25); I2: 25.9 ± 7.9 (37); I3: 27.7 ± 8.2 (26) WMD (I1 v I2): 7.8 (3.9 to 11.7)	
Vernon et al (2009) [37] Chiropractic	Tension type headache, (n = 20) Mean age: I1: 29 ± 9.8; I2: 29.4 ± 10.1; I3: 34 ± 11.6; I4: 43 ± 4.5	I1: amitriptyline and MT (4) I2: amitriptyline and sham MT (5) I3: sham amitriptyline and MT (6) I4: sham amitriptyline and sham MT (5) Chiropractic MTafter 4 weeks of amitriptyline, 3 times/week for 6 weeks and then once per week for 4 weeks. Follow-up 4, 10, 14 weeks	A treatment table with a head piece that was capable of a small downward displacement (drop-piece). Drop-piece was quickly engaged simulating the thrust. Before brief preparatory soft tissue massage.	Days of headache reduction in the last 28 days of the trial (headache diary)	I1: -8.4 ± 7.5 (4) I2: 3.1 ± 5.4 (5) I3: 2.0 ± 6.3 (6) WMD (I1 v I2): -11.5 (-21.6 to – 1.4)	Combined treatment of chiropractic and amitriptyline showed significant and clinical relevant results in headache reduction
Waagen et al (1986) [38] **Chiropractic**	Chronic low back pain (> 3 weeks), (n = 29) Mean age: I1: 25.2; I2: 24.3	I1: MT (11) I2: sham MT (18) Two of three times weekly for 2 weeks Follow-up after 2 weeks	Lumbar drop-piece on the chiropractic adjusting table to minimal tension. Adjustment by applying gentle pressure over posterior superior iliac spines.	Pain (VAS) Function: lumbar spine function tests	Pain: *immediate* (mean differences between pre-post) I1: 13 (9); I2: 7 (10) *2 weeks*; Pain: I1: 23 (9); I2: 6 (10) ASLR: I1: 6 ± 8.7 (9); I2: -13.5 ± 10.3 (8); WMD: 19.5 (9.7 to 29.4) Flexion; I1: 0.34 ± 0.9 (9); I2: 0.95 ± 2.2 (8); MD: -0.6 (-2.3 to 1.1) Extension; I1: 1.2 ± 1.2 (9); I2: -0.5 ± 2.1 (8); WMD: 1.7 (-0.04 to 3.4)	MT is effective for relieving pain compared to sham MT
Walsh and Polus (1999) [39] Crossover study Chiropractic	Premenstrual syndrome (PMS), (n = 45) Mean age: I1: 35 ±7.4; I2: 36 ±7.0	I1: first high velocity, low amplitude MT plus soft tissue therapy second sham treatment (28) I2: first sham treatment second high velocity, low amplitude MT plus soft tissue therapy (17) Three times over a period of ten days. Follow-up after 3 menstrual cycles.	The sham treatment used a Activator Adjusting Instrument (Activator Methods Inc., Phoenix, Ariz)	PMS symptoms (PMS-cator disc)	PMS symptoms I1: 34.9 ± 25.3 (25) I2: 43.11 ± 26.2 (25) WMD: -8.2 (-22.8 to 6.4)	For the total group, there was a decrease in the mean global scores in the treatment phase compared with both the baseline and the sham phases

Table 1 Study characteristics *(Continued)*

Whittingham and Nilsson (2001) [40]	Cervicogenic headache, (n = 105)	I1: first manipulation, second no treatment, third sham manipulation (56)	Sham manipulation was delivered with a deactivated pettibon instrument	Active cervical ROM (goniometer)	*6 weeks* Right Rotation	Spinal manipulation of the cervical spine increases active range of motion
	Mean age:	I2: first sham manipulation, second manipulation, third no treatment (49)			I1: 67 ± 9.0 (56); I2: 57 ± 9.8 (49)	
Crossover study	I1:39.4 ±11.6; I2:41.9 ±12.5				WMD: 10.0 (6.4 to 13.6)	
Chiropractic		4 study phases in 12 weeks			Left Rotation; I1: 67 ± 9.0 (56); I2: 56 ± 9.8 (49) WMD: 11.0 (7.4 to 14.6)	
		Follow-up 3, 6, 9 and 12 weeks			Right lateral flexion; I1: 46 ± 8.2 (56)	
					I2: 39 ± 7.7 (49); WMD: 7.0 (3.9 to 10.1); Left lateral flexion; I1: 44 ± 9.0 (56); I2: 39 ± 9.1 (49); WMD: 5.0 (1.5 to 8.5)	
					12 weeks Right Rotation	
					I1: 70 ± 8.0 (53); I2: 73 ± 9.1 (49)	
					WMD: -3 (-6.4 to 0.4)	
					Left Rotation; I1: 69 ± 8.0 (53)	
					I2: 72 ± 11.2 (49); WMD: -3 (-6.8 to 0.8); Right Lateral Flexion; I1: 47 ± 8.0 (53); I2: 40 ± 9.8 (49); WMD: 7.0 (3.5 to 10.5); Left Lateral Flexion; I1: 45 ± 8.0 (53); I2: 47 ± 9.1 (49); WMD: -2.0 (-5.4 to 1.4)	

MT: manipulative therapy, CI: confidence interval, RD: risk difference, ROM: range of motion, VAS-score: visual analogue scale (100 mm), I1: intervention one, I2: intervention two, I3: intervention three, I4: intervention 4, WMD: weighted mean difference, LFM: low force mimic, NRS: numeric rating scale, FEV1: forced expiratory volume 1 second, FVC: forced vial capacity, RAW: airway resistance, ODI: Oswestry Disability Index, PMS: premenstrual syndromes, WOMAC: Western Ontario and McMaster Universities Osteoarthritis Index, SF-36: Short Form Health Survey, RMQ: Roland Morris Back Pain Questionnaire, ASLR: Active Straight Leg Raising test.

	Random sequence generation (selection bias)	Allocation concealment (selection bias)	Blinding of participants and personnel (performance bias)	Blinding of personnel /care providers (selection bias)	Blinding of outcome assessment (detection bias)	Incomplete outcome data (attrition bias)	Selective reporting (reporting bias)	Group similarity at baseline (selection bias)	Co-interventions (performance bias)	Compliance (performance bias)	Intention-to-treat-analysis (risk of bias)	Timing of outcome assessments (detection bias)
Brantingham 2003	?	−	+	−	−	+	?	−	+	?	−	+
Cleland 2005	+	+	+	−	+	+	?	+	+	+	+	+
Ghroubi 2007	?	?	?	−	?	+	?	+	?	?	+	+
Hawk 2002	+	+	+	−	+	+	?	−	+	+	−	+
Hawk 2005	+	+	−	−	−	+	?	+	?	+	−	+
Hondras 1999	+	+	?	−	?	+	?	+	?	+	−	+
Kokjohn 1992	?	?	+	−	+	+	?	?	+	+	−	+
Learman 2009	+	−	−	−	−	+	−	+	?	?	+	−
Licciardone 2003	+	+	?	−	?	−	?	+	−	+	?	+
Mansilla- Ferragut 2009	+	−	?	−	?	+	?	+	+	+	+	+
Nielsen 1995	+	+	−	−	−	+	?	−	−	+	−	+
Noll 2008	?	?	?	−	?	+	+	−	+	+	+	+
Sanders 1990	+	−	−	−	−	+	?	−	+	+	−	+
Santilli 2006	+	+	?	−	?	+	?	−	?	+	−	+
Senna 2011	+	+	+	−	+	−	?	+	?	?	−	+
Vernon 2009	+	+	?	−	?	−	?	+	?	?	?	+
Waagen 1986	−	−	+	−	?	−	?	−	?	+	−	+
Walsh 1999	?	?	+	−	+	−	?	+	?	?	−	+
Whittingham 2001	+	−	−	−	+	+	?	+	?	?	−	+

Figure 2 Risk of bias summary: review authors' judgments about each risk of bias item for each included study.

scored negative or unknown in 14 studies (74%) [22,25-28,30,32,34-40]. Patients were successfully blinded in seven studies (37%) [22,23,25,28,36,38,39]. Selective outcome reporting, blinding of outcome assessors and co-interventions were the items most often judged as unclear. No firm conclusions could be drawn from the funnel plots that were suggestive of publication bias (Figure 3).

Effect of manipulative therapy

The overall quality of the body of evidence is summarized in Table 2. We found moderate level of evidence for immediate effects of MT compared to sham for adults on pain. The subgroup analysis showed also moderate level of evidence for patients with musculoskeletal complaints on pain. All other levels of evidence were considered low to very low (Table 2).

Pain

Data of seven studies could be pooled [23,24,27,28,31,36,37], six studies did not provide data for calculating SMD or WMD [22,25,29,30,34,38]. Figure 4 shows that there is low level of evidence (high RoB, imprecision) that MT provided statistically significantly better pain relief than sham MT on all time points SMD -0.58 (95% CI – 0.88 to – 0.29) [23,24,28,31,36,37], and at short-term follow-up SMD - 0.37 (95% CI – 0.69 to – 0.04) [24,27,36,37]. We found moderate level of evidence (imprecision) that MT provided better pain relief than sham MT immediate after treatment SMD -0.68 (95% CI -1.06 to -0.32) [23,28,31]. There is low level of evidence from one study (inconsistency, imprecision) that MT is better than sham at long term follow-up SMD -1.31 (95% CI -1.87 to -0.75) [36]. The effects were considered clinically relevant on all time points, immediate after treatment and at long term follow-up.

Subgroup analyses

The largest subgroup concerned patients with musculoskeletal disorders. In these patients there is moderate level of evidence (imprecision) that MT provided statistically significant and clinically relevant better pain relief than sham MT immediately after treatment SMD -0.73 (95% CI, -1.21 to -0.25) [23,31]. We found low level of evidence (high RoB, imprecision) for pain relief at short term follow-up SMD -0.52 (95% CI -0.87 to -0.17) [24,36,37], and low level of evidence (inconsistency, imprecision) at long term follow-up SMD -1.31 (95% CI -1.87 to -0.75) [36]. Moreover, there is low level of evidence (high RoB, imprecision) on all time points SMD -0.71 (95% CI -1.02 to -0.39) [23,24,31,36,37]. Two studies (213 participants) presented dichotomous data [26,35], and showed that MT provided better pain relief than sham: RD 0.27 (95% CI 0.11 to 0.42). These differences are considered clinically relevant.

Considering patients with low back pain, there is only low level of evidence (high RoB, imprecision) that MT showed statistically significantly better pain relief than sham MT (126 participants) at short term follow-up SMD -0.47 (95% CI -0.82 to -0.11) [24,36].

For neck pain patients, there is low level of evidence (inconsistency, imprecision) that MT provides better pain relief than sham immediately after treatment SMD -0.73 (95% CI -1.21 to -0.26) [23,31].

For non-musculoskeletal disorders, two low RoB studies (181 participants) with primary dysmenorrhea demonstrated a non-significant effect in favor of MT on pain

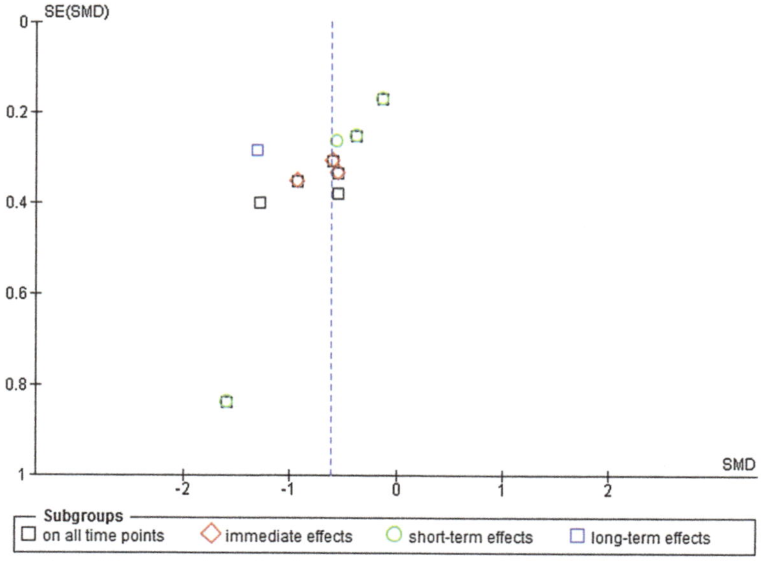

Figure 3 Funnel plot of comparison: MT versus sham for the outcome pain. Negative values favour MT.

Table 2 Summary of the overall quality of the body of evidence

Type of outcome measure (population)	Time frame	(Number of studies) Number of participants	Summary of the quality of the evidence	Reasons for downgrading
Pain (variety of complaints)	On all time points	(7RCTs) 389	Low evidence: MT provides better pain relief than sham	Risk of bias/imprecision
	Immediate	(3RCTs) 117	Moderate evidence: MT provides better pain relief than sham	Incons
	Short-term	(4RCTs) 272	Low evidence: MT provides better pain relief than sham	Risk of bias/imprecision
	Long- term	(1RCT) 62	Low evidence: MT provides better pain relief than sham	Incons./imprecision
Pain (musculoskeletal disorders)	On all time points	(5RCTs) 208	Low evidence: MT provides better pain relief than sham	Risk of bias/imprecision
	Immediate	(2RCTs) 73	Moderate evidence: MT provides better pain relief than sham	imprecision
	Short-term	(3RCTs) 135	Low evidence: MT provides better pain relief than sham	Risk of bias/imprecision
	Long- term	(1RCT) 62	Low evidence: MT provides better pain relief than	Incons./imprecision
Pain (neck pain)	Immediate	(2RCTs) 73	Low evidence: MT does not provide better pain relief than sham	Incons./imprecision
Pain (low back pain)	Short-term	(2RCTs) 126	Low evidence: MT provides better pain relief than sham	Risk of bias/imprecision
Pain (primary dysmenorrhea)	On all time points	(2RCTs) 181	Low evidence: MT does not provide better pain relief than sham	incons./imprecision
Pain (chiropractor)	On all time points	(3RCTs) 190	Very low evidence: MT does not provide better pain relief than sham	Risk of bias/incons./ imprecision
Pain (physical therapist)	On all time points	(3RCTs) 137	Low evidence: MT performed by physical therapist provides better pain relief than sham	Risk of bias/imprecision
Pain (physician)	On all time points	(1RCT) 62	Low evidence: MT performed by a physician therapist provides better pain relief than sham	incons./imprecision
Disability (muscoloskeletal disorders)	Short term	(6RCTs) 355	Very low evidence: MT does not provide better relief of disability than sham	Risk of bias/incons./ imprecision
Perceived (asthma) recovery (chronic asthma)	Short term	(1RCTs) 31	Very low evidence: MT does not provide better perceived (asthma) recovery than sham	Risk of bias/incons./ imprecision

incons. = inconsistency.

Study or Subgroup	manipulation Mean	manipulation SD	manipulation Total	sham manipulation Mean	sham manipulation SD	sham manipulation Total	Weight	Std. Mean Difference IV, Random, 95% CI
1.5.1 on all time points								
Cleland 2005	26.1	17.2	19	43.5	19.5	17	11.5%	-0.93 [-1.62, -0.24]
Ghroubi 2007	49.4	16.8	32	58.4	28.8	32	16.8%	-0.38 [-0.87, 0.12]
Hondras 1999	-10.1	14.8	68	-8	16.6	69	22.6%	-0.13 [-0.47, 0.20]
Kokjohn 1992	-18.7	19.4	23	-7.8	15.7	21	13.6%	-0.60 [-1.21, 0.00]
Mansilla- Ferragut 2009	0.7	0.4	19	0.9	0.3	18	12.3%	-0.55 [-1.21, 0.11]
Senna 2011	29.4	5.5	12	33.2	7.3	18	10.5%	-0.56 [-1.30, 0.19]
Senna 2011	23.5	8	13	38.3	12.8	19	9.8%	-1.30 [-2.08, -0.51]
Vernon 2009	-8.4	7.5	4	3.1	5.4	5	2.9%	-1.60 [-3.24, 0.04]
Subtotal (95% CI)			**190**			**199**	**100.0%**	**-0.58 [-0.88, -0.29]**
Heterogeneity: Tau² = 0.07; Chi² = 12.10, df = 7 (P = 0.10); I² = 42%								
Test for overall effect: Z = 3.88 (P = 0.0001)								
1.5.2 immediate effects								
Cleland 2005	26.1	17.2	19	43.5	19.5	17	29.3%	-0.93 [-1.62, -0.24]
Kokjohn 1992	-18.7	19.4	23	-7.8	15.7	21	38.3%	-0.60 [-1.21, 0.00]
Mansilla- Ferragut 2009	0.7	0.4	19	0.9	0.3	18	32.4%	-0.55 [-1.21, 0.11]
Subtotal (95% CI)			**61**			**56**	**100.0%**	**-0.68 [-1.06, -0.31]**
Heterogeneity: Tau² = 0.00; Chi² = 0.70, df = 2 (P = 0.70); I² = 0%								
Test for overall effect: Z = 3.56 (P = 0.0004)								
1.5.3 short-term effects								
Ghroubi 2007	49.4	16.8	32	58.4	28.8	32	27.7%	-0.38 [-0.87, 0.12]
Hondras 1999	-10.1	14.8	68	-8	16.6	69	42.5%	-0.13 [-0.47, 0.20]
Senna 2011	29.4	5.5	25	33.2	7.3	37	26.1%	-0.57 [-1.08, -0.05]
Vernon 2009	-8.4	7.5	4	3.1	5.4	5	3.7%	-1.60 [-3.24, 0.04]
Subtotal (95% CI)			**129**			**143**	**100.0%**	**-0.37 [-0.69, -0.04]**
Heterogeneity: Tau² = 0.04; Chi² = 4.44, df = 3 (P = 0.22); I² = 32%								
Test for overall effect: Z = 2.22 (P = 0.03)								
1.5.4 long-term effects								
Senna 2011	23.5	8	25	38.3	12.8	37	100.0%	-1.31 [-1.87, -0.75]
Subtotal (95% CI)			**25**			**37**	**100.0%**	**-1.31 [-1.87, -0.75]**
Heterogeneity: Not applicable								
Test for overall effect: Z = 4.59 (P < 0.00001)								

Test for subgroup differences: Chi² = 8.35, df = 3 (P = 0.04), I² = 64.1%

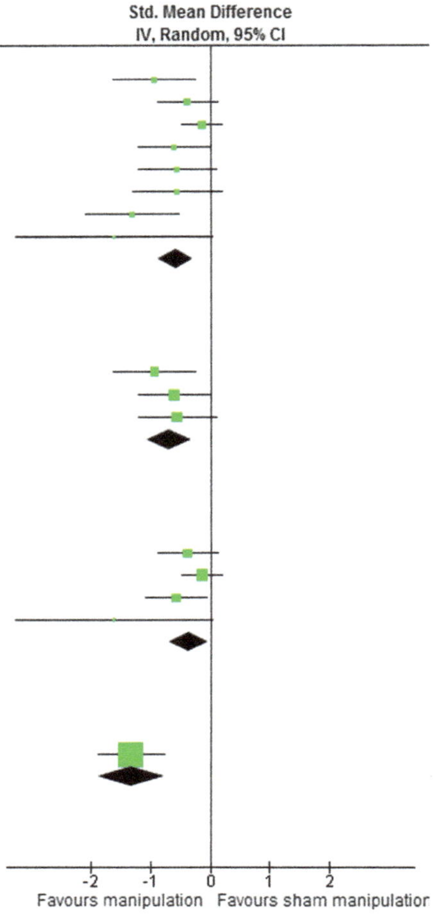

Figure 4 Forest plot of all studies comparing MT versus sham on pain.

relief WMD -5.31 (95% CI -13.62 to 2.99) [27,28]. There is low level of evidence that MT is no better than sham on pain relief in patients with dysmenorrhea.

Stratification for profession, yielded in no significant differences between the professions. MT performed by physicians provided somewhat lager effect sizes than the other professions (Figure 5), however, these results were based on one low RoB study [36].

Sensitivity analyses

Sensitivity analyses did not change our main findings. Only at short term follow-up the level of evidence changed from low level of evidence for pain relief to moderate level of evidence for no significant differences between the groups. The pooled effect size (SMD) decreased from -0.37 (-0.69 to -0.04) to -0.30 (-0.72 to 0.11) [27,36].

For the subgroup musculoskeletal disorders, the level of evidence changed from low level of evidence for pain relief to moderate level of evidence for pain relief on all points. The SMD changed from 0.71 (-1.02 to -0.39) to -0.81 (95% CI -1.17 to -0.45) [23,31,36].

Disability

Pooling was not possible because of statistical heterogeneity. There is very low level of evidence (high RoB, inconsistency, imprecision) that MT has no statistically significant effect on disability [22,24-26,30,36].

Perceived recovery

One study with high risk of bias (31 patients with chronic asthma) evaluated perceived (asthma) recovery [32]. There is very low level of evidence (high RoB, inconsistency, imprecision) that MT has no statistically significant effect on perceived (asthma) recovery [32].

Quality of life

Two studies (164 participants all with low back pain), one with low RoB, were included in the meta-analyses [35,36]. Data from two other studies could not be used [25,26]. There is very low level of evidence (high RoB, inconsistency, imprecision) that there is no statistically significant effect on quality of life MD 1.22 (95% CI, -7.24 to 9.67).

Study or Subgroup	manipulation Mean	SD	Total	sham manipulation Mean	SD	Total	Weight	Std. Mean Difference IV, Random, 95% CI
1.4.1 independent on profession								
Cleland 2005	26.1	17.2	19	43.5	19.5	17	11.5%	-0.93 [-1.62, -0.24]
Ghroubi 2007	49.4	16.8	32	58.4	28.8	32	16.8%	-0.38 [-0.87, 0.12]
Hondras 1999	-10.1	14.8	68	-8	16.6	69	22.6%	-0.13 [-0.47, 0.20]
Kokjohn 1992	-18.7	19.4	23	-7.8	15.7	21	13.6%	-0.60 [-1.21, 0.00]
Mansilla- Ferragut 2009	0.7	0.4	19	0.9	0.3	18	12.3%	-0.55 [-1.21, 0.11]
Senna 2011	29.4	5.5	12	33.2	7.3	18	10.5%	-0.56 [-1.30, 0.19]
Senna 2011	23.5	8	13	38.3	12.8	19	9.8%	-1.30 [-2.08, -0.51]
Vernon 2009	-8.4	7.5	4	3.1	5.4	5	2.9%	-1.60 [-3.24, 0.04]
Subtotal (95% CI)			**190**			**199**	**100.0%**	**-0.58 [-0.88, -0.29]**
Heterogeneity: Tau² = 0.07; Chi² = 12.10, df = 7 (P = 0.10); I² = 42%								
Test for overall effect: Z = 3.88 (P = 0.0001)								
1.4.2 chiropracter								
Hondras 1999	-10.1	14.8	68	-8	16.6	69	52.9%	-0.13 [-0.47, 0.20]
Kokjohn 1992	-18.7	19.4	23	-7.8	15.7	21	37.1%	-0.60 [-1.21, 0.00]
Vernon 2009	-8.4	7.5	4	3.1	5.4	5	9.9%	-1.60 [-3.24, 0.04]
Subtotal (95% CI)			**95**			**95**	**100.0%**	**-0.45 [-1.02, 0.11]**
Heterogeneity: Tau² = 0.13; Chi² = 4.32, df = 2 (P = 0.12); I² = 54%								
Test for overall effect: Z = 1.58 (P = 0.11)								
1.4.3 physical therapist								
Cleland 2005	26.1	17.2	19	43.5	19.5	17	24.6%	-0.93 [-1.62, -0.24]
Ghroubi 2007	49.4	16.8	32	58.4	28.8	32	48.2%	-0.38 [-0.87, 0.12]
Mansilla- Ferragut 2009	0.7	0.4	19	0.9	0.3	18	27.2%	-0.55 [-1.21, 0.11]
Subtotal (95% CI)			**70**			**67**	**100.0%**	**-0.56 [-0.90, -0.22]**
Heterogeneity: Tau² = 0.00; Chi² = 1.61, df = 2 (P = 0.45); I² = 0%								
Test for overall effect: Z = 3.20 (P = 0.001)								
1.4.4 physician								
Senna 2011	23.5	8	13	38.3	12.8	19	48.7%	-1.30 [-2.08, -0.51]
Senna 2011	29.4	5.5	12	33.2	7.3	18	51.3%	-0.56 [-1.30, 0.19]
Subtotal (95% CI)			**25**			**37**	**100.0%**	**-0.92 [-1.64, -0.19]**
Heterogeneity: Tau² = 0.12; Chi² = 1.80, df = 1 (P = 0.18); I² = 44%								
Test for overall effect: Z = 2.48 (P = 0.01)								
Test for subgroup differences: Chi² = 1.03, df = 3 (P = 0.79), I² = 0%								

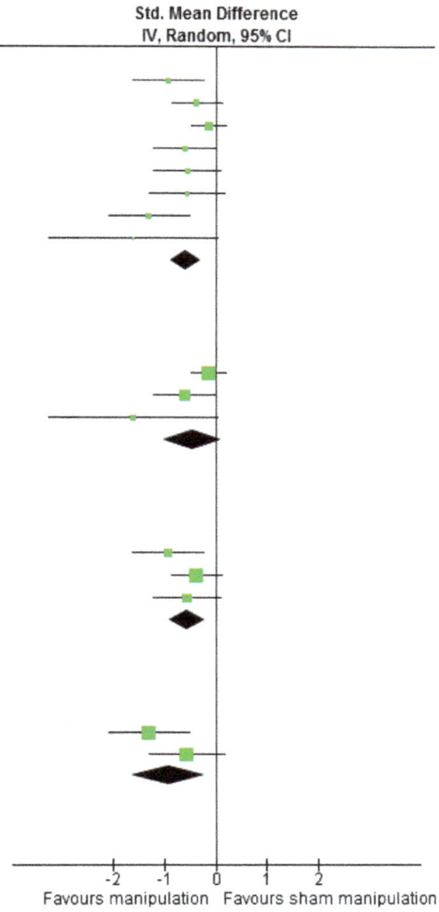

Figure 5 Forest plot comparing MT versus sham MT on pain stratified for profession.

Range of motion

Four studies (179 participants with musculoskeletal complaints), three with high RoB [22,38,40], evaluated range of motion (ROM) after MT [22,31,38,40]. Statistical pooling was not possible because of lack of data or heterogeneity on outcome. There is very low level of evidence (high RoB, inconsistency, imprecision) that MT is not more effective on ROM.

Pulmonary functions

Pulmonary functions were evaluated in two studies (66 participants) [32,33]. Statistical pooling was not possible because lack on data [32]. There is low level of evidence (high RoB, imprecision) that MT does not provide better pulmonary functions.

Adverse events

Eleven studies (58%) did not report about adverse events [22,24-26,28-30,34,38-40] while four studies reported no adverse events [23,31,32,35]. Adverse events in the MT group (9 participants) were limited to minor aggravation of neck pain or headache, muscle soreness, stiffness, tiredness, and local discomfort [27,33,36,37]. Also in the sham MT group some adverse events were reported (6 participants). These consisted of elevated blood pressure in the morning, mild heart palpitations and little muscle soreness [27,33]. None of the studies registered any serious complications in either the experimental or control group.

Discussion

There is low to moderate level of evidence that MT has a significant effect on pain relief in adults with a variety of complaints and in the subgroup of patients with musculoskeletal disorders. Performing sensitivity analysis, including only studies with low Rob, did not change our main findings. Ideally we need interventions with immediate effects that preferably lead to long-term clinically relevant benefits. In this study we found benefit for MT, especially in patients with musculoskeletal disorders. The pooled effect estimates were considered clinically relevant.

A recent systematic review showed that musculoskeletal conditions were the most frequent indications for receiving spinal manipulation, with low back and neck pain being the most common ones [1]. Non-musculoskeletal conditions comprised a very small percentage of indications [1].

It appears reasonable that when MT is used there should be evidence for its efficacy with minimal or no harm. Only a few minor adverse events were reported in the included studies. There were no serious complications such as strokes. Sensitivity/subgroup analyses on the risk of specific manipulation techniques related to adverse events were not possible. Our findings are in agreement with earlier studies, which cast doubt about a causal relation between manipulation and stroke [11,12]. However, it must be acknowledged that the included trials were much too small to pick up more rare serious adverse events (if present).

Interestingly, this review found also some adverse events in the sham MT group [27,33]. Sham manipulation consisted of light touch at the same anatomic thoracic and occipital regions in the same position as the real manipulations [33], and low force maneuver at the left L2-L3 vertebral level in side lying position with bilateral flexion of the hips and knees [27]. Light touch is not expected to create physiological or biomechanical changes, therefore, we cannot explain these events. It seems that low force chiropractic techniques of at least 200 Newton may also produce some treatment effects and that these are indistinguishable from the real MT. To improve reporting of (minor) adverse events, we propose the usage of (validated) questionnaires, at all follow-up visits. An anonymous registration for practitioners in a database should be considered.

To our knowledge, there are no comparable systematic reviews that evaluated MT versus sham MT in adults with a variety of complaints. Therefore, we compared our results with systematic reviews, which evaluate MT on specific patient groups. An earlier systematic review on the effectiveness of MT for chronic low back pain patients found very low quality evidence that MT is equally effective than sham MT for short-term pain relief [15]. Their results were based on three RCTs [24,30,38], all included in this review. We added two more RCT, one with low RoB [29,36], resulting in a different conclusion: low evidence that MT showed statistically significantly better pain relief than sham MT. Our findings are in agreement with Gross et al 2010, who found low quality evidence for the use of thoracic manipulation for immediate pain relief in patients with neck pain [42]. A systematic review of spinal manipulations for patients with dysmenorrhea indicated that there was no evidence to suggest that spinal manipulation was effective in treating dysmenorrhea compared to sham, which is in line with our results [16]. Another Cochrane review for asthma reported from data of two trials [32,43] examining chiropractic MT compared to sham MT, that there are no significant differences between groups for lung function and quality of life measures [17]. One of the included trials concerned young (6 to 8 years) children and therefore was excluded from our systematic review [43].

Limitations of our review include the diversity of professions (chiropractor, physical therapist, osteopath or physician) who delivered the manipulations. Nevertheless, our subgroup analyses showed no clear differences in effect between different professions, but the power is low and the conclusion is based on 2 or 3 small studies. Another limitation is the diversity of sham manipulations. These varied from manipulations with a deactivated Activator instrument, a spring loaded piston activated instrument to low force mimic maneuvers or manual contact. A sham manipulation should produce the smallest possible treatment effect; because any manual intervention inevitably may produce some type of physiologic or biomechanical effect [44]. It is important that sham treatments are credible for the patient, equalizing the effect of expectation of improvement between groups, are valid, so that the patient can adequately be blinded. In this systematic review, adequate blinding of participants was performed in only seven studies [22,23,25,28,36,38,39]. Unclear and inadequate blinding may have affected and enlarged our pooled effect sizes. Moreover, blinding may be affected in patients previously exposed to manipulation.

Four studies used a cross-over design [29,32,39,40]. In crossover studies, participants will be aware eventually of the type of manipulations they received leading to probable bias and this may affect the outcome. Moreover, the effects of spinal manipulation cannot be reversed and are therefore likely to be carried over into the next cycle. However, these studies were not included in the meta-analyses and therefore, could not have affected our pooled results.

Most of our studies included less than 25 participants in their smallest study group. These studies could be considered as underpowered. Also, the overall power of the statistical pooling was limited. The total number of participants was less than 400 for continuous outcomes and 300 for dichotomous outcomes in all of our meta-analyses. Consequently, the level of evidence was downgraded. Our sensitivity analyses were comparable with the original analyses and showed that no other factors might have influenced the overall pooled effects.

Based on personal communication during the review process, two studies did not meet the inclusion criteria of manipulative therapy [25,26]. When asked, the original authors stated that no thrust was given. However, as we were unable to consequently contact all corresponding authors, we chose to base the study selection on the published reports and refrained from removing these studies from the manuscript. Nevertheless, excluding these studies [25,26] would not have affected our results as these were not included in the meta-analysis.

As in each systematic review, the possibility of publication bias cannot be omitted, and is more likely in small studies with non-significant results. Although, our funnel plots did not suggest that this was an issue in this review, relevant studies, hidden in unknown databases are difficult to locate and may not have been included. To reduce these biases, we performed a thorough search in multiple electronic databases and performed reference and hand-searching without language restrictions.

Conclusion

Implications for practice

MT produces pain relief immediate after treatment, at short- and long term follow-up, but no effects are found on disability and perceived (asthma) recovery. Clinicians could refer to MT for pain relief as a treatment goal. For patients with pulmonary diseases, no significant or clinical relevant effects were found.

Implications for research

The quality of evidence varied from very low to moderate, indicating that further research is likely to have an impact on the confidence in the estimate of effect and is likely to change this estimate. There is a need for future low risk of bias RCTs with large sample sizes that evaluate the effect immediate after treatment and at short- and long term follow-up not only on pain but also on disability and perceived recovery. Moreover there is a need for evaluating the effect of these procedures on specific subgroups of patients with musculoskeletal disorders. Adverse events should be reported more consequently.

Competing interests

The authors declare that they have no competing interests.

Authors' contributions

Contributors: GGMSP, KV, APV conceived and designed the study. GGMSP, ET determined eligibility of search results and scored risk of bias. GGMSP, ET, SK, MB extracted data from included studies. GGMSP, ET, APV analyzed and interpreted the data. GGMSP drafted the manuscript. BWK commented on a draft-version of the manuscript. All authors critically revised the manuscript and approved the final version to be published. This article was commissioned and externally peer reviewed. All authors read and approved the final manuscript.

Author details

[1]University of Applied Sciences AVANS, Research Group Diagnostics, PO Box 90116, Breda, RA 4800, The Netherlands. [2]Department of General Practice, Erasmus Medical Centre, University Medical Center, PO Box 2040, Rotterdam, CA 3000, The Netherlands. [3]Rotterdam University of Applied Sciences, Rotterdam, Department physical therapy, Museumpark 40, Rotterdam, CX 3015, The Netherlands.

References

1. Hurwitz EL: **Epidemiology: spinal manipulation utilization.** *J Electromyogr Kinesiol* 2012, **22:**648–654.
2. Evans DW, Lucas N: **What is 'manipulation'? A reappraisal.** *Man Ther* 2010, **15:**286–291.
3. Evans DW: **Mechanisms and effects of spinal high-velocity, low amplitude thrust manipulation: previous theories.** *J Manipulative Physiol Ther* 2002, **25:**251–262.
4. Ianuzzi A, Khalsa PS: **Comparison of human lumbar facet joint capsule strains during simulated high- velocity, low- amplitude spinal manipulation versus physiological motions.** *Spine J* 2005, **5:**277–290.
5. Bialosky JE, Bishop MD, Price DD, Robinson ME, George SZ: **The mechanisms of manual therapy in the treatment of musculoskeletal pain: a comprehensive model.** *Man Ther* 2009, **14:**531–538.
6. Pickar JG: **Neurophysiological effects of spinal manipulation.** *Spine J* 2002, **2:**357–371.
7. van de Veen EA, de Vet HC, Pool JJ, Schuller W, de Zoete A, Bouter LM: **Variance in manual treatment of nonspecific low back pain between orthomanual physicians, manual therapists, and chiropractors.** *J Manipulative Physiol Ther* 2005, **28:**108–116.
8. Albuquerque FC, Hu YC, Dashti SR, Abla AA, Clark JC, Alkire B: **Craniocervical arterial dissections as sequelae of chiropractic manipulation: patterns of injury and management.** *J Neurosurg* 2011, **115:**1197–1205.
9. Wand BM, Heine PJ, O'Connell NE: **Should we abandon cervical spine manipulation for mechanical neck pain? Yes.** *BMJ* 2012, **344:**e3679. doi:10.1136/bmj.e3679.
10. Haldeman S, Kohlbeck FJ, Mcgregor M: **Risk factors and precipitating neck movement causing vertebrobasilar artery dissection after cervical trauma and spinal manipulation.** *Spine* 1999, **24:**785–794.
11. Rothwell DM, Bondy SJ, Williams JI: **Chiropractic manipulation and stroke a population- based case- control study.** *Stroke* 2001, **32:**1054–1060.
12. Cassidy JD, Boyle E, Côté P, He Y, Hogg-Johnson S, Silver FL: **Risk of vertebrobasilar stroke and chiropractic care: results of a population-based case–control and case-crossover study.** *Spine* 2008, **33**(Suppl 4):S176–S183.
13. Cassidy JD, Bronfort G, Hartvigsen J: **Should we abandon cervical spine manipulation for mechanical neck pain? No.** *BMJ* 2012, **344:**e3680. doi:10.1136/bmj.e3680.
14. Cagnie B, Vinck E, Beernaert A, Cambier D: **How common are side effects of spinal manipulation and can these side effects be predicted?** *Man Ther* 2004, **9:**151–156.
15. Rubinstein SM, van Middelkoop M, Assendelft WJ, de Boer MR, van Tulder MW: **Spinal manipulative therapy for chronic low-back pain: an update of a Cochrane review.** *Spine* 2011, **36:**E825–E846.
16. Proctor ML, Hing W, Johnson TC, Murphy PA: **Spinal manipulation for primary and secondary dysmenorrhoea.** *Cochrane Database Syst Rev* 2006, **9**, CD002119.
17. Hondras MA, Linde K, Jones AP: **Manual therapy for asthma.** *Cochrane Database Syst Rev* 2005, **18**, CD001002.
18. ***Cochrane Handbook for Systematic Reviews of Interventions*** **Version 5.1.0 [updated March 2011].** In *The Cochrane Collaboration.* Edited by Higgins JPT, Green S; 2011. Available from www.cochrane-handbook.org.
19. van Tulder MW, Suttorp M, Morton S, Bouter LM, Shekelle P: **Empirical evidence of an association between internal validity and effect size in randomized controlled trials of low-back pain.** *Spine* 2009, **34:**1685–1692.
20. Cohen J: *Statistical Power Analysis for the Behavioural Sciences.* 1st edition. New York, San Francisco, London: Academic; 1988.
21. Guyatt GH, Oxman AD, Vist GE, Kunz R, Falck-Ytter Y, Alonso-Coello P: **GRADE: an emerging consensus on rating quality of evidence and strength of recommendations.** *BMJ* 2008, **336:**924–926.
22. Brantingham JW, Williams AM, Parkin-Smith GF, Weston P, Wood T: **A controlled, prospective pilot study of the possible effects of chiropractic manipulation in the treatment of osteo-arthritis of the hip.** *Eur J Chiropract* 2003, **51:**149–166.
23. Cleland JA, Childs MJD, McRae M, Palmer JA, Stowell T: **Immediate effects of thoracic manipulation in patients with neck pain: a randomized clinical trial.** *Manual Ther* 2005, **10:**127–135.
24. Ghroubi S, Elleuch H, Baklouti S, Elleuch MH: **Les lombalgiques chroniques et manipulations vertébrales. Étude prospective à propos de 64 cas. Chronic low back pain and vertebral manipulation.** *Ann Readapt Med Phys* 2007, **50:**570–576.

25. Hawk C, Long CR, Reiter R, Davis CS, Cambron JA, Evans R: **Issues in planning a placebo-controlled trial of manual methods: results of a pilot study.** *J Altern Complement Med* 2002, **8**:21–32.
26. Hawk C, Long CR, Rowell RM, Gudavalli MR, Jedlicka J: **A randomized trial investigating a chiropractic manual placebo: a novel design using standardized forces in the delivery of active and control treatments.** *J Altern Complement Med* 2005, **11**:109–117.
27. Hondras MA, Long CR, Brennan PC: **Spinal manipulative therapy versus a low force mimic maneuver for women with primary dysmenorrheal: a randomized, observer-blinded, clinical study.** *Pain* 1991, **81**:105–114.
28. Kokjohn K, Schmid DM, Triano JJ, Brennan PC: **The effect of spinal manipulation on pain and prostaglandin levels in women with primary dysmenorrhea.** *J Manipulative Physiol Ther* 1992, **15**:279–285.
29. Learman KE, Myers JB, Lephart SM, Sell TC, Kerns J, Cook CE: **Effects of spinal manipulation on trunk proprioception in subjects with chronic low back pain during symptom remission.** *J Manipulative Physiol Ther* 2009, **32**:118–126.
30. Licciardone JC, Stoll ST, Fulda KG, Russo DP, Siu J, Winn W: **Osteopathic manipulative treatment for chronic low back pain; a randomized controlled study.** *Spine* 2003, **13**:1355–1362.
31. Mansilla- Ferragut P, Fernández-de-las Peñas C, Alburquerque-Sendín F, Cleland JA, Boscá- Gandía JJ: **Immediate effects of atlanta-occipital joint manipulation on active mouth opening and pressure pain sensitivity in women with mechanical neck pain.** *J Manipulative Physiol Ther* 2009, **32**:101–106.
32. Nielsen NH, Bronfort G, Bendix T, Madsen F, Weeke B: **Chronic asthma and chiropractic manipulation: a randomized clinical study.** *Clin Exp Allergy* 1995, **25**:80–88.
33. Noll DR, Degenhardt BF, Johnson JC, Burt SA: **Immediate effects of osteopathic manipulative treatment in elderly patients with chronic obstructive pulmonary disease.** *J Am Osteopath Assoc* 2008, **108**:251–259.
34. Sanders GE, Reinert O, Tepe R, Maloney P: **Chiropractic adjustive manipulation on subjects with acute low back pain: visual analog pain scores and plasma beta-endorphin levels.** *J Manipulative Physiol Ther* 1990, **13**:391–395.
35. Santilli V, Beghi E, Finucci S: **Chiropractic manipulation in the treatment of acute back pain and sciatica with disc protrusion: a randomized double-blind clinical trial of active and simulated spinal manipulations.** *Spine J* 2006, **6**:131–137.
36. Senna MK, Machaly SA: **Does maintained spinal manipulation therapy for chronic nonspecific low back pain result in better long-term outcome?** *Spine* 2011, **18**:1427–1437.
37. Vernon H, Jansz G, Goldsmith CH, McDermaid C: **A randomized, placebo-controlled clinical trial of chiropractic and medical prophylactic treatment of adults with tension-type headache: results from a stopped trial.** *J Manipulative Physiol Ther* 2009, **32**:344–351.
38. Waagen GN, Haldeman S, Cook G, Lopez D, DeBoer KF: **Short term trial ofchiropractic adjustments for the relief of chronic low back pain.** *Manual Med* 1986, **2**:63–67.
39. Walsh MJ, Polus BI: **A randomized, placebo-controlled clinical trial on the efficacy of chiropractic therapy on premenstrual syndrome.** *J Manipulative Physiol Ther* 1999, **22**:582–585.
40. Whittingham W, Nilsson N: **Active range of motion in the cervical spine increases after spinal manipulation (toggle recoil).** *J Manipulative Physiol Ther* 2001, **24**:552–555.
41. Couto IBV: **Efeito agudo da manipulacao em pacientes com dor lombar cronica: estudo piloto (Effect of the manipulation in patients with chronic low back pain: a pilot study) [Portuguese].** *Fisioterapia em Movimento (FISIOTER MOVIMENTO)* 2007, **20**:57–62.
42. Gross A, Miller J, D'Sylva J, Burnie SJ, Goldsmith CH, Graham N, Haines T, Brønfort G, Hoving JL: **Manipulation or mobilisation for neck pain.** *Cochrane Database Syst Rev* 2010, **20**, CD004249.
43. Balon J, Aker PD, Crowther ER, Danielson C, Cox PG, O'Shaughnessy D: **A comparison of active and simulated chiropractic manipulation as adjunctive treatment for childhood asthma.** *N Engl J Med* 1998, **339**:1013–1020.
44. Meeker WC, Haldeman S: **Chiropractic: a profession at the crossroads of mainstream and alternative medicine.** *Ann Intern Med* 2002, **136**:216–237.

Survey based investigation into general practitioner referral patterns for spinal manipulative therapy

Annabel Kier[1*], Matthew George[2] and Peter W McCarthy[1]

Abstract

Background: In the UK Physiotherapy, Chiropractic and Osteopathy are all statutory regulated professions. Though guidelines have supported the use of Spinal Manipulative Therapy (SMT) for low back pain (LBP), General Practitioners (GP) referral patterns to the 3 registered professions that perform SMT are generally unknown.

Method: A short questionnaire was designed and piloted. Demographic information, patient referral to SMT and the GPs own personal utilisation of SMT were obtained. 385 GP's were contacted representing approximately 20% of the GP's in Wales Autumn 2007.

Results and discussion: 182 (50.8%) completed questionnaires were returned.
Profile characteristics: 2/3 of respondents were male, 79% were 40 years old or older (statistically reflective of the total population of GPs in Wales at that time) and 62% had 20 years or less in practise. *Personal use of SMT by GP's*: 48 respondents had sought SMT treatment and a further 56% of those that had not previously sought SMT indicated that they would consider doing so. *Patient referral to SMT by GP's:* 131 respondents (72%) had referred patients to SMT and of those who had not a further 13% would consider referring. The general referral pattern and utilisation pattern was Physiotherapy: Osteopathy: Chiropractic. 21% who had never referred patients neither had, nor would consider it for themselves. A small subgroup appeared to manage personal choice differently from patient referral: 5 individuals who had not referred patients either had or would consider it for themselves and 23 of the group that would refer patients neither had nor would seek it for themselves.

Conclusions: This limited investigation indicates that GP's do practise consistently with guidelines on back pain and utilise SMT as a care option. Although the main option for referral was physiotherapy, slightly over 40% of respondents who expressed a preference would refer to either osteopathy or chiropractic, or both in preference to physiotherapy. There was a small proportion that did not and would not refer patients for SMT regardless of personal use of SMT; these suggested use of acupuncture. Further investigation is needed to determine the alternatives to SMT offered to patients and the decision-making criteria for patient referral to subtypes of SMT practitioner.

Keywords: Spinal manipulative therapy, Referral and personal usage by general practitioners

* Correspondence: annabel.kier@southwales.ac.uk
[1]Welsh Institute of Chiropractic, University of South Wales, Treforest, Pontypridd CF38 2TE, UK
Full list of author information is available at the end of the article

Background

There has been a widened use of Complementary and Alternative Medicine (CAM) over the last two decades [1-7]. One area where this change is most noticeable is that of Low Back Pain (LBP).

LBP is a commonly experienced symptom, which approximately 38% of adults will have in any one year [8]. Of these, 1 in 4 LBP sufferers experience significantly disabling symptoms resulting in a considerable cost to society in particular and a significant proportion of the caseload is dealt with in primary care thus challenging both the health care system and the General Practitioner (GP). Recent research outcomes and guidelines have supported the use of Spinal Manipulative Therapy (SMT) for this condition [9-15]. Although SMT is available in the UK from a small number of GPs the main provision is accessed via 3 statutory registered professions, Chiropractors, Osteopaths and certain qualified Physiotherapists [16]: statutorily regulated by the General Chiropractic Council (GCC), the General Osteopathic Council (GOC) and The Health Professions Council (HPC- Physiotherapists), respectively. Although these three professions have traditionally appeared to have little common ground, anecdotally it appears that some degree of synergy exists between them regarding the management of back pain, as referenced in the guidelines: even though there may be differences in the choice and utilisation of certain manipulative procedures, rehabilitation and exercise protocols [16]. The engagement of services from these private practitioners by the National Health Service (NHS) is still an ardently debated topic [17]. This work has the potential to act as a baseline study for future investigations endeavouring to determine the impact of change on engagement of these services for Low Back pain.

Although the situation regarding direction of GPs to services by guidelines specifically for LBP has been present for a number of years [11], the proportion of GPs who either do, or would consider referring patients to SMT practitioners, in compliance with the low back pain guidelines, is unknown. Similarly there is little information regarding GP's referral preference towards a specific type of SMT or the GP's personal utilisation of SMT and whether these two aspects are linked.

Method

A short questionnaire was designed and initially piloted internally for face/construct validity within the university and a sample of GPs (personal connection). The questionnaire requested information regarding a GP's age, sex, years spent practising, patient referral to SMT as well as the GPs own personal utilisation of SMT. Where there may not have been a need/wish to seek SMT, the GP was asked to answer the question hypothetically. No other personal information was requested. A covering letter containing information and invitation to complete the questionnaire as well as a stamped and addressed return envelope was sent to each selected individual. Anonymity of participants was maintained by the destruction of all returned envelopes once they had been opened and separated from the questionnaire, thereby eliminating the potential of identifying participants from the postmark.

The Primary Care Trust (PCT), PCT sub-division and GP name and address information was obtained from www.specialistinfo.com (2007) [18], an internet directory of over 36,800 hospital consultants and over 38,000 GPs in the UK. Any qualified GP practising in Wales at the time of the study and whose name was listed on the website was eligible for inclusion the study. A selection of 358 GPs from all 22 Primary Care Trusts in Wales were approached for the study representing approximately 20% of the then 1749 practising GP's in Wales during Autumn 2007 who were available on the chosen database. Potential participants were selected by sampling each GP name from alternating sub-divisions of the PCTs until the required number were selected. The selection process was otherwise random, with no consideration made for other factors such as male:female ratio. The study had received approval by the Welsh Institute of Chiropractic research unit ethical review group of the Chiropractic division, University of Glamorgan. In order to reduce bias in terms of SMT selection, no indication of the involvement of a chiropractic teaching facility remained on any of the literature. The return address was to the Faculty of Health, Sports and Science.

The data is presented as either raw numerical or frequency distributions. Limited statistical analysis was performed using Chi^2 test to compare the distributions across groups.

Results

Of the original 358 posted questionnaires, 187 were returned, however 5 were disregarded as void due to completion errors. The remaining 182 (50.8%) were analysed and are reported below.

Profile characteristics

Two thirds 118 (64.8%) of the 182 respondents, were male compared to 64 (35.2%) female. Seventy nine percent of respondents (143/182) were forty years of age or older (105 male and 39 female) in contrast to twenty one percent younger than 40 years of age (13 males and 25 female). Regarding years of experience in practice, sixty two percent had twenty or less years experience (71 male and 42 female) and thirty eight percent had more than twenty years experience (47 male and 22 female).

Personal use of SMT by GP's

48 respondents' forming 26.4% of the 182 GPs who returned the completed questionnaire had personally sought treatment from a SMT practitioner: of which 32 were male in the 30–59 age range, mainly in the 40–49 and 50–59 age groups, and 16 were female between 20–59 years of age, mainly in the 30–39, 40–49 and 50–59 age groups (there was no difference between these populations: Chi^2 $p>0.1$).

The remaining 134 GPs of the 182 returned for analysis, had not previously sought SMT. Of this group, 75 (56%: comprising of 45 males and 30 females) responded that they would consider seeking treatment from a SMT practitioner in the future. The males were mostly in the 40–59 year age range; whereas the females were mostly in the 30–39 age range suggesting age was not an influencing factor in this group. In total, 123 (68%) GPs indicated that they either had personally sought or would consider seeking SMT, leaving 59 (32%) that neither had, nor would consider, seeking SMT treatment in the future, this group appeared no different from the main population in relation to gender or age range (Chi^2 $p>0.1$).

Patient referral for SMT by GP's

131 respondents (72%), 88 males and 43 females, indicated that they had referred a patient to a SMT practitioner. Of these, 31 of the males and 14 of the females had themselves utilised SMT with an additional 40 males and 23 females indicating they would personally consider utilizing SMT in the future. However of this subgroup of GP's, in apparent contrast to their treatment of patients, 17 of the 88 males and 6 of the 43 females had not personally used, and responded that they would not consider utilising SMT themselves in the future. Unfortunately, the structure of the questionnaire did not allow any analysis of the number of GPs who had referred patients but would not do so in the future. For those categories where a data was available (age and gender), none of these distributions varied significantly from the population statistics of those GPs who responded to the questionnaire (Chi^2 $p>0.1$).

Of the 51 (29%) remaining GPs (30 male and 21 female) who had not previously referred a patient to a SMT practitioner, 13 (7%), comprising 6 males and 7 females, indicated they would consider referring a patient to a SMT practitioner in the future (Chi^2 $p>0.1$). This left 38 (21%) of the respondents (24 males and 14 females) who indicated that they have not and would not consider referral of their patients to a SMT practitioner.

Therefore, of the 182 respondents, 144 (79%) indicated that they already had or would consider referring a patient to a SMT practitioner. For outline of all subdivisions see Table 1.

Choice of SMT practitioner in context of personal usage by GPs

When asked to name the type of therapist that GPs had personally sought or would consider seeking SMT treatment from, the results were as follows: physiotherapist 22% / osteopath 16% / chiropractor 13%. Interestingly, those who had previously sought SMT treatment appeared to distribute significantly differently ($P<0.01$) to those who had expressed a preference but had not already experienced SMT treatment (Table 2). Where preference was indicated, the order was found to be similar for both males and females. A further 23% responded that they had no preference and would choose to seek help from either of the 3 professions listed. 24% of respondents were selective in a different manner in that they elected to choose 2 of the 3 options; with osteopathy being favoured in combination with either chiropractic or physiotherapy. A small subgroup (n=4) indicated that they would choose SMT from a profession other than those proposed in this study (this population was not included in Table 2).

Choice of SMT practitioner by GP's in context of patient referral

A similar ratio to that above was found for GP's referral preference for their patients: physiotherapist 19% / osteopath 11% / chiropractor 7%. Interestingly 42% (of respondents who had reported a preference: n=127) did so by choosing either osteopath, chiropractor or both from the 3 options offered. A further subgroup of responses (30%) was most reflective of the NICE guidelines by indicating they have or would refer/recommend their patients to (any) either of the 3 professions. In conclusion, some GP respondents were very specific in their choice of which SMT practitioner they would refer their patients to. As with personal use, some opted for 2 of the 3 professions. In this case the preferred combinations favoured osteopathy (with either chiropractic or physiotherapy: see Table 2). A small subgroup of 3: (not included in Table 2) gave unsolicited information in that they would refer to someone other than SMT practitioners and all indicated Acupuncture as their choice. Though personal comments were not actively sought on the questionnaire one respondent indicated that choice of referral would depend on the practitioner and not the profession, thereby highlighting that personal knowledge of the practitioner was considered at least as important as type of SMT practitioner. Another practitioner emphasised that though they neither utilise for themselves nor refer patients, the option of self-referral is made clear to their patients.

Discussion

On the whole the results of this small study suggest that 140 (77%) of the 182 GP respondents had either already

Table 1 Preference regarding SMT (referral and/or personal usage)

Respondents	Number of completed questionnaires	Have used SMT previously	Have not used	Have not used but would consider using SMT	Total having either used SMT or would consider its use personally	Those GPs who have either used SMT (*or would consider using SMT*) personally			GPs that have not used and would not seek SMT personally (non-users)	GPs that have not used SMT personally (*and GPs who would not consider use of SMT*)		Total of those who either have (*or would consider*) referring patients to SMT
						Have referred patients to SMT	Have not referred patients to SMT but would consider referring patients in the future	Have not referred nor would consider referring to SMT		Have referred or would consider referring patients to SMT	Have not referred and would not consider referring to SMT	
Male	118	32	86	45	77	31+(*40*)=71	1+(*4*)= 5	0+(*1*)= 1	41	17+(*1*)=18	23	105+(*7*)= 112
Female	64	16	48	30	46	14+(*23*)=37	0+(*5*)= 5	2+(*2*)= 4	18	6+(*2*)= 8	10	48+(*10*)= 58
Total	182	48	134	75	123	45+(*63*)=108	1+(*9*)= 10	2+(*3*)= 5	59	23+(*3*)=26	33	153+(*17*)=170

Analysis of results from respondents to the questionnaire and the subdivisions relating to gender, personal utilisation off and patient referral to SMT. In the sections describing the groups that either have or have not previously used SMT, the data presented outside the parentheses refers to those who have experienced and within parentheses relates to those who have not yet experienced SMT.

Table 2 GP's previous and potential future personal usage of SMT

	Expressed preference for personal use		Total expressing personal preference	Expressed preference for Patient referral/ recommendation		Total expressing preference for referral
	Previously	Future		Previously	Future	
Osteopathy	10(21%)	10(13%)	***20(16%)***	15(11%)	1(8%)	***16(11%)***
Chiropractic	13(27%)	3(4%)	***16(13%)***	9(7%)	1(8%)	***10(7%)***
Physiotherapy	9(19%)	18(24%)	***27(22%)***	18(14%)	8(62%)	***26(18%)***
No preference	6(13%)	22(29%)	***28(23%)***	35(27%)	1(8%)	***36(25%)***
Osteopathy /Chiropractic	6(13%)	7(9%)	***13(11%)***	28(21%)	1(8%)	***29(20%)***
Chiropractic/ Physiotherapy	0	4(5%)	***4(3%)***	9(7%)	0	***9(6%)***
Osteopathy/Physiotherapy	3(6%)	9(12%)	***12(10%)***	13(10%)	1(8%)	***14(10%)***
Other	1(2%)	2(3%)	***3(2%)***	4(3%)	0	***4(3%)***
n=	*48*	*75*	***123***	*131*	*13*	***144***

Preference for services: either used previously or not used previously with the caveat that they may do so in the future- regarding SMT and patient referral or recommendation. Percentages are presented for comparison, please note the numbers have been rounded to integers and so may not summate to 100%.

referred patients to SMT practitioners or would consider doing so in the future. Should this be a true representation of the picture across GPs in Wales, the results indicate that over 3 quarters of the GP population were practising consistently with the current guidelines [14]. However, this study's focus on SMT might have under-represented the whole story as a proportion of GPs may refer to other modalities covered by the guidelines, which were not specifically asked for in this study. Although Physiotherapy was the SMT provider of choice for most GPs who expressed a preference, there was a reasonably large proportion (42%) that indicated preference for either osteopathy or chiropractic, or both.

The sample size of this present study is admittedly small, which may have affected some of the statistical analysis of the small sub-groups. Although the total GP population in the region at the time was 1749, the sample reported here was obtained consistently with sampling procedures used in similar studies such as Corbett et al. in 2009 [19]. The literature varies regarding what constitutes a "good" or appropriate survey response rate. Variables such as population size, how the response is collected (interview, phone calls or mail-out) and whether a survey relates to individuals or organizations, appear to affect the response, as well as response rate [20]. In this case, the overall response rate was 50.8%, which although could be considered good [19] some would think it adequate [20], and others unacceptable with one issue being non-response error [21,22]. Although, as a population, GP response rate to questionnaires has been interpreted as being generally low by McAvoy & Kaner [23], due to factors such as lack of information, perceived relevance and or feedback, our study appears to have a high response rate. This might suggest that the topic is one of interest to GPs within this catchment area. In addition to topic, attempts were also made to circumvent elements of potential bias by not mentioning any professional affiliation in the questionnaire, the accompanying literature or mail address.

Regarding response bias, although the data presented here appears to show differences in distribution regarding gender and age, these do generally appear reflective of the total population at the time [24]. For instance, there were nearly twice the number of male respondents to this present survey than female; as at the time the population of GPs in Wales was approximately 60% male [24], therefore, this response would not appear to be too biased in relation to gender. Most male respondents were between 40–59 year of age and most females were between 30–39 years old, which is also in line with the general population statistics for Welsh GPs in 2007–9 [24]. Regarding the whole sample of respondents, 79% were 40 years of age or older, comprising 3 times as many males as females. The statistics available do not allow completely accurate comparison (the data presented as 30–44 and 45-above: [24]), however in the population, 62% were above 45 yrs of age, of which there were approximately 2.4 times as many males to females. In comparison, those less than 40 years of age were represented by double the amount of females compared to males: again the population statistics show 1.3 times the number of females to males [24].

Of the whole sample, 62% had less than 20 years experience, and numerically, was approximately equally distributed between the sexes. In contrast, approximately twice the number of males to females had had greater than 20 years experience. Of the 48 respondents that had utilised SMT, one third were female, which was proportionate with the male:female distribution in the overall response. As there is no information available regarding which point in their lives the participants sought their care, it is impossible to elaborate upon this in relation to trends regarding health care sought in the general population. In hindsight this may have been interesting to pursue and should potentially be considered for any future surveys of this kind.

A higher percentage of males (74% of the males) had referred patients to SMT compared to females (65%) in apparent contrast to previous studies that showed that female general practitioners tend to refer to CAM more than their male counterparts [4,25,26]. Although there is no data available, this finding might simply relate to the disproportionate distribution of males and females in the older age range of GPs. Of the small proportion of individuals (n=38/182: 21%) who would not consider referring patients for SMT, 33 neither have, nor would consider utilising SMT for themselves. Although this appears inconsistent with the guidelines, it does potentially indicate a level of personal choice being reflected in the decision making process concerning patient referral to SMT. Although there are no other studies of this exact nature for direct comparison, research performed prior to guideline direction on SMT reported a correlation between personal use and referral to CAM therapies by medical practitioners [4,27-32]. Furthermore, Brien et al. [31] reported that most GP's would consider referral via NHS contract to CAM therapies where there are no other therapeutic options for their patients. Various factors, including clinical evidence, appear to increase the likelihood of referral, but in particular the individual GP's positive attitude to and experience of CAM, including a trusting relationship with the CAM practitioner and the patients attitude toward CAM were reported as major factors in the decision making process. In the Brien et al. [31] study, 71.4% of the respondents indicated that they had referred a patient to a CAM practitioner with a further 7% indicating that they would consider it in the future, results which compare favourably with those reported here.

Of the remaining 5 of those 38 respondents in this study who would not refer to SMT, it was not unexpected to find 2 had experienced it for themselves. However, it was interesting and unexpected to find that the remaining 3 of the 5 would consider SMT for themselves, although they would not refer their patients. Therefore it appears that there are a number of respondents in each category suggesting they would manage patients with LBP contrary to their own personal choice. Albeit a small proportion, this would indicate that personal choice does not always affect compliance with guidelines or the inclination to refer. The exact reasoning for these differences was not explored here.

Though the National Institute for Health and Care Excellence (NICE) guidelines are exactly that, advice given on what is considered best practice at the time; it is open to personal interpretation by a practitioner based on their assessment and perception of the individual needs and choice of a patient. Having said that, many of the GPs surveyed in this study, appear to be following the guidelines. 96% (118 of 123) of those that had sought or would consider seeking SMT for themselves would refer patients as would 44% (26 of 59) of those GPs who have not and would not consider seeking SMT for themselves. Unfortunately, however, it is not possible to assess whether the proportion referring to SMT may have been affected by the presence of guidelines.

A number of studies have investigated the compliance of various physician groups to National and International guidelines [33-37]. Though not exhaustive, Table 3 lists several factors that may influence the physician's decision making process, besides any previous positive/negative communication with SMT practitioners [4,30,38-43].

It has been suggested that the basis for lack of compliance to guidelines includes factors such as; concerns about loss of autonomy, guidelines being "too rigid", oversimplification of the guidelines and their production being "motivated by a desire to cut costs" [36,37,44]. In addition, although a GP may have been in agreement with the guidelines, these are not necessarily congruent with patients' wishes. Non-adherence to guidelines and contradictory information supplied to patients by other professionals should also be considered important barriers to guideline adherence [33,36,37].

The understanding of why and to which SMT or CAM practitioner GPs may refer is neither transparent nor necessarily consistent across the profession. It has been suggested that unnecessary jargon could and does negatively affect communication and, therefore, the GP – CAM- and possibly SMT- practitioner relationship [38,43,45]. It is worth noting that the study presented here also allowed GPs to indicate their tendency to refer to combinations of SMT practitioner. Although, the underlying reasoning for a GP's selection of SMT practitioner cannot be deduced from this survey, personal

Table 3 Factors that might influence a GP's responses to a questionnaire regarding complementary and alternative medicine

Age	Family behaviour	Personal views
Availability - SMT providers	Finances of patient	Public/Private sector
Colleagues' attitudes	Gender of provider	Space/facilities
Education	Liability/legal issues	Specialisation
Ethnicity	Management	(The) State
Evidence	Media	Status of provider
Experience - in years	Practice size	Strategic reasons
Familiarity - with SMT	Patient preference	Time

Factors that might have influenced the questionnaire responses from the GP respondents in this study. The information derives from a previous study that assessed CAM rather than SMT specifically. (Adapted from Hirschkorn & Bourgeault, [43]).

conversations and anecdote points to the availability of physiotherapy on the NHS being an important factor; as osteopathy and chiropractic care are mostly found in the private sector. Therefore, patients may benefit from greater inter-profession dialogue and enhanced patient choice available from the NHS: complying with best practice regarding patient-centred care. Currently, the main issues which can impede this process are those of lack of quantity of qualified and registered practitioners, lack of understanding of low back pain subgroups and appropriate referral mechanisms to discussed treatment modalities [46]. A further limitation of the study would be the lack of information underlying the individual GP's choices regarding personal utilisation of and patient referral for SMT. Should a follow up study be conducted inclusion of such considerations would be recommended.

Conclusion

The results presented here indicate that a high proportion of the GP's responding to this questionnaire did or would refer patients for SMT, which is in contrast to anecdotal belief amongst some SMT practitioners and previous research findings [47]. This study found that when referrals occur to a specific profession, the majority of patient referrals were to physiotherapists. This result mirrors a previously reported outcome from a study of GPs' perception regarding which of the three types of SMT were considered to be most useful: physiotherapy> osteopathy >chiropractic [48].

Although limited, this survey has allowed for an insight into the GP's utilisation and referral patterns to practitioners of SMT in Wales. Further investigation is needed to determine the alternatives to SMT offered to patients and the decision-making criteria for patient referral to subtypes of SMT practitioner.

Abbreviations

CAM: Complementary and alternative medicine; LBP: Low back pain; GP: General practitioner; SMT: Spinal manipulative therapy; GCC: General chiropractic council; GOC: General osteopathic council; HPC: Health professions council; NHS: National health service; PCT: Primary health care trust; NICE: National institute for health and clinical excellence.

Competing interests

The authors declared that they have no competing interests.

Authors' contributions

MG compiled initial idea of area of interest and partook in the development of the questionnaire. Also participated in the initial write up of the data collected. AK assisted in development of the idea and design of questionnaire. Supervised the initial write up of this data, authored the final paper and in-depth analysis of data collected. PWM assisted in development of the initial questionnaire design, co-authored the final paper and in-depth analysis of data collected. All authors read and approved the final manuscript.

Disclosure

All authors are either chiropractors or teaching at a chiropractic institution.

Author details

[1]Welsh Institute of Chiropractic, University of South Wales, Treforest, Pontypridd CF38 2TE, UK. [2]Private Practice, Worthing BN11 1PS, UK.

References

1. White A, Ernst E: **Economic analysis of complementary medicine: a systematic review.** *Complement Ther Med* 2000, **8**:111–118.
2. Harris P, Rees R: **The prevalence of complementary and alternative medicine use among the general population: a systematic review of the literature.** *Complement Ther Med* 2000, **8**:88–96.
3. Thomas KJ, Nicholl JP, Coleman P: **Use and expenditure on complementary medicine in England: a population based survey.** *Complement Ther Med* 2001, **9**:2–11.
4. Lewith GT, Hyland M, Gray SF: **Attitudes to and use of complementary medicine among physicians in the United Kingdom.** *Complement Ther Med* 2001, **9**:167–172.
5. Emslie MJ, Campbell MK, Walker KA: **Changes in public awareness of, attitudes to, and use of complementary therapy in North East Scotland: surveys in 1993 and 1999.** *Complement Ther Med* 2002, **10**:148–153.
6. Schmidt K, Jacobs PA, Barton A: **Cross-cultural differences in GPs' attitudes towards complementary and alternative medicine.** *Complement Ther Med* 2002, **10**:141–147.
7. Haetzman M, Elliott AM, Smith BH, Hannaford P, Chambers WA: **Chronic pain and the use of conventional and alternative therapy.** *Fam Pract* 2003, **20**:147–154.
8. Bishop A, Foster N, Thomas E, Hay E: **How does the self-reported clinical management of patients with low back pain relate to the attitudes and beliefs of health care practitioners? A survey of UK general practitioners and physiotherapists.** *Pain* 2008, **135**:187–195.
9. Meade TW, Dyer S, Browne W, Townsend J, Frank AO: **Low back pain of mechanical origin: randomised comparison of chiropractic and hospital outpatient treatment.** *Br Med J* 1990, **300**(6737):1431–1437.
10. Meade TW, Dyer S, Browne W, Frank AO: **Randomised comparison of chiropractic and hospital outpatient management for low back pain: results from extended follow up.** *Br Med J* 1995, **311**(7001):349–351.
11. Royal College of General Practitioners: *Clinical guidelines for the management of acute low back pain*; 1999. Available http://www.chiro.org/LINKS/GUIDELINES/FULL/Royal_College/index.html.
12. NICE Clinical guidelines IPG 183; 2006. http://www.nice.org.uk/nicemedia/live/11204/51670/51670.pdf.
13. Department of Health: *Musculoskeletal Services Framework*; 2006. available at http://www.susanoliver.com/pdf/MSF_Final.pdf.
14. NICE Clinical guidelines CG88; 2009. available at http://www.nice.org.uk/nicemedia/live/11887/44343/44343.pdf.
15. Koes BW, van Tulder M, Chung-Wei CL, Macedo LG, McAuley J, Maher C: **An updated overview of clinical guidelines for the management of non-specific low back pain in primary care.** *Eur Spine J* 2010, **19**:2075–2094.
16. Harvey E, Burton AK, Moffett JK, Breen A: **Spinal manipulation for low-back pain: a treatment package agreed by the UK chiropractic, osteopathy and physiotherapy professional associations.** *Man Ther* 2003, **8**:46–51.
17. Hartvigsen J, Foster NE, Croft PR: **We need to rethink front line care for back pain.** *Br Med J* 2011, **342**:d3260.
18. Filed under Wales, Practices within PCT's; 2008. www.specialistinfo.com (specialist info.com/a_directory_gp2.php).
19. Corbett M, Foster NE, Ong BN: **GP attitudes and self-reported behaviour in primary care consultations for low back pain.** *Fam Pract* 2009, **26**:359–364.
20. Babbie E: *Survey research methods.* Belmont, CA: Wadsworth; 1990.
21. Schutt RK: *Investigating the social world; the process and practice of research.* 2nd edition. Thousand Oaks, CA: Pine Forge Press; 1999.
22. Hager MA, Wilson S, Pollak TH, Rooney PM: **Response rates for mail surveys of nonprofit organizations: a review and empirical test.** *Nonprofit and Voluntary Sector Quarterly* 2003, **32**:252–267.
23. McAvoy BR, Kaner EF: **General practice postal surveys: a questionnaire too far?** *Br Med J* 1996, **313**:732.

24. Swain K: *General Medical Practitioners in Wales 2002 to 2012, First release.* SDR 47/2013 The Health and Social Care Information Centre. Available from: http://wales.gov.uk/topics/statistics/headlines/health2013/general-medical-practitioners-2002-2012/?lang=en.
25. Schachter L, Weingarten MA, Kahan EE: **Attitudes of family physicians to nonconventional therapies: a challenge to science as the basis of therapeutics.** *Archive of Family Medicine* 1993, **2:**1268–1270.
26. Botting DA, Cook R: **Complementary medicine: knowledge, use and attitudes of doctors.** *Complement Ther Nurs Midwifery* 2000, **6:**41–47.
27. Reilly DT: **Young doctors' views on alternative medicine.** *Br Med J* 1983, **287**(6388):337–339.
28. Borkan J, Neher JO, Anson O, Smoker B: **Referrals for alternative therapies.** *J Fam Pract* 1994, **39:**545–550.
29. Wharton R, Lewith G: **Complementary medicine and the general practitioner.** *Br Med J* 1986, **2920**(6534):1497–1500.
30. Jump J, Yarbrough L, Kilpatrick S, Cable T: **Physicians' attitudes toward complementary and alternative medicine.** *Integrative Medicine* 1998, **1:**149–153.
31. Brien S, Howells E, Leydon GM, Lewith G: **Why GPs refer patients to complementary medicine via the NHS: a qualitative exploration.** *Primary Health Care Research & Development* 2008, **9:**205–215.
32. Sewitch MJ, Cepoiu M, Rigillo N, Sproule D: **A literature review of health care professional attitudes toward complementary and alternative medicine.** *Practice Review* 2008, **13:**139–154.
33. Hayward RSA, Guyatt GH, Moore K-A, McKibbon KA, Carter AO: **Canadian physicians' attitudes about and preferences regarding clinical practice guidelines.** *Can Med Assoc J* 1997, **156:**1715–1723.
34. Bishop P, Badii M, Wing P: **Implementation of clinical practice guidelines in workers compensation board patients with acute mechanical back pain: a prospective randomized trial.** *Spine J* 2002, **2**(5, Supplement):62–63.
35. Barry CA: **The role of evidence in alternative medicine: contrasting biomedical and anthropological approaches.** *Soc Sci Med* 2006, **62:**2646–2657.
36. Fullen BM, Maher T, Bury G, Tynan A, Daly LE, Hurley DA: **Adherence of Irish general practitioners to European guidelines for acute low back pain: a prospective pilot study.** *Eur J Pain* 2007, **11:**614–623.
37. Chenot JF, Scherer M, Becker A, Donner-Banzhoff N, Baum E, Leonhardt C, Keller S, Pfingsten M, Hildebrandt J, Basler H-D, Kochen MM: **Acceptance and perceived barriers of implementing a guideline for managing low back in general practice.** *Implementation Science* 2008, **3:**7–12.
38. Brussee WJ, Assendelft WJJ, Breen AC: **Communication between general practitioners and chiropractors.** *J Manipulative Physiol Ther* 2001, **24:**12–16.
39. Astin JA, Marie A, Pelletier KR, Hansen E, Haskell WL: **A review of the incorporation of complementary and alternative medicine by mainstream physicians.** *Arch Intern Med* 1998, **158:**2303–2310.
40. Berman BM, Bausell RB, Hartnoll SM, Beckner M, Bareta J: **Compliance with requests for complementary-alternative medicine referrals: a survey of primary care physicians.** *Integrative Medicine* 1999, **2:**11–17.
41. Hasan MY, Das M, Behjat S: **Alternative medicine and the medical profession: views of medical students and general practitioners.** *East Mediterr Health J* 2000, **6:**25–33.
42. Perkin MR, Pearcy RM, Fraser JS: **A comparison of the attitudes shown by general practitioners, hospital doctors and medical students towards alternative medicine.** *J R Soc Med* 1994, **87:**523–525.
43. Hirschkorn KA, Bourgeault IL: **Conceptualizing mainstream health care providers' behaviourism relation to complementary and alternative medicine.** *Soc Sci Med* 2005, **61:**157–170.
44. Clerc I, Ventelou B, Guerville M-A, Paraponaris A, Verger P: **General practitioners and clinical practice guidelines: a re-examination.** *Medical care research and review* 2011, **68:**504–518.
45. Langworthy JM, Birkelid J: **General practice and chiropractic in Norway: how well do they communicate and what do GP's want to know?** *J Manipulative Physiol Ther* 2001, **24:**576–581.
46. Foster NE: **Barriers and progress in the treatment of low back pain.** *BMC Med* 2011, **9:**108. doi:10.1186/1741/-7015-9-108. http://www.biomedicalcentral.com/1741-7015/9/108.
47. Bishop PB, Wing PC: **Knowledge transfer in family physicians managing patients with acute low back pain: a prospective randomized control trial.** *Spine J* 2006, **6:**282–288.
48. Breen A, Carrington M, Collier R, Vogel S: **Communication between general and manipulative practitioners: a survey.** *Complement Ther Med* 2000, **8:**8–14.

9

Comparison of non-surgical treatment methods for patients with lumbar spinal stenosis: protocol for a randomized controlled trial

Michael Schneider[1*], Carlo Ammendolia[2], Donald Murphy[3,4], Ronald Glick[5], Sara Piva[1], Elizabeth Hile[1], Dana Tudorascu[6] and Sally C Morton[7]

Abstract

Background: Lumbar spinal stenosis is the most common reason for spinal surgery in older adults. Previous studies have shown that surgery is effective for severe cases of stenosis, but many patients with mild to moderate symptoms are not surgical candidates. These patients and their providers are seeking effective non-surgical treatment methods to manage their symptoms; yet there is a paucity of comparative effectiveness research in this area. This knowledge gap has hindered the development of clinical practice guidelines for non-surgical treatment approaches for lumbar spinal stenosis.

Methods/design: This study is a prospective randomized controlled clinical trial that will be conducted from November 2013 through October 2016. The sample will consist of 180 older adults (>60 years) who have both an anatomic diagnosis of stenosis confirmed by diagnostic imaging, and signs/symptoms consistent with a clinical diagnosis of lumbar spinal stenosis confirmed by clinical examination. Eligible subjects will be randomized into one of three pragmatic treatment groups: 1) usual medical care; 2) individualized manual therapy and rehabilitative exercise; or 3) community-based group exercise. All subjects will be treated for a 6-week course of care. The primary subjective outcome is the Swiss Spinal Stenosis Questionnaire, a self-reported measure of pain/function. The primary objective outcome is the Self-Paced Walking Test, a measure of walking capacity. The secondary objective outcome will be a measurement of physical activity during activities of daily living, using the SenseWear Armband, a portable device to be worn on the upper arm for one week. The primary analysis will use linear mixed models to compare the main effects of each treatment group on the changes in each outcome measure. Secondary analyses will include a responder analysis by group and an exploratory analysis of potential baseline predictors of treatment outcome.

Discussion: Our study should provide evidence that helps to inform patients and providers about the clinical benefits of three non-surgical approaches to the management of lumbar spinal stenosis symptoms.

Trial registration: ClinicalTrials.gov identifier: NCT01943435

Keywords: Lumbar spinal stenosis, Spine, Rehabilitation, Physical therapy, Chiropractic, Non-surgical treatment

* Correspondence: mjs5@pitt.edu
[1]School of Health and Rehabilitation Sciences, Department of Physical Therapy, University of Pittsburgh, Pittsburgh, PA, USA
Full list of author information is available at the end of the article

Introduction

Background

Nearly 20% of the U.S. population will be 65 years of age or older by the year 2030 and about 34% of them will suffer from some type of osteoarthritis [1]. Lumbar Spinal Stenosis (LSS) is a chronic condition that is caused by degenerative changes in the lumbar spine, which is highly prevalent in the older adult population. Radiographic and clinical data from the Framingham cross-sectional study support a 30% prevalence of degenerative LSS in older adults [2].

The term LSS encompasses a number of conditions that decrease the total area of the central spinal canal, lateral recess, or intervertebral foramen. Although there may be visual evidence of narrowing of these osseous structures on x-ray, MRI or CT scans, symptomatic LSS is characterized by neurogenic claudication and/or radiculopathy [3]. Interestingly, the severity of bony narrowing measured on MRI or CT does not correlate with the severity of patient symptoms [4,5], including the hallmark symptom of the clinical syndrome: significant leg pain that typically worsens with ambulation.

Given the association of LSS symptoms and walking, it is no surprise that individuals with LSS often experience significant functional limitation of walking and associated disability [6]. Ambulation is a key component of overall health, independent living, and fall prevention. Impaired walking is associated with obesity, heart disease, peripheral artery disease, diabetes, and cognitive decline. Both the volume and intensity of walking ability are significantly lower in patients with LSS compared to patients with hip and knee osteoarthritis [7]. Additionally, individuals with LSS have a risk of falling that is comparable to patients with severe knee osteoarthritis [8,9]. The impact of spinal problems on physical function is greater than or similar to the burden on physical function caused by congestive heart failure, cancer, total knee and hip arthroplasty [10]. For all of these reasons, LSS should be considered a high priority condition for clinical research.

Most of the scientific literature on the clinical management of LSS has focused on invasive procedures such as injections and surgery. There is a paucity of literature on usual medical care, chiropractic, physical therapy, and other non-surgical interventions. Patients with recalcitrant symptoms and severe LSS appear to fare better with surgery. The largest clinical trial to date that compared surgical versus non-surgical care for LSS concluded that patients with symptomatic LSS who were treated operatively had greater improvement in pain and function [11]. However, the results from this trial also showed that about a third of patients in the non-operative group had significant improvements in pain and function lasting up to 4 years. This is strong evidence that a subset of LSS patients clearly show improvement without any surgical intervention.

While the most current systematic review of all non-operative treatment options for LSS identified 21 randomized trials, none provided moderate or high quality evidence for any specific treatment option [12]. Instead, low quality evidence from single trials suggests that: 1) epidural injections improve pain and function better than home exercise or in-patient physical therapy; and 2) exercise provides benefit for leg pain and function when compared to no treatment. Another systematic review of epidural injections for the non-surgical treatment of chronic low back pain includes some studies related to treatment of LSS [13]. This systematic review found a total of 10 randomized trials and 11 observational studies; yet only one small randomized trial and two observational studies were specifically related to LSS. In the randomized trial, epidural injections provided significant relief to only 55-65% of the LSS patients.

These reviews of the literature point to a serious lack of research evidence about most non-surgical treatments for LSS. Therefore, this trial is designed to study the comparative effectiveness of three common non-surgical approaches to the management of LSS: 1) usual medical care; 2) clinic-based manual therapy and individualized exercise; and 3) community-based group exercise. We hypothesize that subjects randomized to receive either clinic-based manual therapy/individualized exercise or community-based group exercise will have better outcomes than those randomized to usual medical care. We also hypothesize that the individualized clinic-based individualized approach will lead to better outcomes than the community-based group approach. However, it would be an important finding if we found that both approaches were equally effective due to the potential cost savings of group exercise over clinic-based health care.

This trial is designed to provide clinically relevant evidence that will help to inform the choices confronting clinicians and patients with LSS when faced with the decision about which type of non-surgical treatment to utilize. There is also a paucity of evidence that takes into account what clinical outcomes are important from the patient's perspective. This is consistent with the goal of all patient centered outcomes research, which is to determine which treatment works best, for whom, and under what circumstances [14].

Methods/design

Participants

We will recruit 180 community-dwelling older adults from the Pittsburgh metropolitan area to participate in our clinical trial. Eligibility for participation requires both anatomical and clinical evidence of LSS; potential participants must share diagnostic imaging results (MRI,

CT, etc.) showing bony narrowing, while also presenting with signs/symptoms consistent with the clinical syndrome of LSS (neurogenic claudication).

After informed consent, patients who are willing to be randomized and wish to be considered for participation will first undergo a baseline physical examination and screening process to determine if they meet the study's eligibility criteria.

Inclusion criteria

- Age 60 years or older
- Clinical history and diagnostic imaging evidence of lumbar spinal stenosis (LSS)
- Ability to read/write English
- Limitation of walking tolerance related to LSS (neurogenic claudication)
- Ability to attend 2 intervention session per week for 6 weeks
- Ability to engage in mild exercise
- Ability to walk 50 feet without the need for an assistive device
- Willing to be randomized to one of the 3 treatment groups

Exclusion criteria

- History of metastatic cancer
- Cauda equina symptoms including saddle paresthesia
- Previous lumbar surgery for LSS or lumbar spinal fusion
- History of severe peripheral artery disease or Ankle Brachial Index < 0.8
- Have been told by a physician that they should not engage in physical exercise
- History of neurologic (e.g., cervical myelopathy, stroke) or neuro-degenerative (e.g., Parkinson's disease) other than LSS that affects the subject's ability to walk
- Cannot complete a self-paced walking test (SPWT) for any reason other than symptoms related to LSS (e.g. chest pain, severe hip or knee arthritis, dizziness, etc.)
- Cannot complete SPWT without need for an assistive device

Our inclusion/exclusion criteria are designed to include patients who have a walking intolerance due to neurogenic claudication, and to rule out patients with vascular claudication or other conditions as causes of their limitation of walking. To screen for vascular conditions we will use the Ankle Brachial Index (ABI), which is a simple clinical screening test for peripheral artery disease (PAD). It is performed by using a hand-held Doppler ultrasonic device and sphygmomanometer to record the systolic pressures over the posterior tibial and brachial arteries. The ABI is calculated by dividing the lower extremity by the upper extremity systolic pressure, with the normal ratio being >0.9 [15]. A study of patients with atypical claudication due to either LSS or PAD found good sensitivity/specificity for differentiating PAD in patients with a low ABI [16]. We will exclude patients with an ABI less than 0.8 from participation in our study, for the rationale that they may have a vascular (versus neurogenic) cause of their claudication symptoms.

Research design

This is a prospective, randomized, controlled single-center trial to compare three non-surgical treatment approaches for patients with LSS. We will recruit 180 community dwelling older adults (age 60 years and older) from the Pittsburgh metropolitan area to participate in this study. The study began in November 2013 and will continue for three years until October 2016. Recruitment strategies will include: direct mailings, advertisements on city busses, informational brochures at the offices of spine surgeons and primary care offices, information articles about our study in senior newspapers and other publications, and informational lectures given at community senior centers and health fairs.

People interested in our study will first be screened by telephone. Potentially eligible persons will be scheduled for a baseline assessment visit for confirmation of eligibility. After obtaining informed consent and confirmation of meeting the inclusion criteria, 180 participants will then be randomized with equal probability to one of three intervention arms: 1) usual medical care; 2) clinic-based individualized exercise and manual therapy; or 3) community-based group exercise. The intervention period will last a total of six weeks in each arm. Outcomes will be measured at two follow-up assessment visits; two weeks after intervention (2 month follow-up) and four months after intervention (6 month follow-up).

Interventions

Our choice of interventions was informed by reviews of literature combined with input from patients, providers and our community stakeholders. This led us to choose the three intervention arms listed above. All intervention arms will utilize pragmatic protocols that allow for shared decision making with the patient.

Interviews with primary care physicians, physical medicine & rehabilitation (PM&R) physicians, surgeons, as well as community-dwelling older adults indicated that the "usual medical care" approach to the non-surgical management of LSS is a combination of: advice to stay active, use of oral medications to control pain, mood, and/or inflammation, and judicious referral for spinal injections. The most current lumbar spinal stenosis guideline from the North American Spine Society (NASS) suggests that spinal injections provide short term relief of symptoms, but states there is insufficient evidence for making any recommendations about pharmacological treatment [17].

The most current systematic review of non-surgical treatments for LSS concluded there was a paucity of chiropractic and physical therapy clinical trials [12]. The NASS lumbar spinal stenosis guideline concludes that there is insufficient evidence to make any recommendation for or against physical therapy, spinal manipulation, or exercise for the treatment of LSS [17]. Interviews with physical therapists and chiropractors revealed there were common LSS treatment themes, including the use of spinal de-weighting or traction, spine and hip mobilization, and individualized exercise. Two of the co-investigators (CA, DM) have developed clinical protocols that combine both manual therapy and therapeutic exercises into a pragmatic treatment approach for LSS. Two physical therapists and two chiropractors have been trained by these co-investigators to treat our research subjects with these clinical protocols.

We engaged in discussions about LSS with a number of older adults at community centers in the Pittsburgh metropolitan area, as well as patients with LSS in treatment at local chiropractic and physical therapy clinics. They expressed frustration with the ways in which LSS impacted their daily routines, especially with respect to interference with their ability to perform specific physical activities that involved walking or standing. Many of them had joined community-based exercise programs to help them stay physically fit and active. Several health insurance companies have begun to cover the costs of group exercise programs for their Medicare Advantage subscribers. These group exercise and healthy aging classes are aimed at helping older adults become and/or stay physically fit. These programs are offered at varying levels of difficulty, commensurate with the baseline level of fitness activity of the participant. In general, all of these group exercise classes focus on light non-impact aerobics, overall flexibility and low intensity strength training.

The three intervention arms of this study will utilize a pragmatic *effectiveness* design, using protocols that allow for some individualized variation, rather than comparing strict mono-therapy approaches in an *efficacy* design. Our approach is designed to provide more generalizable results by simulating the real-world delivery of these treatment methods. Each of the treatment arms will be conducted in out-patient or community settings. Subjects with a diagnosis of LSS will be randomized to one of 3 possible treatment groups, which are described in detail below. The duration of treatment will be the same for all groups (6 weeks) but the frequency will vary. The medical care group will receive 3 examination visits over 6 weeks; subjects in the other two groups will receive interventions twice per week for a total of 12 visits over 6 weeks. The procedures and protocols within each treatment group were informed by reviews of the literature, as well as by interviews with patients and providers.

Group 1: usual medical care

Participants will see a board certified physical medicine physician for a history and examination, after which a determination will be made about a course of treatment that is individualized to the needs of each patient. The physician will be permitted to prescribe any one or combination of the following categories of oral medications, based upon the individual clinical presentation of each subject:

- Non-steroidal anti-inflammatory: such as ibuprofen, celocoxib, diclofenac, or misoprostol
- Adjunctive analgesics: such as acetaminophen, tramadol, pregabalin, or gabapentin
- Anti-depressant agents: such as nortriptyline, duloxetine, sertraline, trazodone, or mirtazapine

The physician will also have the option to refer patients for spinal injections, which can be performed at two cooperating pain clinics in Pittsburgh. The type of spinal injections may be either epidural steroid injections or transforaminal nerve blocks; at the discretion of the pain management physician performing the procedure. In addition to oral medications and/or spinal injections, all subjects would be given advice to stay active, along with basic principles of proper posture and some simple home stretching exercises.

Group 2: Clinic-based individualized exercise and manual therapy

Participants in this arm will be treated by a chiropractor or physical therapist, using a pragmatic individualized approach, following the parameters of a clinical protocol that includes the use of the following procedures:

- Light aerobic exercise on a stationary bicycle.
- Distraction-manipulation: a form of manually-assisted segmental lumbar traction manipulation using a specialized treatment table.
- Neural mobilizations: rhythmic stretches of the sciatic and femoral nerves based on the hypothesis that movement of the neural tissues has a mechanical effect on the local neurodynamics [18].
- Hip, sacroiliac and lumbar facet mobilizations: manual mobilizations applied to improve segmental mobility in these joints.

- Soft tissue mobilizations of lumbopelvic and lower extremity muscles: these include manual pressure over taut bands/myofascial trigger points and post-isometric (contract-relax) stretching techniques.
- Home Exercise: patients are advised to use a stationary bike daily, and taught how to perform neural mobilization self-stretches, as well as individualized stretches and core strengthening exercises at home.

Group 3: Community-based group exercise

Participants in this arm will attend group exercise classes designed specifically for older adults and taught by a certified physical fitness instructor. These classes will take place in two large community centers in Pittsburgh that offer programs for older adults. Participants can choose between a class that provides chairs for support while seated/standing or another class for people who are comfortable standing without any support. Each class includes of a variety of exercises designed to increase muscular strength, range of movement, and activity for daily living skills. There is a minimal amount of low impact cardiovascular exercise combined with the use of small hand-held weights, elastic tubing and gym balls for gentle resistance exercise. The participants in these classes are monitored carefully for any signs of physical discomfort and are told to go at their own pace, resting whenever necessary. No specific body region is targeted with these exercise classes. The goal is to provide participants with gentle strengthening, balance training, and generalized fitness training for the entire body. Some of the specific exercises included in these classes are: ankle/wrist rotations, partial squats, leg and knee extension/flexion, strength training of the upper arm and chest muscles with elastic tubing, and coordination drills with a gym ball (bouncing, throwing and catching).

Outcome measures

Our choice of primary outcome measures was informed by input from our community stakeholders and patients with LSS. They stressed the importance of maintaining their independence and their quality of life through improvements in physical function and activity. Suggestions for patient-centered outcomes included improvements in gait, mobility, walking capacity and general physical activity. We have specifically included several of these patient-centered outcome measures, such as measurements of physical activity and walking capacity, into our research design. We will analyze the effectiveness of various treatment options on all of the outcomes that patients have directly informed us are important to them.

The primary self-reported outcome measure will be the Swiss Spinal Stenosis Questionnaire (SSS); a validated 12-item condition-specific instrument for patients with LSS [19]. The SSS is a patient self-reported measure of pain and physical function. Higher scores represent worse symptoms and lower physical function. The 12 items are divided into two subscales; Symptom Severity (further divided into a pain and neuro-ischemic domain) and Physical Function.

The primary performance-based outcome measure will be the Self-Paced Walk Test (SPWT), which is a validated measure of walking capacity in patients with LSS [20]. This test involves having the patient walk comfortably at his/her own pace on a level surface until s/he must rest due to symptoms of back or leg pain. A research assistant follows the patient and measures the total time and distance walked. Patients are not permitted to use an assistive device during the SPWT. We will exclude patients who can walk for a total of 30 minutes without the need to stop, in order to prevent a ceiling effect.

The secondary outcome measure is physical activity measured by a portable activity monitor, the SenseWear Armband (SWA) (Body Media Inc, Pittsburgh, PA). The SWA is a small device that is worn on the upper arm and collects information from multiple sensors: a triaxial accelerometer; heat flux; skin temperature; and galvanic signal [21]. The information is integrated and processed by software using proprietary algorithms utilizing subjects' demographic characteristics (gender, age, height, and weight) to provide minute-by-minute estimates of physical activity. Subjects will wear the SWA on the back of the right arm 24 hours/day for 7 consecutive days (except during shower or water activities) to obtain 5 complete days of data. Figure 1 provides a diagram of the study flow.

Additional measurements

Subjects in this study will complete a series of questionnaires and clinical examination procedures at baseline that will provide additional variables. These variables will give us additional data that allows for the option of an exploratory analysis of any individual or cluster of baseline features that might be predictors of treatment response.

The questionnaires will include the following:

- Demographics: including age, gender, race/ethnicity, smoking status, etc.
- Modified Co-Morbidity Disease Index [22]: subjects will be asked to indicate if they have been diagnosed by a physician with any of 19 medical conditions.
- Fall History Form [23]: subjects will be asked about any falls over the past year, and any current fear of falling.
- Oswestry Low Back Pain Disability Index [24]: A validated 10-item instrument for assessing the

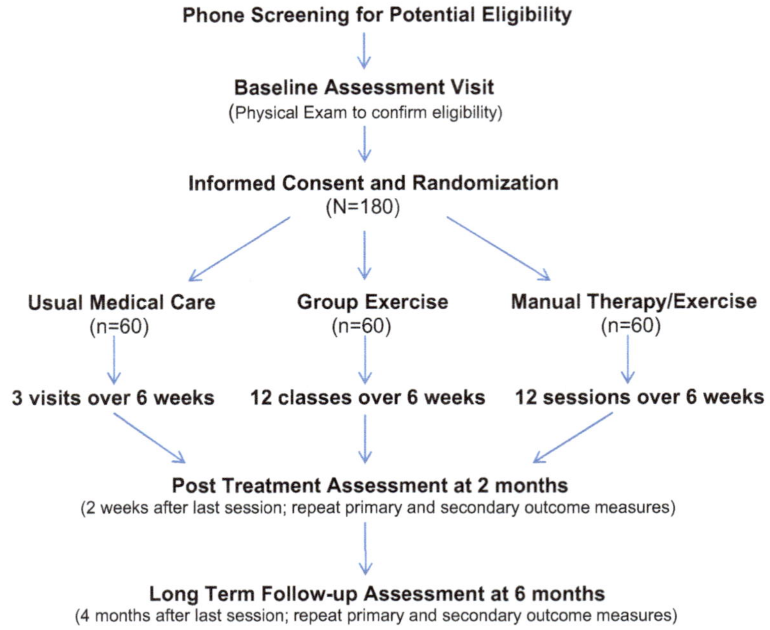

Figure 1 Study flow diagram. Primary outcome measures of self-reported pain/function and physical performance are the Swiss Spinal Stenosis questionnaire [19] and the Self-Paced Walking Test [20]. Secondary outcome measure of physical activity is the SenseWear armband (BodyMedia, Pittsburgh, PA) worn for 1 week.

degree of self-reported impairment of activities of daily living related to low back pain.

- Balance: the Activities-Specific Balance Confidence (ABC) Scale [25] will be administered: a validated questionnaire assessing the patient's level of self-confidence about not losing their balance while performing 16 upright activities of varying difficulty. Additionally, patients will be asked to provide a global rating of their balance, and to rate change at each outcomes visit.
- Tampa Scale for Kinesiophobia [26]: A validated 11-item self-report measure for assessing fear of movement and injury in low back pain patients.
- Depression [27]: We will use the short-form version of the PROMIS depression scale.
- Treatment Expectation [28]: We will use the 6-item credibility and expectancy questionnaire that was modified for use in patients with chronic low back pain.

Clinical examination procedures will include:

- Lumbar spine, hip and knee joint palpation and ranges of motion.
- Height, weight and blood pressure measurements.
- Ankle Brachial Index: systolic blood pressures at brachial and tibial arteries [15,16].
- Neurological exam: lower extremity deep tendon reflexes, manual muscle testing for strength, Babinski test, assessment of pinprick and vibratory sensation.
- Neurodynamic exam including straight leg raise (sciatic nerve and its roots) and femoral nerve stretches (femoral nerve and its roots).
- Self-Paced Walking test [20]: distance and time walked until test must be self-terminated due to symptoms, or 30 minutes, whichever occurs first.
- Balance and Mobility: A modified version of the Short Physical Performance Battery [29] will be administered, in which two of the original subscales (4-meter walking speed and timed chair stands) are combined with an expanded timed standing balance assessment.

Statistical analysis

Outcome measures and primary analysis

The primary outcome variables are the Swiss Spinal Stenosis (SSS) score and Self-Paced Walking Test (SPWT) measured at 2 months (2 weeks after intervention); both will be analyzed similarly. We will also assess these outcomes at 6 months. The outcomes and all baseline characteristics will be summarized with descriptive statistics, separated by treatment group. Analysis of variance (ANOVA) will be used to assess the unadjusted associations between each outcome variable and treatment group membership. A multivariable linear regression model will be used to assess the significance of treatment for each group while adjusting for baseline variables that are at least marginally significant univariately ($p < 0.10$) and other variables that are selected a-priori for clinical significance (e.g. age). All analysis for treatment group comparisons will use an intention-to-treat approach.

Power analysis

A 30% difference between groups on the primary outcome measures will be considered a clinically important difference. A sample size of 150 subjects equates to over 90% power to detect a difference of 9.9 points on the SSS score (with a SD of 6.1 based on preliminary data). In addition, this sample size also yields sufficient power to fit a regression model that detects a statistical difference in the proportion of variability explained; more specifically, a sample size of 150 achieves 81% power to detect an R-square of 5% attributed to two independent variables (representing the two degrees of freedom in the three levels of treatment) and assuming the control variables account for an additional 20% of the variability. We will recruit an additional 30 subjects to account for an anticipated drop-out rate of 15%. This gives us a total sample size of 180 subjects ($n = 60$ per group).

Secondary analysis

We will also perform a responder analysis using dichotomous outcomes, consistent with the recommendations published by the Initiative on Methods, Measurement, and Pain Assessment in Clinical Trials (IMMPACT) [30,31]. Our responder analyses will compare the percentages of subjects who achieve meaningful outcomes between treatment groups on SSS score and SPWT (distance walked). Per IMMPACT recommendations, subjects who achieve at least 30% and 50% decreases in outcome measures are considered to show "moderate improvement" and "substantial improvement", respectively. Differences in the proportion of responders versus non-responders between the groups will be assessed using Chi-square tests. Multiple logistic regression models will be used to assess the association of each of these dichotomized outcomes (>30% followed by >50%) by group, adjusted for covariates. The covariates will be chosen based upon univariate logistic regression ($p < 0.10$) and clinical relevance.

Missing data

If a substantial number of subjects are found to have missing data, we will first determine the causes of why data are missing. These possibilities could be missing completely at random, missing at random, or not missing at random [32]. We will compare characteristics between subjects that have observed data at follow up with those that have missing values. In the case where data is missing at random or completely at random, multiple imputation will be used to substitute for the missing values using a pre-specified model. Once the imputed datasets have been created (we will use $M = 5$ imputations) the proposed analysis will be performed on each of the new datasets and the estimates of interest will be combined [33].

In the case of not missing at random, the missing data mechanism must be modeled in order to obtain unbiased parameter estimates. The missing not at random assumes the missingness is directly related to the value of the missing data. In that case, methods specifically designed to handle the missing not at random mechanism will be used such as Pattern Mixture Models (PMM) [34]. With the PMM, we can simultaneously model whether a subject is a completer (has the data at both time points) versus a non-completer (does not have the data at both time points). We would include an indicator variable for the non-completers as a predictor in the regression model of our outcome measure and examine its interaction with the study covariates. The results of all missing data analysis will be presented in the primary paper for our study. Statistical analysis will be performed using SAS 9.3 (SAS Institute Inc., Cary, NC, USA).

Randomization and blinding

Randomization will be performed by the research coordinator after the baseline screening examination using a computerized randomization algorithm. We will use an adaptive allocation algorithm to balance the three groups on important baseline variables. The randomization scheme is based on a minimization algorithm proposed by Stigsby and Taves [35]. The approach is to balance on multiple baseline prognostic factors using a rank-based method. The balancing baseline variables used will be: Swiss Spinal Stenosis Score; Self-Paced Walking Test (distance walked); Age; and Credibility Expectancy Questionnaire score.

Single blinding will be achieved by having an independent physical therapist perform all baseline exams and post-intervention reassessments. The examining therapist will not be treating any of the subjects or aware of their group assignments. Blinding of the treating clinicians and subjects is not possible because they will obviously be aware of the treatment arm to which they have been assigned.

Ethical considerations

This study will be conducted in accordance with the declaration of Helsinki and all ethics regulations, policies and guidelines of the National Institutes of Health. The Institutional Review Board of the University of Pittsburgh has reviewed and approved this study (PRO12120422). Written informed consent will be obtained from all patients included in the study. Patients will be informed that they are free to leave the study, without explanation and without any negative consequences on their future treatment. Every precaution will be taken to protect the privacy of research subjects and the confidentiality of their personal information. All personal patient details will be rendered anonymous before data entry, by referring to all patient records and data only by their assigned research number. There are no known additional risks associated with patient participation in the study, other than the normal risks associated with these common treatments.

Discussion

Patients with severe symptoms will often require surgical decompression; LSS is the most frequent indication for spinal surgery in the U.S. for patients over the age of 65 years [36]. Clearly, not all LSS patients require surgery and therefore we are only recruiting patients with mild to moderate symptoms who are not surgical candidates. This leads to some important research questions:

- Among the commonly used non-surgical approaches to treat LSS, which ones are most effective at reducing pain and improving walking capacity?
- How much impact does successful treatment have on improving physical activity?
- What are the benefits/risks associated with the various non-surgical treatments for LSS?
- Are there baseline physical examination and case history findings that are predictors of treatment response?

As noted in the introduction section of this article, there is a serious evidence gap about the effectiveness of these various non-surgical treatment approaches. The seriousness of this gap is highlighted by these recommendations from the evidence-based clinical guideline for LSS recently published by the North American Spine Society [17]:

- There is insufficient evidence to make a recommendation for or against the use of pharmacological treatment in the management of LSS.
- There is insufficient evidence to make a recommendation for or against the use of physical therapy or exercise as stand-alone treatments for degenerative LSS.
- There is insufficient evidence to make a recommendation for or against the use of spinal manipulation for the treatment of LSS.

There is essentially insufficient evidence for every common non-surgical treatment approach except epidural steroid injections; and these injections only have one randomized trial showing evidence of modest effectiveness. This puts patients and providers in an uncomfortable position of uncertainty about which approach to non-surgical management is best for which patient. This study is designed to provide evidence to help remove some of this clinical uncertainty experienced by providers who must recommend these treatments. It is also designed to measure outcomes that are important to patients, including measures of physical activity and walking capacity; two of the most patient-centered outcomes reported to us by patients with LSS and their care-givers.

Conclusions

This study will be one of the first of its kind: comparing the clinical effectiveness of three common non-surgical approaches to the management of patients with LSS. We have also designed this study with input from patients with LSS and other community stakeholders. Our research design is also innovative because all treatment groups involve "real-life" management strategies, using pragmatic protocols that can be adapted to individual patients' needs.

Abbreviations

ABI: Ankle-brachial index; LSS: Lumbar spinal stenosis; PAD: Peripheral artery disease; PM&R: Physical medicine and rehabilitation; SPWT: Self-paced walking test; SSS: Swiss spinal stenosis questionnaire.

Competing interests

The authors declare that they have no competing interests.

Authors' contributions

MS initiated the study and had the primary responsibility of writing the grant application and applying for funding. CA and DM are clinical chiropractic experts in the non-surgical management of LSS and developed the clinical treatment protocols for the manual therapy/exercise group. SP and EH are academic physical therapy experts who have clinical and research experience working with older adults, including the use of the SenseWear device to monitor physical activity and the assessment of mobility and falls. They helped to select the outcome measures and refine the exercise protocols. They will also lead the analyses of physical activity, mobility, and falls. RG is a clinical medical expert who is board certified in physical medicine and rehabilitation. He was involved with the design of the usual medical care arm of the study. DT and SM are biostatisticians who performed the power analysis, programmed the randomization algorithm, and will analyze all data at the end of the study. All authors read, revised, and approved this final manuscript, as well as the original grant proposal.

Acknowledgements

We would like to acknowledge the dedication and hard work of our research coordinator Christine McFarland and lead research assistant Kris Gongaware. In addition, we would like acknowledge Christy Tomkins-Lane for sharing her previous research experiences in developing the self-paced walking test and her collaborative input with us on this and other lumbar spinal stenosis research projects.

Funding

This study has received funding from the Patient Centered Outcomes Research Institute (PCORI) as a comparative effectiveness trial.

Author details

[1]School of Health and Rehabilitation Sciences, Department of Physical Therapy, University of Pittsburgh, Pittsburgh, PA, USA. [2]Institute of Health Policy, Management and Evaluation, University of Toronto, Toronto, Ontario, Canada. [3]Clinical Director, Rhode Island Spine Center, Providence, RI, USA. [4]Department of Family Medicine, Alpert Medical School of Brown University, Providence, RI, USA. [5]Departments of Physical Medicine, Family Medicine,

and Psychiatry, University of Pittsburgh, Pittsburgh, PA, USA. [6]School of Medicine, Biostatistics, Clinical and Translational Science Institute, University of Pittsburgh, Pittsburgh, PA, USA. [7]Department of Biostatistics, Graduate School of Public Health, University of Pittsburgh, Pittsburgh, PA, USA.

References

1. Hootman JM, Helmick CG, Brady TJ: **A public health approach to addressing arthritis in older adults: the most common cause of disability.** *Am J Public Health* 2012, **102**(3):426–433.
2. Kalichman L, Cole R, Kim DH, Li L, Suri P, Guermazi A, Hunter DJ: **Spinal stenosis prevalence and association with symptoms: the Framingham study.** *Spine J* 2009, **9**:545–550.
3. Binder DK, Schmidt MH, Weinstein PR: **Lumbar spinal stenosis.** *Semin Neurol* 2002, **22**(2):157–166.
4. Wiesel SW, Tsourmas N, Feffer HL, Citrin C, Patronas N: **A study of computer-assisted tomography: the incidence of positive CAT scans in an asymptomatic group of patients.** *Spine* 1984, **9**(6):549–551.
5. Boden SD, Davis D, Dina T, Patronas N, Wiesel SW: **Abnormal magnetic-resonance scans of the lumbar spine in asymptomatic subjects.** *J Bone Joint Surg* 1990, **72**(3):403–408.
6. Sugioka T, Hayashino Y, Konno S, Kikuchi S, Fukuhara S: **Predictive value of self-reported patient information for the identification of lumbar spinal stenosis.** *Fam Pract* 2008, **25**(4):237–244.
7. Winter CC, Brandes M, Muller C, Schubert T, Ringling M, Hillmann A, Rosenbaum D, Schulte TL: **Walking ability during daily life in patients with osteoarthritis of the knee or the hip and lumbar spinal stenosis: a cross sectional study.** *BMC Musculoskelet Disord* 2010, **11**:233.
8. Kim HJ, Chun HJ, Han CD, Moon SH, Kang KT, Kim HS, Park JO, Moon ES, Kim BR, Sohn JS, Shin SY, Jang JW, Lee KI, Lee HM: **The risk assessment of a fall in patients with lumbar spinal stenosis.** *Spine* 2011, **36**(9):E588–E592.
9. Muraki S, Akune T, Oka H, En-Yo Y, Yoshida M, Nakamura K, Kawaguchi H, Yoshimura N: **Prevalence of falls and the association with knee osteoarthritis and lumbar spondylosis as well as knee and lower back pain in Japanese men and women.** *Arthritis Care Res* 2011, **63**(10):1425–1431.
10. Fanuele JC, Birkmeyer N, Abdu W, Tosteson T, Weinstein JN: **The impact of spinal problems on the health status of patients: have we underestimated the effect?** *Spine* 2000, **25**(12):1509–1514.
11. Weinstein JN, Tosteson T, Lurie J, Tosteson A, Blood E, Herkowitz H, Cammisa F, Albert T, Boden SD, Hilibrand A, Goldberg H, Berven S, An H: **Surgical versus non-operative treatment for lumbar spinal stenosis: four-year results of the spine patient outcomes research trial.** *Spine* 2010, **35**(14):1329–1338.
12. Ammendolia C, Stuber K, de Bruin LK, Furlan AD, Kennedy CA, Rampersaud YR, Steenstra IA, Pennick V: **Non-operative treatment for lumbar spinal stenosis with neurogenic claudication: a systematic review.** *Spine* 2012, **37**(10):E609–E616.
13. Conn A, Buenaventura R, Datta S, Abdi S, Diwan S: **Systematic review of caudal epidural injections in the management of chronic low back pain.** *Pain Physician* 2009, **12**(1):109–135.
14. Slutsky JR, Clancy CM: **AHRQ's effective health care program: why comparative effectiveness matters.** *Am J Med Qual* 2009, **24**(1):67–70.
15. McDermott MM, Criqui MH, Liu K, Guralnik JM, Greenland P, Martin GJ, Pearce W: **Lower ankle/brachial index, as calculated by averaging the dorsalis pedis and posterior tibial arterial pressures, and association with leg functioning in peripheral arterial disease.** *J Vasc Surg* 2000, **32**(6):1164–1171.
16. Jeon CH, Han SH, Chung NS, Hyun HS: **The validity of ankle-brachial index for the differential diagnosis of peripheral arterial disease and lumbar spinal stenosis in patients with atypical claudication.** *Eur Spine J* 2012, **21**(6):1165–1170.
17. Kreiner DS, Shaffer W, Baisden J, Gilbert T, Summers J, Toton J, Hwang SW, Mendel RC, Reitman CA: **An evidence-based clinical guideline for the diagnosis and treatment of degenerative lumbar spinal stenosis (update).** *Spine J* 2013, **13**(7):734–743.
18. Ellis RF, Hing WA: **Neural mobilization: a systematic review of randomized controlled trials with an analysis of therapeutic efficacy.** *J Man Manip Ther* 2008, **16**(1):8–22.
19. Pratt RK, Fairbank JC, Virr A: **The reliability of the shuttle walking test, the Swiss Spinal Stenosis Questionnaire, the Oxford Spinal Stenosis Score, and the Oswestry Disability Index in the assessment of patients with lumbar spinal stenosis.** *Spine* 2002, **27**(1):84–91.
20. Tomkins CC, Battié MC, Rogers T, Jiang H, Petersen S: **A criterion measure of walking capacity in lumbar spinal stenosis and its comparison with a treadmill protocol.** *Spine* 2009, **34**(22):2444–2449.
21. Cole PJ, LeMura LM, Klinger TA, Strohecker K, McConnell TR: **Measuring energy expenditure in cardiac patients using the body media armband versus indirect calorimetry: a validation study.** *J Sports Med Phys Fitness* 2004, **44**(3):262–271.
22. Rigler SK, Studenski S, Wallace D, Reker DM, Duncan PW: **Comorbidity adjustment for functional outcomes in community-dwelling older adults.** *Clin Rehabil* 2002, **16**:420–428.
23. Tinetti ME, Richman D, Powell L: **Falls efficacy as a measure of fear of falling.** *J Gerontol* 1990, **45**(6):239–243.
24. Fairbank JC, Couper J, Davies JB, O'Brien J: **The Oswestry low back pain disability questionnaire.** *Physiotherapy* 1980, **66**(8):271–273.
25. Powell LE, Meyers AM: **The Activities-specific Balance Confidence (ABC) Scale.** *J Gerontol A Biol Sci Med Sci* 1995, **50**(1):M28–M34.
26. Woby SR, Roach NK, Urmston M, Watson PJ: **Psychometric properties of the TSK-11: a shortened version of the Tampa scale for kinesiophobia.** *Pain* 2005, **117**(1–2):137–144.
27. Choi SW, Reise SP, Pilkonis PA, Hays RD, Cella D: **Efficiency of static and computer adaptive short forms compared to full-length measures of depressive symptoms.** *Qual Life Res* 2010, **19**(1):125–136.
28. Smeets RJ, Beelen S, Goossens M, Schouten E, Knottnerus J, Vlaeyen J: **Treatment expectancy and credibility are associated with the outcome of both physical and cognitive-behavioral treatment in chronic low back pain.** *Clin J Pain* 2008, **24**:305–315.
29. Vasunilashorn S, Coppin AK, Patel KV, Lauretani F, Ferrucci L, Bandinelli S, Guralnik JM: **Use of the short physical performance battery score to predict loss of ability to walk 400 meters: analysis from the InCHIANTI study.** *J Gerontol A Biol Sci Med Sci* 2009, **64**(2):223–229.
30. Dworkin RH, Turk DC, Wyrwich KW, Beaton D, Cleeland CS, Farrar JT, Haythornthwaite JA, Jensen MP, Kerns RD, Ader DN, Brandenburg N, Burke LB, Cella D, Chandler J, Cowan P, Dimitrova R, Dionne R, Hertz S, Jadad AR, Katz NP, Kehlet H, Kramer LD, Manning DC, McCormick C, McDermott MP, McQuay HJ, Patel S, Porter L, Quessy S, Rappaport BA, *et al*: **Interpreting the clinical importance of treatment outcomes in chronic pain clinical trials: IMMPACT recommendations.** *Pain* 2008, **9**(2):105–121.
31. Dworkin RH, Turk DC, McDermott MP, Peirce-Sandner S, Burke LB, Cowan P, Farrar JT, Hertz S, Raja SN, Rappaport BA, Rauschkolb C, Sampaio C: **Interpreting the clinical importance of group differences in chronic pain clinical trials: IMMPACT recommendations.** *Pain* 2009, **146**(3):238–244.
32. Rubin DB: **Inference and missing data.** *Biometrika* 1976, **63**(3):581–592.
33. Graham JW, Olchowski AE, Gilreath TD: **How many imputations are really needed? Some practical clarifications of multiple imputation theory.** *Prev Sci* 2007, **8**:206–213.
34. Hedecker D, Gibbons RD: **Application of random-effects pattern mixture models for missing data in longitudinal studies.** *Psych Methods* 1997, **2**:64–78.
35. Stigsby B, Taves DR: **Rank-minimization for balanced assignment of subjects in clinical trials.** *Contemp Clin Trials* 2010, **31**(2):147–150.
36. Deyo RA, Mirza S, Martin B, Kreuter W, Goodman D, Jarvik J: **Trends, major medical complications, and charges associate with surgery for lumbar spinal stenosis in older adults.** *JAMA* 2010, **303**(13):1259–1265.

10

Prognostic accuracy of clinicians for back, neck and shoulder patients in routine practice

Dave Newell[1*], Jonathan Field[2] and Nita Visnes[3]

Abstract

Background: Chronicity amongst musculoskeletal patients remains a considerable burden and predicting outcomes in these patients has proven difficult. Although a large number of studies have investigated a range of predictors of outcome few have looked at the practitioners' ability to discern those that improve from those most likely to fail to improve. This study aimed to investigate the ability of chiropractors to predict patient outcomes.

Methods: Prediction and outcome data were collected from 440 consecutive patients with back, neck or shoulder pain accepted for chiropractic care within 5 linked private practices.

Predictions by chiropractors were compared to patient outcomes as measured by Bournemouth Questionnaire (BQ) scores, pain NRS scores and patient global impression of change (PGIC) collected at 4 and 12 weeks following the initial consultation.

Results: Overall, chiropractors appear unable to accurately predict poor outcomes in their patients particularly in the longer term. Although some conditions (neck) faired a little better in some cases with some trends in short term pain scores being associated with the clinicians prediction, this was marginal. Subgrouping by practitioners or duration did not improve the performance of these predictions

Conclusions: Chiropractors generally fail to reliably predict poor treatment outcome of patients at initial consultation.

Keywords: Prognosis, Practitioner, Prediction, Outcome, Chiropractic

Background

Musculoskeletal disorders (MSD) remain a burden both in terms of suffering and economics with European economies paying up to €240 billion a year in health and work related costs [1]. Up to 80% of the population will suffer from MSDs at some point in their life [2] and at least 100 million people reported chronic musculoskeletal pain in 2008 [3]. Some types of MSD are more prevalent than others. For example, the department of health found that 13-15% of unemployed individuals in Britain between 16 and 64 years of age cite back pain as their reason to be out of work with 5% of employed back pain sufferers having taken time of work in the past month due to pain. It is estimated that annually British businesses lose 4.9 billion work days due to back pain with UK total costs associated with MSDs of around £7 billion [4]. The need to return patients to work and satisfactory resolution of these types of disorders is clearly imperative and The Work Foundation [1] states that *'return to work and maintaining work productivity should be explicit clinical targets, and in this respect, the benefits of early diagnosis, appropriate intervention and effective rehabilitation in managing MSDs are clear'*.

The ability to identify patients likely to respond differentially to care is important to enable the provision of targeted advice and care [5]. This has been described by the Cochrane collaboration as the number one priority in back pain research [6]. Despite a large number of studies looking at prognostic factors associated with poor outcome in those attending chiropractors, few robust predictors have emerged with controversy surrounding those that have been found [7-9]. However, it is possible that clinicians have an additional insight into the likelihood of recovery or otherwise of MSD patients attending seeking their care. If true practitioners do indeed have an insight into their patients prognosis this

* Correspondence: dnewell@aecc.ac.uk
[1]AECC-Anglo European College of Chiropracti, 14-15 Parkwood Road, BH5 2DF, UK
Full list of author information is available at the end of the article

could potentially enable an exploration of the factors behind this prognostic ability as a direction for future work.

Previous research suggests the ability of clinicians in general to predict accurately the likely response of patients to care is uncertain [10]. Hill et al. [11] reported that clinicians (General practitioners, physiotherapists and pain management specialists) using intuition alone to make risk estimations for LBP patients had little agreement compared to a formal screening tool (Start Back Tool) and low inter-clinician agreement. In contrast, Jellema et al. [5] implies that general practitioners ability to assess risk does not dramatically differ from the Örebro Musculoskeletal Pain Screening Questionnaire, the Low Back Pain (LBP) Perception Scale and a clinical prediction rule created for the study. The only other study reporting associations between the clinicians' prediction and LPB patients' outcome was where the primary goal of the study was to generate a clinical prediction rule (CPR). Here, the physiotherapist predictions performed poorly in comparison to the CPR which itself generated AUCs considered to poor, despite the clinicians predictions still adding some utility in the final model [12].

Few if any studies have investigated the ability of chiropractors to predict outcomes in their patients. Given that most LBP patients attending chiropractic care report a good outcome, identifying those who will do poorly as early as possible may allow greater utility for clinicians and researchers in providing more targeted approaches [8]. This study aimed therefore to explore how well chiropractors are able to identify which patients are more likely to fail to recover while undergoing a course of chiropractic care.

Methods

Subjects

Patients with low back, neck or shoulder pain, over 16 years of age and seeking care for the first time from UK chiropractors and were eligible. Patient consent to use their anonymised data for research purposes was achieved via a tick box during routine on line collection of clinical baseline and outcome reporting. The chiropractor's experiences ranged from 2 to 20 years and were aged between 24 and 45 with two being female. Inclusion criteria were; accepted for chiropractic treatment and consented to being sent e-mails as part of an electronic patient reported outcome measures (Care Response) system in these clinics.

Procedure

Chiropractors were asked to record on a form (immediately after the first consultation) whether they thought patients were less likely than average to report a good outcome following a course of care. Patient data collected as normal practice activity was analysed. The data collected at baseline on paper forms at the practice included gender, age (years) , complaint (body area diagram), and duration of complaint (less than 4 weeks, less than 4 weeks recurring and greater than 4 weeks), total Bournemouth Questionnaire (BQ) [13] scores (0–70; higher is worse), pain NRS (0–10) and practice attended.

Patients were then further contacted by either post or email with requests to complete the BQ, pain NRS and patient global impression of change (PGIC) questionnaires at 4 week and 12 week follow up. The PGIC consisted of a question and 6 possible responses as follows:

"How would you describe your pain/complaint now, compared to how you were when you completed the questionnaire before your first visit to this clinic?"

ϑ Very much improved
ϑ Much improved
ϑ Slightly improved
ϑ No change
ϑ Slightly worsened
ϑ Much worsened
ϑ Worse than ever

The setting was 5 UK clinics and involved the practices of 6 separate chiropractors.

Data analysis

We used a primary (BQ Total) and two secondary (Pain NRS, PGIC) measures of outcome and chose to treat the chiropractors predictions as a univariate predictive model, calculating, odds ratios for not improving if the chiropractor assigned a likelihood of poor recovery, positive and negative likelihood ratios, the percentage of variation in outcome explained by the model (Nagelkerke) and area under the curve (AUC) via ROC analysis. This involved using chiropractors' baseline classification of patient status against status of the patient as defined by the outcomes at 4 and 12 week follow-up points. Area under the curve figures were interpreted as follows; .90-1 = excellent, .80-.90 = good, .70-.80 = fair, .60-.70 = poor, .50-.60 = fail.

Categorisation of patient self-reported status at 4 and 12 week follow up was determined by using the reported minimal clinically important change for the total BQ as a cut off for non-improvement for back (≤ 46%) [14] and neck (≤ 35%) pain [15]. For the pain NRS a cut off of ≤29% [16] indicated non improvement while for the PGIC a cut off of <6 points indicated non improvement [7]. Subgroup analysis was carried out where numbers allowed, using; patient complaint, chiropractic practice and complaint duration as stratifying variables. All analysis was carried out using SPSS (v21).

Ethics

This research was ethically approved by the Anglo European College of Chiropractic undergraduate ethics panel in May 2011.

Results

Four hundred and forty patients with complete data were included in the analysis at baseline. Respondents at 4 and 12 week follow up were 255 (58%) and 182 (41%) respectively. Tables 1 and 2 illustrate the demographic characteristics and baseline/follow up scores respectively. Back and neck pain patients showed similar profiles in terms of duration and baseline pain and BQ scores. In contrast most shoulder pain patients had higher chronicity.

Table 3 illustrates the mean percentage change of the continuous outcome measures between baseline and follow up points. Generally, a greater than 50% drop in total BQ and pain scores are observed in all 3 conditions at 4 weeks follow up. This deteriorates slightly for back pain patients, plateaus for neck pain and substantially further improves for shoulder pain at 12 weeks follow up. Changes both in total BQ and pain scores show similar values with changes in pain being generally higher that changes in total BQ with shoulder pain patients improving the most.

Table 4 illustrates these changes as dichotomised around the measures respective MCIC values. For both dichotomised pain and total BQ, similar proportions of LBP patients failed to improve at both 4 and 12 week follow up with around 20 to 25% not improving at 12 weeks. A lower proportion of around 10% fail to improve in the neck pain group by the same time. Of note is the fact that nearly all of the shoulder patients improved by the 12th week with only 4% not improving, although this was only calculated with dichotomous pain scores as there is no validated MCIC for the BQ and shoulder pain.

In slight contrast, the proportions of patients failing to improve as defined by the dichotomised PGIC were somewhat higher for all conditions being around a third at 4 weeks. These proportions remained similar at 12 weeks for back pain, falling slightly for neck pain and dramatically for shoulder pain following a similar pattern to the previous dichotomised outcomes.

Tables 5, 6, 7 report the analysis of the accuracy of the clinicians judgment in correctly identifying those patients failing to improve at 4 and 12 weeks follow up, as defined by 3 outcomes, total BQ, NRS pain and PGIC, dichotomised at their respective MCICs.

In general both the ability of the clinician to predict outcome (Odds Ratio (OR), Nagelkerke) and the discriminative ability of this prediction in separating those patients that did not improve from those that did (+ve and -ve Likelihood ratio, AUC) were extremely poor regardless of the outcome measure used. Although there were some notable minor improvements in these values for the short term (4 weeks) prediction of neck and shoulder patients, the likelihood ratios still indicated no discriminative power, with AUCs still falling into the 'poor' or 'fair' category. All other AUC values are considered to be in a 'failed' category in their ability to predict or discriminate actual outcomes. Interestingly, the mean NRS continuous scores were significantly higher at 4 weeks follow up in the non-improved compared to the improved patients as categorised by the clinician at baseline. However, the PGIC at 4 weeks follow up and both the NRS and PGIC continuous scores at 12 weeks follow up were no different between the predicted categories.

Table 1 Demographic characteristics split by complaint

Variable	Back	Neck	Shoulder
Age (Mean (SD))	44.0 (15.0)	45.7 (15.5)	45.5 (15.9)
Gender (% Female)	52	51	46
Treatments at 1 month	4.6 (1.7)	4.6 (1.5)	4.6 (1.4)
Duration (%)			
< 1 month	31	32	17
< 1 month recurring	23	21	17
> 1 month	46	46	65

Table 2 Baseline and follow up measures split by complaint

	Back	Neck	Shoulder
Baseline (n=440)	**n=312**	**n=71**	**n=57**
Pain NRS (Mean (SD))	5.9 (2.2)	5.6 (2.4)	5.7 (2.3)
BQ total (Mean (SD))	36.3 (15.1)	34.2(16.6)	32.7 (14.9)
Week 4 (n=255)	**n=173**	**n=45**	**n=37**
Pain NRS (Mean (SD))	2.1 (2.0)	1.8 (2.0)	2.2 (1.8)
BQ total (Mean (SD))	11.9 (13.3)	11.8 (11.4)	11.3 (10.6)
Week 12 (n=182)	**n=124**	**n=35**	**n=23**
Pain NRS (Mean (SD))	2.1 (2.4)	1.6 (2.1)	1.2 (1.8)
BQ total (Mean (SD))	12.2 (14.0)	10.4 (12.9)	7.9 (10.4)

Table 3 Change (%) in BQ total and pain NRS scores split by complaint

	Back	Neck	Shoulder
Week 1- 4	**n=173**	**n=45**	**n=37**
BQ total	62.4 (42.2)	62.7 (32.1)	56.9 (40.5)
Pain NRS	62.8 (36.5)	65.3 (37.0)	58.6 (39.7)
Week 1- 12	**n=124**	**n=35**	**n=23**
BQ total	59.6 (53.3)	67.5 (34.8)	74.3(31.3)
Pain NRS	56.3 (62.1)	68.0 (41.7)	81.2 (26.3)

Table 4 Proportion (%) of patients not improving as defined by cut off values for BQ total, pain NRS and PGIC scores split by complaint

	Back (n=nI/I)	Neck (n=nI/I)	Shoulder (n=nI/I)
BQ total*			
Week 4	26.3 (45/128)	21.2 (9/36)	nc
Week 12	26.8 (33/91)	14.3 (5/30)	nc
Pain NRS**			
Week 4	17.4 (29/143)	15.9 (7/38)	16.7 (6/30)
Week 12	20.2 (25/99)	11.8 (4/31)	4.3 (1/22)
PGIC***			
Week 4	30.6 (53/120)	26.7 (12/33)	37.8 (14/23)
Week 12	27.4 (34/90)	22.9 (8/27)	21.7 (5/18)

*(≤ 47% (Back), ≤ 36% (Neck)), **(≤ 30%), ***(≤ 5 points), nc=not calculated as no MCIC, nI/I= not improved/Improved.

When the primary outcome scores were stratified by the individual practitioners or the duration of the condition this predictive and discriminative ability was no better than the previous analysis with all the AUC values falling into the 'failed' category apart from a single practitioner who scored 'poor' at 4 and 12 weeks. Because of the reduction in numbers of patients failing to improve due to stratification of the BQ scores to less than 5 individuals in some cases we performed the same analysis using the secondary PGIC outcome which had larger numbers of non-improved patients at each time point. This analysis found the same lack of predictive and discriminative power of the practitioners initial judgement found using the primary measure.

Table 5 Utility of chiropractors' prediction of patients not improving as categorised by MCIC in BQ total* scores split by complaint

	Back	Neck	Shoulder
Week 4			
N	**173**	**45**	
OR (95% CI)	1.7 (0.8 to 3.8)	3.2 (0.7 to 15.0)	nc
Nagelkerke R^2	0.01	0.07	nc
+ve Likelihood ratio	0.0	0.0	nc
−ve Likelihood ratio	**	**	nc
AUC	0.5 (0.4 to 0.6)	0.6 (0.4 to 0.8)	nc
Week 12			
N	**124**		
OR (95% CI)	1.7 (0.6 to 4.9)	§	nc
Nagelkerke R^2	0.01	§	nc
+ve Likelihood ratio	0.0	§	nc
−ve Likelihood ratio	**	§	nc
AUC	0.5 (0.4 to 0.7)	§	nc

*(≤ 47% (Back), ≤ 36% (Neck)), nc=not calculated as no MCIC, **unable to calculate as divided by 0, § unable to calculate due to less than 5 in one cell, AUC=Area under curve.

Table 6 Utility of chiropractors' prediction of patients not improving as categorised by MCIC in pain NRS* scores split by complaint

	Back	Neck	Shoulder
Week 4			
N	**173**	**45**	**37**
OR (95% CI)	1.3 (0.5 to 3.3)	1.4 (0.2 to 8.9)	5.5 (0.8 to 36.0)
Nagelkerke R^2	0.00	0.01	0.15
+ve Likelihood ratio	0.0	0.0	0.0
−ve Likelihood ratio	**	**	**
AUC	0.5 (0.4 to 0.6)	0.5 (0.3 to 0.8)	0.7 (0.5 to 0.9)
Week 12			
N	**124**		
OR (95% CI)	3.1 (1.1 to 9.3)	§	§
Nagelkerke R^2	0.05	§	§
+ve Likelihood ratio	0.0	§	§
−ve Likelihood ratio	**	§	§
AUC	0.6 (0.4 to 0.7)	§	§

*(≤ 30%), nc=not calculated as no MCIC, **unable to calculate as divided by 0, § unable to calculate due to less than 5 in one cell, AUC=Area under curve.

Discussion

Analysis of the ability of chiropractors to predict their own patents' outcome status suggests that practitioners are overall at best poor and at worst fail. Given that prognosis in this condition does not involve a life threatening outcome, one might argue that the AUC categorisation of

Table 7 Utility of chiropractors' prediction of patients not improving as categorised by PGIC* scores split by complaint

	Back	Neck	Shoulder
Week 4			
N	**173**	**45**	**37**
OR (95% CI)	1.1 (0.5 to 2.5)	4.0 (0.9 to 17.8)	1.3 (0.3 to 5.2)
Nagelkerke R^2	0.00	0.10	0.00
+ve Likelihood ratio	0.0	2.8	0.0
−ve Likelihood ratio	**	0.7	**
AUC	0.5 (0.4 to 0.6)	0.6 (0.4 to 0.8)	0.5 (0.3 to 0.7)
Week 12			
N	**124**	**35**	**23**
OR (95% CI)	2.2 (0.8 to 6.1)	0.5 (0.05 to 4.9)	0.5 (0.04 to 5.5)
Nagelkerke R^2	0.03	0.02	0.02
+ve Likelihood ratio	0.0	0.0	0.0
−ve Likelihood ratio	**	**	**
AUC	0.6 (0.4 to 0.7)	0.5 (0.3 to 0.8)	0.6 (0.3 to 0.8)

*(≤ 5 points), **unable to calculate as divided by 0, AUC=Area under curve.

the discriminative performance of clinicians might be more lenient, i.e. 'poor' becomes 'fair' and 'fail' becomes 'poor'. Despite this, the accuracy of the initial clinician predictions remains predominantly poor. The only other studies to investigate clinician prediction of recovery from low back pain stated that GP's risk estimation was comparable to other prognostic indicators as measured at baseline, although the AUC was reported as only 0.6 and physiotherapists were poorer than a clinical prediction rule which itself scored as poor in terms of AUCs [6,12]. Most other studies investigating prognostic accuracy of physicians have centred on cancer survival with a large systematic review finding only weak evidence to support clinician's estimates alone as predictors of survival [17]. Predicting other important health outcomes also appears difficult with a recent study investigating the prognostic accuracy of occupational therapist advice regarding return to work times revealing consistent and marked underestimation of recovery by these health workers [18]. However, the literature is not unanimous in its lack of support of clinician based prediction. For example, Reiso et al. [19] found that GPs ability to predict the period of certified sickness absence was high and good prediction was most strongly associated with type of diagnosis. However, the frequent lack of definitive diagnoses in the conditions dealt with in this study, most being categorised as nonspecific, has made prognosis considerably more problematic. Additionally, that the duration of sick certification investigated by the study was potentially under the control of the GP, could be considered a confounding factor. Although a small number of factors associated with poor prognosis have arisen from the MSD literature, particularly low back pain studies, they fail to explain much of the variance reported in outcome. In particular, even fewer robust indicators of prognosis have arisen amongst patients seeking manual therapy and it may not be so surprising why the clinicians in this study struggle to accurately judge outcomes amongst their patients given that extensive research into potential predictive factors of outcome have found so few in this particular MSD population.

Of those that have been reported, reviews of prospective studies reveal a variety of prognostic factors. For example longer pain duration has emerged as a generic prognostic factor amongst MSD patients generally and in low back pain patients in particular [20-22]. However, in this study practitioners were no more accurate in predicting outcomes in chronic (> 1 month) as compared to acute (< 1 month) patients. In addition many studies have indicated psychological factors as important in prognosis of MSD and this is may also be true of chiropractic patients [23] although this remains a matter of controversy [8]. Other factors such as socioeconomic, gender, age and activity have been less reliably related to prognosis in neck pain, with research being indecisive in particular regarding age as a risk factor for poor prognosis [24].

Of interest beyond the primary question of this study are the differences and similarities between the method of determining outcomes and the outcomes of the conditions studied. Generally both dichotomised BQ and pain NRS based determination of improvement or otherwise produce similar proportions of patients at both follow up points. Of note is the fact that after 12 weeks around one 20 to 25% of patients remained unimproved for back and neck pain patients. This concurs with previous research that notes that, contrary to commonly held notions, a significant proportion of these patients do not recover entirely [25]. On the other hand those presenting with shoulder pain and in this study, more chronic shoulder pain, seemed to recover remarkably well with the proportion categorised as not improved continuing to fall significantly beyond the first month, unlike with back and neck pain.

Interestingly, the PGIC global measure consistently categorised a greater proportion of patients as not improved at both follow up points across all conditions compared to BQ and pain NRS categorisations. It is possible this may reflect the way this measure may be thought about by patients where it allows any number of factors to be brought into a patients' judgement of their improvement as opposed to a single measure such as pain or even a multidimensional measure such as the BQ. These differences may certainly warrant further investigation.

There are clear limitations to this study. Firstly, the question we asked the practitioners was 'Whether they thought patients were less likely than average to report a good outcome following a course of care'. In meetings with the practitioners involved prior to the study this judgement was discussed in relation to patients' response on the BQ, as the practitioners were familiar with the routine use of this questionnaire in their practice on a day to day basis. However, the question did not explicitly highlight a particular outcome measure. In order to increase the robustness of our conclusion, we therefore used 3 outcome measures dichotomised around published cutoff scores, with the BQ as the primary outcome. Given that similar if not identical findings were generated from all 3 outcomes it would tend to support the conclusion that practitioners fail to predict patient outcome and is less likely to be an idiosyncrasy of the outcome measure we used or a mismatch between the practitioners perception of the original question and the final outcome measure.

Secondly, we chose to analyse the association between practitioner prediction and patient self-reported outcome in a manner reminiscent of diagnostic test validity despite the fact that this was a prospective study.

Normally, diagnostic test validity studies would ideally require minimal time periods between gold standard and new test data collection. In view of this, we also calculated the risk of improvement based on the chiropractor's initial prognosis, typically a method appropriate to prospective studies. Although this provides a further measure of association, risk normally implies some causative impact of the risk factor on the outcome, whereas in our case there is no expectation that the practitioner's prognosis would impact the actual outcome, although we did not know whether the practitioner had explicitly stated their prognosis to the patients and it is possible that if they had done so, this may have influenced outcome.

Thirdly, chiropractors in this study were not asked to predict patients' reports of their outcome at any specific time point but in general and it is possible that had they been asked specifically how patients may report themselves at 1 or 3 months, prognostic accuracy would have been found to be higher.

Lastly, this study used outcome data collected as a normal part of practice activity returned by post or email by patients. It is not possible to exclude the possibility that those who did not respond to the request to complete the PROMs would have answered differently. However the proportion reporting a good outcome in this sample is similar to other studies from this group of practices which achieved a higher response rate by including a telephone follow up of non-responders making it less likely that the results quoted here are subject to non-response bias [26].

Conclusion

In this study chiropractors were found not to be able to accurately predict treatment outcomes of patients prior to treatment at 1 or 3 months follow up, for any of the conditions, chronicity of condition and regardless of the use of multiple measures to determine outcome. The results of this study imply that practitioners insight into a patients likely outcome is not sufficient alone as a prognostic tool. Given the controversy inherent in the prediction literature to define robust predictors of prognosis it maybe that barring generic factors such as duration it will remain up to the practitioner to do their best in how they articulate potential prognosis to the patient. Luckily given that most MSD patients tend to improve in the relatively short term erring on the side of optimism may be the best policy.

Competing interests

The authors declare that they have no competing interests.

Authors' contributions

DN and JF conceived of the study. NV and JF collected the data and contributed to the final manuscript. DN analysed the data, wrote the draft and edited the final manuscript. All authors read and approved the final manuscript.

Author details

[1]AECC-Anglo European College of Chiropracti, 14-15 Parkwood Road, BH5 2DF, UK. [2]Private practice, Bournemouth, UK. [3]AECC, Bournemouth, UK.

References

1. Becan S, Quadrello T, McGee R, Mahdon M, Vavrovsky A, Barham L: *Fit for Work Europe – A Focus on Musculoskeletal Disorders (MSDs).* Europe: The Work Foundation; 2011.
2. WHO Scientific group: **The burden of musculoskeletal conditions at the start of the new millennium.** *WHO Technical Report Series* 2003, **919**.
3. Veale A, Woolf A, Carr A: **Chronic musculoskeletal pain and arthritis: Impact attitudes and perceptions.** *Ir Med J* 2008, **101**(7):208–210.
4. **The British Pain Society-F AQ. 2007/08.** http://www.britishpainsociety.org/media_faq.htm] Health and Safety Executive: **Health and Safety Statistics 2007/08** [www.hse.gov.uk/statistics/lfs/0708/swit6w12.htm]
5. Jellema P, Vander Windt DA, Vander Horst HE, Stalman WA, Bouter LM: **Prediction of an unfavourable course of low back pain in general practice: comparison of four instruments.** *Brit J Gen Pract* 2007, **57**:15–22.
6. Bouter LM, Pennick V, Bombardier C: **Cochrane back review group.** *Spine* 2003, **28**:1215–1218.
7. Newell D, Field J: **Who will get better? Predicting clinical outcomes in chiropractic practice.** *Clin Chiropr* 2007, **10**:179–186.
8. Leboeuf-Yde C, Rosenbaum A, Axén I, Lövgren PW, Jørgensen K, Halasz L, Eklund A, Wedderkopp N: **The Nordic Subpopulation Research Programme: prediction of treatment outcome in patients with low back pain treated by chiropractors–does the psychological profile matter?** *Chiropr Osteopat* 2009, **17**:14.
9. Bolton JE, Hurst H: **Prognostic factors for short-term improvement in acute and persistent musculoskeletal pain consulters in primary care.** *Chiropr Man Ther* 2011, **19**(1):27–21.
10. Kapoor S, Shaw W, Pransky G, Patterson W: **Initial patient and clinician expectations of return to work after acute onset of work-related low back pain.** *J Occup Environ Health* 2006, **48**(11):1173–1180.
11. Hill JC, Kanchan V, Dunn KM, Main CJ, Hay EM: **Comparing the STarT back screening tool's subgroup allocation of individual patients with that of independent clinical experts.** *Clin J Pain* 2010, **26**(9):783–787.
12. Hancock M, Maher C, Latimer J, Herbert R, Mc A: **Can rate of recovery be predicted in patients with acute low back pain? Development of a clinical prediction rule.** *J Eur J Pain* 2009, **13**:51–55.
13. Bolton JE, Breen AC: **The Bournemouth Questionnaire: a short-form comprehensive outcome measure. I. Psychometric properties in back pain patients.** *J Manipulative Physiol Ther* 1999, **22**:503–510.
14. Hurst H, Bolton JE: **Assessing the clinical significance of change scores on subjective outcome measures.** *J Manipulative Physiol Ther* 2004, **27**(1):26–35.
15. Bolton JE: **Sensitivity and specificity of outcome measures in patients with neckpain: Detecting clinically significant improvement.** *Spine* 2004, **29**(21):2410–2417.
16. Ostelo RJ, Deyo R, Stratford P, Waddell G, Croft P, Von Korf M, Bouter L, De Vet H: **Interpreting change scores for pain and functional status in low back pain towards international consensus regarding minimal important change.** *Spine* 2008, **33**(1):90–94.
17. Chow E, Harth T, Hruby G, Finkelstein J, Wu J, Danjoux C: **How accurate are physicians' clinical predictions of survival and the available prognostic tools in estimating survival times in Terminally Ill cancer patients? a systematic review.** *Clin Oncol* 200, **13**(3):209–18.
18. Roy S: *The Prognostic Accuracy of Return to Work Timescales as Advised by Occupational Physicians.* 2011. MSc. Manchester (Accessed Oct, 2012) http://www.medicine.manchester.ac.uk/oeh/postgraduate/msc/2011/Roy_Sujay.pdf.
19. Reiso H, Gulbrandsen P, Brage S: **Doctors' prediction of certified sickness absence.** *Fam Pract* 2004, **21**(2):192–8.
20. Childs JD, Fritz JM, Flynn TW, Irrgang JJ, Johnson KK, Majkowski GR, *et al*: **A clinical prediction rule to identify patients with low back pain most likely to benefit from spinal manipulation: a validation study.** *Ann Intern Med* 2004, **141**(12):920–928.
21. Leboueuf-Yde C, Grønstvedt A, Borge JA, Lothe J, Magnesen E, Nilsson Ø, Røsok G, Stig L, Larsen K: **The Nordic Back Pain Subpopulation Program: demographic and clinical predictors for outcome in patients receiving**

chiropractic treatment for persistent low-back pain. *J Manipulative Physiol Ther* 2004, **27**(8):493–502.
22. Axen I, Jones JJ, Rosenbaum A, Lovgren PW, Halasz L, Larsen K, *et al*: **The Nordic Back Pain Subpopulation Program: validation and improvement of a predictive model for treatment outcome in patients with low back pain receiving chiropractic treatment.** *J Manipulative Physiol Ther* 2005, **28**(6):381–385.
23. Field JR, Newell D, McCarthy PW: **Preliminary study into the components of the fear-avoidance model of LBP: change after an initial chiropractic visit and influence on outcome.** *Chiropr Osteopath* 2010, **1**(2):18–27.
24. Borghouts JA, Koes BW, Bouter LM: **The clinical course and prognostic factors of non-specific neck pain: a systematic review.** *Pain* 1998, **77**(1):1–13.
25. Hestbaek L, Leboeuf-Yde C, Manniche C: **Low back pain: what is the long-term course? A review of studies of general patient populations.** *Eur Spine J* 2003, **12**(2):149–65.
26. Field J, Newell D: **Relationship between STarT Back Screening Tool and Prognosis for Low Back Pain patients receiving Spinal Manipulative Therapy.** *Chiropr Man Ther* 2012, **20**:17.

The effect of spinal manipulative therapy on experimentally induced pain: a systematic literature review

Mario Millan[1,2*], Charlotte Leboeuf-Yde[2,3,4], Brian Budgell[5] and Michel-Ange Amorim[1,6]

Abstract

Background: Although there is evidence that spinal manipulative therapy (SMT) can reduce pain, the mechanisms involved are not well established. There is a need to review the scientific literature to establish the evidence-base for the reduction of pain following SMT.

Objectives: To determine if SMT can reduce experimentally induced pain, and if so, if the effect is i) only at the level of the treated spinal segment, ii) broader but in the same general region as SMT is performed, or iii) systemic.

Design: A systematic critical literature review.

Methods: A systematic search was performed for experimental studies on healthy volunteers and people without chronic syndromes, in which the immediate effect of SMT was tested. Articles selected were reviewed blindly by two authors. A summary quality score was calculated to indicate level of manuscript quality. Outcome was considered positive if the pain-reducing effect was statistically significant. Separate evidence tables were constructed with information relevant to each research question. Results were interpreted taking into account their manuscript quality.

Results: Twenty-two articles were included, describing 43 experiments, primarily on pain produced by pressure (n = 27) or temperature (n = 9). Their quality was generally moderate. A hypoalgesic effect was shown in 19/27 experiments on pressure pain, produced by pressure in 3/9 on pain produced by temperature and in 6/7 tests on pain induced by other measures. Second pain provoked by temperature seems to respond to SMT but not first pain. Most studies revealed a local or regional hypoalgesic effect whereas a systematic effect was unclear. Manipulation of a "restricted motion segment" ("manipulable lesion") seemed not to be essential to analgesia. In relation to outcome, there was no discernible difference between studies with higher vs. lower quality scores.

Conclusions: These results indicate that SMT has a direct local/regional hypoalgesic effect on experimental pain for some types of stimuli. Further research is needed to determine i) if there is also a systemic effect, ii) the exact mechanisms by which SMT attenuates pain, and iii) whether this response is clinically significant.

Background

Pain

Pain is defined as an unpleasant sensory and emotional experience associated with actual or potential tissue damage [1]. It originates in specific receptors, named nociceptors, which are classified according to the type of damage to which they respond; thus, mechanosensitive, thermosensitive, chemosensitive and polymodal nociceptors.

From the peripheral nociceptors, noxious stimuli are transmitted to the dorsal horn of the spinal cord [2]. There, afferent fibers synapse in the superficial laminae of the dorsal gray matter of the spinal cord [3]. Cells in the superficial laminae serve as an integration centre and relay system for many sensations. Most cells of the grey matter involved in nociception send axons across the midline of the spinal cord to ascend to the thalamus. From there, they project upwards, eventually to the

* Correspondence: mariomillan@live.fr
[1]EA 4532 CIAMS, UFR STAPS, University Paris-Sud, Paris, France
[2]The Research Department, The Spine Centre of Southern Denmark Hospital Lillebælt, Lillebælt, Denmark
Full list of author information is available at the end of the article

cortex of the brain. However, impulses are not only transmitted to the cerebral cortex. There are also other pathways and mechanisms that may participate in analgesic influences at the spinal and supraspinal levels.

When a noxious stimulus occurs, there may be a "first pain", conducted by Aδ fibers, and a "second pain", due to temporal sensory summation (TSS) and conducted by nociceptive C-fibers. "First pain" is described as sharp and "pricking". The propagation of this stimulus is relatively quick and it is felt in a well-defined part of the body surface [2]. "Second pain", which is transmitted more slowly, is often described as dull and aching, and it is poorly localized. This pain tends to last beyond the termination of an acute noxious stimulus. Sources, pathways, perception of and treatment of the two types of pain are very different [4].

Modulating pain

The infliction of pain is not always experienced in a linear manner according to the strength and nature of the stimulus. Pain sensations can be very different from one individual to another, and also intra-individual variations can occur, so that identical types of damage do not necessarily result in an identical amount and type of pain. One reason for this is that pain can be modulated, both to increase and decrease.

One modulating system, central sensitization, tends to increase pain sensation [5], particularly in people who have more long-lasting pain, making them more sensitive to "new" pain impulses than they would have been under normal circumstances.

Another endogenous modulating system is afferent or segmental inhibition, meaning that one external stimulus can block an ongoing pain sensation by having higher priority in reaching the brain [4].

Descending antinociceptive systems provide yet another modulating mechanism. These originate largely in the mesencephalon and have synaptic connections with neurons in the medulla and the spinal cord. This means that nociceptive information may be blocked or attenuated before it reaches higher centers [6]. This system is also tightly connected to a descending pain facilitating pathway that has the same general sites of origin (mesencephalon and medulla) but with the opposite effect.

Finally, there are also other intrinsic mechanisms for physiological modulation of pain, such as subjective assessment and motivational-affective modulation [7], which act by raising pain thresholds via endogenous opioids and other substances. These mechanisms, at times, preferentially alter sensory and/or affective aspects of pain perception, and the associated modulation of pain-evoked neural activity occurs in limbic and/or sensory brain regions, suggesting multiple endogenous pain-modulating systems [8]. Thus, pain can be increased or decreased by mere expectations or, even, abolished by feelings of, for example, fear.

Treating back pain with spinal manipulative therapy

Although back pain is common and frequently distressing, and many therapies have arisen to treat it, musculoskeletal pain remains difficult to diagnose and treat. Spinal manipulative therapy (SMT) is one common treatment for musculoskeletal pain. One class of SMT involves a high-velocity, low-amplitude (HVLA) manipulation frequently used by chiropractors. HVLA treatments are mechanical events. They cause slight momentary deformations of the spine and surrounding soft tissues, and often elicit a cracking sound thought to be brought about by cavitation of spinal facet joints [9-11]. It is common to differentiate manipulation from mobilization. In the latter case, the joint is not taken beyond its passive limit. Rather mobilization can be described as a passive and perhaps repetitive stretch. Manipulation, on the other hand, carries the vertebrae beyond the normal physiological range of movement without exceeding the boundaries of anatomic integrity [11]. However, the distinction between manipulation and mobilization is probably not that clear, and it has been shown that cavitation is not necessary for SMT to exert a clinical effect [12-16]. The term SMT can therefore be used to describe various types of manual therapy (MT).

The possible mechanisms of spinal manipulative therapy in back pain

Clinical experience indicates that both HVLA and mobilization, and also other types of manual therapy (MT), can have an immediate effect on pain. The literature also suggests that SMT has a direct neurological pain-reducing effect, by evoking one or possibly several of the physiologic pain-modulating mechanisms described briefly above. Indeed, there could be a combination of mechanisms or a number of these acting on different causes of pain. In this article we shall concentrate on the possible direct effect of SMT on pain. There are three possible levels of this hypothesized direct effect of SMT on pain, i.e. local, regional or central.

Local pain reducing effect

One theory is that SMT would have a pain-reducing effect primarily at the level of the manipulation, i.e. at a specific spinal level. In all, this phenomenon would probably be the result of a mix of different mechanisms. For example, SMT may mechanistically act to decrease the sensitivity of the muscle spindles and/or the various segmental sites of a reflex pathway [17].

Regional pain reducing effect

Another possibility is that SMT could have a regional effect, although still at the spinal level of the manipulative input. Some authors suggest an effect on the dorsal horn of the spinal cord [18] or on the periaqueductal grey area [19-21]. SMT is also thought to affect reflex neural outputs to both muscle and visceral organs by affecting both paraspinal muscle reflexes and motoneuron excitability [22].

Central pain reducing effect

Recently, it has been hypothesized that SMT reduces the potential for central sensitization by inhibiting TSS ("second pain") [23]. One mechanism underlying the effects of SMT may be the ability of manipulation to alter central sensory processing by removing subthreshold mechanical or chemical stimuli from paraspinal tissues [22].

Conflicting literature

Also a comprehensive model of mechanisms of manual therapy in the treatment of musculoskeletal pain has been suggested [24] consisting of a cascade of neurophysiological responses from the peripheral and central nervous systems which are then responsible for the clinical outcomes. In other words, the literature offers many possible mechanisms and combinations of mechanisms to explain the pain-reducing effect of SMT. In fact, there is a lot of information available in the literature on this topic. However, the literature is difficult to grasp and conflicting because it consists of a mixture of discussions, hypotheses, and studies employing different designs, methods and outcome variables. Therefore, there is a need for systematic and critical literature reviews in order to establish the evidence-base for various theories relating to the direct or indirect reduction of pain following SMT. A first step might be to establish the weight of evidence in relation to whether pain is indeed dampened by the application of SMT to the spinal structures.

Aims and objectives

Therefore, in this systematic critical literature review we shall examine the effect of spinal manipulation on experimentally induced pain in healthy study subjects concentrating on the possible direct effects of SMT on pain at three levels, i.e. local, regional or systemic. Because different types of pain may travel through different pathways, these were studied separately.

The specific research questions were:

1- Does SMT reduce pain provoked by pressure?
2- Does SMT reduce pain provoked by temperature?
3- Does SMT reduce pain provoked by methods other than pressure and temperature?
4- Does SMT reduce experimentally induced pain at the spinal segment where it is performed?
5- Does SMT reduce experimentally induced pain in the spinal region where it is performed?
6- Does SMT have a systemic (global) effect on experimentally induced pain?

Methods

In order to obtain answers to the questions above, we undertook a systematic critical literature review, which commenced with a systematic literature search of PubMed, Mantis, and the Cochrane Library using specific search terms. These search terms were: Spinal manipulation pain: ("manipulation, spinal"[MeSH Terms] OR ("manipulation"[All Fields] AND "spinal"[All Fields]) OR "spinal manipulation"[All Fields] OR ("spinal"[All Fields] AND "manipulation"[All Fields])) AND ("pain"[MeSH Terms] OR "pain"[All Fields]) ; Chiropractic manipulation pain: ("manipulation, chiropractic"[MeSH Terms] OR ("manipulation"[All Fields] AND "chiropractic"[All Fields]) OR "chiropractic manipulation"[All Fields] OR ("chiropractic"[All Fields] AND "manipulation"[All Fields])) AND ("pain"[MeSH Terms] OR "pain"[All Fields]) ; Spinal manipulation experimental pain: ("manipulation, spinal"[MeSH Terms] OR ("manipulation"[All Fields] AND "spinal"[All Fields]) OR "spinal manipulation"[All Fields] OR ("spinal"[All Fields] AND "manipulation"[All Fields])) AND experimental[All Fields] AND ("pain"[MeSH Terms] OR "pain"[All Fields]) ; and Chiropractic manipulation experimental pain: ("manipulation, chiropractic"[MeSH Terms] OR ("manipulation"[All Fields] AND "chiropractic"[All Fields]) OR "chiropractic manipulation"[All Fields] OR ("chiropractic"[All Fields] AND "manipulation"[All Fields])) AND experimental[All Fields] AND ("pain"[MeSH Terms] OR "pain"[All Fields]).

Inclusion and exclusion criteria (see Additional file 1) were applied by the first author to the titles and abstracts of the studies identified in the search. Once most selected articles were retrieved, a citation search was made based on the retrieved articles' reference lists. All articles selected were reviewed separately by two different authors blinded to each other's evaluations. Each author separately extracted data from every article according to a checklist. Data were later compared in order to minimize extraction errors. The fourth author would arbitrate any disagreement between the two reviewers. An ongoing search was performed until December 31, 2011 and the review process was repeated when new articles were found.

A table was constructed in order to describe the selected articles, as shown in Table 1.

Articles are presented consecutively by year of publication and identified by a number corresponding to its reference in the first column of each table. As we were unable to locate a suitable quality check-list for this type of research, a second set of criteria was developed in order to evaluate the quality and risk of bias in this type of research. We designed this checklist based on concepts presented in the PRISMA statement [25], the CONSORT statement [26] and Cochrane guidelines [27] bearing in mind that there can be no general recipe for such work, as review procedures have to be topic

Table 1 Descriptive items used in a systematic critical literature review on the effect of SMT on pain

Reference	Year	Authors	Title	Location	Setting	n° of subjects	n° males
[37]	2011	Josue Fernández-Carnero, Joshua A. Cleland and Roy La Touche Arbizu	Examination of motor and hypoalgesic effects of cervical vs thoracic spine manipulation in patients with lateral epicondyalgia: a clinical trial.	Spain	University	18?	8
[42]	2011	V. Maduro de Camargo, F. Alburquerque-Sendín, F. Bérzin, Vinicius Cobos Stefanelli, D. P. Rodrigues de Souza and C. Fernández-de-las-Peñas,	Immediate effects on electromyographic activity and pressure pain thresholds after a cervical manipulation in mechanical neck pain: a randomized controlled trial.	Brazil	University	37	21
[23]	2011	Mark D. Bishop, Jason M. Beneciuk, Steven Z. George;	Immediate reduction in temporal sensory summation after thoracic spinal manipulation.	USA	University	90	24
[28]	2010	Benjamin Soon, Annina B. Schmid, Elias J. Fridriksson, Elizabeth Gresslos, Philip Cheong and Anthony Wright;	A crossover study on the effect of cervical mobilization on motor function and pressure pain threshold in pain-free individuals.	Australia	University	24	13
[29]	2010	Oliveira-Campelo NM, Rubens-Rebelatto J, Martín-Vallejo FJ, Alburquerque-Sendí N F, Fernández-de-Las-Peñas C.	The immediate effects of atlanto-occipital joint manipulation and suboccipital muscle inhibition technique on active mouth opening and pressure pain sensitivity over latent myofascial trigger points in the masticatory muscles.	Spain Brazil	Osteopathic school and university	122	31
[44]	2010	Elaine Willett, Clair Hebron and Oliver Krouwel	The initial effects of different rates of lumbar mobilizations on pressure pain thresholds in asymptomatic subjects.	UK	University	30	8
[38]	2009	P. Mansilla-Ferragut, C. Fernández-de-las Peñas, F Alburquerque-Sendin, J. A. Cleland and JJ Boscá-Gandia	Immediate effects of atlanto-occipital joint Manipulation on active mouth opening and pressure pain sensitivity in women with mechanical neck pain.	Spain	Osteopathic school	37	0
[30]	2009	Oliver Thomson, Lesley Haig, Hazel Mansfield	The effects of high-velocity low-amplitude thrust manipulation and mobilization techniques on pressure pain threshold in the lumbar spine.	Sweden UK	Stockholm College Osteopathic School British College	50	29
[43]	2009	Oliver Krouwel , Clair Hebron, Elaine Willett	An investigation into the potential hypoalgesic effects of different amplitudes of PA mobilizations on the lumbar spine as measured by pressure pain thresholds.	UK	University	30	9

Table 1 Descriptive items used in a systematic critical literature review on the effect of SMT on pain *(Continued)*

Reference	Year	Authors	Title	Location	Setting	n° of subjects	n° males
[18]	2009	Joel E. Bialosky, Mark D. Bishop, Michael E. Robinson, Giorgio Zeppieri Jr, Steven Z. George	Spinal manipulative therapy has an immediate effect on thermal pain sensitivity in people with low back pain: a randomized controlled trial.	USA	University	36	10
[19]	2008	J. Fernández-Carnero, Cesar Fernández-de-las-Peñas, and Joshua A. Cleland	Immediate hypoalgesic and motor effects after a single cervical manipulation in subjects with lateral epicondyalgia.	Spain USA	Universities and Osteopathic school Madrid	10	5
[39]	2008	C. Fernández-de-las-Peñas, C. Alonso-Blanco, J. A. Cleland, C. Rodriguez-Blanco and F.Alburquerque-Sendin	Changes in pressure pain thresholds over C5-C6 zygapophyseal joint after a cervicothoracic junction manipulation in healthy subjects.	Spain USA	Universities and Osteopathic school Madrid	30	13
[20]	2007	M. Ruiz-Sáez, C. Fernández-de-las-Peñas, C. Rodriguez Blanco, R. Martinez-Segura and R. Garcia-León	Changes in pressure pain sensitivity in latent myofascial trigger points in the upper trapezius muscle after a cervical spine manipulation in pain-free subjects.	Spain	Osteopathic school	72	27
[31]	2007	Fernández-de-las-Peñas C, Pérez-de-Heredia M, Brea-Rivero M, Miangolarra-Page JC.	Immediate effects on pressure pain threshold following a single cervical spine manipulation in healthy subjects.	Spain	Universities	15	7
[34]	2007	Hamilton L, Boswell C, Fryer G	The effects of high-velocity, low-amplitude manipulation and muscle energy technique on suboccipital tenderness.	Australia	University	90	29
[36]	2006	George SZ, Bishop MD, Bialosky JE, Zeppieri G Jr, Robinson ME.	Immediate effects of spinal manipulation on thermal pain sensitivity: an experimental study.	USA	University	60	20
[40]	2004	P.Mohammadi, A. Gonsalves, Chris Tsai, T. Hummel and Thomas Carpenter	Areas of capsaicin-induced secondary hyperalgesia and allodynia are reduced by a single chiropractic adjustment: preliminary study.	USA Germany	Universities	20	14
[35]	2004	Fryer G, Carub J, McIver S.	The effect of manipulation and mobilization on pressure pain thresholds in the thoracic spine.	Australia	University	96	39
[21]	2001	M. Sterling, G. Jull, A. Wright	Cervical mobilization: concurrent effects on pain, sympathetic nervous system activity and motor activity.	Canada	University	30	14
[32]	1998	Bill Vicenzino, David Collins and Anthony Wright	An investigation of the Interrelationship between manipulative therapy-Induced hypoalgesia and sympathoexcitation.	Australia	University	24	11
[33]	1996	Bill Vicenzino, David Collins and Anthony Wright	The initial effects of a cervical spine manipulative physiotherapy treatment on the pain and dysfunction of lateral epicondyalgia.	Australia	University	15	7
[41]	1984	Terrett AC, Vernon H.	Manipulation and pain tolerance. A controlled study of the effect of spinal manipulation on paraspinal cutaneous pain tolerance levels.	Canada	Chiropractic college	50	?

T° = temperature.

Table 1 Descriptive items used in a systematic critical literature review on the effect of SMT on pain *(Continued)*

n° females	Ages	Treatment groups	How was pain produced	How was pain measured	When was pain measured	Description of study subjects	Approval ethics committee
9	44.8 SD, 9.2 (30–60)	- Cervical manipulation - Thoracic manipulation	Pressure	Electronic digital algometer	Before and after	Faculty of the Health Science	Yes
16	18 – 42	- SMT C5-C6 - Control	Pressure	Analogue algometer	Before and after	University workers	Yes
66	22.9 + −2.7	- SMT - Cervical exercises - Control	T° and pressure	Algometer	Before and Immediately after	Students	No
11	34 +/−12	- Mobilization - Manual contact control - Control	Pressure	Digital algometer	Before and after	Students	Yes
91	18-30	- Manipulation - Soft tissue - Control	Pressure	Mechanical algometer	Before and 2 min post treatment	Students	Yes
22	33.05 (18–57)	- 2 Hz - 1 Hz - Quasi stable	Pressure	Electronic algometer	Base + 48 h + 48 h	11 naive physiotherapists 19 non naive	Yes
37	35 +/−8	- SMT - Control	Pressure	Mechanical algometer	Before and after	Volunteers, general population	Yes
21	27	- unilateral HVLAT - Spinal lumbar mobilization - Sham laser procedure	Pressure	Pressure algometer	Before and after	Students	Yes
21	26,43 (SD 4,92)	- Large oscillation (force applied) - Small oscillation quasi static	Pressure	Digital algometer	Baseline before and + 24, + 24	13/30 physiotherapy naives	Yes
26	32.38 (12.63)	- SMT - Biking - Back extension exercise	T°	Numerical scale	Before and Immediately after	Students with low back pain	No
5	42 (SD6)	- Manipulative session - Manual contact intervention	T° and pressure	Electronic algometer	Before and after	Patients	Yes

Table 1 Descriptive items used in a systematic critical literature review on the effect of SMT on pain *(Continued)*

n° females	Ages	Treatment groups	How was pain produced	How was pain measured	When was pain measured	Description of study subjects	Approval ethics committee
17	26 (SD 5)	- Manipulative thrust right side C7-T1 - Manipulative thrust left side C7-T1 - Sham-manual procedure	Pressure	Algometer	Before and after	General population	Yes
46	31 (SD10)	- Manipulative - Sham-manual	Pressure	Mechanical algometer	Baseline before 1, 5 and 10 min after	Volunteers, general population	Yes
8	21 + −2	- Manipulation - Placebo - Control	Pressure	Mechanical algometer	Before 5 min after intervention 3 sessions separated by 48 h	Students	Yes
61	23 +/−5	- SMT (C0- C1) - Muscle energy technique - Control	Pressure	Electronic algometer	Before and after	Students	Yes
40	24.03(SD 3.2°	- SMT - Lumbar ext exercise - Bicycle riding	T°	Medoc neurosensory analyzer	Before and 5 min after	Students	Yes
6	27 (21–37)	- SMT - Non-SMT	Cutaneous capsaicin	Visual Analogue Scale	Before and 20 min after after	Healthy volunteers, mostly naive to SMT	Yes
57	19-34	- SMT T2-T4 - Mobilisation - Control	Pressure	Electronic algometer	Before and after	Students	Yes
16	35.7 (SD 14.92)	- SMT - Placebo - Control	Pressure / T°	Visual Analogue Scale, electronic algometer	Before and after	Patients pain +3 months C5/6	Yes
13	49.0 (27–70)	- Mobilization C5-C6 - Manual contact placebo - Nothing	Pressure / T°	Visual Analogue Scale, digital algometer	Before and after	Patients epicond 6.2 +/− 5.1 months	Yes
8	44 +/−2	- Treatment - Placebo - Control	Pressure	Visual Analogue Scale digital algometer	Before and after	Patients epicond 8 +/− 2 months	Yes
?	28.6	- Thoracic manipulation - Control group	Electrical induction	Thresholds	Before and after	Chiropractic students	No

specific. The items selected for the quality checklist and their rationale have been described in Additional file 2. The risk of bias was assessed following the criteria suggested by the method guidelines for systematic reviews of trials of treatments for neck and back pain by Furlan et al [27] (see items 1, 2, 4, 6, 9, and 11 in Additional file 2). Additional items were mainly adapted from PRISMA [25] (see items 3, 5, 7, 8, 10, 12, and 13). Finally, the outcomes were noted for each experiment as a positive effect, negative effect, or no effect.

Classifying articles by their quality

Each article selected was checked for each quality item. By consensus, we decided to give one point for every criterion, except for the 4 items that we considered as most important: a- unbiased/blind/naïve study subjects (item 1), b- random allocation (item 3), c- blinded assessment (item 9), and d- losses and exclusions (item 11). Each of these was assigned two points.

A summary quality score was calculated but no cutoff-point was defined for acceptable or unacceptable level of quality. This allowed us (and the readers) to use the quality scores and the information on each individual quality item as a guide for whether articles would be considered more or less credible. In other words, the quality assessment was meant to be flexible.

A post hoc comparison was made between results of the two quality scores (the total score and the score for the most important criteria). Using thresholds set at 12/18 and 4/8 points, respectively, the distributions of studies with positive and non-positive outcomes were compared for the two scales and in relation to whether the studies were of higher or lower quality.

Data synthesis

The data tables were used, in a systematic fashion, to obtain answers to our research questions. This was done by highlighting relevant information to facilitate a visual representation (green = positive outcome, red = non-positive outcome) to make interpretation easier. Finally, studies were sorted in descending order starting with those with the highest total quality score out of 18. Results were thereafter interpreted and reported in a narrative fashion. If high and low quality studies generally obtained similar outcomes, we assumed that the poorer quality studies provided supporting evidence for the better studies. If, however, it was mainly the poorer quality studies which obtained positive findings, particularly if the assessors were not blinded or the study subjects could have been biased, then we would be more cautious in our interpretation of the results.

Because we decided not to use a scoring system to establish level of quality, we have not defined discrete levels of evidence.

Results

In all, 1279 titles satisfying the inclusion criteria were identified in the initial PubMed search. Other database search results were as follows: a- Spinal manipulation pain: 1276 results in Pubmed, 10 in Mantis and 9 Cochrane Reviews. b- Chiropractic manipulation pain: 806 results in Pubmed, 2 in Mantis and 5 Cochrane Reviews. c- Spinal manipulation experimental pain: 63 results in Pubmed, 0 in Mantis and 13 Cochrane Reviews. d- Chiropractic manipulation experimental pain: 28 results in Pubmed, 0 in Mantis and 0 Cochrane Reviews. Only 5 articles were added after an additional search of reference lists.

All articles found in the Mantis and Cochrane databases were already identified via the Pubmed searches. Of the 1279 references, 116 were retrieved in full text for further scrutiny.

Description of studies

Upon scrutinizing the full texts, 22 articles were found to fulfill the inclusion criteria. They described 43 experiments: 27 with pain produced by pressure, 9 by temperature, 3 by capsaicin, 2 examined spontaneous pain, 1 used a stretch test to produce pain and 1 used electrically induced pain. All were controlled trials published in English. Detailed information is presented in Table 1 and briefly summarized below.

Three research groups were responsible for 13 publications. They did not seem to have repeatedly used the same study samples but appeared to have reported on different study populations for the various studies. In most cases (n = 18), experiments were carried out totally or partially in universities. The number of subjects ranged from 10 to 122. Six articles used patients as study subjects; most of the others included non-clinical populations, often students. There were no studies with animals fulfilling our inclusion criteria.

Most of experiments (n = 20) used external control groups. Twelve of them used three groups: a treatment, a placebo and a control group in which no action was taken - noted in tables as "nothing" (studies [21,23,28-35]). Studies [18,36] used bicycle exercise as their control activity. Seven studies ([19,20,37-41]) used a sham procedure as their control treatment, whereas study [42] compared the treatment group to a control group without a sham procedure. Two studies used only internal control groups; [43] and [44] compared three different types of mobilization.

Data synthesis: Quality of studies

There were no disagreements between reviewers on the scoring of the manuscripts based on the checklists. Table 2 summarizes the quality items for each article. The quality and risk of bias assessment of studies reviewed revealed them to be relatively homogeneous, with the summary scores ranging between 8 and 16 out of 18 points, with mean and median summary scores of 12.2 and 13, respectively.

Of the various quality items that we scrutinized, all studies fulfilled the criteria on the validity of the outcome variable, all had measured the pain before and after the intervention, all had provided some estimate of the results in tables, graphs or text, and all had tested their results for statistical significance. The ANOVA was used for factorial designs in all studies in order to test how variables interacted or combined.

Other checklist items were not always fulfilled. Of the four quality criteria that we considered particularly important, namely unbiased/blind/naïve study subjects (item 1), random allocation (item 3), blinded assessment (item 9), and losses and exclusions (item 11), the first two were commonly satisfied (in 15 and 17 papers, respectively), whereas using unbiased/blind/naïve study subjects and accounting for losses and exclusions were ignored in many studies (present in 7 and 5, respectively). Five of the reviewed articles ([18,23,36,43,44]) should be considered with care since their assessments of outcomes were not blinded.

Seven articles did not mention if the allocation of study subjects to each group was randomized. As it was not our intention to penalize unfairly articles that used a randomized allocation without mentioning it, we identified the numbers of individuals in each group in these reports (see Table 3). Articles [19,32,33] did not provide the number of subjects in each experimental group. The others (except [30]) showed a more even distribution than one could expect with a proper randomization procedure. We therefore assumed that the fact that authors did not discuss the randomization procedure, in most cases, reflected the fact that it had not occurred.

In our review, we did not set a threshold for acceptable/unacceptable quality but displayed the articles in descending order from the highest to the lowest score. Nevertheless, in Table 2a, we compared the spread of articles when using the total score (18 point scale, see Table 2) and the scale based on four high-priority items (8 point scale, see Table 2b). With levels of "acceptance" provisionally set at 12/18 and 4/8, respectively, all articles, with one exception, obtained the same classification of acceptable or not, regardless of the system used. We interpreted this concordance as a confirmation of the robustness of the quality and risk of bias assessment.

In addition to the quality issues identified in this review, the authors themselves have in some instances discussed the limitations of their own studies (see Table 4).

A meta-analysis was not attempted because the heterogeneity of studies on pain provoking methods, units of measurements, areas of the body where experiments were performed, and local, regional of systemic assessments of the effects of SMT.

Data synthesis: Answers to research questions

Herein, each research question is dealt with one at a time, and for each, we refer to a table summarizing the results in order of quality of the study. If one study contains several experiments, they have all been reported individually in the appropriate section of the review. Table 5 presents studies grouped by their results, showing in the upper panels those that presented a hypoalgesic action and, in the lower panels, those that did not. Papers are also separated by the research question, i.e. local, regional or systemic effect. Table 6 summarizes for each article the effect of SMT on pain, the site where SMT was performed and the location of the pain. This table also shows values reported, whether the effect was local, regional or systemic, whether the effects were ipsilateral or contralateral, whether an effect occurred above or below the site of manipulation, and the type of pain induced.

In the majority of experiments (28/43), SMT reduced pain. Outcomes were not dependent on whether quality scores were high or low. These studies demonstrate a clear hypoalgesic effect of SMT (see Table 5a). For specific results, see below.

1. Does SMT reduce experimentally induced pain provoked by pressure? There were 27 experiments performed on pressure pain. Nineteen of these showed manipulation to increase pressure pain thresholds (PPT). There was no obvious link between the reported polarity of the effect and the quality of the studies. Changes produced by SMT were in general statistically significant. Differences in PPT values (before/after SMT), when reported as percentages ranged between 4.8% (in [28]) and 44.2% (in [19]). Other units of measurement were also used making it difficult to summarize with a single parameter the size of the effect. For detailed information, see Tables 6 and Additional file 3.
2. Does SMT reduce experimentally induced pain provoked by temperature? There were 9 experiments on pain induced by temperature, only 3 of which showed a hypoalgesic action for SMT: studies [18,23,36] found that SMT relieves pain provoked by temperature and therefore transmitted by C-fibers. The other experiments (n = 6) did not show significant differences in relation to SMT. Three of these tested first pain (Aδ fiber system) and the other three tested TSS (C-fiber system). There was no obvious link with the quality of studies. For values and detailed information, see Table 6 and Additional file 4.
3. Does SMT reduce experimentally induced pain provoked by methods other than pressure and

Table 2 Quality criteria of articles selected for a systematic critical literature review on the effect of SMT on pain

Article	Is the assessment blinded?		Is there a control on psychological characteristics of subjects?		The validity of the outcome variable:		When was it measured?		Is the random procedure mentioned?		Number of experiments (pain + SMT)		Study subjects:
	Yes = 2 pts No = 0 point	Points	Yes = 1 point No = 0 point	Points	Pilot study = 1 pts or ,Ref are given = 1 pt or, it's reproducible = 1 pt Nothing = 0 pt	Points (max 1 pt)	before and after = 1 point only after = 0 point	Points	Yes = 2 pts No = 0 point	Points	> 1 = 1 point 1 = 0 point	Points	Naive to tx and blind (sham manip) = 2 pts Naive or blind = 1 point Not naive and not blind = 0 pt
[39]	Yes	2	No	0	Ref given	1	Before and after	1	Yes	2	3	1	Blind
[21]	Yes	2	No	0	Reproducible	1	Before and after	1	Yes	2	3	1	Naive and blind
[31]	Yes	2	No	0	Ref given	1	Before and after	1	Yes	2	3	1	Blind
[42]	Yes	2	No	0	Ref given	1	Before and after	1	Yes	2	3	1	Blind
[29]	Yes	2	No	0	Ref given	1	Before and after	1	Yes	2	3	1	Naive
[44]	No	0	No	0	Ref given	1	Before and after	1	Yes	2	3	1	Naive and blind
[38]	Yes	2	No	0	Ref given	1	Before and after	1	Yes	2	3	1	Blind
[34]	Yes	2	No	0	Ref given	1	Before and after	1	Yes	2	3	1	Naive
[35]	Yes	2	No	0	Ref given	1	Before and after	1	Yes	2	3	1	Naive
[37]	Yes	2	No	0	Ref given	1	Before and after	1	Yes	2	3	1	Nothing
[28]	Yes	2	No	0	Ref given	1	Before and after	1	Yes	2	3	1	Naive and blind
[43]	No	0	No	0	Ref given	1	Before and after	1	Yes	2	3	1	Naive and blind
[20]	Yes	2	No	0	Ref given	1	Before and after	1	Yes	2	3	1	Blind
[40]	Yes	2	No	0	Reproducible	1	Before and after	1	Yes	2	2	1	Naive and blind
[18]	No	0	Yes	1	Ref given	1	Before and after	1	Yes	2	2	1	Nothing
[19]	Yes	2	No	0	Ref given	1	Before and after	1	No	0	3	1	Blind
[32]	Yes	2	No	0	Ref given	1	Before and after	1	No	0	3	1	Naive and blind
[30]	Yes	2	No	0	Ref given	1	Before and after	1	No	0	3	1	Blind to sham laser
[36]	No	0	Yes	1	Ref given	1	Before and after	1	Yes	2	10	1	Nothing
[41]	Yes	2	No	0	Ref given	1	Before and after	1	Yes	2	1	0	Nothing
[33]	Yes	2	No	0	Ref given	1	Before and after	1	No	0	3	1	Naive and blind
[23]	No	0	Yes	1	Ref given	1	Before and after	1	No	0	2	1	Nothing

T° = temperature.

Table 2 Quality criteria of articles selected for a systematic critical literature review on the effect of SMT on pain *(Continued)*

Study subjects:	SMT performed by:		Is the SMT well described?		Are losses and exclusions reported?		Experimental conditions		Estimates given		Are differences tested for statistical significance?		Total of points
Points	Same person = 1 point Experienced person (> 5 years) = 1 point	Points (max 2 pts)	Yes = 1 point No = 0 point	Points	Yes = 2 pts No = 0 point	Points	same day or T° controlled or same time = 1 point different day and T° or time not controlled = 0 point	Points	Yes = 1 point No = 0 point	Points	Yes = 1 point No = 0 point	Points	Min = 0 Max = 18
1	Same and experienced	2	Yes	1	Yes	2	Same day	1	Yes	1	Yes	1	16
2	Same and experienced	2	Yes	1	No	0	Same day	1	Yes	1	Yes	1	15
1	Experienced	1	Yes	1	Yes	2	T controlled	1	Yes	1	Yes	1	15
1	Same and experienced	2	Yes	1	No	0	Same day	1	Yes	1	Yes	1	14
1	Same and experienced	2	Yes	1	No	0	Same day	1	Yes	1	Yes	1	14
2	Same and experienced	2	Yes	1	Yes	2	More 48 H, no control T°	0	Yes	1	Yes	1	14
1	Same and experienced	2	Yes	1	No	0	Same day	1	Yes	1	Yes	1	14
1	Same and experienced	2	Yes	1	No	0	Same day?	1	Yes	1	Yes	1	14
1	Same and experienced	2	Yes	1	No	0	Same day?	1	Yes	1	Yes	1	14
0	Same and experienced	2	Yes	1	No	0	Same day	1	Yes	1	Yes	1	13
2	Experienced	1	Yes	1	No	0	More 48 H, no control T°	0	Yes	1	Yes	1	13
2	Same	1	Yes	1	Yes	2	More 3 days, no control T°	0	Yes	1	Yes	1	13
1	Experienced	1	Yes	1	No	0	Same day	1	Yes	1	Yes	1	13
2	Experienced	1	Yes	1	No	0	More 7 days, no control T°	0	Yes	1	Yes	1	13
0	Nothing	0	Yes	1	Yes	2	Same day	1	Yes	1	Yes	1	12
1	Same and experienced	2	Yes	1	No	0	More 48 H, no control T°	0	Yes	1	Yes	1	11
2	Nothing	0	Yes	1	No	0	More 3 days, control T°	1	Yes	1	Yes	1	11
1	Nothing	0	Yes	1	No	0	Same day	1	Yes	1	Yes	1	10
0	Nothing	0	Yes	1	No	0	Same day	1	Yes	1	Yes	1	10
0	Nothing	0	Yes	1	No	0	Same day	1	Yes	1	Yes	1	10
2	Nothing	0	No	0	No	0	More 3 days, no control T°	0	Yes	1	Yes	1	9
0	Nothing	0	yes	1	No	0	Highly controlled	1	Yes	1	Yes	1	8

Table 2a A comparison between total scores obtained from two different scales (8 point scale and 18 point scale)

Article	Score Max = 8	Score Max = 18
[39]	6	16
[31]	7	15
[21]	6	15
[42]	5	14
[29]	5	14
[44]	6	14
[38]	5	14
[35]	5	14
[34]	5	14
[28]	6	13
[43]	6	13
[20]	5	13
[40]	6	13
[37]	4	13
[18]	4	12
[19]	3	11
[32]	4	11
[30]	3	10
[36]	2	10
[41]	4	10
[33]	4	9
[23]	0	8

Articles scoring ≤ 4/8 or ≤ 12/18 are shown in red.

temperature? Only 7 tests were performed using methods other than pressure and temperature to induce pain. Six of these revealed a statistically significant hypoalgesic effect induced by SMT. There did not seem to be a link with the quality of studies. For values and detailed information, see Tables 6 and Additional file 5.

4. Does SMT reduce experimentally induced pain in the spinal segment where it is performed? Twenty experiments investigated whether SMT reduces experimentally induced pain in the spinal segment where it is performed. Twelve of them showed a hypoalgesic effect. The other eight presented no significant effects. Of these, study [28] tested the hypoalgesic action of an anterior-posterior mobilization and not a lateral maneuver, as is usually the case in SMT. In study [20], there was no effect immediately after SMT, but an effect was demonstrable five and ten minutes later. In studies [19,31] differences between sides were studied, but no difference was found. Outcomes did not relate to the quality score. For detailed information, see Tables 5 and 6.
5. Does SMT reduce experimentally induced pain in the same region where it is performed? Nine experiments reported a regional effect of SMT on pain. Only one study failed to obtain a hypoalgesic effect. In this, thoracic manipulation was used as a sham treatment versus cervical manipulation to evaluate the action on elbow PPT. There did not seem to be a link between treatment effects reported and the quality of studies. For detailed information, see Table 5 and 6.
6. Does SMT have a systemic effect on experimentally induced pain? Nine experiments evaluated this hypothesis. None of them had blinded assessors, which makes the results uncertain. Five of them demonstrated a systemic action of SMT on pain, but four of them did not show significant differences between treatment groups. Three of these four (studies [18,23,36]) evaluated first pain transmitted by Aδ fibers. There did not seem to be a link between treatment effects reported and the quality of studies. For detailed information, see Tables 5 and 6.

Additional observations

1. No article presented any data on the duration of the pain reduction. Studies [43,44] concluded that the hypoalgesic effect was unrelated to the amplitude of the manual procedure, whereas [30] concluded that mobilization had a stronger effect than manipulation.

2. Four studies ([29,35,36,40]) applied the SMT to a point on the spine thought to be in need of treatment, i.e. at what was considered to be a dysfunctional spinal segment (manipulable lesion/fixation/subluxation), whereas in all other studies the exact location of SMT was predetermined without reference to local signs or symptoms. However, hypoalgesic results were observed regardless of whether the treatment was provided in a "clinical" fashion, i.e. where the patient would have what the clinician considered a dysfunctional segment, or if the manipulation was given in a predetermined area.

3. In two studies ([20,29]) the investigators searched for so-called trigger points.

4. Five articles ([19,31,37,39,42]) assessed whether the effect of SMT was only on the ipsilateral side of the impulse or if it was also noted on the contra-lateral side. None of the trials found a side-specific effect.

5. Several reports (N = 9) made reference to the "crack" ([18-20,23,29,37-39,42]), which is thought to occur when a joint is cavitated [14]. If no cavitation was obtained, a second manipulation would be given. There was no obvious difference in results between studies that concentrated on the crack and those that did not. However, none studied that issue specifically, making it impossible to know whether all study subjects were "cracked" or not.

Table 2b Four main quality criteria of articles from literature review on effect of SMT on pain – maximum score 8 points

Article	Is the assessment blinded?		Is the randomization procedure mentioned?		Study subjects:		Were losses and exclusions reported?		Total points
	Yes = 2 pts	Points	Yes = 2 pts	Points	Naive to tx and blind	Points	Yes = 2 pts	Points	Max = 8 Min = 0
[31]	Yes	2	Yes	2	Blind	1	Yes	2	7
[28]	Yes	2	Yes	2	Naive and blind	2	No	0	6
[44]	No	0	Yes	2	Naive and blind	2	Yes	2	6
[43]	No	0	Yes	2	Naive and blind	2	Yes	2	6
[40]	Yes	2	Yes	2	Naive and blind	2	No	0	6
[21]	Yes	2	Yes	2	Naive and blind	2	No	0	6
[39]	Yes	2	Yes	2	Blind	1	Yes	2	6
[42]	Yes	2	Yes	2	Blind	1	No	0	5
[29]	Yes	2	Yes	2	Naive	1	No	0	5
[38]	Yes	2	Yes	2	Blind	1	No	0	5
[20]	Yes	2	Yes	2	Blind	1	No	0	5
[34]	Yes	2	Yes	2	Naive	1	No	0	5
[35]	Yes	2	Yes	2	Naive	1	No	0	5
[37]	Yes	2	Yes	2	Nothing	0	No	0	4
[18]	No	0	Yes	2	Nothing	0	Yes	2	4
[32]	Yes	2	No	0	Naive and blind	2	No	0	4
[33]	Yes	2	No	0	Naive and blind	2	No	0	4
[41]	Yes	2	Yes	2	Nothing	0	No	0	4
[30]	Yes	2	No	0	Blind to sham laser	1	No	0	3
[19]	Yes	2	No	0	Blind	1	No	0	3
[36]	No	0	Yes	2	Nothing	0	No	0	2
[23]	No	0	No	0	Nothing	0	No	0	0

Articles scoring ≤4/8 pts.

6. Regarding whether the effect could be noticed above or below the segment where the SMT was performed, results lacked consistency. In two of the studies ([23,39]), an effect was noted below the area of treatment. Studies [39,44] showed an effect above the area of treatment, whereas two of the studies ([36,37]) did not detect an effect above or below the relevant segment.

7. Outcomes were not affected by whether the control group received a sham treatment or no treatment at all.

Table 3 Distribution of subjects in study groups in articles where allocation procedure was not specified

Article	Total of subjects	SMT groups	Control group	No treatment
[23]	60	30	30	30
[39]	30	10	10	10
[19]	10	?	?	?
[31]	15	7	8	-
[33]	18	?	?	?
[30]	50	19	18	13
[32]	24	?	?	?

8. In 10 of the experiments (5 articles), patients with current pain were included ([18,19,21,32,33]). Three of these experiments ([19,21,32]) found increased PPT values after SMT. Article [33] showed relief of pain on stretching painful muscles after SMT but not relief of spontaneous pain, whereas article [21] reported that spontaneous pain was diminished by SMT. Articles [18,19] evaluated temperature-induced pain with similar results, that is to say there was a hypoalgesic action on second pain [18], no action on first pain [18] and no action in 2 trials on TSS.

Discussion

Summary of results

At the time of conducting this review, only one earlier systematic review was available on this subject. It examined 11 articles but was unable to draw conclusions regarding treatment effects [45]. For the present review, however, it was possible to identify 22 relevant articles, which made it possible to draw several conclusions in relation to the possible pain-reducing effect of SMT.

Table 4 Limitations to own studies given by authors of articles reviewed for the effect of SMT on pain

	Limitations given by authors
[37]	Short term effect. Unable to project results on duration.
	Small sample of patients.
	Did not include control group.
[42]	4 different muscle situations assessed (rest, isotonic contraction and 2 isometric contractions) (Is it enough?)
	Duration (only immediate effect assessed).
	Pop sound may have a placebo effect.
[23]	Healthy subjects.
	Unable to describe duration of effects.
[28]	Pain-free patients.
	Style, contacts or force used in the mobilization procedures.
[29]	Duration. Unable to project results on duration.
	Widespread to other areas?
	Subthreshold pain stimulation, what about real pain?
	Latent trigger points, subjects who may not be typical population.
	Control group did not receive an intervention; maybe pop sound has a placebo effect.
[44]	Lack of control and placebo groups.
	Short term effect. Unable to project results on duration.
	Did not take into account subject innate stiffness.
[38]	Short term effect. Unable to project results on duration.
	Placebo effect of cavitation.
	Only women.
[30]	Algometer was not very precise.
[43]	-
[18]	Assessment not blind.
	Chronic low back pain.
	Temporal summation as an indirect measure of central sensitization has been proven only in animals.
[19]	Short term effect. Unable to project results on duration.
	Possible placebo effect of cavitation.
	Small sample of patients.
[39]	Short term effect. Unable to project results on duration.
	Not patients.
	Possible placebo effect of cavitation.
	PPT
[20]	Short term effect. Unable to project results on duration.
	Placebo effect of cavitation.
	Healthy people, not patients.
[31]	Short term effect. Unable to project results on duration.
	Possible placebo effect of cavitation.
	Healthy people, not patients.

Table 4 Limitations to own studies given by authors of articles reviewed for the effect of SMT on pain *(Continued)*

[36]	Short term effect. Unable to project results on duration.
	Possible placebo effect of cavitation.
	Healthy people, not patients.
	No control, no sham group.
[40]	-
[21]	-
[32]	-
[33]	-
[41]	-
[35]	-
[34]	-

Thus our results indicate clearly that such an effect is achievable.

However, differences in effect exist according to whether the outcome is tested locally, regionally or systemically. An effect was clearly shown locally and regionally, whereas an effect is less clear in more distant parts of the body. Also the outcome differs according to the method of pain induction; pain induced by pressure, electricity, stretching of painful tissue, dermal irritation, and spontaneous pain all respond to SMT, whereas temperature-induced pain does not always respond.

Methodological considerations of our own review

One limitation of this review is that there is no generally accepted and validated quality check list for the type of experimental studies which we examined and so we had to select our own quality criteria, based on some basic methodological concepts important to our research questions. Such a check list can be modified, which could affect the overall quality assessment. According to our quality scoring system, studies scored between 8 and 16 points out of a possible 18. However, in order to discriminate better between studies, a more detailed scale could have resulted in different scores, which could perhaps have separated studies into more obviously "good" and "bad". However, the relevance, if any, of these quality items in relation to outcome, is not known and, in fact, the quality scores were not clearly associated with outcomes.

The strengths of this review are that the search for relevant articles was free of language bias, that the constituent articles were reviewed independently by two reviewers, that the results can be considered in relation to the quality of studies, that there was no arbitrary threshold for acceptable quality [46], that the check list tables are sufficiently detailed to allow readers to perform their own analysis of the information provided, and that there was a relatively large number of studies, making it possible to examine several research questions.

Table 5 Effect of SMT on experimentally induced pain by localization of pain reduction

	Systemic effect	Regional effect	Local or same metamere
SMT relieved pain	[23]* -Cervical SMT/hand- foot T°	[42] – C5-C6 SMT / deltoid PPT	[37]- C5-C6 SMT/ Elbow PPT
	[44]* -Lumbar Mob/hand PPT	[29] – Atlantooccipital SMT/masseter PPT	[44] – Lumbar mob/ L2 L5 (foot) PPT
	[43]* - Lumbar SMT/ deltoid PPT	[38] - Atlantooccipital SMT/sphenoid PPT	[19] - C5-C6 SMT/ Elbow PPT
	[18]* -Lumbar SMT/hand- foot PPT	[30] - Lumbar SMT/ 1st segment below PPT	[20] – C3-C4 SMT/ Trapezius PPT 5′
	[18]* -Lumbar SMT/hand- foot T°	[43]* - Lumbar SMT/ L3 PPT	[20] – C3-C4 SMT/ Trapezius PPT 10′
	[36]* -Lumbar SMT/hand- foot T°	[39] – C7-T1 SMT/ C5-C6 PPT	[31] - C5-C6 SMT/ Elbow PPT
		[39] – C7-T1 SMT/ C5-C6 PPT	[21] - C5-C6 SMT/ Elbow PPT
		[40] – Areas of stroking allodynia thorax SMT/ forearm	[21] - C5-C6 SMT/ Elbow spontaneous pain
		[40] – Mechanical hyperalgesia thorax SMT/ forearm	[32]- C5-C6 SMT/ Elbow PPT
		[40] – Spontaneous pain thorax SMT/ forearm	[33] - C5-C6 SMT/ Elbow PPT
			[33] –C5-C6 SMT/ Elbow stretch test
			[41]- Thoracic SMT/ spinous process electricity
			[35]- Thoracic SMT/ Thoracic PPT
SMT **did not** relieve pain	[23]* - Cervical SMT/hand- foot 1st Pain T°	[37] – T5-T8 SMT (sham SMT)/ Elbow PPT	[42] – C5-C6 SMT / Trapezius PPT
	[23]* - Cervical SMT/hand- foot PPT		[28]** – C5-C6 Mob(AP)/ C5-C6 PPT
	[18]* – Lumbar SMT/hand- foot 1st Pain T°		[19] - C5-C6 SMT/ Elbow Cold
	[36]* –Lumbar SMT/hand- foot 1st Pain T°		[19] - C5-C6 SMT/ Elbow Hot
			[20]*** C3-C4 SMT/ Trapezius PPT0′
			[32] - C5-C6 SMT/ Elbow Temp PPT
			[33] –C5-C6 SMT/ Elbow spontaneous pain
			[34]- C0-C1SMT/ C2 PPT

*Assessment not blinded.
**This was an anterior-posterior mobilization, not lateral as SMT.
***PPT measured just after SMT, but there was a hypoalgesic effect at 5′ and 10′.
T° = temperature.
PPT = pressure pain thresholds.

Methodological considerations for the studies under review

This review identified some common methodological problems, such as lack of blinded assessment that could weaken the evidence in these experimental studies. We considered one of the most important points to be that the assessor was blinded, to avoid expectation bias. Some studies ignored this issue. This aspect affected our interpretation of the systemic effect of SMT, as all five articles (10 trials) dealing with the systemic effects of SMT lacked a blinded assessor.

It is also important that the results be truthfully presented, and not exaggerated in some way, meaning that any subjects or data excluded from analysis should be accounted for. This was often ignored.

Another challenge was that of the control group. Ideally, the SMT should be matched against a suitable sham treatment and control procedure, and this was done in 12 studies. This is difficult with physical procedures, but several of the other 10 studies tried to make the best of the situation by selecting naive study subjects, and in some cases different types of treatment were compared (such as treatment in two areas of the spine), in which case no sham treatment would be necessary. However, whether a proper sham treatment was used or not, there were no obvious differences in the results, possibly indicating that the effect is very obvious and not affected to a large extent by expectations.

Potential confounders of these effects would be anxiety in general and fear of pain, known moderators of treatment outcomes in clinical practice. However, according to the three articles in which anxiety and fear of pain were studied, there were no statistically significant correlations between pain-related cognition, pain thresholds and the hypoalgesic response to SMT, indicating that the psychological aspect, considered to be so important in the perception of pain, perhaps does not come into play during experimental studies of this type.

Table 5a Effect of SMT on experimentally induced pain by localization of pain reduction in relation to the quality of studies

	Systemic effect	Regional effect	Local or same metamere
SMT relieved pain	[23]* -Cervical SMT/hand- foot T°	[42] – C5-C6 SMT / deltoid PPT	[37] – C5-C6 SMT/ Elbow PPT
	[44]* -Lumbar Mob/hand PPT	[29] – Atlantooccipital SMT/masseter PPT	[44] – Lumbar mob/ L2 L5 (foot) PPT
	[43]* - Lumbar SMT/ deltoid PPT	[38] - Atlantooccipital SMT/sphenoid PPT	K - C5-C6 SMT/ Elbow PPT
	[18]* -Lumbar SMT/hand- foot PPT	[30] - Lumbar SMT/ 1st segment below PPT	[20] – C3-C4 SMT/ Trapezius PPT 5′
	[18]* -Lumbar SMT/hand- foot T°	[43]* - Lumbar SMT/ L3 PPT	[20] – C3-C4 SMT/ Trapezius PPT 10′
	[36]* -Lumbar SMT/hand- foot T°	[39] – C7-T1 SMT/ C5-C6 PPT	[31] - C5-C6 SMT/ Elbow PPT
		[39] – C7-T1 SMT/ C5-C6 PPT	[21] - C5-C6 SMT/ Elbow PPT
		[40]– Areas of stroking allodynia thorax SMT/ forearm	[21]- C5-C6 SMT/ Elbow spontaneous pain
		[40] – Mechanical hyperalgesia thorax SMT/ forearm	[32]- C5-C6 SMT/ Elbow PPT
		[40] – Spontaneous pain thorax SMT/ forearm	[33] - C5-C6 SMT/ Elbow PPT
			[33] –C5-C6 SMT/ Elbow stretch test
			[41]- Thoracic SMT/ spinous process electricity
			[35]- Thoracic SMT/ Thoracic PPT
SMT **did not** relieve pain	[23]* - Cervical SMT/hand- foot 1st Pain T°	[37] – T5-T8 SMT (sham SMT)/ Elbow PPT	[42] – C5-C6 SMT / Trapezius PPT
	[23]* - Cervical SMT/hand- foot PPT		[28]** – C5-C6 Mob(AP)/ C5-C6 PPT
	[18]* – Lumbar SMT/hand- foot 1st Pain T°		[19]- C5-C6 SMT/ Elbow Cold
	[36]* –Lumbar SMT/hand- foot 1st Pain T°		[19] - C5-C6 SMT/ Elbow Hot
			[20]*** – C3-C4 SMT/ Trapezius PPT0′
			[32] - C5-C6 SMT/ Elbow Temp PPT
			[33] –C5-C6 SMT/ Elbow spontaneous pain
			[34]- C0-C1SMT/ C2 PPT

X- : Studies scoring ≤ 12 points on 18 point scale **and** ≤ 4 points on 8 point scale.
X- : Study scoring ≤ 4 points on 8 point scale and more than 12 points on 18 point scale.
X *: Studies where the assessor was not blinded.
** This was an anterior-posterior mobilization, not lateral as is usually the case in SMT.
*** Pressure pain thresholds measured just after spinal manipulation, but there was a hypoalgesic effect at 5′ and 10′.
T° = temperature.
PPT = pressure pain thresholds.

Comparison with another systematic review

Some of our results were corroborated by a newly published high quality review on this very topic [47]. This other review included 15 of our articles but, as they did not put a restriction on duration of symptoms in symptomatic people, they also incorporated 5 articles not included in our review. They defined effects as occurring "locally" or in "remote" areas, and pooled the results in all studies for the effects of PPT. They found the effects on PPT to be small in both areas but nevertheless statistically significant. When the data were separated for local and remote effect significance was only noted for the remote effect. They did not study any other pain–inducing method nor did they take into consideration the quality of studies, although they did perform a quality assessment.

Discussion of findings

Pain provoked by pressure, electricity, stretching of painful tissue, dermal irritation, or spontaneous pain all respond to SMT.

Experimental pain provoked by pressure was the most common method used to assess the effect of manipulation (27 out of 43 experiments). Unfortunately, the reports did not use the same units for reporting increased tolerance to pressure, making it difficult to compare outcomes, but SMT was shown to increase PPT values between 4.8% and 44.6%. That the algometer, used for this purpose, is a highly reliable method to measure pain [48] suggests that these results are robust. However, they cannot necessary be compared between studies because of different experimental situations.

Table 6 Detailed findings from literature review on effect of SMT on pain

Art	Effect of SMT on pain	Site of SMT/pain	Values	Local/regional/ systemic effect	Same/opposite side	Above/below	Pain form
[37]	The application of a cervical SMT, but not thoracic SMT, resulted in immediate bilateral hypoalgesic effect in patients with lateral epicondylitis.	SMT C5-C6 and T5-T8 /PPT both epicondyles	**Changes PPT in KiloPascals (differences)** PPT Cervical Thoracic affected side 88.6 (35.1%) 18.6 (0.8%) unaffected side 95.6 (25.4%) -40.5 (−0.9%)	Effect within the same segment.. Used SMT caudal level as placebo with no effect.	No significant differences between L and R side	Effect within the same segment. Used SMT caudal level as placebo with no effect.	Pressure
[42]	On deltoid, small effect at the same segment. Didn't work on trapezius and C5	SMT C5-C6 right / PPT upper trapezius, deltoid and C5 spinous process	**Changes PPT in Kg/cm^2 (differences)** PPT SMT Control Trapezius ipsilateral 0.2 0.3 Trapezius contralateral 0.4 0.1 Deltoid ipsilateral 0.3 -0.2 Deltoid contralateral 0.2 -0.2 C5 spinous process 0.1 -0.1	Small effect within the same segment	Comparison of sides baseline in table 2, but no differences p>.523 Bilateral increases of PPT	-	Pressure
[23]	SMT reduced TSS (temporal sensory summation) but not PPT	Lower cervical and upper thoracic region / T° on hand + popliteal fossa	PPT increased for all groups (not only SMT) from pre to post SMT (F=9.6, partial N^2=0.10)= SMT produced a significant reduction in TSS (p=.003)	Averages of lower extremity values were higher than upper extremity values	-	SMT worked at the same level or below	Pressure and Temperature (T°)
[28]	No effect	Cervical mobilization left C5-C6 / PPT left and right articular pillar of C5-C6	**Differences PPT pre/post treatment** Kpa F=0.168 p=0.168 Treatment 15.98 (+/− 4.8%) Manual contact 4.61 (+/− 0.2%) No contact 12.29 (+/− 3.5%)	No effect at same segment	-	-	Pressure
[29]	Small immediate increase of PPT	SMT atlantooccipital/ PPT on trigger points in the masseter and temporalis muscles	Differences before/after SMT in Kg/cm^2: SMT = 0.29 (10%) Soft mobilization = 0.00 control= 0.019	Regional effect of atlantooccipital SMT and effect on trigeminal area	-	-	Pressure
[44]	Hypoaglesia significant at test site and without differences between the rates of mobilization	Lumbar mobilization/L2 dermatome(thigh), L5 (foot), hand and L5 paraspinal	Mean of changes: 19,6% paraspinal muscles 14,2% L2 dermatome 13,4% L5 dermatom 12% hand (this suggest that changes are systemic)	lumbar hypoalgesia was greater than distal (P=0.0028)	-	SMT more effective on lumbar dermatomes than more cephalad dermatomes	Pressure
[38]	Small effect regionally	SMT atlantooccipital/ PPT over both sides of sphenoid bone (V)	PPT effect on group and time F=14.4 (p<0.001) SMT = 3.5 kg/cm^2 control = – 0.1 kg/cm^2	Regional level.	-	-	Pressure
[30]	Mobilization had a stronger effect on pain than SMT	SMT 1 segment below marked PPT (lumbar)	Mobilization = small increase (0.434 kg/cm^2 d= 0.78) SMT = decrease (−0.173 d= 0.36) Control = small decrease (−0.105 d= 0.25) but ANOVA further revealed non signification between groups.	Local and systemic effect but PPT values increase in a caudal direction	-	-	Pressure

Table 6 Detailed findings from literature review on effect of SMT on pain *(Continued)*

[43]	No differences between amplitudes (p= 0.864)	lumbar mobilization/ 1- right erector spinae (L3) 2- left patella (L3 dermatome) 3- proximal lateral sruface of left 5th metatarsal (S1 dermatome) 4- deltoid	PPT A B C 1 18.73% 14.57% 15.48% 2 17.93% 9.93% 10.67% 3 10.53% 15.57% 8.81% 4 19.06% 18.60% 11.69%	Local and systemic effect	-	-	Pressure
[18]	Significant changes in temporal summation, only for SMT	Lumbar SMT/ temporal summation on plantar surface (non dominant) and palmar surface (non dominant). Aδ fibers mediated pain sensitivity in non dominant forearm and calf	**Lumbar (local response)**: A- Aδ fibers sensibility: no differences between groups at 47°C(p= .73), or 49°C (p= . 96) No effect of time at 47°C (p= .31) or 49°C (p= . 94) No changes in Aδ fibers B- temporal summation: F= 3,41 (p= . 05), different by group assignment = Changes in temporal summation **Cervical (general response)**: A- No changes in Aδ fibers B- temporal summation: SMT group F= 6,78 (p= . 40), all groups had a decrease in temporal summation = Changes in temporal summation	Systemic effect, except for first pain.	-	-	T°differences Numeric Rating Scale (0–100) Before/after: Bike = −3,7 LE Exercise = 2,5 SMT= 19,9
[19]	Effect demonstrated for PPT but not for T°	SMT C5-C6 dominant side (right) / PPT , thermal pain thresholds (HPT - CPT) on lateral epicondyles (both sides)	**Differences SMT Control** PPT ipsilateral 121.5 (44.2%) 13.3 (4.4%) PPT contralateral 74.4 (17.7%) 6.1(1.7%) HPT ipsilateral (°C) 1.2 (2.9%) 0.7 (2.2%) HPT contralateral 1.5 (4.1%) -0.9 (1.9%) CPT ipsilateral −0.25(9.2%) -1.5 (9.6%) CPT contralateral 0.9 (18.1%)-1.0 (17.4%)	Same segment	Bilateral increase of PPT. No significant changes for T°	-	Pressure and T°
[39]	SMT changes PPT in both R and L C5-C6 zygapophyseal joints in healthy subjects	SMT C7-T1 / PPT C5-C6 zygapophyseal joints	Differences on PPT before/after: **Right side** SMT dominant: 53.1 SMT non-dominant: 80.7 Placebo: -2.7 **Left side** SMT dominant: 45.9 SMT non-dominant: 48.0 Placebo: -3.9	Effect at regional level	SMT changes PPT in both R and L C5-C6 zygapophyseal. joints in healthy subjects	SMT is also effective above and below of segment treated	Pressure
[20]	SMT changes pressure pain sensitivity in triggers points in the upper trapezius	SMT C3-C4 / PPT upper trapezius trigger points (TrPs)	**Differences pre/post SMT in Kg/cm^2 D**ifference Placebo SMT Pre post −0.06 d=0.35 0.08 d=0.4 Pre - 5' -0.2 d=1.1 0.1 d=0.5 Pre - 10' -0.22 d=1.1 0.12 d=0.44	Regional level	-	-	Pressure
[31]	SMT changes pressure pain sensitivity in epicondyles	SMT C5-C6 both sides / PPT on lateral epicondyles (both sides)	**Differences in Kg/cm^2** SMT ipsilateral 0.8 (35.5%) SMT contralateral 0.5 (24.8%) Placebo Ipsilateral 0.003(0.5%) Placebo contralateral 0.006 (0.4%) Control ipsilateral 0.003(0.5%) Control contralateral 0.006 (2.1%)	Same segment	No differences between L and R sides	-	Pressure

Table 6 Detailed findings from literature review on effect of SMT on pain *(Continued)*

[36]	SMT produces hypoalgesia in lumbar area but not in cervical (control) but no effect on 1st pain	Lumbar SMT/ TSS in plantar surface (non dominant) and palmar surface (non dominant). Aδ fibers mediated pain sensitivity in non dominant forearm and calf	Lumbar Innervated NRS Change 47°C 13.2 (17.2) 12.9 (17.9) 23.5 (17.3) NRS Change 49°C 1.2 (20.2) 6.3 (22.4) 12.1 (19.7) Cervical Innervated NRS Change 47°C −3.0 (13.7) 0.3 (11.6) 0.3 (10.2) NRS Change 49°C 1.9 (9.0) -0.4 (10.1) 1.7 (10.8) NRS= Numeric rating scale	Effect at regional level but not at systemic level	-	Effect at the same level, but not above	T°
[40]	Allodynia and hyperalgesia decrease with SMT	Non specific thoracic SMT / left and right forearm (capsaicin)	Pre-SMT Post-SMT Pre-sham Post-Sham Hyperalgesia(cm^2) 53 31 39 56 Allodynia (cm^2) 40 18 28 40 Spontaneous pain (ratings) 4.9 3.3 3.9 4.2	SMT decreases allodynia at regional level	-	-	Capsaicin
[21]	Effect on PPT	SMT C5-C6 / PPT over symptomatic segment, T°PT	PPT increases p: < 0.05 +/– 0.? % control +/– 2.?% placebo +/– 22.55 SMT VAS didn't work	Regional level	-	-	Pressure
[32]	Mobilization has an effect on pressure pain, not on temperature	Mobilization C5-C6 / PPT both elbows	PPT increases p: < 0.05 +/– –4.? % control +/– –7.?% placebo +/– 29 % SMT TPT didn't work	Regional level.	-	-	Pressure and T°
[33]	Increase of PPT	SMT cervical C5-C6 / PPT both elbows	**Changes pre/post treatment** SMT +/– 26% Placebo +/– –12% Control +/– 0.2%	Regional level.	-	-	Pressure
[41]	Elevation of pain tolerance in manipulated group	Thoracic manipulation/ Electric thresholds left and right articular pillar	**Intensity of current in mAmp** SMT Control Baseline 1.37 1.62 30" 2.05 1.46 2 min 2.43 1.46 5 min 2.70 1.56 10 min 3.30 1.86	Local level.	-	-	Electrical induction
[34]	No significant differences	SMT C0-C1/ PPT C2	preHVLA-HVLA -5′ -39.37 (76.07) Kpa (SD) preHVLA-HVLA-30′ -15.89 (87.50) preMET-MET-5′ -42.03 (62.37) preMET-MET-30′ -30.00 (69.53) preControl-Control-5′ -15.88 (83.62) preControl-Control-30′ -16.12 (62.49)	Local level.	-	-	Pressure
[35]	Mobilization and manipulation both produced a statistically significant increase in PPT in the thoracic spines of asymptomatic subjects. Mobilization more than SMT.	Thoracic manipulation T1-T4/ PPT on most tender thoracic vertebra	**Differences PPT pre/post treatment** Kpa (SD) Manipulation Mobilisation Control Pre-intervention 243.70 (95.22) 204.6 (85.52) 218.71 (82.91) Post-intervention 244.64 (91.59) 216.51 (90.50) 47.13 (96.87) Difference 0.94 (35.07) 11.88 (31.83) 28.42 (39.68)	Local level.	-	-	Pressure

T° = temperature.
PPT = pressure pain thresholds.
HPT = hot pain threshold.
CPT = cold pain threshold.

Nevertheless, it is not clear whether these changes are clinically significant. One author [44] referred to Moss [49], who stated that a 15% improvement in pressure pain tolerance is clinically important, but this statement rests on previous studies which dealt with osteoarthritic pain [50] and pain in an emergency service [51], not experimental pain. Therefore, the cut-off point at which the reduction of artificially induced pain has reached a clinically significant level is not known.

In addition, it cannot be concluded that the effect of SMT, as seen in these studies, would be as large in "naturally" painful areas. Therefore, it is not certain that the degree of pain reduction detected in experimental studies can be extrapolated to other situations.

Apart from pressure and temperature, other sources of pain were: capsaicin to irritate the skin followed by skin stroking to evoke allodynia, hyperalgesia induced by mechanical means, and spontaneous pain. In these instances also, SMT was generally able to reduce pain.

Pain provoked by temperature does not always respond to SMT.

Nine trials from five papers examined the effects of SMT on temperature induced pain. In 3 of the 6 tests examining second pain, an effect was found but none of the 3 trials evaluating first pain could demonstrate such an effect. This indicates that SMT may have an effect on C-fiber mediated "second pain" but not on the more acute "first pain" mediated by A-delta fibers. This finding may help to resolve the mechanisms by which SMT reduces pain.

How broadly does the effect extend?

Almost all authors discussed the possibility of a systemic effect of SMT but this was tested in only 5 studies (9 experiments). The results were clearly positive, although two of the authors concluded that local effects were stronger than more distant ones. However, none of these studies used a blinded assessor, and so the reported results must be treated with caution.

Nine experiments out of the ten that studied the regional effect were positive (see Table 5). However, in the reviewed articles, it was difficult to differentiate between strictly local vs. more regional effects. The definition of regional is uncertain if following the dermatomes, as they are known to differ from the text-book mappings [52] and the origins and distributions of cutaneous nerves differ from person to person. Thus, a negative outcome in one person may simply be due to that person having an unusual pattern of nerve distribution. Despite this, most studies showed a positive effect with relatively few study subjects. This could indicate either that negative results were removed from the analyses or that the effect is consistent.

Imprecise dermatomal mapping makes it difficult not only to separate clearly local from regional effects but also regional from systemic effects. Interestingly, the application of spinal manipulation at the atlanto-occipital region was found to have an effect on the masseter muscle, despite that muscle being supplied by the trigeminal nerve, which does not exit in the upper cervical spine. We therefore described this experiment under "regional" rather than "local" but it could perhaps equally well have been described it as "systemic".

Concerning the action of SMT on pain produced above or below the manipulated segment, only a few studies dealt with this and no consistent findings emerged. It would be necessary to test this issue specifically, in order to work out whether manipulation-induced impulses travel up or down the spinal cord or whether both occur.

Five studies investigated whether the hypoalgesic effect was mainly on the side of the manipulation or if it also appeared on the opposite side. These studies consistently demonstrated a bilateral effect.

Some clinical concepts

Although this review was based on experimentally induced pain, four findings emerged that could have a bearing on clinical practice, or at least on the concepts on which clinical practice is based. Manipulation of a "restricted motion segment", sometimes referred to as a "manipulable lesion", was not required for the "treatment" to have an effect. Additionally, the side of the manipulation was irrelevant. However, the results from this review can only be considered from a clinical point of view, if SMT has a similar effect on pain in a clinical context, which was not investigated in this study.

Finally, although a hypoalgesic effect was shown, it is not known how long this effect lasts; long enough for a person with pain to be able to regain a normal movement pattern or only long enough to give an impression of improvement? Other effects of the SMT were not studied in this review; effects such as improved biomechanics or reduced inflammation of disturbed tissues [53].

Implications in relation to research

There is a need to establish a coordinated global research strategy on the subject of SMT and pain relief. It seems unnecessary to conduct further research on simply whether SMT has an effect on pain or not. Rather, future work should focus on more precise questions such as why SMT does not affect first pain, and which mechanisms are involved in relieving pain locally, regionally and systemically. The magnitude and duration of effects also need to be defined. Consideration needs to be given to the most appropriate research designs for addressing different questions.

There could also be more consistency in outcome measures, and closer attention should be paid to important design elements such as blinded assessment, random allocation, appropriate control groups and, if possible, the recruitment of naïve subjects.

Implications in relation to education and clinical practice

Some of the findings in this review do not support the imperative of specificity, i.e. precise identification of a manipulable lesion and the exact level and side of the manipulation.

Conclusions

This systematic critical review of the literature confirms an effect of spinal manipulative therapy (SMT) on experimentally induced pain in human beings. This hypoalgesic effect seems to be local/regional and more consistent for pain provoked by pressure than by temperature. Further and better research is needed to determine if there is a systemic effect, to determine the exact mechanisms by which SMT relieves pain, the clinical importance and duration of the hypoalgesic effect.

Additional files

Additional file 1: Inclusion and exclusion criteria in a survey of the effect of spinal manipulative therapy on experimentally induced pain [2,46,54-60].

Additional file 2: The items selected for the quality checklist and their rationale.

Additional file 3: Effects of SMT on pressure pain thresholds (PPT).

Additional file 4: Effects of SMT on pain produced by temperature.

Additional file 5: Effects of SMT on pain produced by methods other than pressure or temperature.

Competing interests

Authors declare there are no conflicts of interest.

Authors' contributions

All authors instigated this review. MM and CLY designed the check-lists, reviewed the literature and wrote the first draft. BB and MAA provided expertise on the topic, assisted with the literature review and provided critical comments to the first draft. All authors reviewed the final manuscript and approved the final version.

Acknowledgements

Søren O'Neill, DC for helping at the stage of conception and generously sharing his insights into technical matters.

Author details

[1]EA 4532 CIAMS, UFR STAPS, University Paris-Sud, Paris, France. [2]The Research Department, The Spine Centre of Southern Denmark Hospital Lillebælt, Lillebælt, Denmark. [3]Institut Franco-Européen de Chiropratique, Paris, France. [4]Institute of Regional Health Services Research, Faculty of Health Sciences, University of Southern Denmark, Odense, Denmark. [5]Canadian Memorial Chiropractic College, Toronto, ON, Canada. [6]Institut Universitaire de France, Paris, France.

References

1. *International Association for the Study of Pain Taxonomy.* http://www.iasp-pain.org/AM/Template.cfm?Section=Pain_Defi. . .isplay.cfm&ContentID=1728#Pain.
2. Kandel ESJ, Jessell T: ***Principles of neural science**, vol.* Internationalth edition. Fourth edn: McGraw-Hill; 2000.
3. Tandon OP, Malhotra S, Tandon S, D'Silva I: **Neurophysiology of pain: insight to orofacial pain.** *Indian J Physiol Pharmacol* 2003, **47**(3):247–269.
4. Wall M: **Wall and Melzack's textbook of pain.** In *5th edn.* Edited by Mahon SM. Elservier; 2006:3–201.
5. Ji R, Kohno T, Moore KA, Woolf CJ: **Central sensitization and LTP: do pain and memory share similar mechanisms?** *Trends Neurosci* 2003, **26**(12):696–705.
6. Mense S, Gerwin R: **Central nervous mechanisms of muscle pain: ascending pathways, central sensitization, and pain-modulating systems.** In *Muscle Pain: Understanding the Mechanisms.* Springer; 2010:126–-144.
7. Rhudy JL, Williams AE, McCabe KM, Nguyen M, Rambo P: **Affective modulation of nociception at spinal and supraspinal levels.** *Psychophysiology* 2005, **42**(5):579–587.
8. Villemure C, Bushnell MC: **Cognitive modulation of pain: how do attention and emotion influence pain processing?** *Pain* 2002, **95**(3):195–199.
9. Walter H: **The biomechanics of spinal manipulation.** *J Bodyw Mov Ther* 2010, **14**(3):280–286.
10. Maigne J-Y, Vautravers P: **Mechanism of action of spinal manipulative therapy.** *Joint Bone Spine* 2003, **70**(5):336–341.
11. Vernon H, Mrozek J: **A revised definition of manipulation.** *J Manipulative Physiol Ther* 2005, **28**(1):68–72.
12. Flynn T, Fritz J, Wainner R, Whitman J: **The audible pop is not necessary for successful spinal high-velocity thrust manipulation in individuals with low back pain.** *Arch Phys Med Rehabil* 2003, **84:**1057–1060.
13. Flynn T, Childs J, Fritz J: **The audible pop from high-velocity thrust manipulation and outcome in individuals with low back pain.** *J Manipulative Physiol Ther* 2006, **29:**40–45.
14. Cramer G, Ross K, Pocius J, Cantu J, Laptook E, Fergus M, Gregerson D, Selby S, Raju P: **Evaluating the relationship among cavitation, zygapophyseal joint gapping, and spinal manipulation: an exploratory case series.** *J Manipulative Physiol Ther* 2011, **34**(1):2–14.
15. Cleland J, Flynn T, Childs J, Eberhart S: **The audible pop from thoracic spine thrust manipulation and its relation to short-term outcomes in patients with neck pain.** *J Man Manipulative Ther* 2007, **15**(3):143–154.
16. Bialosky JE, Bishop MD, Robinson ME, George SZ: **The relationship of the audible pop to hypoalgesia associated with high-velocity, low-amplitude thrust manipulation: a secondary analysis of an experimental study in pain-free participants.** *J Manipulative Physiol Ther* 2010, **33**(2):117–124.
17. Clark B, Goss D, Walkowski S, Hoffman R, Ross A, Thomas J: **Neurophysiologic effects of spinal manipulation in patients with chronic low back pain.** *BMC Musculoskelet Disord* 2011, **12**(1):170.
18. Bialosky JE, Bishop MD, Robinson ME, Zeppieri G Jr, George SZ: **Spinal manipulative therapy has an immediate effect on thermal pain sensitivity in people with low back pain: a randomized controlled trial.** *Phys Ther* 2009, **89**(12):1292–1303.
19. Fernández-Carnero J, Fernández-de-las-Peñas C, Cleland J: **Immediate hypoalgesic and motor effects after a single cervical spine manipulation in subjects with lateral epicondylalgia.** *J Manipulative Physiol Ther* 2008, **31**(9):675–681.
20. Ruiz-Sáez M, Fernández-de-las-Peñas C, Blanco C, Martínez-Segura R, García-León R: **Changes in pressure pain sensitivity in latent myofascial trigger points in the upper trapezius muscle after a cervical spine manipulation in pain-free subjects.** *J Manipulative Physiol Ther* 2007, **30**(8):578–583.
21. Sterling M, Jull G, Wright A: **Cervical mobilisation: concurrent effects on pain, sympathetic nervous system activity and motor activity.** *Man Ther* 2001, **6**(2):72–81.
22. Joel GP: **Neurophysiological effects of spinal manipulation.** *Spine J* 2002, **2**(5):357–371.
23. Bishop MD, Beneciuk JM, George SZ: **Immediate reduction in temporal sensory summation after thoracic spinal manipulation.** *Spine J* 2011, **11**(5):440–446.
24. Bialosky JE, Bishop MD, Price DD, Robinson ME, George SZ: **The mechanisms of manual therapy in the treatment of musculoskeletal pain: a comprehensive model.** *Man Ther* 2009, **14**(5):531–538.
25. Liberati A, Altman D, Tetzlaff J, Mulrow C, Gøtzsche P, Ioannidis J, Clarke M, Devereaux P, Kleijnen J, Moher D: **The PRISMA statement for reporting systematic reviews and meta-analyses of studies that evaluate health care interventions: explanation and elaboration.** *J Clin Epidemiol* 2009, **62**(10):e1–e34.

26. Moher D, Hopewell S, Schulz K, Montori V, Gøtzsche P, Devereaux P, Elbourne D, Egger M, Altman D: **CONSORT 2010 explanation and elaboration: updated guidelines for reporting parallel group randomised trials.** *Int J Surg* 2011, **1**:27–54.
27. Furlan A, Pennick V, Bombardier C, Van Tulder M: **2009 updated method guidelines for systematic reviews in the Cochrane back review group.** *Spine* 2009, **34**(18):1929–1941.
28. Soon B, Schmid A, Fridriksson E, Gresslos E, Cheong P, Wright A: **A crossover study on the effect of cervical mobilization on motor function and pressure pain threshold in pain-free individuals.** *J Manipulative Physiol Ther* 2010, **33**(9):652–658.
29. Oliveira-Campelo N, Rubens-Rebelatto J, Marti N, Vallejo F, Alburquerque-Sendi N, Fernandez-de-Las-Penas C: **The immediate effects of atlanto-occipital joint manipulation and suboccipital muscle inhibition technique on active mouth opening and pressure pain sensitivity over latent myofascial trigger points in the masticatory muscles.** *J Orthop Sports Phys Ther* 2010, **40**(5):310–317.
30. Thomson O, Haig L, Mansfield H: **The effects of high-velocity low-amplitude thrust manipulation and mobilisation techniques on pressure pain threshold in the lumbar spine.** *Int J Osteopathic Med* 2009, **12**:56–62.
31. Fernandez-de-las-Penas C, Perez-de-Heredia M, Brea-Rivero M, Miangolarra-Page J: **Immediate effects on pressure pain threshold following a single cervical spine manipulation in healthy subjects.** *J Orthop Sports Phys Ther* 2007, **37**(6):325–329.
32. Vicenzino B, Collins D, Benson H, Wright A: **An investigation of the interrelationship between manipulative therapy-induced hypoalgesia and sympathoexcitation.** *J Manipulative Physiol Ther* 1998, **21**(7):448–453.
33. Vicenzino B, Collins D, Wright A: **The initial effects of a cervical spine manipulative physiotherapy treatment on the pain and dysfunction of lateral epicondylalgia.** *Pain* 1996, **68**(1):69–74.
34. Hamilton L, Boswell C, Fryer G: **The effects of high-velocity, low-amplitude manipulation and muscle energy technique on suboccipital tenderness.** *Int J Osteopathic Med* 2007, **10**:42–49.
35. Fryer G, Carub J, McIver S: **The effect of manipulation and mobilisation on pressure pain thresholds in the thoracic spine.** *J Osteopathic Med* 2004, **7**(1):8–14.
36. George SZ, Bishop MD, Bialosky JE, Zeppieri G, Robinson ME: **Immediate effects of spinal manipulation on thermal pain sensitivity: an experimental study.** *BMC Musculoskelet Disord* 2006, **7**(1):68.
37. Fernández-Carnero J, Cleland JA, Arbizu RLT: **Examination of motor and hypoalgesic effects of cervical vs thoracic spine manipulation in patients with lateral epicondylalgia: a clinical trial.** *J Manipulative Physiol Ther* 2011, **34**(7):432–440.
38. Mansilla-Ferragut P, Fernández-de-las Peñas C, Alburquerque-Sendín F, Cleland JA, Boscá-Gandía JJ: **Immediate effects of atlanto-occipital joint manipulation on active mouth opening and pressure pain sensitivity in women with mechanical neck pain.** *J Manipulative Physiol Ther* 2009, **32**(2):101–106.
39. Fernández-de-las-Peñas C, Alonso-Blanco C, Cleland J, Rodríguez-Blanco C, Alburquerque-Sendín F: **Changes in pressure pain thresholds over C5-C6 zygapophyseal joint after a cervicothoracic junction manipulation in healthy subjects.** *J Manipulative Physiol Ther* 2008, **31**(5):332–337.
40. Mohammadian P, Gonsalves A, Tsai C, Hummel T, Carpenter T: **Areas of capsaicin-induced secondary hyperalgesia and allodynia are reduced by a single chiropractic adjustment: a preliminary study.** *J Manipulative Physiol Ther* 2004, **27**(6):381–387.
41. Terrett A, Vernon H: **Manipulation and pain tolerance. A controlled study of the effect of spinal manipulation on paraspinal cutaneous pain tolerance levels.** *Am J Phys Med* 1984, **63**(5):217–225.
42. Maduro de Camargo V, Alburquerque-Sendín F, Bérzin F, Cobos Stefanelli V, Rodrigues de Souza D, Fernández-de-las-Peñas C: **Immediate effects on electromyographic activity and pressure pain thresholds after a cervical manipulation in mechanical neck pain: a randomized controlled trial.** *J Manipulative Physiol Ther* 2011, **34**(4):211–220.
43. Krouwel O, Hebron C, Willett E: **An investigation into the potential hypoalgesic effects of different amplitudes of PA mobilisations on the lumbar spine as measured by pressure pain thresholds (PPT).** *Man Ther* 2010, **15**(1):7–12.
44. Willett E, Hebron C, Krouwel O: **The initial effects of different rates of lumbar mobilisations on pressure pain thresholds in asymptomatic subjects.** *Man Ther* 2010, **15**(2):173–178.
45. Vernon H: **Qualitative review of studies of manipulation-induced hypoalgesia.** *J Manipulative Physiol Ther* 2000, **23**:134–138.
46. Chesterton L, Sim J, Wright C, Foster N: **Interrater reliability of algometry in measuring pressure pain thresholds in healthy humans, using multiple raters.** *Clin J Pain* 2007, **23**(9):760–766.
47. Coronado RA, Gay CW, Bialosky JE, Carnaby GD, Bishop MD, George SZ: **Changes in pain sensitivity following spinal manipulation: a systematic review and meta-analysis.** *J Electromyogr Kinesiol* 2012, (0).
48. Chesterton LSS, Wright J, Christine C, Foster NE: **Interrater Reliability of Algometry in Measuring Pressure Pain Thresholds in Healthy Humans, Using Multiple Raters.** *Clin J Pain* 2007, **23**(9):760–766.
49. Moss P, Sluka K, Wright A: **The initial effects of knee joint mobilization on osteoarthritic hyperalgesia.** *Man Ther* 2007, **12**(2):109–118.
50. Bird SB, Dickson EW: **Clinically significant changes in pain along the visual analog scale.** *Ann Emerg Med* 2001, **38**(6):639–643.
51. Bellamy N, Bell MJ, Goldsmith CH, Pericak D, Walker V, Raynauld JP, Torrance GW, Tugwell P, Polisson R: **Evaluation of WOMAC 20, 50, 70 response criteria in patients treated with hylan G-F 20 for knee osteoarthritis.** *Ann Rheum Dis* 2005, **64**(6):881–885.
52. Downs MB, LaPorte C: **Conflicting dermatome maps: educational and clinical implications.** *J Orthop Sports Phys Ther* 2011, **41**(6):427–434.
53. Leach RA: **The chiropractic theories.** In *Fourth edn.* Edited by Darcy P. Lippincott Williams & Wilkins; 2004:131–197–235–246.
54. Schmelz M: **Translating nociceptive processing into human pain models.** *Exp Brain Res* 2009, **196**(1):173–178.
55. Modir J, Wallace M: **Human experimental pain models 2: the cold pressor model.** *Analgesia - Meth Mol Biol* 2010, **617**:165–168.
56. Graven-Nielsen T, McArdle A, Phoenix J, Arendt-Nielsen L, Staehelin Jensen T, Jackson MJ, Edwards RHT: **In vivo model of muscle pain: Quantification of intramuscular chemical, electrical, and pressure changes associated with saline-induced muscle pain in humans.** *Pain* 1997, **69**(1–2):137–143.
57. Graven-Nielsen T, Fenger-Gron LS, Svensson P, Steengaard-Pedersen K, Arendt-Nielsen L, Jensen TS: **Quantification of deep and superficial sensibility in saline-induced muscle pain-a psychophysical study.** *Somatosens Mot Res* 1998, **15**(1):46–53.
58. Modir J, Wallace M: **Human experimental pain models 3: heat/capsaicin sensitization and intradermal capsaicin models.** *Analgesia - Meth Mol Biol* 2010, **617**:169–174.
59. Müller H: **Neuroplasticity and chronification of pain.** *Anästhesiology Intensivmedizin Notfallmed Schmerztherapie* 2000, **35**(05):274–284.
60. Zhuo M: **Central plasticity in pathological pain.** *Novartis Found Symp* 2004, **261**:132–145. discussion 145–5.

12

Evaluation of a modified clinical prediction rule for use with spinal manipulative therapy in patients with chronic low back pain: a randomized clinical trial

Paul E Dougherty[1,2,3*], Jurgis Karuza[2,4,5], Dorian Savino[1] and Paul Katz[6,7]

Abstract

Background: Spinal Manipulative Therapy (SMT) and Active Exercise Therapy (AET) have both demonstrated efficacy in the treatment of Chronic Lower Back Pain (CLBP). A Clinical Prediction Rule (CPR) for responsiveness to SMT has been validated in a heterogeneous lower back pain population; however there is a need to evaluate this CPR specifically for patients with CLBP, which is a significant source of disability.

Methods: We conducted a randomized controlled trial (RCT) in Veteran Affairs and civilian outpatient clinics evaluating a modification of the original CPR (mCPR) in CLBP, eliminating acute low back pain and altering the specific types of SMT to improve generalizability. We enrolled and followed 181 patients with CLBP from 2007 to 2010. Patients were randomized by status on the mCPR to undergo either SMT or AET twice a week for four weeks. Providers and statisticians were blinded as to mCPR status. We collected outcome measures at 5, 12 and 24-weeks post baseline. We tested our study hypotheses by a general linear model repeated measures procedure following a univariate analysis of covariance approach. Outcome measures included, Visual Analogue Scale, Bodily pain subscale of SF-36 and the Oswestry Disability Index, Patient Satisfaction and Patient Expectation.

Results: Of the 89 AET patients, 69 (78%) completed the study and of the 92 SMT patients, 76 (83%) completed the study. As hypothesized, we found main effects of time where the SMT and AET groups showed significant improvements in pain and disability from baseline. There were no differences in treatment outcomes between groups in response to the treatment, given the lack of significant treatment x time interactions. The mCPR x treatment x time interactions were not significant. The differences in outcomes between treatment groups were the same for positive and negative on the mCPR groups, thus our second hypothesis was not supported.

Conclusions: We found no evidence that a modification of the original CPR can be used to discriminate CLBP patients that would benefit more from SMT. Further studies are needed to further clarify the patient characteristics that moderate treatment responsiveness to specific interventions for CLBP.

Trial registration: ISRCTN30511490

Keywords: Clinical prediction rule, Chronic lower back pain, Spinal manipulative therapy, Active exercise therapy, Randomized controlled trial

* Correspondence: paul.dougherty@va.gov
[1]Canandaigua Veterans Affairs Medical Center, Canandaigua, NY, USA
[2]New York Chiropractic College, Seneca Falls, NY, USA
Full list of author information is available at the end of the article

Background

Chronic lower back pain (CLBP) is a significant public health problem in both Veterans and the general population [1,2]. Chronic Lower Back Pain is not only a problem in the US, the recent global burden of disease reports that it is one of the most common causes of years lived with disability [2]. Chronic lower back pain is secondary only to respiratory conditions in reasons for visiting primary care [3]. Despite over 200 treatments for CLBP, the costs of treating CLBP have risen 65% in the last 10 years with no appreciable improvement in patient outcomes [4,5].

One contributory factor is inappropriate management due to poor understanding of prognostic factors [6,7]. This is particularly relevant for primary care providers who must make decisions on management strategies for this very common problem [8]. Spinal Manipulative Therapy (SMT) and Active Exercise Therapy (AET) are two commonly utilized, evidence based, interventions for CLBP [9] however neither has shown superiority [10]. It has been hypothesized that identification of specific characteristics predicting clinical responsiveness to these interventions would improve the outcomes through appropriate management [11].

The desire to identify these specific patient characteristics has led to the development of clinical prediction rules (CPR). A CPR is a clinical tool that quantifies individual contributions that various components of the history as well as the physical examination results make towards the diagnosis, prognosis, or likely response to treatment in an individual patient [12]. The CPR for SMT (CPR SMT) was first reported in 2002 [12] and then a validation study was published in 2004 [13]. This CPR predicted responsiveness in patients with lower back pain (LBP) to SMT [13]. Although this is the most studied of the CPRs, it still has not achieved the level of validation to be recommended for general clinical practice [14]. Furthermore, the previous validation studies of CPR SMT included acute, sub-acute and chronic conditions, and so their generalizability specifically to CLBP is unclear. A recent systematic review stated that there "is a lack of good quality RCTs validating the effects of a clinical prediction rule for low back pain" [15].

The current study evaluates the generalizability of the CPR for SMT to a CLBP population. The current study modified the original CPR for SMT for use with a CLBP population therefore creating a modified CPR for SMT (mCPR) that applies four of the five originally proposed components of the CPR for SMT.

Study hypotheses

Based on previous data, our first hypothesis is that patients in both SMT and AET groups would demonstrate statistically and clinically significant improvements in disability and pain from baseline [9,10]. Our second hypothesis predicts that the mCPR moderates the comparative effectiveness of treatment in the SMT group but not the AET treatment group. Based on the data from Childs et al. [13], we hypothesized that the mCPR modifies the comparative effectiveness of (i.e., the differences between) the two treatment groups. We expect the comparative effectiveness between the two treatment arms for the positive on the mCPR group would be different from the comparative effectiveness between the two treatment arms for the negative on the mCPR group.

Methods

Trial design

The study was a prospective RCT using a stratified permutated block design conducted between 2007 and 2010. Chronic lower back pain patients were recruited and evaluated for their status on a mCPR for responsiveness to SMT. Patients were then randomized to receive either SMT or AET twice a week for four weeks. The protocol received Institutional Review Board approval through the Syracuse/Canandaigua Veterans' Affairs (VA) Medical Centers (MIRB#00367) and through the New York Chiropractic College (NYCC) (IRB#07-01). Trial Registration: ISRCTN30511490- http://www.controlled-trials.com/ISRCTN30511490/.

Participants

Our patients were 181 adults who met the following inclusions criteria. Inclusion: LBP for ≥12 weeks prior to enrollment, pain upon deep palpation of the lumbar erector spinae, LBP from L1 to sacroiliac joint inclusive, live within 50 miles of Rochester, NY, have a baseline >30 mm on the Visual Analogue Scale (VAS) [16] and >20% on the Oswestry Disability Index (ODI) [17]. Patients had to be willing to undergo no new or different treatment during the study intervention and follow up period, although they were allowed to continue any medications.

Exclusion: Radiographic or clinical evidence of cauda equina syndrome, spinal neoplasia or metastatic disease, destructive joint pathology such as rheumatoid arthritis, bowel/bladder dysfunction associated with the LBP, peripheral neuropathy or progressive lumbosacral radiculopathy, progressive myelopathy or neurogenic claudication and spinal surgery within the past six months. Patients were excluded if they had undergone a course of SMT or supervised AET within the six months prior to enrollment into the study and if they could not perform an exercise program based on a New York Heart Association Classification of grade III or IV [18].

To attempt to reduce any variability of the assessment of the mCPR physical examination elements, all study patients were screened by the same clinician, the VA patients were screened in a VA setting and the non-VA patients were screened at a local hospital clinic. Based on the response to the Fear Avoidance Belief Questionnaire (FABQ), subjective symptoms and the physical exam findings, patients were categorized in terms of whether they were positive or negative on the modified clinical prediction rule [13]. Patients within each group were then randomized into either the SMT or AET treatments.

Study settings

This multisite RCT was conducted in Rochester, NY at the VA Outpatient chiropractic and physical therapy clinics and two civilian outpatient chiropractic clinics and two civilian outpatient physical therapy clinics. The SMT interventions were carried out by licensed chiropractors (DC) and the AET interventions were carried out by licensed physical therapists (PT) at both the VA and in the private locations. Prior to initiation of the study the providers (DC and PT) met to discuss evaluation and treatment parameters and a video was made as a resource for all providers to refer to if they had questions.

Interventions

Spinal Manipulative Therapy, as defined in this study, included high velocity low amplitude spinal manipulation and/or flexion distraction therapy or mobilization, and advise on heat/ice all of which are commonly performed by manual therapists [19-21]. The practitioner was allowed to give the patient one of two stretches to do at home, either "cat/camel stretch" or "knee to chest stretch." While this definition differed from the original CPR validation study, it was felt that this allowed for greater generalizability of the SMT arm of the study to those who perform manual therapy.

Active Exercise Therapy included directional preference exercises, lumbar stabilization, general flexibility, and specific training exercises [22-24]. The therapists were given freedom to choose the active care exercise that they felt was best suited to the patient's needs, but could only utilize those exercises that were included in the protocol and no specific limit was given on the number of exercises that could be prescribed. No passive stretching or modalities such as electric stimulation or ultrasound were allowed. Both treatment were performed twice a week for four weeks [25].

Outcomes

The study evaluated improvement in pain using the VAS [16] and the SF-36 pain subscale [26] and disability using the ODI [17] in CLBP patients. The treatment outcomes are described in Table 1. All outcome measures have previously been validated in a CLBP population. Outcome measures were collected at baseline, 5, 12 and 24-weeks post baseline. A face valid open-ended Patient Expectation scale was administered prior to and after randomization to detect potential patient bias associated with the assigned treatment intervention. This scale asked patients to "Circle below on the scale from 0 to 10 how confident you are that the treatment you will be receiving will be successful at reducing your low-back pain." Responses were measured on an 11 point scale anchored by "Not Confident" and "Confident". As an adjunct to the outcomes, we examined the patients' satisfaction at the end of the treatment at the last data collection point, the 24-week follow up visit, by administering a Patient Satisfaction survey [27]. We computed a mean patient treatment satisfaction score for each subject by averaging the ten patient satisfaction questions. Four of the items were reversed scored and were recoded so that the higher the score indicated the more satisfied the subject. The scale was reliable, (Cronbach's alpha = .85). We performed a 2 × 2 analysis of variance on the treatment satisfaction score with the mCPR and treatment arm as the two between subject factors.

Randomization

Randomization to treatments was through a random number producing algorithm. The same screening clinician performed the history and physical exam for all study participants. The screening clinician was blinded to the results of the FABQ, and thus did not assign the status on the rule. The study coordinator administered the baseline questionnaires including: VAS, ODI, SF-36, FABQ and the Patient Expectation scale. The de-identified results of the FABQ and the subjective and objective components of the mCPR were faxed to the evaluator who combined the data and determined the status on the mCPR. Once the status was determined the evaluator utilized the random number algorithm to assign the intervention. The assignment of treatment intervention was then faxed to the study coordinator who scheduled the first visit with the appropriate provider. The screening clinician, the statistician and the treating clinician were all blinded to the status on the mCPR. The patient data on the mCPR was revealed upon completion of the study. At the first treatment visit, the patient was given the second Patient Expectation scale. Patients were recruited through radio ads, posters, and physician recruitment.

Modified clinical prediction rule

The original study validating the CPR for SMT included acute, sub-acute and chronic lower back pain patients; however the median duration of pain for participants was 27 days [13]. Therefore, most of the patients in the original validation were classified as having acute and

Table 1 Summary of outcome measures

Variable	Definition
VAS: Visual Analogue Scale	A patient completed analogue measure that evaluates pain intensity on a 100 mm long horizontal line.
ODI Oswestry Disability Index	The back pain specific, self-rating scale to measure the degree of functional impairment that a subject is experiencing in a number of activities of daily living.
Patient Satisfaction	A self-developed questionnaire based on Cherkin's satisfaction questionnaire.
Patient Expectation	The recovery expectations measured using a time-based, specific single-item tool produced a strong prediction of outcome.
SF-36: Short Form-36 item health survey	A set of generic, coherent, and easily administered physical and mental quality-of-life measures.

sub-acute lower back pain. Given that much of the morbidity associated with back pain is in chronic lower back pain patients, we felt that it was necessary to assess a modification of the rule in an exclusively CLBP population. The original mCPR criteria included: pain <16 days, pain proximal to the knee, internal hip rotation of greater than 35 degrees, hypomobility of one or greater lumbar segments and FABQ work subscale score of less than 19 [12]. The original rule was modified to exclude the criteria concerning pain <16 days, this allowed for only CLBP patients to be included. In order for a patient to be considered positive on the mCPR, they had to have at least three of the four criteria positive from the original rule.

Power analysis

Paralleling Child et al's study [13], we based sample size calculation on our primary outcome disability measure, the ODI. Based on the work of Ostelo et al. [28] a minimally clinically significant outcome for the ODI is 10 points. Our power analysis was based on detecting a difference that size or larger when comparing the effectiveness between the two treatment arms in both the positive on the mCPR group and negative on the mCPR group at each time of measurement which would be necessary in the test of our second hypothesis. We required 112 patients in a balanced design, or 28 patients in each group assuming an α level of 0.05, two tailed test, and a power (1-beta) of .80. Our power analysis for our secondary outcomes, the VAS, and SF-36 pain sub score, required the same or fewer patients to detect the same clinically meaningful differences. Since we treated them as secondary outcomes, we did not perform an alpha correction for the power analysis. Because of difficulties in recruiting patients who were negative on the mCPR and given our randomization strategy we were forced to recruit additional patients who were positive on the mCPR until we reached the minimum number of patients who were negative on the mCPR. Rather than exclude them from the analyses, and thus possibly create a bias, we kept the additional patients who were positive mCRP, which resulted in an excess of patients in the positive mCPR cells.

Statistical analyses

We tested our study hypotheses a repeated measures analysis of variance strategy using Statistical Package for the Social Sciences (SPSS) version 21. The patients' status on the mCPR (negative, positive) and the treatment group the patients were randomized to (SMT, AET) defined the between subject factors. The time of measurement (baseline, 5, 12 and 24-weeks post baseline) defined the within subject repeated measures factor. To control for age and length of pain significant differences and the fact that this was a multi-site study, we included them as covariates in the analyses.

We articulated our hypothesis in terms of main effects and interactions, as defined by our study design, and we employed traditional analyses of covariance tests of significance to test our derived hypothesis. We tested our hypothesis 1, which predicts significant clinical improvement in patients' outcomes in both SMT and AET, by testing the main effect of time. We would expect a significant main effect of time, which would reflect a significant improvement in outcomes from baseline in both treatment groups. We also tested for mean differences between treatment groups in response to treatment over time, which is tested by the treatment × time interaction, to see whether the pattern of improvement was similar in the two treatment groups.

We tested our hypothesis 2, which predicts that the mCPR modifies the comparative effectiveness of (i.e., the differences between) the two treatment groups, i.e., the comparative effectiveness between the treatment arms for the positive on the mCPR group is different from the comparative effectiveness between the treatment arms for the negative on the mCPR group by examining the mCPR × treatment × time of measurement interaction.

We report the effect sizes using partial eta^2. Partial eta^2 is an effect size measurement for analysis of variance with more than one independent variable and conceptually is the proportion of variance in the dependent variable explained by an effect while controlling for other effects.

We used an intention to treat approach that included all enrolled patients who met inclusion criteria regardless of whether they completed the study. Ten patients dropped out. There was no significant difference in the dropout rate across the study groups. We used multiple imputation to handle missing data. We conducted the multiple imputation using SPSS missing values module (version 21) with five imputation runs using an iterative Markov chain Monte Carlo (MCMC) method with a linear regression model and assuming data missing at random.

We included the outcome measures at baseline and followups, subject expectations for treatment effectiveness, and the subject characteristics, with categorical variables dummy coded, as the variables in the multiple imputation.

Results

A total 953 patients were phone screened of which 390 patients were physically screened. A total of 181 CLBP patients were enrolled; 89 were randomized into AET of these 69 (78%) completed the study and 92 to SMT of these 76 (83%) completed the study. (See Figure 1 for details).

Patient characteristics

As seen in Table 2, the sample was predominately white, male, overweight, and with a mean age ranging from 53 to 61 years. Most attended college or graduated from college. While patients who were recruited from and treated in VA clinics accounted for slightly less than half the patients, the percentage of VA patients across groups was not significantly different. Slightly more than one third of the patients self-reported arthritis on their clinical history, and about one third of the patients self-reported a depression diagnosis. We did not find any significant differences between patients who were positive on the mCPR and patients negative on the mCPR with the exception of age and self-report of pain duration. We included these patient characteristics as covariates in the analysis.

Also seen in Table 2, nearly all patients previously sought allopathic medicine treatment for the CLBP and a majority had previously sought chiropractic treatment in all groups.

We next examined patient expectations of the treatment's effectiveness prior to and after randomization to assure that patients who may have had preconceived biases toward one treatment or another would be detected, as this would have the potential to affect treatment responsiveness [29]. We performed a 4 × 2 analyses of variance with the study group as the between subject factor, and the time of the expectation rating (prior to randomization and post randomization before the start of treatment) as the within subject factor. We present the group × time interaction in Table 3. Patients became slightly more positive in their expectations for the treatment's effectiveness after randomization to their treatment arm compared to their expectations prior to randomization (main effect of time, $p = .02$). This increase was similar across the four study groups, as indicated by the absence of a significant study group × time interaction ($p = .43$). This finding indicates that patients did not seem to lower their expectations once they knew which treatment they would be receiving.

Given that this was a multisite study, before combining the data, we tested for the presence of site differences. We ran preliminary analyses that included site of treatment as a between subject factor. We found no significant site of treatment main effects or interactive effects of site of treatment with treatment group, mCPR, or time of measurement on the outcome measures.

With the absence of site of treatment effects, we pooled data across treatment sites. Even so, we included site as a covariate in our analysis.

We performed separate analyses on our three outcome measures, i.e., VAS, ODI, and the SF-36 pain subscales. We present the means and standard deviations for the outcome measures at each point in time in Table 4.

Test of hypothesis 1

We found a significant time of measurement effect for VAS ($p = .05$, partial $eta^2 = .02$), ODI ($p = .001$, partial $eta^2 = .04$), and the SF-36 pain subscale ($p = .003$, partial $eta^2 = .03$). We found no significant treatment arm × time interactions ($p > .50$). The SMT and AET groups both exhibited similar improvements in pain and disability outcomes after treatment. To help interpret the significant main effect of time, we then tested the within-patients linear, quadratic, and cubic contrasts with analysis of variance for each of the three outcome measures. We only found significant linear contrasts for the VAS ($p = .03$), SF-36 pain subscale ($p = .002$) and ODI ($p = .001$) with pain and disability dropping from the baseline to the post treatment follow ups (see Figure 2). The pattern of results support hypothesis 1.

Test of hypothesis 2

We did not find significant mCPR × treatment × time of measurement interactions on the three outcome measures, VAS ($p = .70$), ODI ($p = .76$), and SF-36 pain subscale ($p = .93$). This is contrary to the expected pattern of results and so does not support hypothesis 2. We found no differences in the changes in treatment outcomes between SMT and AET in the positive on the mCPR group and no differences in the changes in

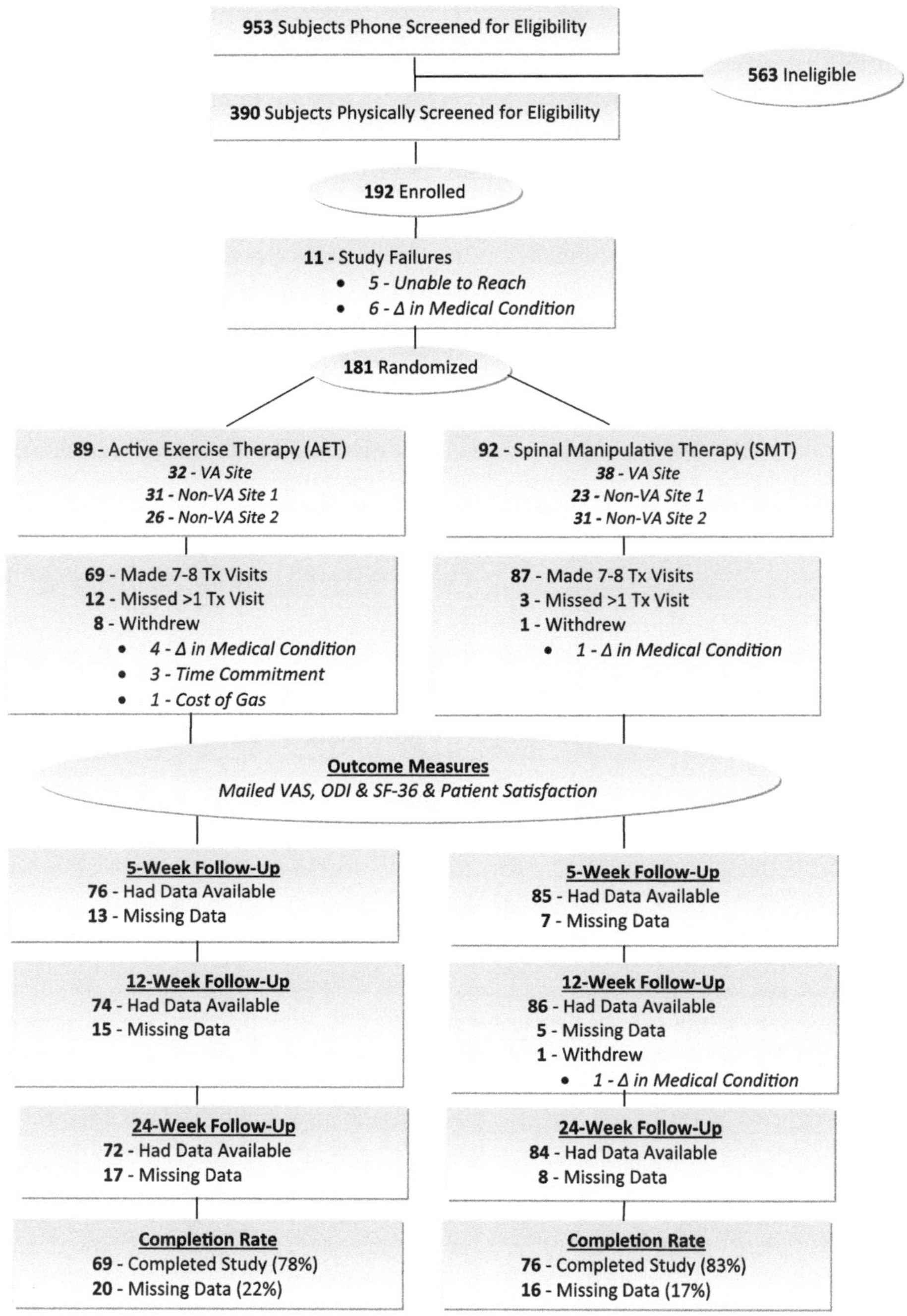

Figure 1 Study flow sheet.

treatment outcomes between SMT and AET in the negative on the mCPR group. We present the adjusted cell means and confidence intervals within the negative on the mCPR and positive on the mCPR groups for each of the follow up time points in Table 5.

Patient satisfaction

We found a significant mCPR x treatment arm interaction ($p = .02$, partial $eta^2 = .03$) on the patients' satisfaction scores. As seen in Table 6, the positive on the mCPR group was equally satisfied with the AET and SMT. In contrast, the negative on the mCPR group was more satisfied with the AET than the SMT.

Harms

Adverse event (AE) and serious adverse event (SAE) data were tracked for each of the treatment groups, AET and SMT. Adverse event data was collected at each

Table 2 Patient demographics

Variable	Study group			
	SMT Negative mCPR N = 32 (St. Dev.)	SMT Positive mCPR N = 60 (St. Dev.)	AET Negative mCPR N = 28 (St. Dev.)	AET Positive mCPR N = 61 (St. Dev.)
Mean Age[a]	61.16 (16.24)	54.12 (16.04)	60.00 (15.00)	53.43 (18.18)
Mean Height (inches)	67.62 (4.14)	67.55 (4.08)	67.29 (3.36)	68.23 (5.82)
Mean Weight (pounds)	206.09 (39.36)	206.22 (49.34)	201.75 (34.07)	192.25 (44.31)
Mean BMI	31.84 (6.75)	31.71 (6.87)	31.34 (4.95)	29.34 (7.36)
Mean Pain Duration (mos)[b]	261.31 (237.90)	140.78 (196.29)	186.62 (188.63)	138.37 (152.13)
Arthritis	56%	40%	39%	38%
Osteoporosis	0%	2%	0%	0%
Depression	37%	45%	25%	28%
Female	25%	38%	24%	36%
White	91%	87%	82%	84%
African American	6%	8%	14%	11%
Hispanic	0%	5%	0%	5%
VA Patients	47%	37%	59%	30%
Education				
Some High School or Less	0%	5%	11%	8%
High School Graduate	41%	20%	18%	21%
Some College	31%	32%	43%	27%
College Graduate	8%	21%	26%	44%
Previous Treatment History				
Allopathic Medicine	87%	75%	93%	77%
Physical Therapy	41%	40%	52%	34%
Chiropractic	62%	55%	67%	52%
Surgery	16%	10%	26%	8%
Injection	12%	13%	26%	19%

[a]difference between positive and negative mCPR groups, $p < .01$.
[b]difference between positive and negative mCPR groups, $p < .01$.

treatment visit and patients also received phone calls during the 5, 12, and 24-week post baseline follow up period. For purpose of this protocol, an AE was defined as any undesirable medical event with new onset or significant exacerbation during the course of the study, regardless of whether or not it was considered to be related to study treatment. Each clinician rated each AE as to severity (a clinical judgment): mild, moderate or severe. An SAE was defined as any AE occurring during the study or within 30 days of conclusion of study participation resulting in any one of the following outcomes: death, life threatening persistent or significant disability/incapacity, hospitalization (when the result of an AE occurring during the study; note, hospitalization for an elective procedure or for treatment of a preexisting condition not worsened during the study was not considered an SAE; admission to the ER for 23 hours or less was not considered a hospitalization), congenital anomaly, important medical event (i.e. an event that in the opinion of the investigator may jeopardize the participant and may require medical or surgical intervention to prevent one of the outcomes listed above). The Data Safety and Management Board (DSMB) met four times during the study (at 25%, 50%, 75%, and final enrollment), the DSMB evaluated the reported AEs and SAEs and found no issues with the reporting of these events and no trends that would require alteration of the study methods. A total of 243 AEs were reported over the course of the study with 54.7% in the AET group and 45.3% in the SMT group. Of the 133 AEs reported in the AET group, the DSMB judged 16 as definitely or probably associated with the intervention. Of the 110 AEs reported in the SMT group, the DSMB judged 14 as definitely or probably associated

Table 3 Patient expectation

	Patient expectation	
	Mean[a]	(±95% CI)
Negative on mCPR SMT (n = 32)		
Pre randomization	5.78	(5.09, 6.47)
Post randomization	6.03	(5.27, 6.79)
Negative on mCPR AET (n = 28)		
Pre randomization	6.14	(5.41, 6.88)
Post randomization	6.79	(5.97, 7.60)
Positive on mCPR SMT (n = 60)		
Pre randomization	6.62	(6.11, 7.12)
Post randomization	7.07	(6.51, 7.62)
Positive on mCPR AET (n = 61)		
Pre randomization	6.46	(5.95, 6.96)
Post randomization	6.47	(5.91, 7.04)

[a]patient expectation for treatment score. The higher the number the more confident the patient was with the treatment. Responses measured on a 11 point scale anchored by 0, not at all confident and 10, very confident.

with the intervention. The majority of AEs that were reported consisted of musculoskeletal soreness and resolved within the study period. During the study period there were 10 SAEs reported after the start of the treatments (5 in the AET group and 5 in the SMT group), the DSMB judged that none of the SAEs were associated with the study intervention.

Table 4 Intention to treat analysis

mCPR status treatment group time of measurement	Outcome measures		
	VAS[a]	ODI[b]	SF-36 Pain[c]
	(St. Dev.)	(St. Dev.)	(St. Dev.)
Negative on mCPR			
SMT (n = 32)			
Baseline	58.44 (15.46)	35.13 (8.55)	5.56 (1.20)
5-weeks	37.51 (28.89)	29.01 (14.66)	6.98 (1.66)
12-weeks	43.29 (24.62)	32.14 (15.77)	6.41 (1.92)
24-weeks	47.61 (25.66)	30.17 (15.69)	6.60 (2.06)
AET (n = 28)			
Baseline	65.36 (16.78)	37.04 (12.57)	5.35 (1.21)
5-weeks	36.50 (33.77)	30.15 (17.71)	6.56 (2.33)
12-weeks	42.00 (33.57)	32.91 (20.82)	6.54 (2.72)
24-weeks	52.54 (27.24)	32.71 (18.64)	6.44 (2.47)
Positive on mCPR			
SMT (n = 60)			
Baseline	61.25 (13.74)	33.62 (9.60)	5.78 (1.22)
5-weeks	34.86 (31.18)	26.71 (15.06)	7.10 (2.22)
12-weeks	40.43 (27.53)	29.64 (18.30)	6.57 (2.55)
24-weeks	38.47 (26.99)	23.16 (15.74)	7.51 (2.71)
AET (n = 61)			
Baseline	55.38 (16.64)	31.44 (10.05)	6.00 (1.52)
5-weeks	26.60 (33.48)	23.73 (17.14)	7.49 (2.57)
12-weeks	36.30 (29.64)	25.94 (19.90)	7.05 (2.98)
24-weeks	42.11 (31.77)	23.52 (18.98)	7.75 (3.08)

[a]the higher the number the higher the reported pain on a 100 point scale.
[b]the higher the number the more disability reported due to pain on a 100 point scale.
[c]the higher the number the *less* self-reported pain on the computed SF-36 pain subscale.

Discussion

Interpretation

Recent literature has highlighted the lack of definitive data to emerge from RCTs evaluating CLBP, with no treatment producing consistently superior outcomes [29-32]. In keeping with this previous literature and supporting our first hypothesis, we found clinically and statistically significant improvements in outcomes from baseline to follow up in the groups receiving SMT and AET, which are both recognized as evidence based interventions for CLBP [10,31].

After an initial promising start in developing treatment based classification in lower back pain, two recent reviews did not identify any studies validating the use of a treatment based classification in CLBP [33,34]. The lack of data on specific patient factors that would moderate the treatment of CLBP is what makes the current study important. Our second hypothesis was that the status on the mCPR would moderate the effectiveness of SMT. If the mCPR moderated the effectiveness of SMT, then we would have expected a significant treatment × mCPR × time interaction. We did not find significant treatment × mCPR × time interaction and so we cannot support our second hypothesis.

Our study results can be compared to the findings of Hancock et al. [35], that found the CPR performed no better than chance in identifying responsiveness to SMT among patients with acute lower back pain. Together the two studies (Hancock and our study) that attempted to apply the CPR to specific populations (Hancock et al. in acute lower back pain and ours in chronic lower back pain) suggest that the CPR, as it is able to be applied, does not seem to moderate the responsiveness to SMT of lower back pain patients, and thus suggesting a limited use of mCPR in clinical judgments of treatment selection for CLBP patients. We are aware of the fallacy of "proving" the null hypothesis of no effect, and so call for additional research to determine the effectiveness of the CPR as a clinical tool in predicting treatment responsiveness in lower back pain patients. Of particular note is the need for additional research to examine the role of other psychosocial factors in the prognosis of CLBP patients [36-39].

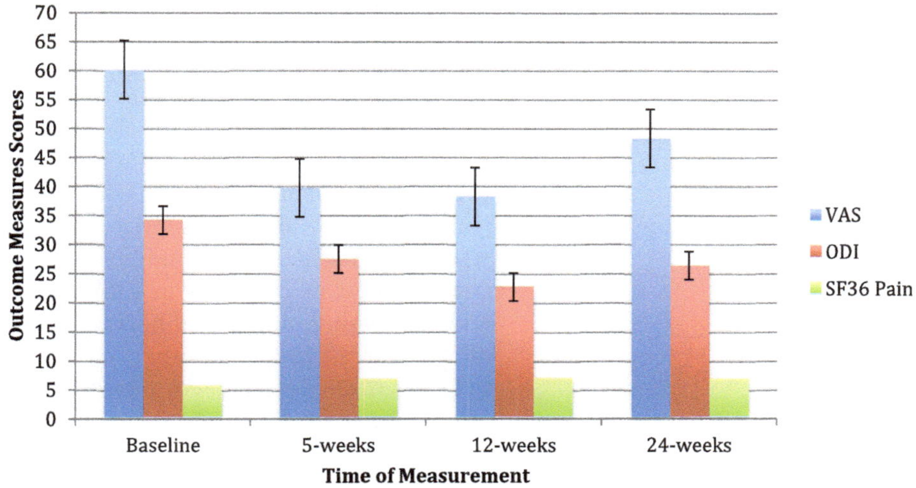

Figure 2 Adjusted Outcome Measures. VAS, ODI, and SF-36 Pain Subscale scores, adjusted for age, duration of pain, and treatment site, and 95% confidence intervals at baseline, post treatment 5, 12 and 24-weeks followup. Linear decrease significant for VAS ($p = .03$), ODI ($p = .001$) and SF-36 Pain Subscale ($p = .002$). The larger the score the more pain as measured by the VAS and disability as measured by the ODI. The larger the score the *less* pain as measured by the SF-36 Pain Subscale.

Limitations

Our study is limited by factors that may need to be addressed in future trials. The first limitation is that we modified a rule that was developed to be utilized in general population of LBP patients. The original rule defined a patient as positive on the rule, if the patient scored positive on four or more of the five criteria, one of which was pain <16 days (acute pain). Since all the patients had CLBP they could not meet the mCPR criteria of pain <16 days (i.e., acute pain). Using the original rule would have been overly restrictive by drastically limiting the universe of positive mCPR patients, who would have had to score positive on all the remaining four rule criteria.

We recognize that our study is limited to two different broadly defined interventions and that this limits the extent to which one can make definitive statements about the individual treatment nuances of each. We purposefully allowed for a more broadly defined SMT treatment, in order to capture more realistically the treatments of clinicians performing manual therapy. Allowing for a more encompassing definition has been seen in other studies, both of these studies allowed the SMT groups to utilize treatments outside of high velocity low amplitude SMT [40,41]. We however, realize that this comes at a price of clouding the impact of specific types of SMT, thus limiting the direct correlation

Table 5 Adjusted difference scores between SMT and AET groups

Time of measurement	Outcome measures		
	VAS[a] (±95% CI)	ODI[b] (±95% CI)	SF-36 pain[c] (±95% CI)
5-week Follow Up			
Negative on mCPR between	7.16 (−20.32, 34.62)	0.75 (−8.84, 10.23)	0.21 (−1.99, 2.42)
Positive on mCPR between	0.81 (−31.21, 32.83)	0.37 (−9.92, 10.66)	−0.03 (−2.84, 2.77)
12-week Follow Up			
Negative on mCPR between	5.36 (−68.25, 78.96)	2.58 (−10.18, 15,34)	−0.66 (−2.30, 0.98)
Positive on mCPR between	2.48 (−11.32, 16.27)	1.93 (−17.08, 20.94)	−0.50 (−2.48, 1.48)
24-week Follow Up			
Negative on mCPR between	−4.26 (−34.82, 26,29)	0.03 (−20.65, 20.70)	0.16 (−1.85, 2.17)
Positive on mCPR between	−8.50 (−48.75, 31.75)	−2.28 (−29.18, 24.62)	0.11 (−2.05, 2.26)

[a]A positive difference score indicates SMT group reported more pain in comparison to the AET group. A negative difference score indicates the AET group reported more pain in comparison to the SMT group. The larger the absolute value, the greater the difference.
[b]t A positive difference score indicates SMT group reported more disability in comparison to the AET group. A negative difference score indicates the AET group reported more disability in comparison to the SMT group. The larger the absolute value, the greater the difference.
[c]A positive difference score indicates SMT group reported less pain in comparison to the AET group. A negative difference score indicates the AET group reported less pain in comparison to the SMT group. The larger the absolute value, the greater the difference.

Table 6 Treatment satisfaction as a function of mCPR and treatment group

mCPR status	Treatment group	
	SMT	AET
	Mean[a] (±95% CI)	Mean (±95% CI)
Negative on mCPR	3.65[a] (3.42, 3.89) st dev = .76 n = 26	4.14 (3.88, 4.04) st dev = .55 n = 21
Positive on mCPR	3.97 (3.80, 4.13) st dev = .58 n = 52	3.96 (3.80, 4.13) st dev = .54 n = 49

[a]responses measured on five point Likert Scales anchored by 1 and 5. The higher the number the more satisfaction.

to the original CPR. Further studies may be used to address which specific aspects of the SMT (manipulative thrust or distraction) were the most effective. Another limitation is that the SMT group did allow for the recommendation of a simple stretching exercise (Cat/camel stretch); although allowing this did increase the generalizability of the study as a whole, it limits that ability to evaluate SMT alone. We also recognize the limitations due to the subjective nature of some of the assessment tools utilized in this study including the use of "deep palpation of erector spinae" and the use of "hypomobility of one or greater segments." These assessment tools have not demonstrated reliability or validity; however they are commonly utilized measures in clinical practice. We acknowledge that the use of these criteria could introduce certain selection bias in the inclusion criteria and the designation of status on the prediction rule; however the study utilized previously reported criteria [12]. To attempt to maintain reliability however, we did use a single screening clinician to perform all baseline screening examinations. Future study should work to identify reliable and valid criteria for identification of pain and hypomobility.

Generalizability

The current trial utilized easily administered tools (spinal mobility, hip motion, symptom characteristics and a simple questionnaire) to attempt to characterize those patients who would respond to one type of treatment over another. In addition, the interventions were designed to be easily generalizable to the typical practice of a manual therapist (PT, DC or Osteopath). This study was designed to apply a modification of a previously defined CPR and see if it was applicable to a different population and a more generalizable treatment method. This study should not be construed to discount the original CPR.

Conclusion

While patients benefited from both SMT and AET, the mCPR did not moderate the effectiveness of SMT, as we hypothesized. Future studies are needed to better understand the specific and non-specific nature of interventions for CLBP [42-45] and also to aid the general practitioner in his/her decision on what intervention may be most appropriate. Further studies are warranted to evaluate the underlying physiological and psychological mechanisms in CLBP in order to better address these underlying abnormalities with the most effective treatment. The results of these studies may help to inform development of a new CPR that would be applicable to CLBP. There is also a need for further studies to evaluate the role of predictive factors for responsiveness for conservative interventions that will be sensitive to the role of non-specific effects of both SMT and AET.

Abbreviations

AE: Adverse Event; AET: Active Exercise Therapy; CLBP: Chronic Lower Back Pain; CPR: Clinical Prediction Rule; CONSORT: Consolidated Standards of Reporting Trials; DC: Doctor of Chiropractic; DSMB: Data and Safety Monitoring Board; FABQ: Fear Avoidance Belief Questionnaire; HRSA: Health Resources and Services Administration; IRB: Institutional Review Board; LBP: Lower Back Pain; MCMC: Markov chain Monte Carlo; mCPR: Modified Clinical Prediction Rule; NYCC: New York Chiropractic College; ODI: Oswestry Disability Index; PT: Physical Therapist; RCT: Randomized Controlled Trial; SAE: Serious Adverse Event; SF-36: Short Form-36 Item Health Survey; SMT: Spinal Manipulative Therapy; SPSS: Statistical Package for the Social Sciences; VA: Veteran's Affairs; VAS: Visual Analogue Scale.

Competing interests

The authors declare that they have no competing interests.

Authors' contributions

All authors contributed to the research design and administration. JK performed the data analysis and PED performed the initial drafting of the manuscript. PED supervised the research and edited the final manuscript. All authors read and approved the final manuscript.

Acknowledgements

The authors would also like to acknowledge the practitioners who provided the clinical intervention for the study: Jim Codarro, PT, Jonathon Egan, DC, MPH, Brian Justice, DC, Andrew Opett, PT, DPT, OCS, CKTP, Scott Spinner, DC, Marcia Miller Spoto, PT, DC, OCS, John Ventura, DC, and Brian Westlake, PT, DPT, MPSPT, Cert. MDT.

Funding

This study was funded by a Department of Health and Human Services, Health Resources and Service Administration (HRSA) Chiropractic Demonstration grant. AWARD NO.: R18HP07641-03-03, GRANT NO.: R18HP07641.

Author details

[1]Canandaigua Veterans Affairs Medical Center, Canandaigua, NY, USA. [2]New York Chiropractic College, Seneca Falls, NY, USA. [3]University of Rochester School of Medicine and Dentistry, Rochester, NY, USA. [4]University of Rochester, Rochester, NY, USA. [5]State University of New York College at Buffalo, Buffalo, NY, USA. [6]University of Toronto, Toronto, ON, Canada. [7]Medical Affairs, Baycrest Geriatric Centre, Toronto, Canada.

References

1. Gironda RJ, Clark ME, Massengale JP, Walker RL: **Pain among veterans of operations enduring freedom and Iraqi Freedom.** *Pain Med* 2006, **7**:339–343.
2. Vos T, Flaxman AD, Naghavi M, Lozano R, Michaud C, Ezzati M, Shibuya K, Salomon JA, Abdalla S, Aboyans V, Abraham J, Ackerman I, Aggarwal R, Ahn SY, Ali MK, Alvarado M, Anderson HR, Anderson LM, Andrews KG, Atkinson C, Baddour LM, Bahalim AN, Barker-Collo S, Barrero LH, Bartels DH, Basanez MG, Baxter A, Bell ML, Benjamin EJ, Bennett D, *et al*: **Years lived with disability (YLDs) for 1160 sequelae of 289 diseases and injuries 1990–2010: a systematic analysis for the Global Burden of Disease Study 2010.** *Lancet* 2012, **380**:2163–2196.
3. Deyo RA, Weinstein JN: **Low back pain.** *N Engl J Med* 2001, **344**:363–370.
4. Martin BI, Deyo RA, Mirza SK, Turner JA, Comstock BA, Hollingworth W, Sullivan SD: **Expenditures and health status among adults with back and neck problems.** *JAMA* 2008, **299**:656–664.
5. Haldeman S, Dagenais S: **A supermarket approach to the evidence-informed management of chronic low back pain.** *Spine J* 2008, **8**:1–7.
6. Fairbank J, Gwilym SE, France JC, Daffner SD, Dettori J, Hermsmeyer J, Andersson G: **The role of classification of chronic low back pain.** *Spine (Phila Pa 1976)* 2011, **36**:S19–S42.
7. Apkarian AV, Baliki MN, Geha PY: **Towards a theory of chronic pain.** *Prog Neurobiol* 2009, **87**:81–97.
8. Grotle M, Foster NE, Dunn KM, Croft P: **Are prognostic indicators for poor outcome different for acute and chronic low back pain consulters in primary care?** *Pain* 2010, **151**:790–797.
9. Chou R, Qaseem A, Snow V, Casey D, Cross JT Jr, Shekelle P, Owens DK: **Diagnosis and treatment of low back pain: a joint clinical practice guideline from the American College of Physicians and the American Pain Society.** *Ann Intern Med* 2007, **147**:478–491.
10. Chou R, Huffman LH: **Nonpharmacologic therapies for acute and chronic low back pain: a review of the evidence for an American Pain Society/American College of Physicians clinical practice guideline.** *Ann Intern Med* 2007, **147**:492–504.
11. Hebert J, Koppenhaver S, Fritz J, Parent E: **Clinical prediction for success of interventions for managing low back pain.** *Clin Sports Med* 2008, **27**:463–479.
12. Flynn T, Fritz J, Whitman J, Wainner R, Magel J, Rendeiro D, Butler B, Garber M, Allison S: **A clinical prediction rule for classifying patients with low back pain who demonstrate short-term improvement with spinal manipulation.** *Spine (Phila Pa 1976)* 2002, **27**:2835–2843.
13. Childs JD, Fritz JM, Flynn TW, Irrgang JJ, Johnson KK, Majkowski GR, Delitto A: **A clinical prediction rule to identify patients with low back pain most likely to benefit from spinal manipulation: a validation study.** *Ann Intern Med* 2004, **141**:920–928.
14. Haskins R, Rivett DA, Osmotherly PG: **Clinical prediction rules in the physiotherapy management of low back pain: a systematic review.** *Man Ther* 2012, **17**:9–21.
15. Patel S, Friede T, Froud R, Evans DW, Underwood M: **Systematic review of randomized controlled trials of clinical prediction rules for physical therapy in low back pain.** *Spine (Phila Pa 1976)* 2013, **38**:762–769.
16. Ohnmeiss DD: **Million visual analog scale.** In *Compendium of Outcome Instruments for Assessment and Research of Spinal Disorders.* Edited by Gatchel RJ. La Grange, Illinois: North American Spine Society; 2001:42–63.
17. Fairbank JC, Couper J, Davies JB, O'Brien JP: **The Oswestry low back pain disability questionnaire.** *Physiotherapy* 1980, **66**:271–273.
18. Sharma S, Firoozi S, McKenna WJ: **Value of exercise testing in assessing clinical state and prognosis in hypertrophic cardiomyopathy.** *Cardiol Rev* 2001, **9**:70–76.
19. Cherkin DC, Deyo RA, Battie M, Street J, Barlow W: **A comparison of physical therapy, chiropractic manipulation, and provision of an educational booklet for the treatment of patients with low back pain.** *N Engl J Med* 1998, **339**:1021–1029.
20. Bronfort G, Goldsmith CH, Nelson CF, Boline PD, Anderson AV: **Trunk exercise combined with spinal manipulative or NSAID therapy for chronic low back pain: a randomized, observer-blinded clinical trial.** *J Manipulative Physiol Ther* 1996, **19**:570–582.
21. Christensen MG, Kollasch MW, Ward R, Webb KR, Day AA, zumBrunnen J: *Job Analysis of Chiropractic: a project report, survey anlaysis, and summary of the practice of chiropractic within the United States.* Greeley: National Board of Chiropractic Examiners; 2005.
22. O'Sullivan PB, Phyty GD, Twomey LT, Allison GT: **Evaluation of specific stabilizing exercise in the treatment of chronic low back pain with radiologic diagnosis of spondylolysis or spondylolisthesis.** *Spine (Phila Pa 1976)* 1997, **22**:2959–2967.
23. Hides JA, Jull GA, Richardson CA: **Long-term effects of specific stabilizing exercises for first-episode low back pain.** *Spine (Phila Pa 1976)* 2001, **26**:E243–E248.
24. Wilke HJ, Wolf S, Claes LE, Arand M, Wiesend A: **Stability increase of the lumbar spine with different muscle groups. A biomechanical in vitro study.** *Spine (Phila Pa 1976)* 1995, **20**:192–198.
25. Haas M, Groupp E, Kraemer DF: **Dose–response for chiropractic care of chronic low back pain.** *Spine J* 2004, **4**:574–583.
26. McHorney CA, Ware JE Jr, Raczek AE: **The MOS 36-Item Short-Form Health Survey (SF-36): II. Psychometric and clinical tests of validity in measuring physical and mental health constructs.** *Med Care* 1993, **31**:247–263.
27. Hertzman-Miller RP, Morgenstern H, Hurwitz EL, Yu F, Adams AH, Harber P, Kominski GF: **Comparing the satisfaction of low back pain patients randomized to receive medical or chiropractic care: results from the UCLA low-back pain study.** *Am J Public Health* 2002, **92**:1628–1633.
28. Ostelo RW, Deyo RA, Stratford P, Waddell G, Croft P, Von KM, Bouter LM, de Vet HC: **Interpreting change scores for pain and functional status in low back pain: towards international consensus regarding minimal important change.** *Spine (Phila Pa 1976)* 2008, **33**:90–94.
29. Iles RA, Davidson M, Taylor NF, O'Halloran P: **Systematic review of the ability of recovery expectations to predict outcomes in non-chronic non-specific low back pain.** *J Occup Rehabil* 2009, **19**:25–40.
30. Hurwitz EL: **Commentary: exercise and spinal manipulative therapy for chronic low back pain: time to call for a moratorium on future randomized trials?** *Spine J* 2011, **11**:599–600.
31. Rubinstein SM, Van MM, Assendelft WJ, De Boer MR, Van Tulder MW: **Spinal manipulative therapy for chronic low-back pain: an update of a Cochrane review.** *Spine (Phila Pa 1976)* 2011, **36**:E825–E846.
32. Gore M, Tai KS, Sadosky A, Leslie D, Stacey BR: **Clinical comorbidities, treatment patterns, and direct medical costs of patients with osteoarthritis in usual care: a retrospective claims database analysis.** *J Med Econ* 2011, **14**:497–507.
33. Kent P, Mjosund HL, Petersen DH: **Does targeting manual therapy and/or exercise improve patient outcomes in nonspecific low back pain? A systematic review.** *BMC Med* 2010, **8**:22.
34. Hebert JJ, Koppenhaver SL, Walker BF: **Subgrouping patients with low back pain: a treatment-based approach to classification.** *Sports Health* 2011, **3**:534–542.
35. Hancock MJ, Maher CG, Latimer J, Herbert RD, McAuley JH: **Independent evaluation of a clinical prediction rule for spinal manipulative therapy: a randomised controlled trial.** *Eur Spine J* 2008, **17**:936–943.
36. Ramond A, Bouton C, Richard I, Roquelaure Y, Baufreton C, Legrand E, Huez JF: **Psychosocial risk factors for chronic low back pain in primary care–a systematic review.** *Fam Pract* 2011, **28**:12–21.
37. Kongsted A, Johannesen E, Leboeuf-Yde C: **Feasibility of the STarT back screening tool in chiropractic clinics: a cross-sectional study of patients with low back pain.** *Chiropr Man Therap* 2011, **19**:10.
38. Hill JC, Whitehurst DG, Lewis M, Bryan S, Dunn KM, Foster NE, Konstantinou K, Main CJ, Mason E, Somerville S, Sowden G, Vohora K, Hay EM: **Comparison of stratified primary care management for low back pain with current best practice (STarT Back): a randomised controlled trial.** *Lancet* 2011, **378**:1560–1571.
39. Grotle M, Vollestad NK, Brox JI: **Clinical course and impact of fear-avoidance beliefs in low back pain: prospective cohort study of acute and chronic low back pain: II.** *Spine (Phila Pa 1976)* 2006, **31**:1038–1046.
40. Haas M, Vavrek D, Peterson D, Polissar N, Neradilek MB: **Dose–response and efficacy of spinal manipulation for care of chronic low back pain: a randomized controlled trial.** *Spine J* 2014, **14**:1106–1116.
41. Bronfort G, Maiers MJ, Evans RL, Schulz CA, Bracha Y, Svendsen KH, Grimm RH Jr, Owens EF Jr, Garvey TA, Transfeldt EE: **Supervised exercise, spinal manipulation, and home exercise for chronic low back pain: a randomized clinical trial.** *Spine J* 2011, **11**:585–598.
42. Steiger F, Wirth B, de Bruin ED, Mannion AF: **Is a positive clinical outcome after exercise therapy for chronic non-specific low back pain contingent upon a corresponding improvement in the targeted aspect(s) of performance? A systematic review.** *Eur Spine J* 2012, **21**:575–598.

43. Machado LA, Kamper SJ, Herbert RD, Maher CG, McAuley JH: **Analgesic effects of treatments for non-specific low back pain: a meta-analysis of placebo-controlled randomized trials.** *Rheumatology (Oxford)* 2009, **48:**520–527.
44. Fregni F, Imamura M, Chien HF, Lew HL, Boggio P, Kaptchuk TJ, Riberto M, Hsing WT, Battistella LR, Furlan A: **Challenges and recommendations for placebo controls in randomized trials in physical and rehabilitation medicine: a report of the international placebo symposium working group.** *Am J Phys Med Rehabil* 2010, **89:**160–172.
45. Dougherty P, Karuza J, Dunn A, Savino D, Katz P: **Spinal manipulative therapy for chronic lower back pain in older veteran's: a prospective, randomized, placebo-controlled trial.** *Geriatric Orthopaedic Surgery and Rehabilitation* in press.

13

Indicating spinal joint mobilisations or manipulations in patients with neck or low-back pain: protocol of an inter-examiner reliability study among manual therapists

Emiel van Trijffel[1,2*], Robert Lindeboom[1], Patrick MM Bossuyt[1], Maarten A Schmitt[2], Cees Lucas[1], Bart W Koes[3] and Rob AB Oostendorp[4,5]

Abstract

Background: Manual spinal joint mobilisations and manipulations are widely used treatments in patients with neck and low-back pain. Inter-examiner reliability of passive intervertebral motion assessment of the cervical and lumbar spine, perceived as important for indicating these interventions, is poor within a univariable approach. The diagnostic process as a whole in daily practice in manual therapy has a multivariable character, however, in which the use and interpretation of passive intervertebral motion assessment depend on earlier results from the diagnostic process. To date, the inter-examiner reliability among manual therapists of a multivariable diagnostic decision-making process in patients with neck or low-back pain is unknown.

Methods: This study will be conducted as a repeated-measures design in which 14 pairs of manual therapists independently examine a consecutive series of a planned total of 165 patients with neck or low-back pain presenting in primary care physiotherapy. Primary outcome measure is therapists' decision about whether or not manual spinal joint mobilisations or manipulations, or both, are indicated in each patient, alone or as part of a multimodal treatment. Therapists will largely be free to conduct the full diagnostic process based on their formulated examination objectives. For each pair of therapists, 2×2 tables will be constructed and reliability for the dichotomous decision will be expressed using Cohen's kappa. In addition, observed agreement, prevalence of positive decisions, prevalence index, bias index, and specific agreement in positive and negative decisions will be calculated. Univariable logistic regression analysis of concordant decisions will be performed to explore which demographic, professional, or clinical factors contributed to reliability.

Discussion: This study will provide an estimate of the inter-examiner reliability among manual therapists of indicating spinal joint mobilisations or manipulations in patients with neck or low-back pain based on a multivariable diagnostic reasoning and decision-making process, as opposed to reliability of individual tests. As such, it is proposed as an initial step toward the development of an alternative approach to current classification systems and prediction rules for identifying those patients with spinal disorders that may show a better response to manual therapy which can be incorporated in randomised clinical trials. Potential methodological limitations of this study are discussed.

Keywords: Manual therapy, Motion assessment, Diagnostics, Decision-making, Reliability, Clinical reasoning, Neck pain, Back pain

* Correspondence: e.vantrijffel@somt.nl
[1]Department of Clinical Epidemiology, Biostatistics & Bioinformatics, Academic Medical Centre, University of Amsterdam, Amsterdam, the Netherlands
[2]Institute for Master Education in Musculoskeletal Therapy, Amersfoort, the Netherlands
Full list of author information is available at the end of the article

Background

Neck and low-back pain are common and costly disorders in adult general populations [1-6]. Manual spinal joint mobilisations and manipulations are widely used treatments in patients with these complaints [7,8]. Although the underlying mechanisms of these treatments are far from understood, spinal joint mobilisations and manipulations are effective as well as cost-effective in patients with non-specific neck and low-back pain although no more effective than other treatment modalities [9-14].

Traditionally, manual therapy has a strong focus on the diagnostics, treatment, and evaluation of spinal joint function by emphasising the use of passive physiological and accessory movements [15-17]. Passive intervertebral motion (PIVM) assessment is used to judge the quantity and quality of functions of spinal motion segments and is assumed to play an important role in diagnostically classifying patients and selecting treatment [18]. Dutch, New Zealand, and USA manual therapists indeed believe that passive spinal mobility testing is important for deciding on manual mobilisation or manipulation as a treatment option [19,20]. Moreover, a recent international, multidisciplinary survey showed that PIVM assessment is the most commonly used impairment outcome measure in patients with neck pain [21].

In order to yield accurate and uniform decisions about treatment options for patients, test results need to be reliable [22]. Reliability is a component of reproducibility along with agreement and reflects the extent to which test results can diagnostically discriminate between patients despite measurement errors [23,24]. Agreement, on the other hand, concerns the possibility of examiners to obtain the same test results on different measurement occasions [25]. Systematic reviews have consistently shown poor inter-examiner reliability for spinal physical tests, and for PIVM assessment in particular [26-30]. However, the large majority of studies investigating the reliability of physical tests and PIVM assessment can be regarded as test research following a single-test or univariable approach, thus neglecting the multivariable character of the diagnostic process as opposed to diagnostic research [31].

Physiotherapists conduct a diagnostic process by collecting data through interview and physical examination and by generating hypotheses as to why a problem exists in order to reach a decision about appropriate patient management [32,33]. During this diagnostic process, manual therapists indeed seem to apply, amongst others, a hypothetico-deductive way of clinical reasoning [34,35]. PIVM assessment is usually conducted after history-taking, questionnaires, and other physical tests and is indicated after interpreting earlier clinical information and formulating specific hypotheses about spinal joint dysfunction [35]. Moreover, Canadian manual therapists reported to decide on manual mobilisation or manipulation based on their whole clinical assessment and clinical reasoning in a patient [36]. It is therefore reasonable to assume that the diagnostic process in manual therapy has a multivariable character.

Over the last three decades, many systems have been developed for classifying patients with spinal disorders, in particular for those with low-back pain [37]. A systematic review found 28 systems for classifying chronic low-back pain alone and it was concluded that there was insufficient evidence to support or recommend any particular system for use in clinical description, determining prognosis, or predicting response to treatment [38]. Some systems were tested for their inter-examiner reliability, but evidence was either conflicting or moderate to strong for poor reliability [27]. On the other hand, using clusters of tests for diagnosing sacroiliac joint dysfunction yielded acceptable reliability [39-41]. However, the majority of these systems either lack evidence for their reliability, only use certain parts of the clinical examination (e.g. only physical tests), are prescriptive in their application, do not include PIVM assessment, are not related to manual therapy interventions, or do not direct towards treatment decisions. Some systems [42,43] were developed as treatment-based classification algorithms for subgrouping patients with low-back pain and were strongly based on factors derived from several clinical prediction rules [44-47]. However, these rules lack validation, and methodological and statistical issues regarding their development have been raised [48]. In contrast to the field of classification systems for low-back pain, the development and number of systems for classifying neck pain patients lie far behind. Besides a treatment-based classification system for physiotherapy interventions [49], clinical prediction rules have been derived to identify factors that predict response to spinal manipulation in patients with neck pain but with identical problems as in the rules for low-back pain as mentioned above [50-55]. In a systematic review, Gemmell and Miller [56] found poor inter-examiner reliability of multitest regimens using only physical tests for identifying manipulable spinal lesions in chiropractic. Including pain scores and medical history next to manual examination of spinal motion segments resulted in high accuracy in identifying neck pain patients [57]. To summarise, however, the value of the diagnostic process as a whole to classify patients with neck or low-back pain in order to decide whether or not spinal mobilisations or manipulations are indicated remains unclear.

This is the protocol of a study that aims to determine the inter-examiner reliability among Dutch manual therapists of indicating spinal joint mobilisations or manipulations in patients with neck or low-back pain based on a multivariable, hypothesis-based diagnostic reasoning and decision-making process. Secondly, using univariable logistic regression analysis of concordant decisions about indications, we will explore which demographic, professional, and clinical factors can explain variation in reliability of therapists' decisions with specific attention to the contribution of PIVM assessment.

Methods

Design

This study will be conducted as a repeated-measures design in which pairs of manual therapists independently examine a consecutive series of patients with neck or low-back pain presenting in primary care physiotherapy in the Netherlands. Primary outcome measure is therapists' decision about whether or not spinal manual therapy (SMT) is indicated in each patient, alone or as part of a multimodal treatment. SMT is defined here as either spinal joint mobilisations or manipulations, or both. Therapists will largely be free to conduct the full diagnostic process as they are routinely used to.

Participants

Consecutive patients aged 18 years or older presenting with a primary complaint of neck or low-back pain, either referred to primary care physiotherapy by their general practitioner or medical specialist, or by self-referral, will be eligible for participation in the study. Neck pain is defined as pain in the region between the superior nuchal line, the external occipital protuberance, the spines of the scapula, the superior border of the clavicula, and the suprasternal notch, with or without radiation to the head, trunk, or upper limbs [58]. Patients will not be eligible when headache or dizziness is their dominant complaint. Low-back pain is defined as pain or discomfort localised below the costal margin and above the inferior gluteal folds, with or without radiation to the lower limbs [59]. All patients who are assumed to have non-specific or (non-serious) specific neck or low-back pain with a potential indication for SMT will be included. Patients who are not able to speak or read Dutch fluently will be ineligible. Patients will receive verbal and written information on all aspects of the study and will be asked to provide written consent at their inclusion. The Central Committee for Research involving Human Subjects (CCMO, the Hague, the Netherlands) decided that a full evaluation of the study protocol by a medical ethical committee was not required because patients will undergo a diagnostic process similar to routine daily practice.

Examiners

Examiners will be manual therapists working at least 20 hours a week in their private practices in the Netherlands and registered by the Dutch Association for Manual Therapy or the Royal Dutch Society for Physical Therapy. From a database of those graduated from the Institute for Master Education in Musculoskeletal Therapy (SOMT: Stichting Opleidingen Musculoskeletale Therapie, Amersfoort, the Netherlands), 14 pairs of manual therapists will be invited to participate. Each pair works together in the same practice and practices will be selected based on their ability to logistically organise the study. We aim to include therapists who vary in years of clinical experience in manual therapy. Therapists will attend an information session followed by a two-hour training session in which procedures for digitally registering data are explained and practised. They will not receive additional training in history-taking, physical examination procedures, or using questionnaires. Pairs of therapists will be strictly requested not to discuss their experiences during the study with each other until their last patient has been included. Gender, age, years of clinical experience in manual therapy, highest diploma, practice setting, weekly amount of work related to spinal disorders (hours), teaching experience (yes/no), and participation in research (yes/no) will be recorded as professional characteristics from the participating therapists.

In each practice, a third colleague will function as a research assistant to coordinate the inclusion and flow of patients. Research assistants will be instructed with respect to applying the inclusion criteria, the order of assigning patients to therapists, and assuring blinding procedures.

Procedures

From eligible patients, demographic (gender, age, marital status, working status) and clinical (type of complaints (neck or low-back pain), duration of complaints (days), radiation (yes/no), traumatic origin (yes/no), comorbidity (yes/no)) data will be recorded as baseline data by the local research assistant. In addition, baseline pain and disability will be determined using the Numeric Pain Rating Scale (NPRS 0–10, higher scores indicate higher pain intensity), and the Quebec Back Pain Disability Scale (QBPDS 0–100, higher scores indicate higher disability) for low-back pain patients and the Neck Disability Index Dutch Language Version (NDI-DLV 0–50, higher scores indicate higher pain and disability) for neck pain patients, respectively. The NPRS is a reliable and valid scale to measure pain intensity in adults [60]. The Dutch version of the QBPDS is a reliable and valid instrument for measuring disability in low-back pain patients [61] and the Dutch version of the NDI is recommended for measuring pain and disability in patients with neck pain [62].

All baseline data will be available to each therapist before he or she starts the diagnostic process. The first therapist of each pair will be the treating therapist to whom the patient was assigned to, so the order in which both therapists act as the first examiner will vary according to the practice's planning. The first therapist will screen all consecutive patients with neck or low-back pain for the presence of red flags [63]. In accordance with guidelines in the Netherlands [64], patients suspected of having serious (spinal or non-spinal) pathology will not enter the study which will be recorded. Patients will then undergo a full history-taking by the first therapist. The therapist will record his or her findings as well as proposed hypotheses about patient's health status by formulating explicit objectives for further examination. The therapist will then choose the diagnostic procedures (e.g. observation, physical tests, performance tests, questionnaires) that he or she plans to perform in the patient. After performing each procedure, its outcome will be recorded. If PIVM assessment is indicated, therapists will use three-dimensional coupled movements in flexion and extension directions for each individual motion segment [65]. Movements will be judged on mobility (hypermobile-normal-hypomobile), resistance perceived by the therapist during the movement (increased resistance or stiffness yes/no), resistance perceived by the therapist at the end of the movement (end-feel) (increased resistance or stiffness at the end of the movement yes/no), and pain provocation (yes/no). Therapists will perform a maximum of three repetitions for each movement per direction per spinal motion segment to afford the best stiffness discriminability [66].

The therapist will then be asked to record whether he or she has made any changes to the original examination objectives as well as to specify these changes, and a diagnostic conclusion in terms of specific or non-specific neck or low-back pain is given. Finally, the therapist will make the decision about whether or not SMT is indicated in the patient and, when indicated, it will also be stated whether mobilisations or manipulations, or both, are indicated, and to which spinal motion segments these techniques would be targeted. In addition, the therapist will rate his or her level of certainty of the primary decision about the indication on a bipolar seven-point scale ranging from −3 (completely uncertain) to 3 (completely certain). It will also be recorded which other interventions he or she believes would further be indicated in the patient. However, at this point, no actual treatment will be provided.

After the first therapist has performed the full examination, he or she will leave the examination room and the patient will be given a 10 minute break. After checking whether all data have been registered, the research assistant then guides the second therapist into the room and makes sure that there is no visual or verbal contact between the two therapists. The second therapist will then conduct the full diagnostic process, excluding the screening for red flags, whilst being unaware of the outcomes of the first examination. Patients will be requested not to mention any outcomes or conclusions from the first examination. Both therapists will record all their findings and data into a fit-for-purpose software program. The research assistant will check whether all data have been entered by both therapists.

Statistical analysis

Demographic and clinical baseline characteristics of patients will be summarised using descriptive statistics. Absolute and relative frequencies are used to describe categorical data. Ordinal data relating to patients' pain and disability will be described with their median and interquartile range. Normally distributed numerical data will be summarised by their mean and standard deviation. In case of non-normality, median and interquartile range are presented. Examination objectives as formulated by therapists will be classified by one researcher (EvT) according to the framework of the World Health Organization's *International Classification of Functioning, Disability and Health* (ICF) [67] to describe patients' functioning in terms of impairments of neuromusculoskeletal and movement-related functions, activity limitations and participation restrictions, and personal and environmental factors. Diagnostic procedures will be listed and described with their frequencies, and also outcomes of PIVM assessment, changes to the original examination objectives, diagnostic conclusions, and examiners' level of certainty of their decision about the treatment indication will be summarised. Concordance between the formulated examination objectives concerning spinal joint motion function and the actual use of PIVM assessment will be presented as frequencies.

For each pair of therapists, 2×2 tables will be constructed and reliability for the dichotomous positive or negative decisions about whether or not SMT is indicated will be calculated as chance-corrected reliability using Cohen's kappa [68]. As recommended by Cicchetti and Feinstein [69] and Byrt et al. [70], observed agreement (%), prevalence of positive decisions (mobilisations and/or manipulations indicated) relative to the total number of indications, prevalence index (PI), bias index (BI), and specific agreement (%) in positive (p_{pos}) and negative (p_{neg}) decisions will be calculated in order to evaluate whether kappa was influenced by high prevalence of positive or negative decisions, or by systematic bias between examiners. PI reflects the difference between the proportion of agreement on positive indications as compared to that of negative indications. PI ranges between 0 and 1, and is high when the prevalence of concordant positive (or negative) indications is high, chance agreement is consequently also high, and kappa is reduced accordingly (prevalence effect) [71]. BI provides a quantification of the extent to which examiners disagree on the proportions of positive (or negative) indications. BI also ranges between 0 and 1, and is high when the difference between the discordant indications is high, chance agreement is consequently low, and kappa is inflated accordingly (bias) [71]. P_{pos} and P_{neg} are the proportions of agreement on positive and negative indications, respectively, relative to the total number of positive and negative indications, respectively, from both therapists. Overall kappa (95% CI) will be calculated as a generalized chance-corrected reliability across all pairs of therapists. See Additional file 1 for formulas.

In addition, for each pair of therapists, separate 2×2 tables will be presented for judgements about the indication for PIVM assessment and for judgements about mobility, end-feel, and pain provocation obtained from PIVM assessment (four tables in total). Observed agreement, prevalence of positive decisions, PI, BI, p_{pos}, p_{neg}, and overall kappa (95% CI) will also be calculated. Analyses will be conducted using DAG_Stat [72].

Kappa (95% CI) is interpreted in accordance with value labels as assigned by Landis & Koch [73]: <0.00: poor, 0.00-0.20: slight, 0.21-0.40: fair, 0.41-0.60: moderate, 0.61-0.80: substantial, 0.81-1.00: almost perfect. We arbitrarily assume a lower bound of the 95% CI around overall kappa of 0.60 to indicate acceptable reliability.

Univariable logistic regression analysis will be performed to explore which demographic, professional, and clinical factors contributed to the reliability of therapists' decision-making. Firstly, patients' demographic and clinical factors at baseline will concern their gender, age, type of complaints, duration of complaints (less or more than three months), radiation, traumatic origin, comorbidity, pain intensity, and disability. Such factors are associated with variation in diagnostic accuracy [74], but evidence in the context of reliability is lacking. Secondly, therapists' professional factors will include their clinical experience and weekly amount of work related to spinal disorders. Weekly amount of work related to spinal disorders was positively associated with perceived importance and confidence related to the use and interpretation of PIVM assessment [20] and may, therefore, contribute to variation in diagnostic decision-making. In addition, other clinical factors will be explored involving PIVM assessment (indicated or not, and judgements on mobility, resistance, and pain provocation), the diagnostic conclusion (specific or non-specific neck or low-back pain), therapists' level of certainty of their decision about the treatment indication, and the concordance between examination objectives and the use of PIVM assessment. Factors will be entered in the model as single covariates with the concordant decisions, either positive or negative, as the dependent variable. Concordant decisions will be coded as 1 while the discordant decisions will be coded 0. Therapists' experience and work related to spinal disorders will be entered as mean scores from each pair. A p-value <0.05 indicates a statistically significant association between a factor and a concordant decision about whether or not SMT is indicated.

With a sample size of 165, a two-sided 95% CI around kappa would extend ±0.109 from the observed value of kappa, assuming a true value of kappa of 0.70, and a prevalence of positive decisions of 50%. Consequently, each pair of examiners will be asked to include 12 patients. Multiple imputation will be used to handle records with data points missing at random. If, for any reason, data on the primary outcome measure are not available or obtainable from one or both therapists, all data from this patient will be excluded from the analysis and the pair of therapists will be asked to include a new patient. Analyses will be conducted using IBM SPSS Statistics for Windows version 22.

Discussion

The results of this study will provide 1) an estimate of the inter-examiner reliability among manual therapists of indicating SMT in patients with neck or low-back pain based on a multivariable diagnostic reasoning and decision-making process, as opposed to reliability of individual clinical tests, and 2) a first exploration of which demographic, professional, or clinical factors can explain variation in the reliability of therapists' decision-making with specific attention to the contribution of PIVM assessment. We do not aim or hypothesise that reliability from a multivariable approach to clinical diagnostics will be higher than that from individual test diagnostics. Rather, we believe that such an estimate will be a more real resemblance of the reliability among therapists of making decisions in daily practice concerning the distinction between patients who are indicated for SMT and those who are not. In addition, this approach will add to the ongoing discussion of the identification of specific subgroups of patients that may be more likely to respond to SMT and we propose alternative research strategies for establishing treatment effects.

It has been recognised that treatment effects of SMT, or any other physiotherapy modality for that matter, especially in patients with low-back pain, are, on average, small which may be due to heterogeneity of patients obscuring a wide range of individual treatment responses and variation of treatment effects [75]. Ever since the mid-nineties of the last century, identifying subgroups of patients that may benefit more from specific or targeted interventions has had the highest research priority [76-81]. As a result, there has been a proliferation of subgrouping systems aiming to identify people with a particular pathoanatomical condition, a particular prognosis, or those that are more likely to respond favorably to treatment [82]. Primary care clinicians themselves do not believe that low-back pain is one condition and they treat patients differently based on patterns of clinical signs and symptoms [83]. Moreover, they classify patients predominantly based on pathoanatomy, but they show little consensus regarding these related patterns [84]. With the aim to identify patients that may be more likely to show a positive response to spinal manipulation, clinical prediction rules have been derived to identify predictors in patients with neck and low-back pain [44-47,50-55]. Unfortunately, systematic reviews have consistently concluded that there is, as yet, insufficient evidence to support the general application of these rules [85-89]. Another systematic review found significant treatment effects favoring subgroup-specific SMT over a number of comparison treatments for pain and disability at short and intermediate follow-up based on low-quality trials [90]. Foster et al. [75] concluded that no subgrouping approaches have yet passed the tests for clinical value and robustness of evidence, and there is still a long way to go before closer matching of treatments to patient characteristics becomes a clinical reality. Indeed, two decades after the derivation of the Ottawa Ankle Rules [91], their validation and implementation is still an ongoing research process worldwide and it can be assumed that following a similar pathway for far more complex problems such as the treatment of non-specific neck and low-back pain may be even more time-consuming.

When determining treatment effects of SMT, randomised clinical trials currently do not make use of patients' full clinical health profile according to the domains of the ICF for targeting treatment. For instance, Cochrane Reviews consider primary studies including participants only based on their age and the presence of pain with or without radiation [11,13,14]. The resulting heterogeneity among trial participants and the subsequent dilution of treatment effects may be deleterious to SMT as its effectiveness may be underestimated for certain groups of patients. The majority of primary studies in patients with neck pain do not apply well-defined clinical criteria to select patients for SMT and if they do, they use only one physical test, such as a mobility test or a pain provocation test, in order to diagnose neck pain from a mechanical origin [92]. It is stated that clinical tests are not valid or reliable to allow targeting treatment in clinical trials [84]. This is certainly true when the reliability of individual physical tests is considered [26-30]. However, several of the increasingly popular predication rules also contain clinical variables that are unreliable, including PIVM assessment [42,46,88]. Targeting SMT to a more homogeneous group of patients with neck or low-back pain, based on a multivariable diagnostic process resembling daily practice, may outweigh the disadvantages of the current selection procedures in randomised clinical trials.

Awaiting evidence from the further validation of prediction rules and other classification systems, our study could offer an initial step toward a faster and easier development of an alternative approach to the identification of those patients with spinal disorders that may show a better response to SMT based on a multivariable decision process. A satisfactory level of reliability is a prerequisite for incorporating such decision-making into the design of randomised clinical trials for establishing treatment effects of SMT and thereby validating the approach. When reliability (lower bound of 95% CI around kappa) exceeds 0.60 and with BI, arbitrarily, <0.10, patients with neck or low-back pain with a positive indication can be randomised to receive, for instance, either manual mobilisations or manipulations, or both, within a multimodal treatment on the one hand or multimodal treatment without mobilisations or manipulations on the other (Figure 1A). Should reliability be below this cut-off but with p_{pos} (or p_{neg}), arbitrarily, >60%, this strategy can still be used by randomising only those patients of which the indication was agreed upon by two manual therapists (Figure 1B). P_{pos} and p_{neg} here indicate the absolute specific agreement on positive or negative indications, respectively, between therapists [25].

With respect to our second research objective, it is important to note that empirical evidence for sources of bias and variation in reliability studies is lacking contrary to studies of diagnostic accuracy [74,93-95]. Variation arises from differences between studies, for example, in terms of demographic and disease features of study participants, characteristics of examiners, setting, or test protocol. As such, it does not lead to biased estimates of reliability, but it can limit the applicability of study results [94]. Knowledge of factors that explain variation in reliability may inform ways to improve reliability. For instance, examiner training and choosing a group of more heterogeneous study participants have been mentioned as improvement strategies, but both have their limitations and lack supporting evidence [24]. Systematic reviews may reveal subgroups of participants, examiners, or tests that consistently show higher or lower reliability. In systematic reviews, between-study comparisons are conducted to search for these subgroups as sources of variation. However, these comparisons are less valid as they are hampered by the often strong clinical and methodological heterogeneity between studies [96]. In addition, the identification of these sources of variation becomes even more troublesome when reliability is consistently low (or high) across studies. Within-study comparisons are the preferred method to explore variation in reliability. To date, very few studies have been undertaken in the field of manual therapy with this aim and method. Cook et al. [97] investigated factors related to the large variability of forces used during passive accessory intervertebral movements and they found that examiners' age, gender, experience, background and education, and frequency of use did not contribute to this variation. We present simple logistic regression analysis of concordant decisions as a flexible method that can easily be incorporated in any reliability study to explore and

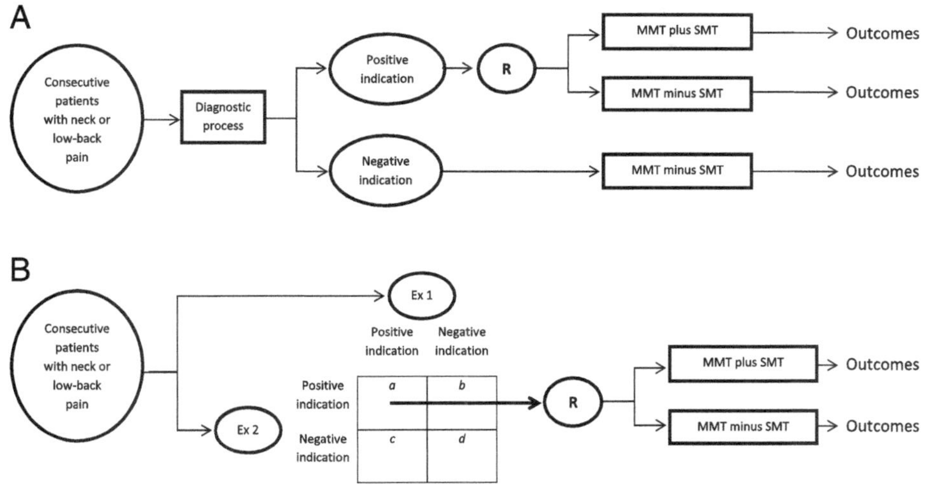

Figure 1 A. Design of an RCT including patients positively indicated for SMT when lower bound of 95% CI around kappa >0.60 and BI <0.10. B. Design of an RCT including only patients positively indicated for SMT by two examiners when kappa <0.60 but p_{pos} (or p_{neg}) >60%.

explain variation in reliability from a large number of demographic, professional, and clinical factors.

Potential limitations of this study

This study protocol presents several new approaches to investigating and analysing decision-making in manual therapy and to reliability research in general. Several of its methods need further discussion in order to appraise their effect on the validity and generalisability of the study's results. First, establishing examination objectives for physical examination by physiotherapists has been used in earlier studies [98,99]. However, the prospective formulation and registration of examination objectives is far from common practice for physiotherapists in the Netherlands [100]. The specific training of our examiners in the formulation and digital registration of these objectives may diminish the generalisability of the estimated reliability of indicating SMT. We encourage that establishing and prospectively registering of examination objectives become an integral part of daily practice in physiotherapy.

Stability of participants' characteristics is a prerequisite for the valid estimation of reliability [23]. However, very few empirical data are available as to the minimum length of the time period between test procedures that ensures that patients' responses to questions and physical tests, such as joint motion assessment, will remain unchanged. Shirley et al. [101] reported that stiffness responses to repeated mechanical posteroanterior loading of lumbar motion segments returned to the pre-testing state within five minutes. On the other hand, a 30-minute recovery period after 30 minutes of *in vitro* creep loading of the lumbar spine was not sufficient to return to the baseline situation [102]. By incorporating a 10 minute break for patients between examinations and limiting the number of movement repetitions during PIVM assessment, we are more confident that underestimation of reliability will be avoided. Research into the natural variation over time within and between individuals regarding joint mobility and other body functions, as well as into the variation induced by the physical examination itself, is needed.

Our sample size calculation strongly depends on the assumed prevalence of positive indications which was based on data from the numerous studies on practice patterns among physiotherapists in the treatment of patients with neck and low back pain [103-113]. Within the large variation in choices of treatment options by therapists, mobilisations and manipulations were only rarely among the most preferred options and their frequency of use ranged from 16% to 83% and from 2% to 37%, respectively. These figures were not substantially different for specific subgroups of manual therapists who reported remarkably low frequencies of use of manipulations in the cervical region [36,114-116]. As we will consider reliability of indicating either mobilisations or manipulations, or both, we assume a 50% prevalence of positive indications. Choosing a higher or lower prevalence would have resulted in a larger required sample [117].

In our sample of manual therapists and patients, we cannot rule out the possibility of a substantially higher (or lower) prevalence of positive indications for SMT. Because of such a skewed distribution of decisions, a distorted interpretation of kappa could then occur. Recently, kappa, as a relative measure of reliability, has been criticised because it can only provide information about the ability to distinguish between patients on a sample level [25]. The authors suggest using the specific agreement parameters (p_{pos} and p_{neg}) as absolute measures to quantify observer variation regarding a certain diagnosis or decision on an individual patient level [25]. No single omnibus index, however, can be satisfactory for all purpose and situations [69,70]. Therefore, we will calculate all recommended parameters from the 2×2 tables to allow full interpretation of reliability and agreement as related to the prevalence of concordant and discordant indications. We will not, however, correct kappa for prevalence effects and bias, for instance by calculating prevalence-adjusted bias-adjusted kappa, because this would generate values of reliability that no longer relate to the original situation [117,118].

We will select pairs of manual therapists as examiners that share a common educational background. With this background from the largest institute for manual therapy education in the Netherlands, they likely form a representative sample from the Dutch population of manual therapists registered with the Dutch Association for Manual Therapy or the Royal Dutch Society for Physical Therapy. Manual therapy education in the Netherlands is strongly embedded within international concepts. In these traditional concepts, especially passive joint motion assessment takes a prominent place [15]. Therefore, we suppose that the results of this study will to a certain extent be generalisable to populations of manual therapists outside the Netherlands. We do, however, suggest that this study be replicated over different countries and concepts to account for local idiosyncrasies in clinical reasoning and decision-making. In addition, for practical reasons, we will choose pairs of manual therapists that work in the same practice. This may inflate reliability and by pairing therapists with different levels of experience, we aim to minimise this potential threat to the validity of the study.

Finally, when analysing the reliability of indicating SMT, we will not distinguish specifically between mobilisations or manipulations. Despite the disparate mechanisms of these interventions [9,119], no evidence is available on whether one or the other, or both, should be preferred in any clinical situation. Results of randomised controlled trials have been conflicting so far [120-123]. New research should focus on the relationship between clinical findings, the choice for either mobilisation or manipulation, and subsequent clinical outcomes.

Additional file

Additional file 1: Formulas for kappa and associated measures.

Abbreviations

ICF: International Classification of Functioning, Disability and Health; PIVM: Passive intervertebral motion; SMT: Spinal manual therapy.

Competing interests

The authors declare that they have no competing interests.

Authors' contributions

EvT is the principal investigator of the study, developed the research questions and methods, obtained ethical approval, and drafted the article. RL, MS, CL, BK, RO assisted in the development of the methods and wrote the study protocol. RL, EvT, PB developed the statistical plan for this protocol. PB, RO supervised the project. All authors assisted with revisions to the study protocol and methods, and approved the final version of the article.

Author details

[1]Department of Clinical Epidemiology, Biostatistics & Bioinformatics, Academic Medical Centre, University of Amsterdam, Amsterdam, the Netherlands. [2]Institute for Master Education in Musculoskeletal Therapy, Amersfoort, the Netherlands. [3]Department of General Practice, Erasmus MC University Medical Centre, Rotterdam, the Netherlands. [4]Scientific Institute for Quality of Healthcare, Radboud University Nijmegen Medical Centre, Nijmegen, the Netherlands. [5]Department of Rehabilitation, Physiotherapy and Manual Therapy, Faculty of Medicine and Pharmacology, Free University of Brussels, Brussels, Belgium.

References

1. Borghouts JAJ, Koes BW, Bouter LM: **Cost-of-illness in neck pain in the Netherlands in 1996.** *Pain* 1999, **80:**629–636.
2. Côte P, Cassidy D, Carroll L: **The Saskatchewan health and back pain survey. The prevalence of neck pain and related disability in Saskatchewan adults.** *Spine* 1998, **23:**1689–1698.
3. Hogg-Johnson S, van der Velde G, Carroll LJ, Holm LW, Cassidy JD, Guzman J, Côte P, Haldeman S, Ammendolia C, Carragee E, Hurwitz E, Nordin M, Peloso P: **The burden and determinants of neck pain in the general population: results of the Bone and Joint Decade 2000–2010 Task Force on Neck Pain and Its Associated Disorders.** *Spine* 2008, **33**(Suppl 4):39–51.
4. Linton SJ, Hellsing AL, Hallden K: **A population-based study of spinal pain among 35–45 year old individuals. Prevalence, sick leave and health care use.** *Spine* 1998, **23:**1457–1463.
5. van Tulder MW, Koes BW, Bouter LM: **A cost-of-illness study of back pain in The Netherlands.** *Pain* 1995, **62:**233–240.
6. Waddell G: **Low back pain: a twentieth century health care enigma.** *Spine* 1996, **21:**2820–2825.
7. Assendelft WJ, Morton SC, Yu EI, Suttorp MJ, Shekelle PG: **Spinal manipulative therapy for low back pain. A meta-analysis of effectiveness relative to other therapies.** *Ann Intern Med* 2003, **138:**871–881.
8. Gross A, Miller J, D'Sylva J, Burnie SJ, Goldsmith CH, Graham N, Haines T, Brønfort G, Hoving JL: **Manipulation or mobilization for neck pain: a Cochrane Review.** *Man Ther* 2010, **15:**315–333.
9. Bialosky JE, Bishop MD, Price DD, Robinson ME, George SZ: **The mechanisms of manual therapy in the treatment of musculoskeletal pain: A comprehensive model.** *Man Ther* 2009, **14:**531–538.
10. Bronfort G, Haas M, Evans R, Leininger B, Triano J: **Effectiveness of manual therapies: The UK evidence report.** *Chiropr Osteopat* 2010, **18:**3.
11. Gross A, Miller J, D'Sylva J, Burnie SJ, Goldsmith CH, Graham N, Haines T, Brønfort G, Hoving JL: **Manipulation or mobilisation for neck pain.** *Cochrane Database Syst Rev* 2010, (Issue 1): Art. No.: CD004249. doi:10.1002/14651858.CD004249.pub3.
12. Michaleff ZA, Lin C-WC, Maher CG, van Tulder MW: **Spinal manipulation epidemiology: Systematic review of cost-effectiveness studies.** *J Electromyogr Kinesiol* 2012, **22:**655–662.
13. Rubinstein SM, van Middelkoop M, Assendelft WJJ, de Boer MR, van Tulder MW: **Spinal manipulative therapy for chronic low-back pain.** *Cochrane Database Syst Rev* 2011, (Issue 2): Art. No.: CD008112. doi:10.1002/14651858.CD008112.pub2.
14. Rubinstein SM, Terwee CB, Assendelft WJJ, de Boer MR, van Tulder MW: **Spinal manipulative therapy for acute low-back pain.** *Cochrane Database Syst Rev* 2012, (Issue 9): Art. No.: CD008880. doi:10.1002/14651858.CD008880.pub2.
15. Farrell JP, Jensen GM: **Manual therapy: A critical assessment of role in the profession of physical therapy.** *Phys Ther* 1992, **72:**843–852.
16. Maher C, Latimer J: **Pain or resistance – the manual therapists' dilemma.** *Austr J Physiotherapy* 1992, **38:**257–260.

17. van Ravensberg CDD, Oostendorp RAB, van Berkel LM, Scholten-Peeters GGM, Pool JJM, Swinkels RAHM, Huijbregts PA: **Physical therapy and manual physical therapy: Differences in patient characteristics.** *J Man Manip Ther* 2005, **13**:113–124.
18. Jull G, Treleaven J, Versace G: **Manual examination: Is pain provocation a major cue for spinal dysfunction?** *Austr J Physiotherapy* 1994, **40**:159–165.
19. Abbott JH, Flynn TW, Fritz JM, Hing WA, Reid D, Whitman JM: **Manual physical assessment of spinal segmental motion: Intent and validity.** *Man Ther* 2009, **14**:36–44.
20. van Trijffel E, Oostendorp RAB, Lindeboom R, Bossuyt PMM, Lucas C: **Perceptions and use of passive intervertebral motion assessment of the spine. A survey of Dutch physiotherapists specializing in manual therapy.** *Man Ther* 2009, **14**:243–251.
21. MacDermid JC, Walton DM, Côté P, Lina Santaguida P, Gross A, Carlesso L: **Use of outcome measures in managing neck pain: An international multidisciplinary survey.** *Open Orthop J* 2013, **7**:440–460.
22. Bartko JJ, Carpenter WT: **On the methods and theory of reliability.** *J Nerv Ment Dis* 1976, **163**:307–317.
23. de Vet HC, Terwee CB, Knol DL, Bouter LM: **When to use agreement versus reliability measures.** *J Clin Epidemiol* 2006, **59**:1033–1039.
24. Streiner DL, Norman GR: *Health measurement scales. A practical guide to their development and use.* 4th edition. Oxford, UK: Oxford University Press; 2008:167–210.
25. de Vet HCW, Mokkink LB, Terwee CB, Hoekstra OS, Knol DL: **Clinicians are right not to like Cohen's κ.** *BMJ* 2013, **346**:f2125.
26. Haneline MT, Cooperstein R, Young M, Birkeland K: **Spinal motion palpation: A comparison of studies that assessed intersegmental end feel vs excursion.** *J Manipulative Physiol Ther* 2008, **31**:616–626.
27. May S, Littlewood C, Bishop A: **Reliability of procedures used in the physical examination of non-specific low back pain: a systematic review.** *Austr J Physiother* 2006, **52**:91–102.
28. Seffinger MA, Najm WI, Mishra SI, Adams A, Dickerson VM, Murphy LS, Reinsch S: **Reliability of spinal palpation for diagnosis of back and neck pain: a systematic review of the literature.** *Spine* 2004, **29**:E413–E425.
29. Stochkendahl MJ, Christensen HW, Hartvigsen J, Vach W, Haas M, Hestbæk L, Adams A, Bronfort G: **Manual examination of the spine: a systematic critical literature review of reproducibility.** *J Manipulative Physiol Ther* 2006, **29**:475–485.
30. van Trijffel E, Anderegg Q, Bossuyt PM, Lucas C: **Inter-examiner reliability of passive assessment of intervertebral motion in the cervical and lumbar spine: a systematic review.** *Man Ther* 2005, **10**:256–269.
31. Moons KG, Biesheuvel CJ, Grobbee DE: **Test research versus diagnostic research.** *Clin Chem* 2004, **50**:473–476.
32. Jones MA, Jensen G, Edwards I: **Clinical reasoning in physiotherapy.** In *Clinical Reasoning in the Health Professions.* 3rd edition. Edited by Higgs J, Jones MA, Loftus S, Christensen N. Edinburgh, UK: Elsevier/Butterworth Heinemann; 2008:245–256.
33. Rothstein JM, Echternach JL, Riddle DL: **The hypothesis-oriented algorithm for clinicians II (HOAC II): a guide for patient management.** *Phys Ther* 2003, **83**:455–470.
34. Rivett DA, Higgs J: **Hypothesis generation in the clinical reasoning behaviour of manual therapists.** *J Phys Ther Educ* 1997, **11**:40–45.
35. van Trijffel E, Plochg T, van Hartingsveld F, Lucas C, Oostendorp RAB: **The role and position of passive intervertebral motion assessment within clinical reasoning and decision-making in manual physical therapy: a qualitative interview study.** *J Man Manip Ther* 2010, **18**:111–118.
36. Carlesso LC, Macdermid JC, Santaguida PL, Thabane L, Giulekas K, Larocque L, Millard J, Williams C, Miller J, Chesworth BM: **Beliefs and practice patterns in spinal manipulation and spinal motion palpation reported by Canadian manipulative therapists.** *Physiother Canada* 2013, **65**:167–175.
37. Riddle DL: **Classification and low back pain: A review of the literature and critical analysis of selected systems.** *Phys Ther* 1996, **78**:708–737.
38. Fairbank J, Gwilym SE, France JC, Daffner SD, Dettori J, Hermsmeyer J, Andersson G: **The role of classification of chronic low back pain.** *Spine* 2011, **36**(Suppl 2):19–42.
39. Arab AM, Abdollahi I, Joghataei MT, Golafshani Z, Kazemnejad A: **Inter- and intra-examiner reliability of single and composites of selected motion palpation and pain provocation tests for sacroiliac joint.** *Man Ther* 2009, **14**:213–221.
40. Kokmeyer DJ, van der Wurff P, Aufdemkampe G, Fickenscher TC: **The reliability of multitest regimens with sacroiliac pain provocation tests.** *J Manipulative Physiol Ther* 2002, **25**:42–48.
41. Robinson HS, Brox JI, Robinson R, Bjelland E, Solem S, Telje T: **The reliability of selected motion- and pain provocation tests for the sacroiliac joint.** *Man Ther* 2007, **12**:72–79.
42. Fritz JM, Brennan GP, Clifford SN, Hunter SJ, Thackeray A: **An examination of the reliability of a classification algorithm for subgrouping patients with low back pain.** *Spine* 2006, **31**:77–82.
43. Stanton TR, Fritz JM, Hancock MJ, Latimer J, Maher CG, Wand BM, Parent EC: **Evaluation of a treatment-based classification algorithm for low back pain: A cross-sectional study.** *Phys Ther* 2011, **91**:496–509.
44. Childs JD, Fritz JM, Flynn TW, Irrgang JJ, Johnson KK, Majkowski GR, Delitto A: **A clinical prediction rule to identify patients with low back pain most likely to benefit from spinal manipulation: A validation study.** *Ann Intern Med* 2004, **141**:920–928.
45. Flynn T, Fritz J, Whitman J, Wainner R, Magel J, Rendeiro D, Butler D, Garber M, Allison S: **A clinical prediction rule for classifying patients with low back pain who demonstrate short-term improvement with spinal manipulation.** *Spine* 2002, **27**:2835–2843.
46. Fritz JM, Whitman JM, Flynn TW, Wainner RS, Childs JD: **Factors related to the inability of individuals with low back pain to improve with a spinal manipulation.** *Phys Ther* 2004, **84**:173–190.
47. Hicks GE, Fritz JM, Delitto A, McGill SM: **Preliminary development of a clinical prediction rule for determining which patients with low back pain will respond to a stabilization exercise program.** *Arch Phys Med Rehabil* 2005, **89**:1753–1762.
48. Cook C: **Key issues for manual therapy clinical practice and research in North America.** *Man Ther* 2013, **18**:269–270.
49. Fritz JM, Brennan GP: **Preliminary examination of a proposed treatment-based classification system for patients receiving physical therapy interventions for neck pain.** *Phys Ther* 2007, **87**:513–524.
50. Cleland JA, Childs JD, Fritz JM, Whitman JM, Eberhart SL: **Development of a clinical prediction rule for guiding treatment of a subgroup of patients with neck pain: Use of thoracic spine manipulation, exercise, and patient education.** *Phys Ther* 2007, **87**:9–23.
51. Cleland JA, Fritz JM, Whitman JM, Heath R: **Predictors of short-term outcome in people with a clinical diagnosis of cervical radiculopathy.** *Phys Ther* 2007, **87**:1619–1632.
52. Puentedura EJ, Cleland JA, Landers MR, Mintken PE, Louw A, Fernándes-de-las-Peñas C: **Development of a clinical prediction rule to identify patients with neck pain likely to benefit from thrust joint manipulation to the cervical spine.** *J Orthop Sports Phys Ther* 2012, **42**:577–592.
53. Schellingerhout JM, Verhagen AP, Heymans MW, Pool JJ, Vonk F, Koes B, de Vet HCW: **Which subgroups of patients with non-specific neck pain are more likely to benefit from spinal manipulation, physiotherapy, or usual care?** *Pain* 2008, **139**:670–680.
54. Thiel HW, Bolton JE: **Predictors for immediate and global responses to chiropractic manipulation of the cervical spine.** *J Manipulative Physiol Ther* 2008, **31**:172–183.
55. Tseng Y-L, Wang WTJ, Chen W-Y, Hou T-J, Chen T-C, Lieu F-K: **Predictors for the immediate responders to cervical manipulation in patients with neck pain.** *Man Ther* 2006, **11**:306–315.
56. Gemmell H, Miller P: **Interexaminer reliability of multidimensional examination regimens for detecting spinal manipulable lesions: a systematic review.** *Clin Chiropr* 2005, **8**:199–204.
57. de Hertogh WJ, Vaes PH, Vijverman V, de Cordt A, Duquet W: **The clinical examination of neck pain patients: the validity of a group of tests.** *Man Ther* 2007, **12**:50–55.
58. Guzman J, Hurwitz EL, Carroll LJ, Haldeman S, Côté P, Carragee EJ, Peloso PM, van der Velde G, Holm LW, Hogg-Johnson S, Nordin M, Cassidy JD: **A new conceptual model of neck pain: linking onset, course, and care. The Bone and Joint Decade 2000–2010 Task Force on Neck Pain and Its Associated Disorders.** *Spine* 2008, **33**(Suppl 4):14–23.
59. Airaksinen O, Brox JI, Cedraschi C, Hildebrandt J, Klaber-Moffet J, Kovacs F, Mannion AF, Reis S, Staal JB, Ursin H, Zanoli G: **Chapter 4 European guidelines for the management of chronic nonspecific low back pain.** *Eur Spine J* 2006, **15**(Suppl 2):192–300.
60. Hawker GA, Mian S, Kendzerska T, French M: **Measures of adult pain. Visual Analog Scale for Pain (VAS Pain), Numeric Rating Scale for Pain (NRS Pain), McGill Pain Questionnaire (MPQ), Short-Form McGill Pain Questionnaire (SF-MPQ), Chronic Pain Grade Scale (CPGS), Short Form-36 Bodily Pain Scale (SF-36 BPS), and Measure of Intermittent and Constant Osteoarthritis Pain (ICOAP).** *Arthritis Care Res* 2011, **63**(Suppl 11):240–252.

61. Schoppink LE, van Tulder MW, Koes BW, Beurskens SA, de Bie RA: **Reliability and validity of the Dutch adaptation of the Quebec Back Pain Disability Scale.** *Phys Ther* 1996, **76:**268–275.
62. Schellingerhout JM, Heymans MW, Verhagen AP, de Vet HC, Koes BW, Terwee CB: **Measurement properties of translated versions of neck-specific questionnaires: A systematic review.** *BMC Med Res Methodol* 2011, **11:**87.
63. Greenhalgh S, Selfe J: *Red flags. A guide to identifying serious pathology of the spine.* Amsterdam/New York: Elsevier/Churchill Livingstone; 2006:5–48.
64. **KNGF Guideline Low-back Pain.** 2013, [http://www.fysionet-evidencebased.nl/index.php/component/kngf/richtlijnen/lage-rugpijn-2013] [In Dutch] Last accessed 30 December 2013.
65. van der El A: *Orthopaedic manual therapy diagnosis. Spine and temperomandibular joints.* London, UK: Jones and Bartlett Publishers; 2010:351–498.
66. Macfadyen N, Maher CG, Adams R: **Number of sampling movements and manual stiffness judgements.** *J Manipulative Physiol Ther* 1998, **21:**604–610.
67. **International classification of functioning, disability and health (ICF).** [http://www.who.int/classifications/icf/en/] Last accessed 30 December 2013.
68. Cohen J: **A coefficient of agreement for nominal scales.** *Educ Psychol Meas* 1960, **20:**37–46.
69. Cicchetti DV, Feinstein AR: **High agreement but low Kappa: II. Resolving the paradoxes.** *J Clin Epidemiol* 1990, **43:**551–558.
70. Byrt T, Bishop J, Carlin JB: **Bias, prevalence and Kappa.** *J Clin Epidemiol* 1993, **46:**423–429.
71. Feinstein AR, Cicchetti DV: **High agreement but low kappa: I. The problems of two paradoxes.** *J Clin Epidemiol* 1990, **43:**543–549.
72. MacKinnon A: **A spreadsheet for the calculation of comprehensive statistics for the assessment of diagnostic tests and inter-rater agreement.** *Comput Biol Med* 2000, **30:**127–134.
73. Landis JR, Koch DG: **The measurement of observer agreement for categorical data.** *Biometrica* 1977, **33:**159–164.
74. Whiting PF, Rutjes AWS, Westwood ME, Mallett S, and the QUADAS-2 Steering Group: **A systematic review classifies sources of bias and variation in diagnostic test accuracy studies.** *J Clin Epidemiol* 2013, **66:**1093–1104.
75. Foster NE, Hill JC, Hay EM: **Subgrouping patients with low back pain in primary care: Are we getting any better at it?** *Man Ther* 2011, **16:**3–8.
76. Borkan JM, Cherkin DC: **An agenda for primary care research on low back pain.** *Spine* 1996, **21:**2880–2884.
77. Borkan JM, Koes B, Reis S, Cherkin DC: **A report from the Second International Forum for Primary Care Research on Low Back Pain. Examining priorities.** *Spine* 1998, **23:**1992–1996.
78. Bouter LM, van Tulder MW, Koes BW: **Methodologic issues in low back pain research in primary care.** *Spine* 1998, **23:**2014–2020.
79. **Clinical research agenda for physical therapy.** *Phys Ther* 2000, **80:**499–513. http://www.ncbi.nlm.nih.gov/pubmed/10792860.
80. Foster NE, Dziedzic KS, van der Windt DAWM, Fritz JM, Hay EM: **Research priorities for non-pharmacological therapies for common musculoskeletal problem: Nationally and internationally agreed recommendations.** *BMC Musculoskelet Disord* 2009, **10:**3.
81. Goldstein MS, Scalzitti DA, Craik RL, Dunn SL, Irion JM, Irrgang J, Kolobe THA, McDonough CM, Shields RK: **The revised research agenda for physical therapy.** *Phys Ther* 2011, **91:**165–174.
82. Kent P, Keating JL, Leboeuf-Yde C: **Research methods for subgrouping low back pain.** *BMC Med Res Methodol* 2010, **10:**62.
83. Kent P, Keating J: **Do primary care clinicians think that nonspecific low back pain is one condition?** *Spine* 2004, **29:**1022–1031.
84. Kent P, Keating J: **Classification in nonspecific low back pain: What methods do primary care clinicians currently use?** *Spine* 2005, **30:**1433–1440.
85. Beneciuk JM, Bishop MD, George SZ: **Clinical prediction rules for physical therapy interventions: A systematic review.** *Phys Ther* 2009, **89:**114–124.
86. May S, Rosedale R: **Prescriptive clinical prediction rules in back pain research: A systematic review.** *J Man Manip Ther* 2009, **17:**36–45.
87. Kent P, Mjøsund HL, Petersen DHD: **Does targeting manual therapy and/or exercise improve patient outcomes in nonspecific low back pain. A systematic review.** *BMC Med* 2010, **8:**22.
88. Stanton TR, Hancock MJ, Maher CG, Koes BW: **Critical appraisal of clinical prediction rules that aim to optimize treatment selection for musculoskeletal conditions.** *Phys Ther* 2010, **90:**843–854.
89. Patel S, Friede T, Froud R, Evans DW, Underwood M: **Systematic review of randomized controlled trials of clinical prediction rules for physical therapy in low back pain.** *Spine* 2013, **38:**762–769.
90. Slater SL, Ford JJ, Richards MC, Taylor NF, Surkitt LD, Hahne AJ: **The effectiveness of sub-group specific manual therapy for low back pain: A systematic review.** *Man Ther* 2012, **17:**201–212.
91. Stiell IG, Greenberg GH, McKnight RD, Nair RC, McDowell I, Worthington JR: **A study to develop clinical decision rules for the use of radiography in acute ankle injuries.** *Ann Emerg Med* 1992, **21:**384–390.
92. Smith J, Bolton PS: **What are the clinical criteria justifying spinal manipulative therapy for neck pain? A systematic review of randomized controlled trials.** *Pain Med* 2013, **14:**460–468.
93. Lijmer JG, Mol BW, Heisterkamp S, Bonsel GJ, Prins MH, van der Meulen JHP, Bossuyt PMM: **Empirical evidence of design-related bias in studies of diagnostic tests.** *JAMA* 1999, **282:**1061–1066.
94. Whiting P, Rutjes AWS, Reitsma JB, Glas AS, Bossuyt PMM, Kleijnen J: **Sources of variation and bias in studies of diagnostic accuracy. A systematic review.** *Ann Intern Med* 2004, **140:**189–202.
95. Rutjes AW, Reitsma JB, di Nisio M, Smidt N, van Rijn JC, Bossuyt PM: **Evidence of bias and variation in diagnostic accuracy studies.** *CMAJ* 2006, **174:**469–476.
96. Scales CD Jr, Canfield SE: **Advanced topics in evidence-based urological oncology: Using results of a subgroup analysis.** *Urol Oncol* 2011, **29:**462–466.
97. Cook C, Turney L, Ramirez L, Miles A, Haas S, Karakostas T: **Predictive factors in poor inter-rater reliability among physical therapists.** *J Man Manip Ther* 2002, **10:**200–205.
98. Riddle DL, Rothstein JM, Echternach JL: **Application of the HOAC II: An episode of care for a patient with low back pain.** *Phys Ther* 2003, **83:**471–485.
99. Thoomes EJ, Schmitt MS: **Practical use of the HOAC II for clinical decision making and subsequent therapeutic interventions in an elite athlete with low back pain.** *J Orthop Sports Phys Ther* 2011, **41:**108–117.
100. Oostendorp RAB, Rutten GM, Dommerholt J, Nijhuis-van der Sanden MW, Harting J: **Guideline-based development and practice test of quality indicators for physiotherapy care in patients with neck pain.** *J Eval Clin Prac* 2013, **13:**194.
101. Shirley D, Ellis E, Lee M: **The response of posteroanterior lumbar stiffness to repeated loading.** *Man Ther* 2002, **7:**19–25.
102. Busscher I, van Dieën JH, van der Veen AJ, Kingma I, Meijer GJM, Verkerke GJ, Veldhuizen AG: **The effects of creep and recovery on the *in vitro* biomechanical characteristics of human multi-level thoracolumbar spinal segments.** *Clin Biomech* 2011, **26:**438–444.
103. Battlé MC, Cherkin DC, Dunn R, Ciol MA, Wheeler KJ: **Managing low back pain: Attitudes and treatment preferences of physical therapists.** *Phys Ther* 1994, **74:**219–226.
104. Carey TS, Freburger JK, Holmes GM, Castel L, Darter J, Agans R, Kalsbeek W, Jackman A: **A long way to go. Practice patterns and evidence in chronic low back pain care.** *Spine* 2009, **34:**718–724.
105. Freburger JK, Carey TS, Holmes GM: **Physical therapy for chronic low back pain in North Carolina: Overuse, underuse, or misuse?** *Phys Ther* 2011, **91:**484–495.
106. Goode AP, Freburger J, Carey T: **Prevalence, practice patterns, and evidence for chronic neck pain.** *Arthritis Care Res* 2010, **62:**1594–1601.
107. Gracey JH, McDonough SM, Baxter GD: **Physiotherapy management of low back pain. A survey of current practice in Northern Ireland.** *Spine* 2002, **27:**406–411.
108. Jette AM, Delitto A: **Physical therapy treatment choices for musculoskeletal impairments.** *Phys Ther* 1997, **77:**145–154.
109. Li LC, Bombardier C: **Physical therapy management of low back pain: An exploratory survey of therapist approaches.** *Phys Ther* 2001, **81:**1018–1028.
110. Liddle SD, Baxter GD, Gracey JH: **Physiotherapists' use of advice and exercise for the management of chronic low back pain: A national survey.** *Man Ther* 2009, **14:**189–196.
111. Mikhail C, Korner-Bitensky N, Rossignol M, Dumas J-P: **Physical therapists' use of interventions with high evidence of effectiveness in the management of a hypothetical typical patient with acute low back pain.** *Phys Ther* 2005, **85:**1151–1167.
112. Mielenz TJ, Carey TS, Dyrek DA, Harris BA, Garrett JM, Darter JD: **Physical therapy utilization by patients with acute low back pain.** *Phys Ther* 1997, **77:**1040–1051.

113. van Baar ME, Dekker J, Bosveld W: **A survey of physical therapy goals and interventions for patients with back and knee pain.** *Phys Ther* 1998, **78**:33–42.
114. Adams G, Sim J: **A survey of UK manual therapists' practice of and attitudes towards manipulation and its complications.** *Physiother Res Int* 1998, **3**:206–227.
115. Jull G: **Use of high and low velocity cervical manipulative therapy procedures by Australian manipulative physiotherapists.** *Aust J Physiother* 2002, **48**:189–193.
116. Hurley L, Yardley K, Gross AR, Hendry L, McLaughlin L: **A survey to examine attitudes and patterns of practice of physiotherapists who perform cervical spinal manipulation.** *Man Ther* 2002, **7**:10–18.
117. Sim J, Wright CC: **The Kappa statistic in reliability studies: use, interpretation, and sample size requirements.** *Phys Ther* 2005, **85**:257–268.
118. Hoehler FK: **Bias and prevalence effects on kappa viewed in terms of sensitivity and specificity.** *J Clin Epidemiol* 2000, **53**:499–503.
119. Zusman M: **There's something about passive movement.** *Med Hypotheses* 2010, **75**:106–110.
120. Hurwitz EL, Morgenstern H, Harber P, Kominski GF, Yu F, Adams AH: **A randomized trial of chiropractic manipulation and mobilization for patients with neck pain: Clinical outcomes from the UCLA neck-pain study.** *Am J Public Health* 2002, **92**:1634–1641.
121. Leaver AM, Maher CG, Herbert RD, Latimer J, McAuley JH, Jull G, Refshauge KM: **A randomized controlled trial comparing manipulation with mobilization for recent onset neck pain.** *Arch Phys Med Rehabil* 2010, **91**:1313–1318.
122. Dunning JR, Cleland JA, Waldrop MA, Arnot C, Young I, Turner M, Sigurdsson G: **Upper cervical and upper thoracic thrust manipulation versus mobilization in patients with mechanical neck pain: A multicenter randomized clinical trial.** *J Orthop Sports Phys Ther* 2012, **42**:5–18.
123. Cook C, Learman K, Showalter C, Kabbaz V, O'Halloran B: **Early use of thrust manipulation versus non-thrust manipulation: a randomized clinical trial.** *Man Ther* 2013, **18**:191–198.

Spinal manipulation and exercise for low back pain in adolescents: study protocol for a randomized controlled trial

Craig Schulz[1*], Brent Leininger[1], Roni Evans[1], Darcy Vavrek[2], Dave Peterson[3], Mitchell Haas[2] and Gert Bronfort[1]

Abstract

Background: Low back pain is among the most common and costly chronic health care conditions. Recent research has highlighted the common occurrence of non-specific low back pain in adolescents, with prevalence estimates similar to adults. While multiple clinical trials have examined the effectiveness of commonly used therapies for the management of low back pain in adults, few trials have addressed the condition in adolescents. The purpose of this paper is to describe the methodology of a randomized clinical trial examining the effectiveness of exercise with and without spinal manipulative therapy for chronic or recurrent low back pain in adolescents.

Methods/design: This study is a randomized controlled trial comparing twelve weeks of exercise therapy combined with spinal manipulation to exercise therapy alone. Beginning in March 2010, a total of 184 participants, ages 12 to 18, with chronic or recurrent low back pain are enrolled across two sites. The primary outcome is self-reported low back pain intensity. Other outcomes include disability, quality of life, improvement, satisfaction, activity level, low back strength, endurance, and motion. Qualitative interviews are conducted to evaluate participants' perceptions of treatment.

Discussion: This is the first randomized clinical trial assessing the effectiveness of combining spinal manipulative therapy with exercise for adolescents with low back pain. The results of this study will provide important evidence on the role of these conservative treatments for the management of low back pain in adolescents.

Trial registration: (ClinicalTrials.gov NCT01096628).

Keywords: Back pain, Pain, Spinal manipulation, Musculoskeletal manipulations, Exercise, Randomized controlled trial, Adolescent

Background

Low back pain prevalence and burden in adolescents

Low back pain (LBP) in adolescents has become increasingly recognized as a public health concern, with an estimated one year prevalence of 34% [1]. Often beginning at a young age, the prevalence of LBP quickly mirrors that of adults by the late teenage years [2]. The natural history of LBP in adolescents is also similar to adults with recurrent symptoms occurring in over one half of patients [3]. Importantly, recurrent LBP in adolescence is highly associated with continued pain in adulthood [4,5].

While the prevalence of LBP steadily increases with age during childhood, the number of adolescents seeking care does not dramatically increase until mid-adolescence [6]. Care-seeking for LBP in childhood is strongly influenced by pain intensity and limitations in daily activities [7]. Approximately one-quarter of adolescents with LBP miss school because of their LBP condition [8].

Although little is currently known regarding the societal cost of LBP in adolescents, the disease burden in adulthood is substantial. The 2010 Global Burden of Disease study ranked LBP as the leading cause of years lived with disability in the world [9]. After respiratory disorders, LBP causes more short-term work absence that any other condition [10]. In the US alone, costs associated with LBP are estimated between $20 and $120

* Correspondence: cschulz@nwhealth.edu
[1]Wolfe-Harris Center for Clinical Studies, Northwestern Health Sciences University, 2501 W 84th St, Bloomington, MN 55431, USA
Full list of author information is available at the end of the article

billion annually and are increasing [11,12]. In addition, there are growing concerns regarding the overutilization and safety of frequently prescribed medical treatments, particularly in light of the lack of evidence to support their effectiveness [13].

Recognizing that LBP begins at an early age and becomes burdensome and costly in adulthood, research focusing on conservative management strategies for adolescents with LBP is urgently needed.

Treatment of adolescent LBP

Whereas multiple randomized trials have examined the effectiveness of commonly used conservative treatments for LBP in adults [14-17], few have been performed in adolescent LBP populations. Three small randomized clinical trials have evaluated exercise as a treatment approach for adolescent LBP [18-20]. Collectively, the published trials to date suggest exercise may be effective in reducing pain and disability in adolescents with LBP, but larger, high quality trials are needed. Interestingly, although spinal manipulative therapy (SMT) is commonly used for children with spine conditions [21], no randomized trials examining the effectiveness of SMT for adolescent LBP have been published to date [22].

Study aims

Our primary aim is to determine the relative clinical effectiveness of 1) exercise with SMT versus 2) exercise alone in 184 adolescents with sub-acute recurrent (2-12 weeks) or chronic (>12 weeks) LBP, measured at 12, 26, and 52 weeks. The primary outcome measure is patient-rated LBP at these time points. Our hypothesis is that the addition of SMT to exercise will reduce pain more than exercise alone.

Our secondary aims are to assess between-group differences in disability, quality of life, improvement, satisfaction, activity level, dynamic lumbar motion, and trunk muscle endurance. In addition, we will assess the participant's perceptions of treatment using qualitative interviews.

Methods/design

Design & setting

This trial began in March 2010, and is a two-site, parallel-group randomized controlled trial. Participants are being recruited at Northwestern Health Sciences University in Bloomington, MN and the University of Western States in Portland, OR. All treatments are provided within university-associated outpatient clinics.

Ethical approval

Ethical approval has been granted by the Institutional Review Boards of the participating institutions (Project ID: 1-77-10-09).

Recruitment

Potential subjects are recruited from the Minneapolis/St. Paul, MN and Portland, OR metropolitan areas using multiple methods. The primary recruitment method is targeted mailings to households with adolescents. Other recruitment methods include internet advertising through Facebook and Craigslist, newspaper advertising, flyers, and targeted referral letters to local physicians specializing in pediatrics or musculoskeletal conditions and coaches of sport programs at local schools.

Participants

Adolescents, age 12 to18, with a history of sub-acute recurrent or chronic low back pain are eligible to participate. The inclusion/exclusion criteria are described in Table 1.

Baseline assessments

Interested individuals are assessed for eligibility and compliance during a scripted telephone interview followed by three distinct baseline evaluations. For participants ages 12-17, written assent is obtained in addition to written informed consent from a legal guardian. Participants 18 years of age provide written informed consent. Individuals complete a clinical health history and physical exam. Plain film radiographs are taken if suspicion of a specific cause of LBP is present. To maintain consistency across sites, study clinicians and investigators, who are blinded to upcoming treatment assignment, meet (in-person and by teleconference) to review each case to determine eligibility. Self-report outcome measures and blinded objective assessments of lumbar spine motion, strength, and endurance are completed at the first two baseline evaluations. An accelerometer is issued to potential participants to monitor their physical activity level for the week prior to treatment assignment. Participants are assigned to study treatments at the third baseline evaluation. The participant's flow through baseline evaluations and treatment is shown in Figure 1.

Treatment allocation & concealment

As participants become eligible, study staff masked to upcoming treatment assignments use a dynamic allocation (rank-order minimization) computer program to assign subjects to treatment [23-25]. Gender, age, pain duration, and intensity are entered into the program to balance patient characteristics between groups.

A computer-generated random allocation sequence secured in sealed, opaque, sequentially numbered envelopes is used to randomize the first six participants at each site to provide a "seed" group of participants for the dynamic allocation program. Envelopes are also used as a back-up in the event the treatment allocation program becomes unavailable.

Table 1 Inclusion and exclusion criteria

Inclusion criteria	Exclusion criteria
• 12 to 18 years old	• Spinal manipulative therapy or exercise therapy in the previous month
• Either:	
◦ Sub-acute recurrent non-specific low back pain defined as current episode of 2 to 12 weeks duration AND an additional 2 week episode of back pain in the past year	• Ongoing treatment for low back pain by other health care providers • Other serious physical or mental health conditions (e.g., uncontrolled diabetes, cancer)
OR	• Contraindications to study treatments including acute disc herniation, clinical
◦ Chronic non-specific low back pain defined as a current episode ≥ 12 weeks duration	• instability of the lumbar spine, or inflammatory arthritides
• Low back pain intensity ≥ 3 on 0 to 10 numerical rating scale	• Benign joint hypermobility syndrome
• Stable prescription medication plan (no changes to prescription medications that affect musculoskeletal pain in the previous month)	

Interventions

All interventions are provided by study staff at Northwestern Health Sciences University and the University of Western States research clinics. The physical nature of the treatments prevents blinding of participants and providers to treatment assignment. Participants are asked not to receive care for their LBP condition from other providers during the active treatment phase (12 weeks). Data regarding non-study care is collected in the self-report questionnaires.

Treatment providers have been trained in protocols to ensure standardized intervention and documentation. To facilitate protocol adherence, clinical records are monitored weekly by research staff. Non-adherent providers and patients are contacted using various methods (e.g., in-person, by phone, or email) to resolve compliance issues.

Exercise therapy (ET)

There are three components to the ET program: self-care education, supervised exercise visits, and home exercise. The overall objectives are to help adolescents manage their LBP and prevent future LBP recurrences. The total number of visits ranges from 8 to 16, depending on the patient's needs (e.g., ability to perform exercises independently). Experienced chiropractors and exercise therapists have been trained and certified to deliver the program.

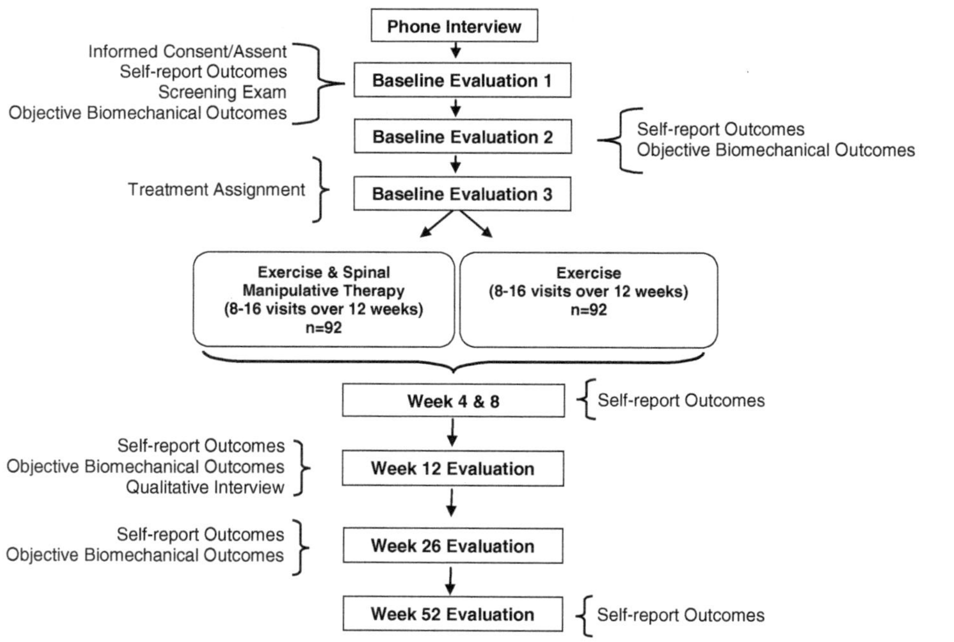

Figure 1 Study flow diagram. Self-report Outcomes: Primary and secondary outcomes (e.g., Pain, Disability). **Objective Biomechanical Outcomes:** Torso muscle strength & endurance; Continuous lumbar motion; Accelerometer readings for 7 consecutive days. **Qualitative Interview:** Face-to-face interviews assessing treatment experience and expectations.

Table 2 Treatment interventions

Intervention	Spinal Manipulative Therapy (SMT)	Exercise Therapy (ET)
Type	• High velocity, low amplitude SMT preferred	**ET Visit**
		Self-care education
	• Other manual therapies if needed	• Supervised exercise
	◦ Low velocity, low amplitude SMT or mobilization	◦ Aerobic warm up
	◦ Flexion-distraction manipulation	
	◦ Drop-table assisted SMT	◦ Stretching (cat/camel, piriformis, hamstring, laying back rotation)
	• Up to 5 minutes adjunct therapies to facilitate SMT:	
	◦ Light soft tissue massage, active and passive stretching, ischemic compression of tender points, ice and heat	◦ Strengthening (bridge, abdominal curl, back extension, side bridge, quadruped, and squats) with changes in body positioning and addition of labile surface (i.e., gym ball) for progressions
		Home Exercise
		• Instructions provided at treatment visits and supplemented by take home materials
Design & delivery format	• Individualized: number of visits, spinal levels treated, SMT and manual therapy technique used and adjunct therapies determined by provider according to patient needs and tolerance	**ET Visit**
		• Supervised
		• Individualized: number of visits, exercise progressions determined by provider
		Home Exercise
		• Unsupervised
Delivery method	• One-on-one treatment visit	**ET Visit**
	• Treatment provided by licensed chiropractor	• One-on-one exercise therapy visit
		• Instructions and supervision provided by licensed chiropractor or exercise therapist
		Home Exercise
		• Instructions provided at treatment visits
		• Instructions supplemented by take home materials (exercise photos, modified *Back in Action* [26] book)
Dose	• 8 to 16 treatment visits	**ET Visit**
	• 10 to 20 minutes per visit	• 8 to 16 visits
	• Maximum frequency: 2 times/week	• 45 minutes per visit
		◦ 10 minutes self-care education
		◦ 5 minutes aerobic exercise warm up
		◦ 30 minutes supervised exercise
		▪ Stretching: 1 set; 3 reps
		▪ cat/camel; 1 rep each side for other stretches
		▪ Strengthening: 2 sets; 16 to 20 repetitions each exercise
		Home Exercise
		• Maximum frequency: 2 times/week

The details of the exercise program are outlined in Table 2. Each visit starts with 10 minutes of self-care education to help patients establish and monitor goals aligned with the exercise program and enhance their understanding of LBP. Participants are taught the importance of movement and activity, pain management techniques, and methods for developing spinal posture awareness during activities of daily living (e.g., lifting, pushing, pulling, sitting, getting out of bed, and using a backpack). Individuals are provided printed instructions and photos of exercises in addition to a modified *Back in Action* [26] binder, which emphasizes movement and restoration of normal function and fitness [27,28]. The supervised exercises begin with a 5-minute, light aerobic warm up, followed by stretching and strengthening exercises (bridge, abdominal crunches, quadruped, side bridge, and back extensions). Participants begin with exercises appropriate for their fitness level and gradually progress in difficulty by changing body position and/or using a labile surface (i.e., gym ball). Participants are encouraged to perform the same exercises at home combined with 20-40 minutes of aerobic activity two times per week.

Exercise therapy combined with spinal manipulative therapy (ET + SMT)

Participants in the ET + SMT group participate in the same ET program described above. In addition, they take part in 8 to 16, 10- to 20-minute sessions of SMT over 12 weeks (Table 2). Previous research has shown that 9 to 12 treatments are more beneficial than 3 to 6 treatments for adults with LBP [29]. The number and frequency of treatments is determined by the individual chiropractor based on patient-rated symptoms and exam findings [30]. SMT is provided by experienced chiropractors following standardized treatment protocols. The preferred treatment consists of a high-velocity, low amplitude thrust SMT. The treating chiropractor has the option to perform other techniques (e.g., flexion-distraction, spinal mobilization, or neuromuscular techniques) [31], as indicated. Light soft tissue techniques (i.e., active and passive muscle stretching, hot and cold packs, and ischemic compression of tender points) may be used as needed to facilitate the manual therapy.

Modification and discontinuation of treatment

Prescription-strength nonsteroidal anti-inflammatory rescue medications are available for patients experiencing severe pain and are prescribed as needed by a study medical doctor. Any patient who demonstrates progressive neurological signs or severe intractable pain is removed from study treatment and referred for orthopedic consultation. Participants who receive medications or are discontinued from treatment will be included in the intention-to-treat analyses.

Outcomes

Patient self-report outcomes are collected at the first two baseline visits and at 4, 8, 12, 26, and 52 weeks after randomization. The self-report outcomes are based on the Pediatric Initiative on Methods, Measurement, and Pain Assessment in Clinical Trials (PedIMMPACT) groups' recommendations [32]. Objective spinal biomechanical outcome measures are collected at the first two baseline visits and at 12 and 26 weeks after study enrollment by examiners blinded to treatment assignment. The participant's physical activity level is assessed at baseline and at weeks 12 and 26. Qualitative interviews are conducted at 12 weeks (end of treatment) to ascertain their perceptions of treatment.

Primary outcome

Pain Patient-rated low back pain at 12, 26, and 52 weeks, measured by the 11-box numerical rating scale, is the primary outcome measure. LBP at 4 and 8 weeks is a secondary outcome. Pain severity is regarded as one of the most important clinical outcomes by adults with spinal pain [33,34] and is recommended as a core outcome by an international group of back pain researchers in addition to the PedIMMPACT group [32,35]. The 11-box numerical rating scale for pain has been shown to perform similarly to the visual analogue scale (VAS) in both pediatric and adult populations [36,37].

Secondary outcomes

Disability Patient-rated disability is assessed using the 18-item Roland-Morris Disability Questionnaire. The 18-item Roland-Morris Disability Questionnaire has been shown to be reliable, valid, and as responsive as the original 24-item Roland-Morris Disability Questionnaire [38,39].

Quality of life Participants rate their quality of life using the 23-item PedsQL instrument, which has been developed to measure physical, emotional, social, and school functioning domains in children 8 to 18 years old. The PedsQL is a reliable, valid, and responsive measure of quality of life [40-43].

Improvement Patient-rated improvement is determined by asking participants to compare their LBP condition to what it was before study treatment on a 9-point scale ranging from no symptoms (100% improvement) to as bad as it could be (100% worse). The caregiver's impression of improvement will also be measured using the same 9-point scale. Improvement is an important outcome that has shown to be responsive [44].

Satisfaction The participant's overall satisfaction with care is assessed with a 7-point scale ranging from completely satisfied (couldn't be better) to completely dissatisfied (couldn't be worse). The caregiver's satisfaction with care is also evaluated using the same scale. Research examining global satisfaction with treatment in pediatric pain trials is lacking and has been identified as an area of great need by the PedIMMPACT group [32].

Adverse events The complete reporting of adverse events in clinical trials has received little attention [45]. To address this, we collect adverse event information at several levels. First, participants are queried about expected adverse events in the self-report questionnaires by choosing from a list generated from previous studies [46,47]. Participants are asked to rate the bothersomeness of each adverse event on a 0 to10 scale (0 = not at all bothersome, 10 = extremely bothersome). In addition, they are asked about new or ongoing adverse events at each treatment visit; these are recorded on standardized treatment notes. Finally, all patients are instructed to a report serious adverse event at any time to study staff (see Data and Safety Monitoring below).

Expectation Participants rate their perception of how helpful they believe each treatment will be on a 1 to 5 scale (1 = Much better, 5 = Much worse) prior to randomization. After randomization, participants are asked to estimate the degree of improvement they expect to have after 12 weeks of care using the 9-point improvement scale described above.

Health care utilization and compliance Patients report the number of visits and care received from non-study health care providers. They also report the number of days they took medication for LBP and performed the study exercises in the past week.

Qualitative outcomes

Qualitative interviews One-on-one interviews are conducted at 12 weeks. A schedule of questions is used to direct the interviews and keep the interviewers on a path consistent with the purpose of the study [48]. The questions begin broadly, asking how patients felt about the treatment they received, whether it met their expectations, and what they liked and disliked. These questions are followed by probe questions to elicit underlying reasons.

Objective biomechanical outcomes

Continuous lumbar motion Lumbar spinal motion is assessed using the Zebris CMS-HS Spine Motion Analyzer (Zebris Inc., Isny im Allgau, Germany), a reliable and accurate measurement system [49,50]. Lumbar flexion-extension, rotation, and side-bending are examined using a modified protocol described by Vogt et al [51].

Torso muscle strength & endurance Endurance of the lower back musculature (trunk flexors, lateral flexors, and extensors) is examined using the protocol described by McGill [52]. The tests have been shown to be a valid and reliable measure of torso muscle endurance [53,54]. Maximum isometric strength of trunk flexors and extensors is measured using a modified standing method described by Jørgensen and Nicolaisen [55,56].

Activity level Participants' physical activity level is assessed by having them wear a GT3X accelerometer (Actigraph, Inc. Pensacola, FL) for 7 consecutive days prior to randomization, then again prior to the week 12 and 26 evaluations. The GT3X accelerometer has been found to be a reliable and valid measure of physical activity level [57].

Analysis plan

For the primary analysis, patient-rated low back pain will be analyzed at 12, 26, and 52 weeks with linear mixed model regression to estimate mean differences between treatment groups at each time point adjusting for baseline covariates (i.e., rank-order minimization variables) and accounting for correlation across measurements within person. Short- and long-term longitudinal effects between groups will also be assessed using mixed model analyses including LBP intensity outcomes from weeks 4 to 12 and weeks 4 to 52, respectively. Due to the longitudinal study design, the primary analysis plan was modified from a one-way analysis of covariance to a linear mixed model approach to allow increased flexibility when specifying a variance-covariance structure and accounting for missing data [58-60]. The analysis plan was modified prior to the completion of data collection and the start of data analysis.

The variance-covariance structure that best fits the data will be used to account for correlation among the repeated measurements within participants [61,62]. Normality assumptions will be evaluated through normal probability plots and transformations used, if necessary. We will test for a site-by-group interaction, but given our standardization plan, we do not expect it to be present. Adjusted mean differences and 95% confidence intervals between groups for short- and long-term effects based on the final models will be presented in tables and line graphs. The need for inclusion of additional covariates to balance baseline group differences will be evaluated in sensitivity analysis. Intention-to-treat analysis will be used; all patients with at least one follow-up measure will be included in the analysis as the methods do not require data at every time point. In the event that missing data is present, the pattern of missingness will be assessed and appropriate imputation and sensitivity analyses will be performed. Responder analyses (i.e., 50, 75, and 100% pain reduction) will be conducted to facilitate the interpretation of the results [63-65].

Power analysis and sample size

The basis for our sample size calculation is the one-way analysis of covariance (ANCOVA), comparing the primary outcome (reported pain level at the 12, 26, and 52 week time points) between groups and adjusting for baseline pain level. We estimated the standard deviation for change in pain using data from the trial by Jones et al [18] (SD = 1.4). A conservative R^2 estimate of 0.2 was used for the sample size calculation. With a power of 0.92 and a 2-group design tested at an alpha level of 0.01, 80 subjects per group are required to detect a pain reduction of 0.8 points (Power and Precision™ 2.0). We will allow for a dropout rate/loss to follow-up of up to 15%. Therefore, 92 patients are required per group, for a total of 184 subjects.

Data and safety monitoring

The Office of Data Management at Northwestern Health Sciences University serves as the data coordinating center responsible for creation of data collection forms, coordination of data transfer, and data management. A Data Safety and Monitoring Committee consisting of study and non-study clinicians and scientists meet annually to review the study. Due to the low risk profiles of the study interventions no interim analyses are planned. Adverse events are classified using the National Institutes of Health Office of Human Subjects Research definitions [66].

Discussion

LBP is a significant health problem not only for adults, but also for children and adolescents. Given the large social and economic costs associated with the condition, identifying effective, conservative management strategies is critical. While SMT and exercise have been shown to be effective in adult populations, high quality research is needed to investigate their effectiveness in adolescent LBP patients.

Only a limited number of interventions for adolescent LBP have been evaluated in clinical trials; consequently, there is no established 'gold-standard' treatment. We chose exercise as a core intervention because of the evidence of effectiveness for adults with LBP [15,16], in addition to the preliminary evidence in adolescent populations [67]. Further, we wanted to encourage active behaviors for the management of pain in an adolescent population. We hypothesized that adding SMT to a promising treatment like exercise will produce greater improvements in LBP than what will be achieved by exercise alone.

Given there have been few studies addressing LBP in adolescents (and there have been no randomized clinical trials of SMT), we designed this trial with sufficient methodological rigor to maintain high internal validity; however, where possible, we also included pragmatic design features to enhance generalizability [68]. Explanatory design aspects of the trial aimed at ensuring high validity and low risk of bias include: the use of multiple baseline assessments to ensure participant compliance; eligibility criteria to exclude individuals unlikely to demonstrate treatment effects (e.g., pain intensity ≥ 3/10); restricted utilization of co-interventions during the intervention phase; structured protocols for the application of the intervention (number of visits, exercise, or SMT techniques used); application of the intervention at university-associated research clinics by clinicians with investigator supervision; and monitoring of participant and provider compliance including strategies to maximize adherence to study protocols. Pragmatic features of the study include: multiple recruitment sources from the general population at multiple sites; flexibility in the application of the intervention (e.g., exercise progressions, type of SMT used) based on individual patient needs and abilities; the use of an active treatment comparison group; the collection of both short- and long-term outcomes; and the plan to use intention-to-treat statistical analysis.

Upon completion, this study will provide high quality scientific evidence regarding SMT and exercise for LBP in adolescents with the potential to alter clinical practice and reduce both the current and future burden of LBP.

Competing interests

The authors declare that they have no competing interests.

Authors' contributions

GB and MH are the co-principal investigators and have been primarily responsible for study conception, design, analysis plan, funding acquisition and implementation. CS, DP, DV, and RE contributed to the conceptualization and design of the study, funding acquisition, and implementation. BL participated in the implementation and management of the trial, drafted the Background, Methods, and Discussion sections of the manuscript, and coordinated manuscript preparation and revision. All authors provided critical evaluation and revision of the manuscript and have given final approval of the manuscript accepting responsibility for all aspects.

Acknowledgements

The trial was funded by the U.S. Department of Health and Human Services Health Resources and Services Administration (HRSA), Bureau of Health Professions (BHPr), Division of Medicine and Dentistry (DMD), grant number R18HP15124. The content and conclusions of this manuscript are those of the authors and should not be construed as the official position or policy of, nor should any endorsements be inferred by the U.S. government, HHS, HRSA, BHPr, or the DMD.

The authors wish to acknowledge the contributions of our dedicated project managers Kayla Kelly and Sarah Kirkpatrick, in addition to the research clinicians and staff.

Author details

[1]Wolfe-Harris Center for Clinical Studies, Northwestern Health Sciences University, 2501 W 84th St, Bloomington, MN 55431, USA. [2]Center for Outcome Studies, University of Western States, 2900 NE 132nd Ave, Portland, OR 97230, USA. [3]Division of Chiropractic Sciences, University of Western States, 2900 NE 132nd Ave, Portland, OR 97230, USA.

References

1. Calvo-Munoz I, Gomez-Conesa A, Sanchez-Meca J: **Prevalence of low back pain in children and adolescents: a meta-analysis.** *BMC Pediatr* 2013, **13**:14.
2. Jeffries LJ, Milanese SF, Grimmer-Somers KA: **Epidemiology of adolescent spinal pain: a systematic overview of the research literature.** *Spine* 2007, **32**:2630–2637.
3. Burton AK, Clarke RD, McClune TD, Tillotson KM: **The natural history of low back pain in adolescents.** *Spine* 1996, **21**:2323–2328.
4. Hestbaek L, Leboeuf-Yde C, Kyvik KO: **Is comorbidity in adolescence a predictor for adult low back pain? A prospective study of a young population.** *BMC Musculoskelet Disord* 2006, **7**:29.
5. Hestbaek L, Leboeuf-Yde C, Kyvik KO, Manniche C: **The course of low back pain from adolescence to adulthood: eight-year follow-up of 9600 twins.** *Spine* 2006, **31**:468–472.
6. Kjaer P, Wedderkopp N, Korsholm L, Leboeuf-Yde C: **Prevalence and tracking of back pain from childhood to adolescence.** *BMC Musculoskelet Disord* 2011, **12**:98.
7. Tiira AH, Paananen MV, Taimela SP, Zitting PJ, Jarvelin MR, Karppinen JI: **Determinants of adolescent health care use for low back pain.** *Eur J Pain* 2012, **16**:1467–1476.

8. Bejia I, Abid N, Ben SK, Letaief M, Younes M, Touzi M, Bergaoui N: **Low back pain in a cohort of 622 Tunisian schoolchildren and adolescents: an epidemiological study.** *Eur Spine J* 2005, **14**:331–336.
9. Vos T, Flaxman AD, Naghavi M, Lozano R, Michaud C, Ezzati M, Shibuya K, Salomon JA, Abdalla S, Aboyans V, Abraham J, Ackerman I, Aggarwal R, Ahn SY, Ali MK, Alvarado M, Anderson HR, Anderson LM, Andrews KG, Atkinson C, Baddour LM, Bahalim AN, Barker-Collo S, Barrero LH, Bartels DH, Basáñez MG, Baxter A, Bell ML, Benjamin EJ, Bennett D, *et al*: **Years lived with disability (YLDs) for 1160 sequelae of 289 diseases and injuries 1990-2010: a systematic analysis for the Global Burden of Disease Study 2010.** *Lancet* 2012, **380**:2163–2196.
10. Woolf AD, Pfleger B: **Burden of major musculoskeletal conditions.** *Bull World Health Organ* 2003, **81**:646–656.
11. Dagenais S, Caro J, Haldeman S: **A systematic review of low back pain cost of illness studies in the United States and internationally.** *Spine J* 2008, **8**:8–20.
12. Martin BI, Deyo RA, Mirza SK, Turner JA, Comstock BA, Hollingworth W, Sullivan SD: **Expenditures and health status among adults with back and neck problems.** *JAMA* 2008, **299**:656–664.
13. Deyo RA, Mirza SK, Turner JA, Martin BI: **Overtreating chronic back pain: time to back off?** *J Am Board Fam Med* 2009, **22**:62–68.
14. Rubinstein SM, Van MM, Assendelft WJ, de Boer MR, van Tulder MW: **Spinal manipulative therapy for chronic low-back pain.** *Cochrane Database Syst Rev* 2011, doi:10.1002/14651858.CD008112.pub2.
15. Hayden JA, van Tulder MW, Malmivaara A, Koes BW: **Exercise therapy for treatment of non-specific low back pain.** *Cochrane Database Syst Rev* 2005, **20**(3): CD000335.
16. van Middelkoop M, Rubinstein SM, Verhagen AP, Ostelo RW, Koes BW, van Tulder MW: **Exercise therapy for chronic nonspecific low-back pain.** *Best Pract Res Clin Rheumatol* 2010, **24**:193–204.
17. Bronfort G, Haas M, Evans R, Leininger B, Triano J: **Effectiveness of manual therapies: the UK evidence report.** *Chiropr Osteopat* 2010, **18**:3.
18. Jones M, Stratton G, Reilly T, Unnithan V: **The efficacy of exercise as an intervention to treat recurrent nonspecific low back pain in adolescents.** *Pediatr Exerc Sci* 2007, **19**:349–359.
19. Ahlqwist A, Hagman M, Kjellby-Wendt G, Beckung E: **Physical therapy treatment of back complaints on children and adolescents.** *Spine* 2008, **33**:E721–E727.
20. Fanucchi GL, Stewart A, Jordaan R, Becker P: **Exercise reduces the intensity and prevalence of low back pain in 12-13 year old children: a randomised trial.** *Aust J Physiother* 2009, **55**:97–104.
21. Barnes PM, Bloom B: **Complementary and Alternative Medicine Use Among Adults and Children: United States, 2007.** *National Health Statistics Reports* 2008, **12**:1–24.
22. Hestbaek L, Stochkendahl MJ: **The evidence base for chiropractic treatment of musculoskeletal conditions in children and adolescents: The emperor's new suit?** *Chiropr Osteopat* 2010, **18**:15.
23. Pocock SJ, Simon R: **Sequential treatment assignment with balancing for prognostic factors in the controlled clinical trial.** *Biometrics* 1975, **31**:103–115.
24. Bracken MB: **On stratification, minimization and protection against types 1 and 2 error.** *J Clin Epidemiol* 2001, **54**:104–105.
25. Stigsby B, Taves DR: **Rank-Minimization for balanced assignment of subjects in clinical trials.** *Contemp Clin Trials* 2010, **31**:147–150.
26. Cherkin DC, Deyo RA, Street JH, Hunt M, Barlow W: **Pitfalls of patient education. Limited success of a program for back pain in primary care.** *Spine* 1996, **21**:345–355.
27. Engers A, Jellema P, Wensing M, van der Windt D, Grol R, van Tulder M: **Individual patient education for low back pain; a systematic review.** In *Low Back Pain in General Practice. Should Treatment be aimed at Psychosocial Factors?*. Edited by Jellema P. Amsterdam, The Netherlands: Febodruk BV; 2005:123–156.
28. Burton AK, Waddell G, Tillotson KM, Summerton N: **Information and advice to patients with back pain can have a positive effect. A randomized controlled trial of a novel educational booklet in primary care.** *Spine* 1999, **24**:2484–2491.
29. Haas M, Groupp E, Kraemer DF: **Dose-response for chiropractic care of chronic low back pain.** *Spine J* 2004, **4**:574–583.
30. Seffinger MA, Najm WI, Mishra SI, Adams A, Dickerson VM, Murphy LS, Reinsch S: **Reliability of spinal palpation for diagnosis of back and neck pain: a systematic review of the literature.** *Spine* 2004, **29**:E413–E425.
31. Peterson DH, Bergmann TF: *Chiropractic Technique: Principles and Procedures.* St. Louis, MO: Mosby; 2011.
32. McGrath PJ, Walco GA, Dworkin RH, Brown MT, Davidson K, Eccleston C, Finley GA, Goldschneider K, Haverkos L, Hertz SH, Ljungman G, Palermo T, Rappaport BA, Rhodes T, Schechter N, Scott J, Sethna N, Svensson OK, Stinson J, von Baeyer CL, Walker L, Weisman S, White RE, Zajicek A, Zeltzer L, PedIMMPACT: **Core outcome domains and measures for pediatric acute and chronic/recurrent pain clinical trials: PedIMMPACT recommendations.** *J Pain* 2008, **9**:771–783.
33. Evans RL, Maiers MJ, Bronfort G: **What do patients think? Results of a mixed methods pilot study assessing sciatica patients' interpretations of satisfaction and improvement.** *J Manipulative Physiol Ther* 2003, **26**:502–509.
34. Evans R, Bronfort G, Schulz C, Maiers M, Bracha Y, Svendsen K, Grimm R Jr, Garvey T, Transfeldt E: **Supervised Exercise with and Without Spinal Manipulation Perform Similarly and Better Than Home Exercise for Chronic Neck Pain: A Randomized Controlled Trial.** *Spine (Phila Pa 1976)* 2012, **37**:903–914.
35. Deyo RA, Battie M, Beurskens AJ, Bombardier C, Croft P, Koes B, Malmivaara A, Roland M, Von Korff M, Waddell G: **Outcome measures for low back pain research. A proposal for standardized use.** *Spine* 1998, **23**:2003–2013.
36. Von Baeyer CL, Spagrud LJ, McCormick JC, Choo E, Neville K, Connelly MA: **Three new datasets supporting use of the Numerical Rating Scale (NRS-11) for children's self-reports of pain intensity.** *Pain* 2009, **143**:223–227.
37. Hjermstad MJ, Fayers PM, Haugen DF, Caraceni A, Hanks GW, Loge JH, Fainsinger R, Aass N, Kaasa S: **Studies comparing Numerical Rating Scales, Verbal Rating Scales, and Visual Analogue Scales for assessment of pain intensity in adults: a systematic literature review.** *J Pain Symptom Manage* 2011, **41**:1073–1093.
38. Stratford PW, Binkley JM: **Measurement properties of the RM-18. A modified version of the Roland-Morris disability scale.** *Spine* 1997, **22**:2416–2421.
39. Macedo LG, Maher CG, Latimer J, Hancock MJ, Machado LA, McAuley JH: **Responsiveness of the 24-, 18- and 11-item versions of the Roland Morris Disability Questionnaire.** *Eur Spine J* 2011, **20**:458–463.
40. Varni JW, Seid M, Kurtin PS: **PedsQL 4.0: reliability and validity of the Pediatric Quality of Life Inventory version 4.0 generic core scales in healthy and patient populations.** *Med Care* 2001, **39**:800–812.
41. Langer MM, Hill CD, Thissen D, Burwinkle TM, Varni JW, DeWalt DA: **Item response theory detected differential item functioning between healthy and ill children in quality-of-life measures.** *J Clin Epidemiol* 2008, **61**:268–276.
42. Varni JW, Seid M, Knight TS, Uzark K, Szer IS: **The PedsQL 4.0 Generic Core Scales: sensitivity, responsiveness, and impact on clinical decision-making.** *J Behav Med* 2002, **25**:175–193.
43. Varni JW, Seid M, Rode CA: **The PedsQL: measurement model for the pediatric quality of life inventory.** *Med Care* 1999, **37**:126–139.
44. Fischer D, Stewart AL, Bloch DA, Lorig K, Laurent D, Holman H: **Capturing the patient's view of change as a clinical outcome measure.** *JAMA* 1999, **282**:1157–1162.
45. Ioannidis JP, Evans SJ, Gotzsche PC, O'Neill RT, Altman DG, Schulz K, Moher D: **Better reporting of harms in randomized trials: an extension of the CONSORT statement.** *Ann Intern Med* 2004, **141**:781–788.
46. Bronfort G, Maiers MJ, Evans RL, Schulz CA, Bracha Y, Svendsen KH, Grimm RH Jr, Owens EF Jr, Garvey TA, Transfeldt EE: **Supervised exercise, spinal manipulation, and home exercise for chronic low back pain: a randomized clinical trial.** *Spine J* 2011, **11**:585–598.
47. Maiers M, Hartvigsen J, Schulz C, Schulz K, Evans R, Bronfort G: **Chiropractic and exercise for seniors with low back pain or neck pain: the design of two randomized clinical trials.** *BMC Musculoskelet Disord* 2007, **8**:94.
48. Newman I, Benz CR: *Qualitative-Quantitative Research Methodology: Exploring the Interactive Continuum.* Carbondale, IL: Southern Illinois University Press; 1998.
49. Portscher M, Vogt L, Pfeifer K, Banzer W: **Reproducibility of lumbar spine kinematics in clinical gait analysis.** *Sportverletz Sportschaden* 2000, **14**:50–54.
50. Himmelreich H, Stefanicki E, Banzer W: **Ultrasound-controlled anthropometry–on the development of a new method in asymmetry diagnosis.** *Sportverletz Sportschaden* 1998, **12**:60–65.
51. Vogt L, Pfeifer K, Portscher AM, Banzer W: **Influences of nonspecific low back pain on three-dimensional lumbar spine kinematics in locomotion.** *Spine* 2001, **26**:1910–1919.
52. Mcgill S: **Evaluating the patient.** In *Low Back Disorders Evidence-Based Prevention and Rehabilitation.* Edited by Mcgill S. Champaign, IL: Human Kinetics; 2002:223–238.
53. McGill SM, Childs A, Liebenson C: **Endurance times for low back stabilization exercises: clinical targets for testing and training from a normal database.** *Arch Phys Med Rehabil* 1999, **80**:941–944.

54. Biering-Sorensen F: **Physical measurements as risk indicators for low-back trouble over a one-year period.** *Spine* 1984, **9:**106–119.
55. Jorgensen K, Nicolaisen T: **Two methods for determining trunk extensor endurance. A comparative study.** *Eur J Appl Physiol* 1986, **55:**639–644.
56. Nicolaisen T, Jorgensen K: **Trunk strength, back muscle endurance and low-back trouble.** *Scand J Rehabil Med* 1985, **17:**121–127.
57. Brage S, Brage N, Wedderkopp N, Froberg K: **Reliability and validity of the computer science and applications accelerometer in a mechanical setting.** *Meas Phys Educ Exerc Sci* 2003, **7:**101–119.
58. Diggle PJ, Heagerty P, Liang KY, Zeger SL: *Analysis of Longitudinal Data.* Oxford, United Kingdom: Oxford University Press; 2002.
59. Krueger C, Tian L: **A comparison of the general linear mixed model and repeated measures ANOVA using a dataset with multiple missing data points.** *Biol Res Nurs* 2004, **6:**151–157.
60. Petkova E, Teresi J: **Some statistical issues in the analyses of data from longitudinal studies of elderly chronic care populations.** *Psychosom Med* 2002, **64:**531–547.
61. Littell RC, Milliken GA, Stroup WW, Wolfinger RD: *SAS System for Mixed Models.* Cary, NC: SAS Publications; 1996.
62. Vonesh EF, Chinchilli VM: *Linear and nonlinear models for the analysis of repeated measurements.* New York, NY: Marcel Dekker, Inc.; 1997.
63. Fritz JM, Hebert J, Koppenhaver S, Parent E: **Beyond minimally important change: defining a successful outcome of physical therapy for patients with low back pain.** *Spine (Phila Pa 1976)* 2009, **34:**2803–2809.
64. Ostelo RW, Deyo RA, Stratford P, Waddell G, Croft P, Von Korff M, Bouter LM, de Vet HC: **Interpreting change scores for pain and functional status in low back pain: towards international consensus regarding minimal important change.** *Spine* 2008, **33:**90–94.
65. Guyatt GH, Juniper EF, Walter SD, Griffith LE, Goldstein RS: **Interpreting treatment effects in randomised trials.** *BMJ* 1998, **316:**690–693.
66. **Guidance on Reviewing and Reporting Unanticipated Problems Involving Risks to Subjects or Others and Adverse Events.** http://www.hhs.gov/ohrp/policy/advevntguid.html.
67. Calvo-Munoz I, Gomez-Conesa A, Sanchez-Meca J: **Physical therapy treatments for low back pain in children and adolescents: a meta-analysis.** *BMC Musculoskelet Disord* 2013, **14:**55.
68. Thorpe KE, Zwarenstein M, Oxman AD, Treweek S, Furberg CD, Altman DG, Tunis S, Bergel E, Harvey I, Magid DJ, Chalkidou K: **A pragmatic-explanatory continuum indicator summary (PRECIS): a tool to help trial designers.** *J Clin Epidemiol* 2009, **62:**464–475.

15

Three-dimensional chiropractor-patient contact loads during side posture lumbar spinal manipulation: a pilot study

Maruti Ram Gudavalli[1*] and Robert M Rowell[2]

Abstract

Background: Patients with low back pain often seek chiropractic care and more than ninety percent of Chiropractors use lumbar side posture manipulation for the treatment of low back pain. During this procedure chiropractors deliver forces by means of hand contact on the patient in a side lying position. The objective of this pilot study was to report on the three-dimensional forces at the hand contact between the chiropractor and the simulated patient (asymptomatic volunteers) during side posture lumbar high velocity low amplitude adjustments.

Methods: In 2005, two licensed chiropractors delivered spinal manipulations to the lumbar spines of the participants. A three-dimensional force transducer (Model # Mini-45, ATI-Industrial Automation, Apex, North Carolina) was used to measure the three-dimensional loads. The force-time histories were analyzed for preloads, peak loads, duration of thrusts to peak load, duration of thrust for completion, rate of loading, and magnitudes of the three forces and the resultant total force delivered by the chiropractor.

Results: The two chiropractors delivered a total of 14 thrusts to the five asymptomatic volunteers. Normal force (Fz) is the dominating force, followed by inferior-superior force (Fx). The lateral force (Fy) occurred in both directions.

Conclusions: This study reports on the three dimensional load (three forces and the total resultant force) characteristics of chiropractor-patient hand contact while delivering a chiropractic high velocity low amplitude (HVLA) manipulation in a side lying position.

Keywords: Manipulation, Biomechanics, Chiropractic, Low back, Spine, Low back pain

Background

Low back pain (LBP) is a major health problem to society in terms of cost and lost work days [1]. LBP will affect as many as 80% of US adults during their life [2]. The cost of LBP treatment in the US was estimated at $85 billion in 2006 [3]. Patients with low back pain seek chiropractic care for pain relief and for return to normal activities. More than ninety percent of Chiropractors use lumbar side posture manipulation for the treatment of low back pain [4]. During this procedure a chiropractor delivers forces by means of hand contact on the patient in a side lying position. These forces are complex three-dimensional forces and are delivered to create forces and moments at the joint of interest thereby creating joint movements. This type of manipulation is defined as High Velocity Low Amplitude-Spinal Manipulation or HVLA-SM.

Much work has been done to quantify the forces delivered during chiropractic spinal manipulation (SM). The need for further research on the biomechanics of spinal manipulation has been identified in position papers [5,6]. Several investigators reported force-time profile characteristics during spinal manipulation for different regions of the spine [7-25]. Most of the studies measured only the normal force (defined by the perpendicular force to the back surface) characteristics of thrusting hand during the delivery of spinal manipulation [7-15,24]. All of these studies looked at the forces generated during SM of the cervical and thoracic spine, and the sacroiliac (SI) joint. These authors found that the peak and preload

* Correspondence: Gudavalli_r@palmer.edu
[1]Biomechanics Core, Palmer Center for Chiropractic Research, 741 Brady street, Davenport, IA 52803, USA
Full list of author information is available at the end of the article

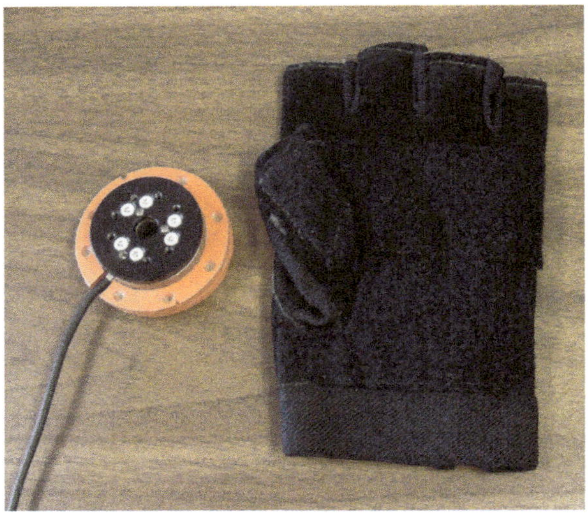

Figure 1 A photograph of the transducer and the glove used in this study.

forces were considerably smaller for HVLA-SM to the cervical spine compared with HVLA-SM to the thoracic spine. Kirstukas et al. [24] quantified forces delivered during unilateral thoracic manipulation using Tekscan pressure mats whereas other investigators [7-15] used Emed pressure sensors to measure pressure and convert it to force. All these studies reported on the preload force, peak force, thrust duration, and rates of loading from the force-time data collected while delivering the spinal manipulation. Triano et al. have done pioneering work on three dimensional (3-D) loads transmitted during spinal manipulation using an inverse dynamics approach with force plate embedded into the treatment table [17-19,21,26]. Van Zoest et al. were the first to report on a measurement method to quantify the three-dimensional forces at the chiropractor-patient hand contact [27,28]. These investigators reported on the 3-D forces during thoracic and sacro-iliac manipulations in the prone position. Their measurement did not include the moment loads at the hand contact.

The objective of this pilot study was to report on the three-dimensional forces at the hand contact between the chiropractor and the simulated patient (asymptomatic volunteers) during side posture lumbar high velocity low amplitude spinal manipulations.

Methods

This project was approved by the Palmer College of Chiropractic Institutional Review Board (IRB # 2005G070). In 2005, informed consent was obtained from five participants with no symptoms of low back pain. The participants were a convenience sample of volunteers from our institution and consisted of 4 males and one female aged 22–51 years old. All participants were informed of the study details and signed the informed consent form. The chiropractors examined the participants for palpatory tenderness, spinal hypomobility, and any contraindication to spinal manipulation. The examination included history, vital signs, review of systems, an orthopedic examination, a brief neurological screen, and a spinal examination. Patients were excluded if contraindications to manipulation were found. Two licensed chiropractors evaluated the spinal segments for hypomobility using palpatory examination and delivered HVLA-SM to the lumbar spine of the participants in a side-lying posture. The participant was positioned in a side-lying (lateral recumbent) posture. The superior or free hip and knee were flexed and adducted across the midline. The chiropractor stabilized the participant by leaning his/her own leg against the participant's superior leg, while holding the participant's superior shoulder. The

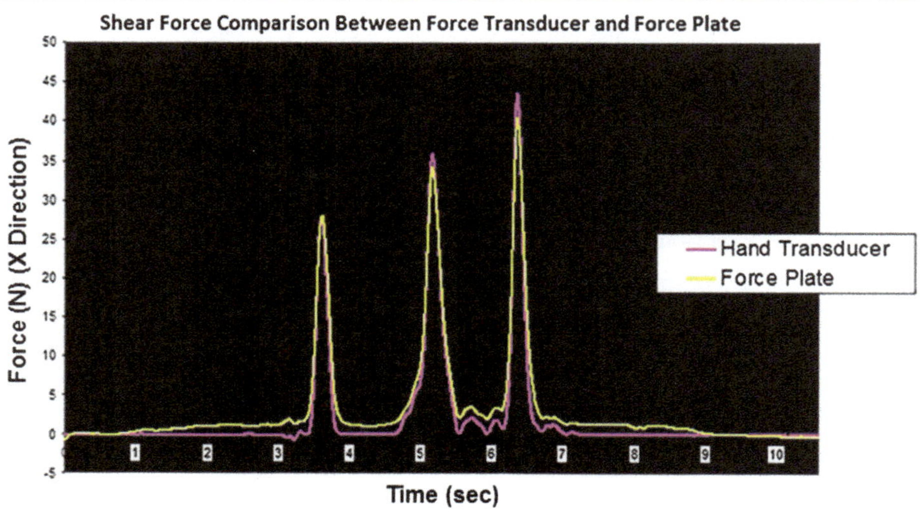

Figure 2 A typical graph comparing transducer and force plate measurements in shear.

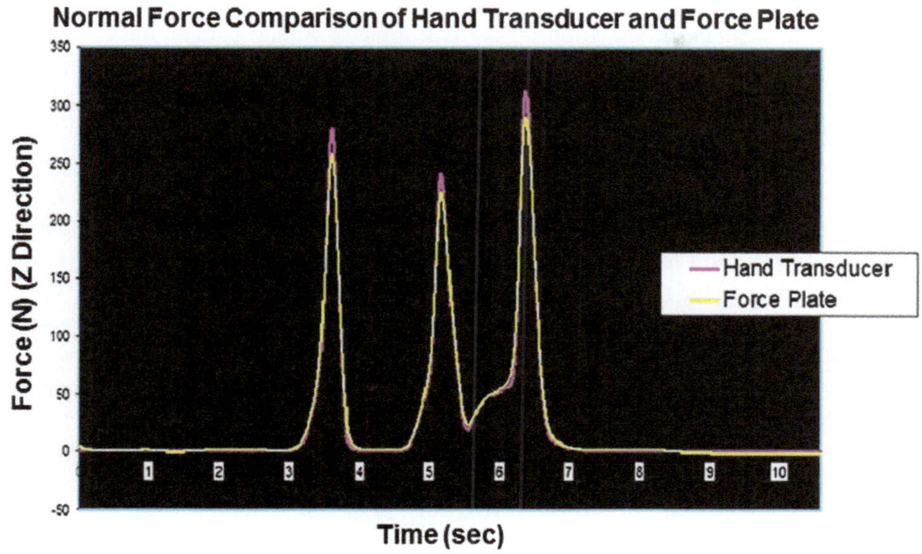

Figure 3 A typical graph comparing transducer and force plate measurements in normal force.

manipulation was applied with the chiropractor's hand by thrusting into the spine or sacroiliac joint. The thrusting load is a quick, short, controlled movement of the shoulder, arm and hand combined with a slight body drop.

A three-dimensional force transducer (Model # Mini-45, ATI-Industrial Automation, Apex, North Carolina) was used to measure the three-dimensional loads (three forces and the resultant total force) (see Figure 1). The transducer was placed between the chiropractor's hand (that was enclosed in a glove) and the participant's back. A thin layer of rubber padding was used between the transducer and the participant's back, and the transducer was attached to the chiropractor's glove using Velcro® brand fasteners. The X-axis was pointed superiorly on the spine, the Y-axis was pointing left laterally, and the Z-axis was pointing posteriorly normal to the back surface. The load-time histories were recorded at a sampling rate of 1000 Hz using custom written Lab View software and a laptop computer connected to the force transducer by means of a PCMCIA card (Keithly Instruments Inc.,Cleveland, Ohio). The transducer was tested to compare the accuracy of force measurements in normal direction as well as shear direction with a Bertec force plate and found to have good agreement (less than 3% differences) between both sensors (Figures 2 and 3).

The force-time histories were plotted using custom written MathCAD software (version 12, Parametric Technologies Corporation, Boston, Massachusetts) and to extract important parameters with user interface. With user interface the following parameters were extracted from the force-time graphs: Preload forces, peak forces, duration of preload, duration of thrusts to peak force, duration of unloading, total duration, rate of loading, and rate of unloading. The extracted data were then exported into an excel spreadsheet for further descriptive analysis using means and standard deviations.

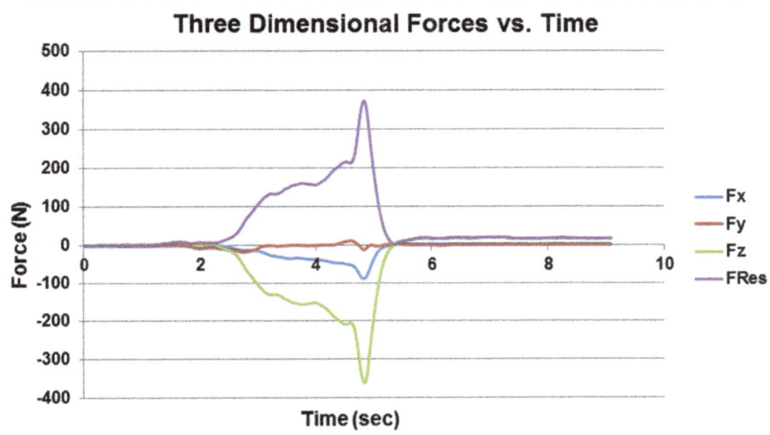

Figure 4 A typical 3-d force-time graphs during the side posture spinal manipulation.

Results

Figure 4 shows typical force-time profiles of the three forces measured during the manipulation. Normal force which is perpendicular to the back surface is the dominant force applied by the chiropractor but shear forces (parallel to the back surface) were also observed.

The two chiropractors delivered a total of 14 thrusts to the five asymptomatic volunteers. Table 1 summarizes descriptively the 3-D forces, durations, and loading rates for all 14 spinal manipulations as well as for the two chiropractors. Normal force (Fz) is the dominating force, followed by inferior-superior force (Fx), and the lateral force (Fy) which occurred in both directions.

Discussion

Van Zoest et al. were the first to report on a measurement method to quantify the three-dimensional forces at the chiropractor-patient hand contact [27,28]. Their study was restricted to three forces at the hand contact and only reported on the forces for thoracic and sacro-iliac spinal manipulations in the prone position. Our study expands to the lumbar spine, the measurement of 3-D forces at the chiropractor-patient interface during side posture lumbar spinal manipulation.

This study demonstrates that shear forces are present at the chiropractor's hand-patient interface while delivering treatments to the lumbar spine. These shear forces have distinct ranges for the two chiropractors. The chiropractor who delivered faster thrusts had higher shear force values. The average normal forces previously reported for sacro-iliac manipulations (222-228 N) were smaller compared to the present study [27,28]. Previous studies have also reported shear forces with large standard deviations similar to our study [27]. The average normal peak forces (328 N) reported on sacro-iliac joint manipulations on three participants by Herzog et al. are comparable to the normal forces measured in the present study [9].

Triano et al. reported on the transmitted 3-D loads to the spine using an inverse dynamics approach [17]. However, they did not report on the chiropractor-patient hand contact loads. The shear forces measured in the present study were smaller compared to the transmitted loads in the lumbar spine reported by Triano et al. using the inverse dynamics approach and force plate measurements [17].

The force measuring system developed and used in this study consisted of a laptop computer and was easily portable. The force-time graphs are displayed for

Table 1 Three-Dimensional spinal manipulation load characteristics

	Both Chiropractors (N = 14)		Chiropractor 1 (N = 6)		Chiropractor 2 (N = 8)	
Fx (N)	Mean	SD	Mean	SD	Mean	SD
Preload	14.6	7.1	19.4	4.9	11.1	6.5
Peak load	25.3	37.5	61.8	26.2	−2.1	10.6
Fy (N)						
Preload	4.8	9.3	7.4	9.2	2.8	9.5
Peak load	−20.6	40.2	−40.4	51.7	−5.8	22.4
Fz (N)						
Preload	96.4	30.7	71.5	22.8	115.1	21.0
Peak load	335.3	71.3	382.2	37.7	300.1	71.5
FRes (N)						
Preload	98.7	29.3	75.5	20.9	116.1	21.7
Peak load	340.3	75.2	392.6	41.0	301.0	72.0
Preload duration (ms)	1966	1022	2976	524	1209	462
Thrust loading Duration(ms)	164	37	144	26	179	39
Thrust unloading duration(ms)	746	316	1046	211	521	134
Total duration(ms)	2876	1240	4166	422	1909	482
Rateof Fz thrust loading(N/s)	1577.9	733.8	2226.3	452.6	1091.6	472.3
Rate of Fz thrust unloading(N/s)	−517.4	203.6	−384.5	119.9	−617.1	200.6
Rateof FRes thrust loading(N/s)	1595.1	749.8	2267.3	442.7	1090.9	475.7
Rate of FRes thrust unloading(N/s)	−522.7	201.9	−394.5	121.3	−618.8	201.4

Fx-Inferior to superior force Fy- Lateral force Fz-Posterior-to-anterior force FRes-Resultant force.
N-Newtons ms-milliseconds N/s- Newtons per second.

viewing immediately after delivering the spinal manipulation. This system has the potential for taking it to any field clinicians' office to gather data and give immediate feedback on the forces delivered.

Limitations and future directions

The transducer is a two centimeter thick metal device with a rubber pad for the comfort of the participant. Unfortunately, tactile feedback is lost because of the transducer between the chiropractor's hand and patients back. Furthermore, this study had only 2 chiropractors and 5 asymptomatic volunteers. Future studies should aim at collecting data from more chiropractors and using more volunteers as well as low back pain patients. This is a preliminary study and provides the basis for such larger studies.

Conclusions

This study reports the three dimensional forces at chiropractor-patient hand contact while delivering a high velocity low amplitude (HVLA) manipulation. This is a preliminary study that showed there are shear forces applied at the chiropractor's hand-patient interface. Future studies should be directed in a systematic way on patients and with more chiropractors. These measurements have an important role in understanding the effects at the spinal joints that are being treated. These studies could also play an important role in the training of future chiropractors.

Competing interests

The authors declare that they have no competing interests.

Authors' contributions

MRG participated in the design of the study, carried out the biomechanical measurements, conducted the statistical analysis, and the drafting and revising of the manuscript. RMR participated in the design of the study and the drafting and revising of the manuscript. Both authors read and approved the final manuscript.

Acknowledgments

We would like to acknowledge the volunteers for their participation. This work was conducted in a facility constructed with support from Research Facilities Improvement Program Grant Number C06 RR15433-01 from the National Center for Research Resources, National Institutes of Health, Bethesda, Maryland.

Author details

[1]Biomechanics Core, Palmer Center for Chiropractic Research, 741 Brady street, Davenport, IA 52803, USA. [2]Diagnosis and Radiology Department, Palmer College of Chiropractic, 1000 Brady street, Davenport, IA 52803, USA.

References

1. Martin BI, Deyo RA, Mirza SK, Turner JA, Comstock BA, Hollingworth W, Sullivan SD: **Expenditures and health status among adults with back and neck problems.** *JAMA* 2008, **299:**656–664.
2. Deyo RA, Weinstein JN: **Low back pain.** *N Engl J Med* 2001, **344:**363–370.
3. Friedly J, Standaert C, Chan L: **Epidemiology of spine care: the back pain dilemma.** *Phys Med Rehabil Clin N Am* 2010, **21:**659–677.
4. Christensen MG, Mark G, Kollash MW, Hyland JK: *Practice Analysis of Chiropractic 2010: A project report, survey analysis, and summary of chiropractic practice in the United States.* Greeley, Colorado: National Board of Chiropractic Examiners; 2010.
5. Brennan PC, Cramer GD, Kirstukas SJ, Cullum ME: **Basic science research in chiropractic: the state of the art and recommendations for a research agenda.** *J Manipulative Physiol Ther* 1997, **20:**150–168.
6. Cramer G, Budgell B, Henderson C, Khalsa P, Pickar J: **Basic science research related to chiropractic spinal adjusting: the state of the art and recommendations revisited.** *J Manipulative Physiol Ther* 2006, **29:**726–761.
7. Forand D, Drover J, Suleman Z, Symons B, Herzog W: **The forces applied by female and male chiropractors during thoracic spinal manipulation.** *J Manipulative Physiol Ther* 2004, **27:**49–56.
8. Herzog W, Leonard TR, Symons B, Tang C, Wuest S: **Vertebral artery strains during high-speed, low amplitude cervical spinal manipulation.** *J Electromyogr Kinesiol* 2012, **22:**740–746.
9. Herzog W, Conway PJ, Kawchuk GN, Zhang Y, Hasler EM: **Forces exerted during spinal manipulative therapy.** *Spine* 1993, **18:**1206–1212.
10. Herzog W, Kats M, Symons B: **The effective forces transmitted by high-speed, low-amplitude thoracic manipulation.** *Spine* 2001, **26:**2105–2110.
11. Herzog W, Zhang YT, Conway PJ, Kawchuk GN: **Cavitation sounds during spinal manipulative treatments.** *J Manipulative Physiol Ther* 1993, **16:**523–526.
12. Herzog W: **The Mechanical Neuromuscular, and Physiologic Effects Produced by Spinal Manipulation.** In *Clinical Biomechanics of Spinal Manipulation.* Edited by Herzong W. New York: Churchill Livingstone; 2000:191–207.
13. Hessell BW, Herzog W, Conway PJ, McEwen MC: **Experimental measurement of the force exerted during spinal manipulation using the Thompson technique.** *J Manipulative Physiol Ther* 1990, **13:**448–453.
14. Kawchuk GN, Herzog W, Hasler EM: **Forces generated during spinal manipulative therapy of the cervical spine: a pilot study.** *J Manipulative Physiol Ther* 1992, **15:**275–278.
15. Kawchuk GN, Herzog W: **Biomechanical characterization (fingerprinting) of five novel methods of cervical spine manipulation.** *J Manipulative Physiol Ther* 1993, **16:**573–577.
16. Triano JJ: **The Mechanics of Spinal Manipulation.** In *Clinical Biomechanics of Spinal Manipulation.* Edited by Herzog W. New York: Churchill Livingstone; 2000:92–190.
17. Triano J, Schultz AB: **Loads transmitted during lumbosacral spinal manipulative therapy.** *Spine* 1997, **22:**1955–1964.
18. Triano JJ, Rogers CM, Combs S, Potts D, Sorrels K: **Developing skilled performance of lumbar spine manipulation.** *J Manipulative Physiol Ther* 2002, **25:**353–361.
19. Triano JJ, Rogers CM, Combs S, Potts D, Sorrels K: **Quantitative feedback versus standard training for cervical and thoracic manipulation.** *J Manipulative Physiol Ther* 2003, **26:**131–138.
20. Triano JJ, Gissler T, Forgie M, Milwid D: **Maturation in rate of high-velocity, low-amplitude force development.** *J Manipulative Physiol Ther* 2011, **34:**173–180.
21. Triano JJ, Scaringe J, Bougie J, Rogers C: **Effects of visual feedback on manipulation performance and patient ratings.** *J Manipulative Physiol Ther* 2006, **29:**378–385.
22. DeVocht JW, Owens EF, Gudavalli MR, Strazewski J, Bhogal R, Xia T: **Force-time profile differences in the delivery of simulated toggle-recoil spinal manipulation by students, instructors, and field doctors of chiropractic.** *J Manipulative Physiol Ther* 2013, **36:**342–348.
23. Gudavalli MR, DeVocht J, Tayh A, Xia T: **Effect of sampling rates on the quantification of forces, durations, and rates of loading of simulated side posture high-velocity, low-amplitude lumbar spine manipulation.** *J Manipulative Physiol Ther* 2013, **36:**261–266.
24. Kirstukas SJ, Backman JA: **Physician-applied contact pressure and table force response during unilateral thoracic manipulation.** *J Manipulative Physiol Ther* 1999, **22:**269–279.
25. Colloca CJ, Cunliffe C, Pinnock MH, Kim YK, Hinrichs RN: **Force-time profile characterization of the McTimoney toggle-torque-recoil technique.** *J Manipulative Physiol Ther* 2009, **32:**372–378.
26. Triano JJ, Descarreaux M, Dugas C: **Biomechanics–review of approaches for performance training in spinal manipulation.** *J Electromyogr Kinesiol* 2012, **22:**732–739.

27. van Zoest GG, Gosselin G: **Three-dimensionality of direct contact forces in chiropractic spinal manipulative therapy.** *J Manipulative Physiol Ther* 2003, **26**:549–556.
28. van Zoest GG, van den Berg HT, Holtkamp FC: **Three-dimensionality of contact forces during clinical manual examination and treatment: a new measuring system.** *Clin Biomech* 2002, **17**:719–722.

Adverse events from spinal manipulation in the pregnant and postpartum periods: a critical review of the literature

Kent Jason Stuber[1*], Shari Wynd[2] and Carol Ann Weis[1]

Abstract

Background: The safety of spinal manipulation during pregnancy and the postpartum periods has been a matter of debate among manual therapists. Spinal manipulative therapy during these periods is a commonly performed intervention as musculoskeletal pain is common in these patients. To date there has not been an evaluation of the literature on this topic exclusively.

Methods: A literature search was conducted on PubMed, CINAHL and the Index to Chiropractic Literature along with reference searching for articles published in English and French in the peer-reviewed literature that documented adverse effects of spinal manipulation during either pregnancy or postpartum. Case reports, case series, and any other clinical study designs were deemed acceptable for inclusion, as were systematic reviews. The appropriate Scottish Intercollegiate Guidelines Network (SIGN) tools were used to rate included articles for quality when applicable.

Results: Five articles identifying adverse events in seven subjects following spinal manipulation were included in this review, along with two systematic reviews. The articles were published between 1978 and 2009. Two articles describing adverse effects from spinal manipulation on two postpartum patients were included, while the remaining three articles on five patients with adverse effects following spinal manipulation were on pregnant patients. Injury severity ranged from minor injury such as increasing pain after treatment that resolved within a few days to more severe injuries including fracture, stroke, and epidural hematoma. SIGN scores of the prospective observational cohort study and systematic reviews indicated acceptable quality.

Conclusions: There are only a few reported cases of adverse events following spinal manipulation during pregnancy and the postpartum period identified in the literature. While improved reporting of such events is required in the future, it may be that such injuries are relatively rare.

Keywords: Chiropractic, Spinal manipulative Therapy, Pregnancy, Postpartum, Adverse effects

Background

Musculoskeletal pain is a common occurrence during pregnancy and the postpartum period. For example, low back pain has been reported to occur as frequently as 50% to 85% of pregnant women [1-4] and at two to three years postpartum, eight to 20% of these women still report persistent symptoms [5,6]. Although low back pain is often accepted as an unavoidable complaint during pregnancy, for some women the pain can be debilitating, interfering with sleep, work and normal activities of daily living [7,8]. However, the etiology of this pain is unknown [9]. It has been suggested that low back pain experienced during pregnancy is multifactoral in nature and some of the proposed mechanisms include, but are not limited to, the influence of altered circulating relaxin levels producing ligamentous laxity [7,10], maternal weight gain and/or biomechanical changes due to pregnancy [7].

In the non-pregnant population, low back pain is a significant cause of pain and disability as well, with 80%

* Correspondence: kstuber@cmcc.ca
[1]Division of Graduate Education and Research, Canadian Memorial Chiropractic College, 6100 Leslie Street, Toronto, ON M2H 3J1, Canada
Full list of author information is available at the end of the article

of the population experiencing an episode during their lifetime [7,11]. Neck pain [12,13] and headaches [14] are also a substantial source of pain and disability in the non-pregnant population [12]. One of the effective treatment options used by manual practitioners for those suffering from low back pain [15,16] cervical spine [16,17] and some headache pain [18,19] is spinal manipulative therapy (SMT). SMT is usually characterized as a localized force of high velocity and low amplitude directed at a spinal segment [1]. Severe adverse effects of SMT are rare in the cervical spine [20-22] and lumbar spine [23].

Manual treatment options for pregnancy-induced pain, such as back pain, have been reported to be limited [1]. However, chiropractors report seeing pregnant patients frequently, and surveys of chiropractors reflect an opinion that SMT is safe for pregnant patients [1,24]. While the safety of SMT for adult and pediatric populations has undergone scrutiny in both public and scientific domains [13,22,25], the safety of SMT in sub-groups of the population including pregnant and postpartum patients has received little attention. This lack of evidence is surprising given the obvious importance of the welfare of the expectant and new mother. Given the hormonal and the coagulability status of peripartum and postpartum individuals, it is possible that SMT is a contraindication to the musculoskeletal complaints associated with pregnancy.

It is accepted that females are more susceptible to increases in joint laxity than men [26-28]. Hormonal causes have been postulated as a potential source for this increase in female joint laxity [29-32]. Relaxin, a polypeptide that is produced by the corpus luteum during pregnancy [32], is one of the implicated hormones. In the pregnant female, relaxin is essential in order to secure the passage of the fetus during parturition in several animal species [33]; it has been associated with a decrease in soft tissue tension especially in preparing the female body for delivery including relaxing the pelvic ligaments, inhibiting spontaneous uterine contractions, ripening of the uterine cervix, and stimulating the mammary glands [34]. Although relaxin increases laxity in the symphysis pubis in preparation for birth, its effects are not solely limited to that joint. In addition, women immediately postpartum are thought to also have this hormone-mediated ligament laxity that might reduce the protective stability of the intervertebral articulations [35].

Hypercoaguable disorders that promote thrombosis have been categorized as thrombophilias [36]. During pregnancy and the postpartum state the risk of thrombophilia increases compared to the non-pregnant state [36,37]. Thromboembolism or pulmonary embolism has been identified as the leading cause of maternal death in the United States [36,37]. These hypercoaguable disorders during pregnancy can be a result of venous stasis, changes in the vessel wall and changes in the composition of blood; also known as Virchow's triad [36].

In the absence of a prospective study of the safety of SMT during the antepartum and postpartum periods, it would be beneficial to survey the scientific literature for the number and types of injuries sustained by pregnant and postpartum patients following spinal manipulation. While systematic reviews of the literature on the use of SMT for pregnancy and related conditions have been conducted [1,11], an exploration of the literature specifically for adverse events associated with SMT and pregnancy has not yet been undertaken. Accordingly, the aim of this study is to critically review the literature for reported cases of iatrogenic injuries following spinal manipulative therapy during the pregnancy and postpartum periods.

Methods

Objective

To collect and synthesize available evidence on adverse events associated with SMT during the pregnancy and postpartum periods.

Search strategy

A literature search was conducted in three different electronic databases: PubMed (including MEDLINE), CINAHL, and the Index to Chiropractic Literature. The date ranges applied were from the beginning of each respective database to October 2011. The following search terms were employed: adverse effects, adverse reactions, adverse events, harm, pregnancy, postpartum, chiropractic, spinal manipulative therapy, spinal manipulation, and manual therapy. These search terms were categorized and combined using Boolean terms (please see Additional file 1: Appendix 1 for the complete search strategy). Reference searching of relevant articles retrieved from the electronic literature search was also undertaken, as was a search of each of the authors' personal collections. Specific inclusion criteria for this review were:

Study designs

All clinical study designs published in peer-reviewed journals. Conference proceedings, cross-sectional and other descriptive designs and narrative reviews were excluded.

Population

Female patients who are either pregnant or postpartum (defined as the period between the delivery of the child and six weeks after the birth) [38].

Intervention

Spinal Manipulative Therapy (SMT) (defined as a manual therapy technique that uses a high velocity low amplitude thrust applied at a spinal motion segment [39] to any region of the spine.

Comparison

Not relevant.

Outcomes

Any adverse events associated with SMT.

Language

Articles in either English or French were considered for inclusion.

Study selection

Two of the authors (KS and SW) independently reviewed the titles and abstracts of the electronic database searches for any that appeared to match the inclusion criteria. The full text versions of any potentially relevant articles were obtained and reviewed by the same two authors using the inclusion criteria described above. Each of the authors compiled a list of articles to include that was compared, and any disagreements were resolved through discussion.

Data collection and rating process

A data extraction sheet was compiled by one of the authors (KS) and relevant data from each included article was entered into the sheet. The appropriate Scottish Intercollegiate Guidelines Network (SIGN) tools were used to rate included articles for quality, although any case reports included in the review were not rated for quality as there is no applicable SIGN tool for case reports. The overall assessment of a paper using a SIGN tool is given one of three scores: "++" indicates the highest level of methodological quality for that study type, fulfilling all or most of the internal validity criteria for that particular study type, "+" indicates some criteria were fulfilled, and "-" indicates that few or none of the criteria were satisfied. Two of the authors (KS and SW) rated the articles using the applicable SIGN tool. One of the authors (KS) was an author on one of the systematic reviews and thus that article was rated by the other two authors (SW and CAW) to avoid potential bias. Where reviewers disagreed, consensus was achieved by discussion.

Analysis

Meta-analysis could not be conducted as only case reports and an observational cohort study were identified; data are summarized in text (percentages).

Results

Figure 1 depicts the flow of articles through the review process [40]. One full text article was excluded because it did not use HVLA spinal manipulation [41]. Five articles that identified possible adverse events in seven subjects following spinal manipulation of a pregnant or

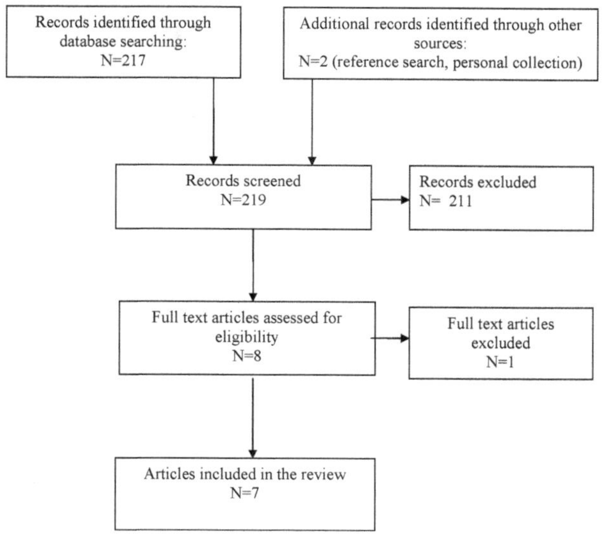

Figure 1 PRISMA Information Flow [40].

post-partum subject were identified from the literature search, along with two relevant systematic reviews [1,11] (the full list of included articles appears in Additional file 2: Appendix 2). The five articles consisted of four case reports [20,21,35,42] and one prospective observational cohort study [43]. The four case reports all detailed adverse events following cervical manipulation, whereas the prospective observational cohort study described three adverse events following lumbar manipulation. The articles were published between 1978 and 2009. Figure 2 describes the four case reports included, while (Additional file 3: Table S1) provides additional details on those case reports. One case report [42] was identified by reference searching. A systematic review of manipulative therapy during pregnancy [1] was identified from the authors' personal collections.

Murphy et al published an observational cohort study in 2009, which evaluated a diagnosis-based decision rule for pregnancy-related lumbopelvic pain [43]. One hundred and fifteen patients began the study and complete data was obtained on 78 subjects. In terms of adverse effects three subjects (3.8%) reported increased pain after treatment; this was reported as resolving for two of these patients in less than 48 hours and in one week for the third patient. The treatments that each patient received depended on their specific diagnosis and it is unsure what diagnosis these patients were given. However nearly all patients (68/78) received some form of manual therapy. No other complications were reported in this study. The overall SIGN rating assigned to this article was "+", indicating acceptable quality although it was limited by a lack of blinding and possible confounders.

Item / Citation	Case description
Ng KPL, Doube A. Stroke after neck manipulation in the post partum period. J NZ Med Assoc 2001; 114(1143): 498.	A 34 year old woman, 5 week post-partum with right sided neck pain after delivery. She received a cervical manipulation by a chiropractor and experienced memory loss within 30 minutes which resolved, the following day she had poor coordination of her right hand, difficulty with articulation, and unsteady gait. MRI demonstrated a right cerebellar infarct with a wedge shaped area of increased T2 signal in the right antero-superior cerebellar cortex. She had a full recovery within one month.
Parkin PJ, Wallis WE, Wilson JL. Vertebral artery occlusion following manipulation of the neck. NZ Med J 1978; 88: 441-443.	A 23 year old woman, 2 weeks post-partum with head and neck pain. She saw a physiotherapist and underwent a provocative test followed by vertical traction with lateral head rotation which resulted in vertigo within seconds and discontinuation of the procedure. Upon standing she became ataxic, and had dysarthria, with right sided numbness of the body. Cerebral angiography demonstrated total occlusion of the left vertebral artery, a small right vertebral artery which filled normally, and a large thrombus in the basilar artery. She was discharged after 2 months of moderate improvement with some residual issues with coordination, sensation, and ataxia, as well as left-sided paralysis of the palate and tongue.
Schmitz A, Lutterbey G, von Engelhardt L, von Falkenhausen M, Stoffel M. Pathological cervical fracture after spinal manipulation in a pregnant patient. J Manipulative Physiol Ther 2005; 28(8): 633-636.	A 37 year old woman, 15 weeks pregnant with neck pain. She saw a general medicine practitioner 5 days prior and underwent a single cervical manipulative treatment and paravertebral injections. She had swelling and neck pain five days later and MRI showed a pathological type II odontoid fracture with ventral displacement producing spinal cord compression and paravertebral hematoma, a tumor was identified in the C2 vertebral body. She was discharged without neurological complications and the pregnancy was undisturbed.
Heiner JD. Cervical epidural hematoma after chiropractic spinal manipulation. Am J Emerg Med 2009; 27: 1023.e1-1023.e2.	A 38 year old woman, 29 weeks pregnant with low back pain. She received a cervical manipulation from a chiropractor and experienced numbness and pain in the neck and arms during the treatment followed by several seconds of transient upper extremity paralysis and lower extremity numbness. MRI showed a right sided epidural hematoma with associated mass effect on the spinal cord. She was discharged 2 weeks later with minimal residual paresthesias along the posterior aspect of the neck.

Figure 2 Case Report Descriptions.

The systematic review by Stuber and Smith in 2008 on spinal manipulation for pregnancy-related lower back pain indicated that no adverse effects were noted in any of the papers that they reviewed, although only one of the articles specifically commented on an absence of adverse events [11]. The systematic review by Khorsan et al published in 2009 identified only the case report by Schmitz et al as having an adverse event resulting from manipulative therapy during pregnancy [1]. Most of the studies included in that review did not report adverse effects at all, although it was noted that three clinical studies indicated that there were no adverse events during their trials. The overall SIGN rating assigned to both of these systematic reviews was "++", indicating good quality.

Discussion

To our knowledge, this is the first critical review of the literature regarding adverse events from spinal manipulation during pregnancy and postpartum and it provides healthcare professionals with a comprehensive evaluation of the available scientific literature. This review revealed adverse affects during spinal manipulation in three studies during pregnancy and two studies in the postpartum period. Of the studies identified, four case studies demonstrated adverse events following cervical manipulation whereas the observational cohort study demonstrated adverse events following lumbar manipulation. The remaining two papers that were identified were systematic reviews. As such reports of adverse events following spinal manipulation in these populations are scarce in the literature.

Mild and transient adverse events were reported as a result of lumbar spinal manipulation [43] whereas the serious adverse events reported in the literature all occurred following cervical spinal manipulation either during pregnancy [20,21] or postpartum [35,42]. Murphy and colleagues found that 3.4% of their pregnant population incurred an injury following manual therapy which resulted in a transient increase in pain after a single session. They found this to be much lower than other studies that have focused on manual therapy in which the rate of injury was approximately one third of the study group [43]. As such they suggested that SMT of the lumbar spine is safe for this population, however a larger sample size would be needed to detect rare complications [43]. This review did not identify any injuries or adverse events that could be associated specifically with either being pregnant or in the postpartum period (such as premature delivery or an abnormally difficult delivery, etc), that is to say that the adverse events identified may have occurred in a non-pregnant patient.

In the non-pregnant population severe complications after cervical spinal manipulation are rare [13,22]. However rare, reported complications include vertebral artery dissection, cord or root injury, epidural hematoma, cervical disc rupture and vertebral fracture [21]. Pregnant and postpartum populations are not immune to this possibility and given the hormonal and coagulability status of pregnant and postpartum patients it is possible that SMT is contraindicated in pregnant and postpartum patients with musculoskeletal complaints. However, this may depend on the spinal regions and complaints being treated as different consideration may need to be given to manipulation of the cervical spine versus the thoracic or lumbopelvic regions.

Most contraindications to spinal manipulation are evident during a careful history and physical exam [21]. Clinicians who use SMT as part of the plan of management for pregnant patients should consider prothrombotic and joint laxity risk factors when deciding whether to undertake such a therapy in order to minimize the risks of potentially dangerous neurological complications [35]. Patients at higher risk for complications, such as those in a post-thrombotic state and possibly those with lax joints, should be treated with additional care and consideration. There is an increased importance to counsel this patient with respect to the risks of SMT [20,35] and these patients should be made aware of the signs and symptoms of possible neurovascular complications [20,35]. However, based on the literature reviewed, it cannot be ascertained as to what role those factors may have actually played in the etiology of the adverse events documented, if any.

Although this study has resulted in very few papers to review, it had strengths including the thorough search of the literature to help reduce bias in the review. The authors searched multiple relevant electronic databases over all possible years represented in those databases, employed a number of broad search terms, performed reference and hand-searching, examined personal libraries, and used multiple authors to determine articles for inclusion in the review and to evaluate and rate the literature.

The major limitation of this critical review was the number of studies available and the hierarchy of evidence that the studies available yielded. The papers identified for this review were case studies and a prospective observational cohort study, both of which are lower levels of evidence. Given the levels and paucity of evidence identified, the possible level of risk to pregnant and postpartum patients undergoing spinal manipulative therapy cannot be measured or stated definitively, nor can it be determined if any such risk level is higher or lower than in the non-pregnant or postpartum populations. However, this does allow for hypothesis generation and should help drive future directions for research. There is a need to design and execute larger and higher quality observational and randomized controlled studies investigating the potential benefits of the use of spinal manipulation as a treatment during pregnancy or postpartum particularly for those with low back pain. Such studies should ensure that any possible adverse events are tracked throughout. One possible option for an observational study design may be a case-crossover study as adverse events from spinal manipulative therapy may be rare in these populations [44,45]. The previous systematic reviews on spinal manipulation as a treatment during pregnancy have highlighted the lower levels of evidence available thus far on the topic [1,11]. Another limitation of this review was including only articles published in English and French.

Conclusions

There are only a handful of reported cases of adverse events following spinal manipulation during pregnancy and the postpartum period in the literature with the severity ranging from mild increases in pain that resolved quickly to significant life-threatening injuries. While improved reporting of such events is required in the future, it may be that such injuries are relatively rare. Clearly future research into efficacy of this treatment for these populations and the rates of occurrence of adverse events is necessary to determine whether or not this is true.

Additional material

Additional file 1: Appendix 1. Search strategy.
Additional file 2: Appendix 2. List of included articles.
Additional file 3: Table S1. Case report details.

Author details
[1]Division of Graduate Education and Research, Canadian Memorial Chiropractic College, 6100 Leslie Street, Toronto, ON M2H 3J1, Canada. [2]Texas Chiropractic College, 5912 Spencer Highway, Pasadena, TX 77505-1699, USA.

Authors' contributions
KJS conceived the study, participated in its design and coordination, conducted the literature search, screened the literature search results, analyzed and interpreted the data, and drafted the manuscript. SW conceived the study, participated in its design, screened the literature search results, and analyzed and interpreted the data. CAW analyzed and interpreted the data and drafted the manuscript. All authors read and approved the final manuscript.

Competing interests
The authors declare that they have no competing interests.

References

1. Khorsan R, Hawk C, Lisi AJ, Kizhakkeveettil A: **Manipulative therapy for pregnancy and related conditions: a systematic review.** *Obstet Gynecol Survey* 2009, **64**:416-427.
2. Skaggs C, Prather H, Gross G, George J, Thompson P, Nelson D: **Back and pelvis pain in an underserved United States pregnant population: A preliminary descriptive survey.** *J Manipulative Physiol Ther* 2007, **30**:130-134.
3. Stapleton D, MacLennan A, Kristiansson P: **The prevalence of recalled low back pain during and after pregnancy: a South Australian population survey.** *Aust N Z J Obstet Gynaecol* 2002, **42**:482-485.
4. Wu H, Meijer O, Uegaki K, Mens J, van Dieen J, Wuisman P, Ostgaard H: **Pregnancy-related pelvic girdle pain (PPP) I: Terminology, clinical presentation and prevalence.** *Eur Spine J* 2004, **13**:575-589.
5. Olsen MF, Gutke A, Elden H, Nordenman C, Fabrisius L, Gravesen M, Lind A, Kjellby-Wendt G: **Self-administered tests as a screening procedure for pregnancy-related pelvic girdle pain.** *Eur Spine J* 2009, **18**:1121-1129.
6. Mogren IM: **Physical activity and persistent low back pain and pelvic pain post partum.** *BMC Public Health* 2008, **8**:417-421.
7. Pennick VE, Young G: **Interventions for preventing and treating pelvic and back pain in pregnancy.** *Cochrane Database of Syst Rev* 2007, **2**: CD001139, DOI:10.1002/14651858.CD001139.pub2.
8. Mogren IM, Pohjanen AI: **Low back pain and pelvic pain during pregnancy: Prevalence and risk factors.** *Spine* 2005, **30**:983-991.
9. Lisi A: **Chiropractic spinal manipulation for low back pain of pregnancy; A retrospective case series.** *J Midwifery Women Health* 2005, **51**:e7-e10.
10. Kristiansson P, Savardsudd K, von Schoultz B: **Back pain during pregnancy.** *A prospective study. Spine* 1996, **2**:702-709.
11. Stuber KJ, Smith DL: **Chiropractic treatment of pregnancy-related low back pain: a systematic review of the evidence.** *J Manipulative Physiol Ther* 2008, **31**:447-454.
12. Natvig B, Ihlebaek C, Grotle M, Brage S, Bruugsgaard D: **Neck pain is often a part of widespread pain and is associated with reduced functioning.** *Spine* 2010, **35**:E1285-E1289.
13. Haldeman S, Carroll L, Cassidy JD: **Findings from The Bone and Joint Decade 2000 to 2010 Task Force on Neck Pain and Its Associated Disorders.** *J Occup Environ Med* 2010, **52**:424-427.
14. Coulter ID, Hurwitz EL, Adams AH: **Patients using chiropractors in North America: who are they, and why are they in chiropractic care?** *Spine* 2002, **27**:291-296.
15. Bishop PB, Quon JA, Fisher CG, Dvorak MF: **The Chiropractic Hospital-based Interventions Research Outcomes (CHIRO) study: a randomized controlled trial on the effectiveness of clinical practice guidelines in the medical and chiropractic management of patients with acute mechanical low back pain.** *Spine J* 2010, **10**:1055-64.
16. McMorland G, Suter E: **Chiropractic management of mechanical neck and low -back pain: a retrospective, outcome-based analysis.** *J Manipulative Physiol Ther* 2000, **23**:307-11.
17. Shekelle PG, Coulter I: **Cervical spine manipulatiion: summary report of a systemic review of the literature and multidisciplinary expert panel.** *J Spin Disord* 1997, **10**:223-8.
18. Nelson C: **Principles of effective headache management.** *Topics Clin Chiro* 1998, **5**:55-61.
19. Bryans R, Descarreaux M, Duranleau M, Marcoux H, Potter B, Ruegg R, Shaw L, Watkin R, White E: **Evidence-based guidelines for the chiropractic treatment of adults with headache.** *J Manipulative Physiol Ther* 2011, **34**:274-89.
20. Heiner JD: **Cervical epidural hematoma after chiropractic spinal manipulation.** *Am J Emerg Med* 2009, **27**:1023. e1-1023.e2.
21. Schmitz A, Lutterbey G, von Engelhardt L, von Falkenhausen M, Stoffel M: **Pathological cervical fracture after spinal manipulation in a pregnant patient.** *J Manipulative Physiol Ther* 2005, **28**:633-636.
22. Cassidy JD, Boyle E, Côté P, He Y, Hogg-Johnson S, Silver FL, Bondy SJ: **Risk of vertebrobasilar stroke and chiropractic care: results of a population-based case-control and case-crossover study.** *J Manipulative Physiol Ther* 2009, **32(Suppl 2)**:S201-8.
23. Oliphant D: **Safety of spinal manipulation in the treatment of lumbar disc herniations: a systematic review and risk assessment.** *J Manipulative Physiol Ther* 2004, **27**:197-210.
24. Stuber K: **The safety of chiropractic during pregnancy: a pilot e-mail survey of chiropractors' opinions.** *Clin Chiro* 2007, **10**:24-35.
25. Humphreys BK: **Possible adverse events in children treated by manual therapy: a review.** *Chiropr Osteopat* 2010, **18**:12.
26. Juul-Kristensen B, Rogind H, Jensen DV, Remvig L: **Inter-examiner reproducibility of tests and criteria for generalized hypermobility and benign joint hypermobility syndrome.** *Rheumatol* 2007, **46**:1835-1841.
27. Beighton P, Solomon L, Soskolne CL: **Articular mobility in an African population.** *Ann Rheum Dis* 1973, **32**:413-418.
28. Carter C, Wilkinson J: **Persistent joint laxity and congenital dislocation.** *J Bone Joint Surg* 1964, **46B**:40-45.
29. Marnach ML, Ramin KD, Ramsey PS, Song SW, Stensland JJ, An KN: **Characterization of the relationship between joint laxity and maternal hormones in pregnancy.** *Am Coll Obstet Gynecol* 2003, **101**:331-335.
30. Björklund K, Nordström ML, Odlind V: **Combined oral contraceptives do not increase the risk of back and pelvic pain during pregnancy or after delivery.** *Acta Obstet Gynecol Scand* 2000, **79**:979-83.
31. Calguneri M, Bird HA, Wright AV: **Changes in joint laxity occurring during pregnancy.** *Ann Rheum Dis* 1982, **41**:126-128.
32. Dragoo JL, Lee RS, Benhaim P, Finerman GA, Hame SL: **Relaxin receptors in the human female anterior cruciate ligament.** *Am J Sports Med* 2003, **31**:577-84.

33. Hansen A, Jensen DV, Larsen E, Wilken-Jensen C, Petersen K: **Relaxin is not related to symptom-giving pelvic relaxation in pregnant women.** *Acta Obstet Gynecol Scand* 1996, **75**:245-249.
34. Skott O, Carter AM: **Relaxin is a vasodilator hormone.** *Am J Physiol Regularory Integrative Comp Care* 2002, **283**:R347-R348.
35. Ng KPL, Doube A: **Stroke after neck manipulation in the post partum period.** *J NZ Med Assoc* 2001, **114**:498.
36. Stella CL, Sibai BM: **Thrombophilia and adverse maternal-perinatal outcome.** *Clin Obstet Gynecol* 2006, **49**:850-860.
37. Drife J: *Thromboembolism. Br Med Bull* 2003, **67**:177-190.
38. Maternal and Newborn Health/Safe Motherhood Unit, World Health Organization: *Postpartum Care of the Mother and Newborn: A Practical Guide. Geneva* 1998.
39. Bergmann T, Peterson D: *Chiropractic Technique: Principles and Procedures.* 3 edition. St. Louis: Elsevier; 2011.
40. Moher D, Liberati A, Tetzlaff J, Altman DG: **Preferred reporting items for systematic reviews 368 and meta-analyses: the PRISMA statement.** *J Clin Epidemiol* 2009, **62**:1006-1012.
41. McPartland JM: **Craniosacral iatriogenesis - side-effects from cranial sacral treatment: case reports and commentary.** *J Bodywork Movement Ther* 1996, **1**:2-5.
42. Parkin PJ, Wallis WE, Wilson JL: **Vertebral artery occlusion following manipulation of the neck.** *NZ Med J* 1978, **88**:441-443.
43. Murphy DR, Hurwitz EL, McGovern EE: **Outcome of pregnancy-related lumbopelvic pain treated according to a diagnosis-based decision rule: a prospective observational cohort study.** *J Manipulative Physiol Ther* 2009, **32**:616-624.
44. Redelmeier DA, Tibshirani RJ: **Interpretation and bias in case-crossover studies.** *J Clin Epidemiol* 1997, **50**:1281-7.
45. Smeeth L, Donnan PT, Cook DG: **The use of primary care databases: case-control and case-only designs.** *Fam Pract* 2006, **23**:597-604.

US chiropractors' attitudes, skills and use of evidence-based practice: A cross-sectional national survey

Michael J Schneider[1*], Roni Evans[2], Mitchell Haas[3], Matthew Leach[4], Cheryl Hawk[5], Cynthia Long[6], Gregory D Cramer[7], Oakland Walters[8], Corrie Vihstadt[2] and Lauren Terhorst[9]

Abstract

Background: Evidence based practice (EBP) is being increasingly utilized by health care professionals as a means of improving the quality of health care. The introduction of EBP principles into the chiropractic profession is a relatively recent phenomenon. There is currently a lack of information about the EBP literacy level of US chiropractors and the barriers/facilitators to the use of EBP in the chiropractic profession.

Methods: A nationwide EBP survey of US chiropractors was administered online (Nov 2012-Mar 2013) utilizing a validated self-report instrument (EBASE) in which three sub-scores are reported: attitudes, skills and use. Means, medians, and frequency distributions for each of the sub-scores were generated. Descriptive statistics were used to analyze the demographic characteristics of the sample. Means and proportions were calculated for all of the responses to each of the questions in the survey.

Results: A total of 1,314 US chiropractors completed the EBASE survey; the sample appeared to be representative of the US chiropractic profession. Respondents were predominantly white (94.3%), male (75%), 47 (+/− 11.6) years of age, and in practice for more than 10 years (60%). EBASE sub-score means (possible ranges) were: attitudes, 31.4 (8–40); skills, 44.3 (13–65); and use, 10.3 (0–24). Survey participants generally held favorable attitudes toward EBP, but reported less use of EBP. A minority of participants indicated that EBP coursework (17%) and critical thinking (29%) were a major part of their chiropractic education. The most commonly reported barrier to the use of EBP was "lack of time". Almost 90% of the sample indicated that they were interested in improving their EBP skills.

Conclusion: American chiropractors appear similar to chiropractors in other countries, and other health professionals regarding their favorable attitudes towards EBP, while expressing barriers related to EBP skills such as research relevance and lack of time. This suggests that the design of future EBP educational interventions should capitalize on the growing body of EBP implementation research developing in other health disciplines. This will likely include broadening the approach beyond a sole focus on EBP education, and taking a multilevel approach that also targets professional, organizational and health policy domains.

Keywords: Evidence-based medicine, Chiropractic, Complementary and alternative medicine, Survey research, Dissemination and implementation, Knowledge translation

* Correspondence: mjs5@pitt.edu
[1]Department of Physical Therapy, School of Health and Rehabilitation Sciences, Clinical and Translational Science Institute, University of Pittsburgh, Pittsburgh, PA, USA
Full list of author information is available at the end of the article

Background

Evidence-based practice (EBP) has been steadily advocated since the mid 1990's [1,2] and has increasingly been adopted as a foundational framework for improving the quality of healthcare delivery systems [3,4]. Despite the growing awareness of EBP, there still remains a large gap between this appreciation of EBP and the actual uptake and application of EBP in clinical settings. This gap between knowledge and awareness of EBP - and actual clinical use of EBP - is found in almost all healthcare fields, including medicine, nursing, and physical therapy [5,6].

Over the past decade the chiropractic profession has also embraced EBP, as evidenced by new EBP educational programs at chiropractic institutions [7-11] and the creation of professional evidence-based chiropractic guidelines [12-16]. However, while the enthusiasm for EBP in chiropractic is encouraging, a key aspect of its success will be whether or not it translates to changes in clinical practice. These changes would include the reduced use of unsupported clinical tests and procedures, as well as increased emphasis on those with an evidence base [17].

Dissemination and implementation research provides the means to bridge the gap between EBP principles and their application in clinical practice. This is accomplished by examining the mechanisms by which research evidence is spread and affects change in healthcare providers' attitudes and beliefs, and by evaluating strategies for changing healthcare professionals' behaviors to include the uptake of evidence-based clinical practices [18].

Chiropractic is one of the largest complementary and alternative medicine (CAM) professions in the United States. An important step for addressing the EBP gap in the chiropractic profession is to first understand chiropractors' attitudes and knowledge related to EBP, as well as the perceived barriers and facilitators to its application. Much of what is currently known is based on studies performed outside the United States. Walker et al. reported the results of an EBP survey showing that most of the 584 Australian chiropractors surveyed held positive attitudes towards EBP, thought EBP was useful, and were interested in improving their EBP skills [19]. However, despite their favorable inclination toward EBP, many Australian chiropractors stated they did not routinely use clinical practice guidelines. The three main barriers to the uptake of EBP identified in this study were: insufficient time, lack of generalizability of evidence to patient population, and inability to apply research findings to individual patients [19]. Similarly, researchers from Canada [20] and Great Britain [21] have found that accessibility to research, knowledge of how to access research, and critical appraisal skills are poor amongst chiropractors.

A study in a sub-specialty of 144 chiropractic orthopedists in the US also found favorable attitudes towards EBP, and a desire for EBP post-graduate continuing education [22]. The most frequently reported barriers to EBP in this study were lack of relevant clinical evidence and lack of time. Facilitators to EBP included internet and database access, online EBP educational materials, critical reviews of chiropractic research, and ability to download full-text articles. The findings of this study are limited however by its small and specialized sample; consequently, the factors associated with the uptake of EBP by the US chiropractic profession still remain poorly understood.

The purpose of this article is to describe the results of a cross-sectional survey of US chiropractors' attitudes, skills and use of research evidence in clinical practice, as well as the barriers and facilitators to use of EBP.

Methods

Study design and setting

This was a cross-sectional survey conducted online between November 17, 2012 and March 5, 2013. The survey was administered electronically through the University of Pittsburgh (UPitt), Pittsburgh, Pennsylvania, using the UPitt web platform.

Ethics

Ethical approval (PRO12060417) was obtained through the University of Pittsburgh's (UPitt) institutional review board (IRB), which granted "exempt status" in June 2012. Informed consent was secured from all subjects on the homepage of the research website, prior to participation in the survey.

Context

The *Distance Education Online Intervention for Evidence-Based Practice Literacy (DELIVER)* project is a two-phase NIH/NCCAM-funded study (R21 AT007547) designed to evaluate the effectiveness of an online EBP educational program on chiropractors' attitudes, skill, and use of EBP. This cross-sectional survey comprised the first phase of the DELIVER study and served as a baseline measure of EBP literacy against which to analyze the effectiveness of an online EBP educational program (second phase).

Participants & recruitment

The survey was open to all Doctors of Chiropractic (DCs) in the US who had internet access and a valid email address. A convenience sample of DCs were recruited primarily by emails forwarded to the membership rosters of several cooperating organizations including the following: American Chiropractic Association, Council on Chiropractic Guidelines and Practice Parameters, Congress of Chiropractic State Associations, Sacro Occipital Research Society International, Activator Methods, US ChiroDirectory, International College of Applied Kinesiology, the Pediatric

Councils of the American Chiropractic Association and International Chiropractors Association.

These organizations provided email-forwarding services through their respective membership lists, which created a potential pool of over 30,000 DCs. The forwarded email message described a unique opportunity to participate in an online survey; participation was incentivized by offering participants the opportunity to enter a drawing to win an Apple iPad™. Recipients of the email were encouraged to forward the message on to their colleagues. Articles announcing the study and inviting readers to participate were published in two national chiropractic publications; Dynamic Chiropractic [23] and the Journal of American Chiropractic Association [24]. Another national chiropractic publication - The American Chiropractor - announced the study by sending an email blast to its national circulation of DCs.

Questionnaire and outcomes

The **E**vidence-**B**ased Practice **A**ttitude and Utilization **S**urv**E**y (EBASE) is a self-administered instrument designed to measure CAM providers' attitudes, skills and use of EBP [25]. The instrument has demonstrated good internal consistency, content validity, and acceptable test-retest reliability [26]. Minor modifications of a few EBASE items were required to ensure the language was appropriate for use with chiropractors [22]. These changes were made in consultation with the survey developer (ML) to ensure the structure and intent of the modified questions were not altered in any manner that would jeopardize the validity of the original survey. Only the demographics section (Part G) required major modifications to be relevant to the chiropractic profession.

Our modified version of the EBASE contains 75 items and is divided into 7 parts (Parts A-G); Parts A-F each address a different EBP construct, and Part G contains demographic items only. Each question within these parts allowed the participant 5 possible responses, which were rated numerically from 1 to 5 for Parts A and B, and from 0 to 4 for Part D. Although there are 7 parts to this survey, only 3 parts generate sub-scores: Parts A (Attitudes), B (Skill), and D (Use). The 4 remaining parts of the EBASE are not scored, including Part C (Training & Education), Part E (Barriers), Part F (Facilitators) and Part G (Demographics). The completion time of the online EBASE is approximately 10–12 minutes (see Additional file 1 for a copy of the modified EBASE survey and the scoring rubric used for calculating the three sub-scores).

Survey administration and data collection

Interested DCs were invited to follow a link to a dedicated UPitt website where they could obtain detailed information about the study procedures and register for the study by submitting an email address. Participants were subsequently emailed a password to enter the survey site, an effort aimed at preventing multiple responses from the same individual. To encourage honest and transparent responses, anonymity was insured by assigning a unique identification number to each registered DC, which was used to identify the respondent's survey data. As participants completed the survey, responses were captured through a secure data capturing feature/system, Web Data Xpress, an interface that allows for direct entry and storage of data within a designated SQL Server database. This method of data capture is resource-efficient and minimizes human error by avoiding the need for manual data entry.

Data analysis

Data were analyzed using SPSS version 22 (SPSS Inc., Chicago, IL, USA). Since this was a cross-sectional survey we calculated descriptive statistics including response frequencies and means for each item in Parts A, B, D, E and F and response frequencies for Parts C and G. The attitudes, skills, and use sub-scores were calculated using the scoring rubric (see Additional file 1) developed with the original EBASE. This involves summing the first eight items of Parts A (response range 1–5; total score range of 8–40), all 13 of the items of Part B (response range 1–5; total score range of 13–65), and the first 6 items of Part D (response range 0–4; total score range of 0–24). Frequency distributions for the group sub-score means for Part A, B and D were also calculated. Higher sub-scores indicate higher self-reported levels of attitudes (Part A), skills (Part B) and use (Part D) of EBP.

Results

Sample Size

A total of 1,314 US chiropractors responded to the survey.

Participant characteristics (Demographics and Education/Training)

Table 1 provides a summary of the frequencies of the demographic characteristics of the participants. The majority of the sample were male (75%), Caucasian (94%), practiced as sole proprietors (72%) and held a Bachelor's or higher level graduate degree in addition to their chiropractic degree (>80%). The average age of our sample was 47 years (range: 24 to 85 years), and the mean number of years in practice was 17 years (range: 0 to 30 years or more).

Only a small minority of the sample indicated that the following topics were major parts of their chiropractic education: coursework about EBP (17%), applying research evidence to clinical practice (13%), and critical thinking/analysis (29%) (Table 2). Eleven percent of the

Table 1 Demographic characteristics of the 1,314 American chiropractors who completed the online evidence-based practice survey

Variable	Characteristic	n (%)
Gender	Male	989 (75.3)
	Female	325 (24.7)
Age	Mean = 46.7 yrs (SD = 11.6); Range = 24-85 yrs	
Race	White	1239 (94.3)
	Black	13 (1.0)
	Asian	33 (2.5)
	Mixed Race/Other	29 (2.2)
Years since chiropractic graduation	0-5	273 (20.8)
	6-10	146 (11.1)
	11-15	187 (14.2)
	16-20	159 (12.1)
	21-25	170 (12.9)
	26-29	144 (11.0)
	30 or more Mean = 17 yrs; Range = 0-30 or more yrs	235 (17.9)
Highest education level	High School	17 (1.3)
	Associate's Degree	214 (16.3)
	Bachelor's Degree	821 (62.5)
	Master's Degree	226 (17.2)
	Doctorate	36 (2.7)
Region of practice	Midwest	380 (28.9)
	Northeast	287 (21.8)
	West	264 (20.1)
	Southeast	245 (18.6)
	Southwest	131 (10.0)
	Non-continental US	7 (0.5)
Geographic setting	Suburban	629 (47.9)
	City	449 (34.2)
	Rural	236 (18.0)
Patients seen daily	0-10	367 (27.9)
	11-20	455 (34.6)
	21-30	259 (19.7)
	31-40	126 (9.6)
	41-50	60 (4.6)
	51 or more Median = 20/day; (IQR = 10-30) Range = 0-100/day	47 (3.6)
Focus of clinical practice	**Musculoskeletal focus**	**869 (66.1)**
	Spine and extremities	742 (56.5)
	Spine	72 (5.5)
	Sports	55 (4.2)
	Non-musculoskeletal focus	**445 (33.9)**
	Family care	192 (14.6)
	Subluxation-based	114 (8.7)
	Wellness/Prevention	105 (8.0)
	Non-musculoskeletal	20 (1.5)
	Pediatrics	14 (1.1)
Clinical role	Sole Proprietor	946 (72.0)
	Partner or group practice	171 (13.0)
	Associate or employee	144 (11.0)
	Hospital-based practice	53 (4.0)
Organizational membership	Unaffiliated	722 (55.0)
	American Chiropractic Assoc. (ACA)	526 (40.0)
	International Chiropractors Assoc. (ICA)	66 (5.0)

SD = Standard Deviation. IQR = Interquartile Range. Yrs = Years.

sample indicated they never had any critical thinking/ analysis included in their chiropractic education. Almost half the sample reported that they had never received any education/training on conducting systematic reviews (48%) or clinical research (42%).

Descriptive results for parts A, B and D (Attitudes, Skills and Use)

Participants held a generally favorable attitude (Part A) toward EBP, with a mean attitude sub-score of 31.4 (range 8–40); while the frequency distribution was skewed to the left, the median sub-score (32.0) was close to the mean (Figure 1). The majority (>75%) of participants gave responses of "agree" or "strongly agree" to most questions (Table 3). There were two individual attitude related items with which a smaller proportion of the respondents agreed: 1) "EBP takes into account a patient's preference for treatment" (42% agree/strongly agree); and 2) "EBP takes into account my clinical experience when making clinical decisions" (65% agree/strongly agree). It was also very interesting to note that the vast majority of our sample (89.5%) agreed or strongly agreed with the statement "I am interested in learning or improving the skills necessary to incorporate EBP into my practice".

For self-reported skills in EBP (Part B) the mean sub-score was 44.3 (range of 13–65) with a left skewed frequency distribution, and a median sub-score (44.0) similar to the mean (Figure 2). For the majority of skill items, more than half of respondents indicated a generally high level ('4' or '5') of self-reported skill in EBP (Table 4); however nearly a third of respondents rated their skills in the mid-range ('3' on 1–5 scale) for 11 of the 13 skill items. The two skills rated poorest were: 1) "conducting clinical research" (66% of respondents) and 2) "conducting systematic reviews" (47% of respondents).

Table 2 Response frequency of Training/Education items (Part C of E-BASE)

PART C Item	None	Seminar (<1 day)	Short course (<1 week)	Minor part of chiropractic education	Major part of chiropractic education	Minor part of diplomate education	Major part of diplomate education	Academic diploma	Informal personal study
Applying research evidence to clinical practice	8.1%	23.4%	5.7%	23.4%	13.1%	3.7%	3.9%	1.8%	17.0%
Critical thinking/critical analysis	10.8%	8.4%	5.3%	21.7%	29.0%	2.7%	3.8%	3.4%	14.9%
Evidence-based clinical practice/evidence-based chiropractic	4.8%	25.5%	5.5%	22.8%	17.0%	5.6%	4.9%	1.8%	12.1%
Conducting systematic reviews or meta-analysis	47.6%	6.3%	6.5%	21.8%	3.7%	1.9%	0.6%	1.2%	10.4%
Conducting clinical research	42.2%	6.3%	6.1%	26.5%	4.0%	2.4%	0.9%	1.8%	9.8%

These are responses to the question "Please indicate the highest level of training/education you have received in the following areas".

The mean sub-score for use of EBP (Part D) was 10.3 (range of 0–24). The frequency distribution was skewed to the right, with a median sub-score of 8.0 (Figure 3). While 36% reported not consulting magazines, laypersons or self-help books for clinical decision making in the previous month, 23% also reported not using research findings to change their clinical practice and 29% did not use an online database to search for practice-based literature or research findings. About 45% of the sample indicated that only a small, very small, or no proportion of their practice was based on clinical research evidence (Table 5).

Descriptive results for parts E and F (Barriers and Facilitators to EBP Uptake)

When presented with a list of potential barriers to EBP uptake (Part E), most (>75%) participants indicated that the majority of the factors were either "not a barrier" or a "minor barrier" (Table 6), with a few notable exceptions. Items rated as being moderate or major barriers to EBP uptake included: 1) 'lack of time' (48%); 2) 'lack of clinical evidence about CAM' (44%); 3), 'lack of industry support' (37%); and 4) 'lack of incentive' (36%). Approximately a quarter of respondents cited insufficient skills for interpreting (27%); locating (23%) and critically appraising research (24%); lack of colleague support for EBP (23%); and lack of relevance to chiropractic practice (24%).

In terms of the perceived usefulness of various factors in facilitating the uptake of EBP (Part F) in clinical practice, over 70% of respondents indicated all 10 items as either "moderately useful" or "very useful" (Table 7). The two items that received the greatest percentage of "very useful" responses were "access to the internet" (78%) and "access to free online databases" (70%). Items

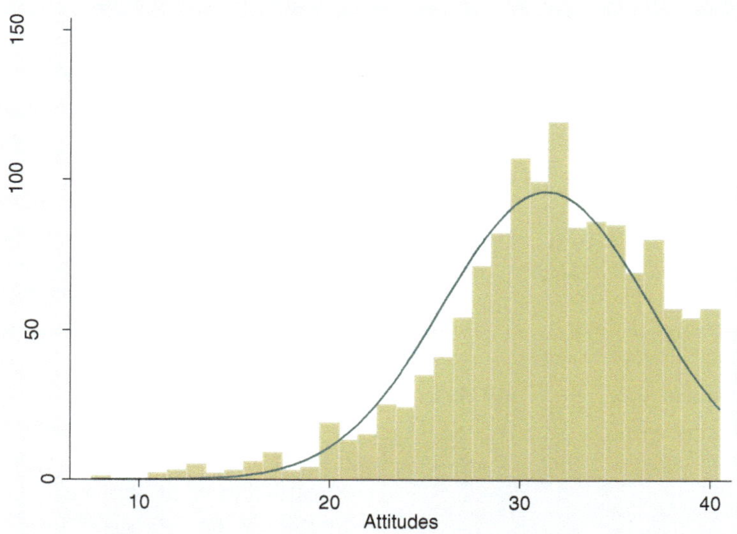

Figure 1 Frequency distribution of Attitudes sub-scores. The Y-axis indicates the number of survey participants and the X-axis indicates the Attitudes subscores. The mean sub-score was 31.4 (sd = 5.5) with a possible range of 8 to 40 (8 items scored 1–5). Median = 32.0 (IQR = 28-35).

Table 3 Response frequency and means of Attitudes toward EBP items (Part A of E-BASE)

Part A Items	Strongly Disagree(1)	Disagree(2)	Neutral(3)	Agree(4)	Strongly Agree(5)	Mean (Range=1-5)
*I am interested in learning or improving the skills necessary to incorporate EBP into my practice	0.9%	2.1%	7.5%	42.8%	46.7%	4.3
*Evidence based practice (EBP) is necessary in the practice of chiropractic	2.1%	3.5%	9.1%	39.6%	45.7%	4.2
*Professional literature (i.e. journals & textbooks) and research findings are useful in my day-to-day practice	0.9%	3.4%	9.6%	53.4%	32.7%	4.1
*EBP improves the quality of my patient's care	2.1%	4.4%	14.4%	43.2%	35.9%	4.1
*EBP assists me in making decisions about patient care	1.2%	3.7%	10.6%	48.6%	35.9%	4.1
Prioritizing EBP within chiropractic practice is fundamental to the advancement of the profession	2.4%	7.8%	13.3%	39.8%	36.7%	4.0
*EBP takes into account my clinical experience when making clinical decisions	2.3%	14.8%	17.7%	41.5%	23.7%	3.7
*The adoption of EBP places an unreasonable demand on my practice **[Note: Item is reverse coded]**	14.4%[5]	43.2[4]	29.1%[3]	10.6% [2]	2.7%[1]	3.6
*EBP takes into account a patient's preference for treatment	5.3%	24.1%	28.5%	27.1%	15.0%	3.2
There is a lack of evidence from clinical trials to support most of the treatments I use in my practice	13.5%	42.2%	17.7%	22.6%	4.0%	2.6

*The sum of the 8 items with asterisks comprises the "Attitudes" sub-score, which ranges from 8-40. See Figure 1 for frequency distribution graph of attitudes sub-scores. These are responses to the question "On a scale ranging from strongly disagree to strongly agree, how would you rate your opinion on the following statements?"

most frequently reported as "not useful" or "slightly useful" included: 1) "access to online tools to assist you to conduct your own critical appraisals of multiple research papers" (30%), and 2) "access to research rating tools that facilitate critical appraisal of single research papers" (26%).

Discussion

This is one of the largest studies to examine chiropractors' perspectives relative to EBP, and to our knowledge, the first national survey to be conducted in the United States. One other EBP study was performed in the US, however the sample was limited to mid-western chiropractors with advanced training in orthopedics [22]. Despite the large absolute sample size of our survey (n = 1,314), it represents only a small relative cross-sectional sample of the American chiropractic profession (n = 60,000) [27-29]. However, the demographic characteristics of our sample (Table 1) are strikingly similar to those reported by three National Board of Chiropractic Examiners' Job Analysis Reports [27-29]. This provides support for the generalizability of our survey results and makes us more confident that we have obtained a representative sample of US chiropractors.

The results suggest that our respondents generally have positive attitudes about evidence-based practice and a high level of self-reported skills in EBP, but only a modest level of EBP uptake in their clinical practices. These results are relatively similar to those reported from a recent EBP survey of Australian chiropractors [19] and are consistent with the observation that passive diffusion of knowledge does not automatically translate into clinical implementation [6]. Further, it emphasizes the need for high quality EBP continuing education programs to meet the needs of the chiropractic profession.

Our participants reported generally positive attitudes toward EBP, with most agreeing that EBP is important for improving practice, patient care, and advancing the profession. Noteworthy was that nearly a third strongly agreed that there is a 'lack of evidence from clinical trials to support most of the treatments I use in my practice'. Similarly, only 42% agreed or strongly agreed that 'EBP takes into account a patient's preference for treatment'. These findings suggest that the basic principles of EBP may be misunderstood by DCs given the original definition of EBP clearly states that clinical expertise, patient values and best available research evidence are all integral components of evidence-based practice [1]. However, these opinions might also reflect what has become a growing recognition across healthcare fields; that clinical research needs to become more patient-oriented, pragmatic and generalizable to "real life" clinical practice [30].

Our sample of DCs reported that their poorest EBP skills were in conducting clinical research and/or systematic reviews; given that this survey was of practicing DCs without academic or research affiliation, this is not surprising. Distinctions have been drawn between the expectation for practitioners to be 'consumers' who 'use' research rather than 'manufacturers' who 'produce' research [31]; future studies should take this into consideration by ensuring that data collection instruments reflect this thinking.

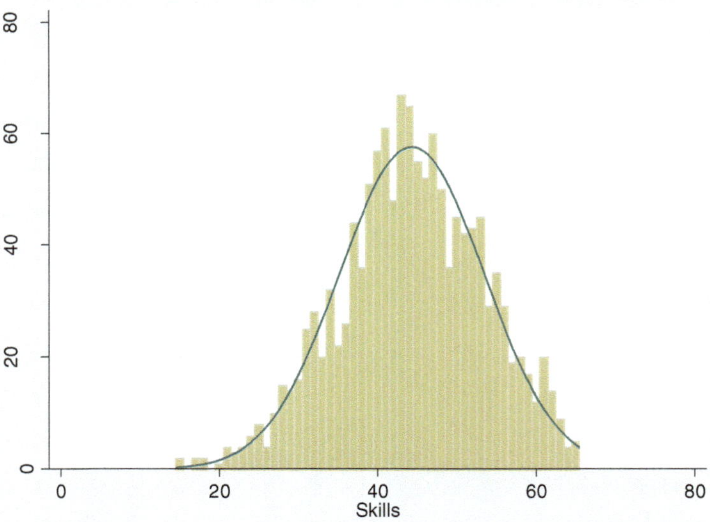

Figure 2 Frequency distribution of Skills sub-scores. The Y-axis indicates the number of survey participants and the X-axis indicates the Skills subscores. The mean sub-score was 44.3 (sd = 9.1) with a possible range of 13 to 65 (13 items scored 1–5). Median = 44.0 (IQR = 39-51).

Most of our sample reported above average skills in EBP, particularly in relation to identifying answerable clinical questions, identifying knowledge gaps in practice, locating professional literature and online database searching. However, nearly a third of respondents rated themselves only in the mid-range on nearly all of the EBP skill items. Some of these skills included the ability to synthesize research evidence, sharing evidence with colleagues, and using the findings from systematic reviews. Interestingly, while almost two-thirds reported above-average to advanced skills in using findings from clinical research, less than half reported the same level of skill in using findings from systematic reviews. This suggests that DCs have a limited understanding of the value and availability of systematic reviews, which is problem shared by many health professionals [32].

The introduction of EBP into the curricula of US chiropractic colleges is a relatively new phenomenon that has largely occurred over the past decade. The National Center for Complementary and Integrative Health (formerly NCCAM) has provided funding through its R25 mechanism to nine CAM colleges - four of them with chiropractic education programs - to develop institutional programs focused on teaching EBP. An

Table 4 Response frequency and means of Skills in EBP items (Part B of E-BASE)

PART B Items	Poor (1)	(2)	(3)	(4)	Advanced(5)	Mean (Range=1-5)
Identifying answerable clinical questions	0.3%	3.0%	18.6%	52.5%	25.6%	4.0
Identifying knowledge gaps in practice	0.4%	3.5%	29.5%	50.0%	16.7%	3.8
Locating professional literature	1.7%	8.6%	25.5%	38.7%	25.5%	3.8
Online database searching	3.7%	12.1%	25.3%	35.2%	23.7%	3.6
Retrieving evidence	3.0%	11.4%	28.5%	38.5%	18.6%	3.6
Critical appraisal of evidence	1.9%	10.6%	31.2%	42.4%	13.9%	3.6
Synthesis of research evidence	3.7%	15.8%	34.6%	36.6%	9.3%	3.3
Applying research evidence to patient cases	1.7%	8.0%	27.2%	48.9%	14.2%	3.7
Using findings from clinical research	1.5%	7.1%	29.1%	47.4%	14.9%	3.7
Sharing evidence with colleagues	4.8%	18.0%	30.6%	33.3%	13.3%	3.3
Using findings from systematic reviews	6.3%	19.2%	30.7%	34.0%	9.8%	3.2
Conducting systematic reviews	17.0%	29.9%	29.9%	18.4%	4.8%	2.6
Conducting clinical research	36.8%	29.5%	20.9%	10.3%	2.5%	2.1

The sum of all 13 items comprises the "skills" sub-score, which ranges from 13-65. See Figure 2 for frequency distribution graph of skills sub-scores. These are responses to the question "On a scale from 1 to 5, with 1 being poor and 5 being advanced, how would you rate your skills in the following areas"?

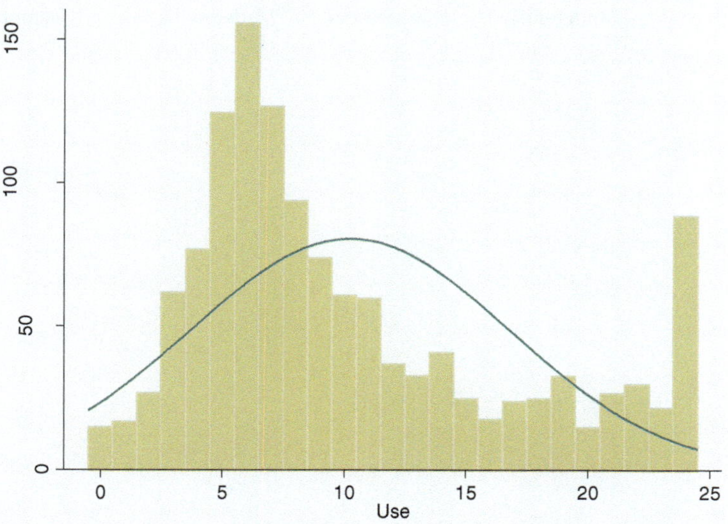

Figure 3 Frequency distribution of Use sub-scores. The Y-axis indicates the number of survey participants and the X-axis indicates the Use subscores. The mean sub-score was 10.3 (sd = 6.5) with a possible range of 0 to 24 (6 items scored 0–4). Median value = 8.0 (IQR = 6-14).

overarching goal of these R25 research education grants was to provide CAM faculty and students with the skills they need to apply a rigorous evidence-based perspective to their training and practice. Adding research literacy and EBP competencies to the curricula at these CAM colleges has led to changes in their institutional cultures, such as increased faculty use of EBP case studies in the classroom and student-led research/journal clubs [33-35]. However, with approximately two thirds of our sample receiving their chiropractic training 11 to 30 years ago, it is

Table 5 Response frequency and means of Use of EBP items (Part D of E-BASE)

PART D Item	None (0)	Very small (1-25%) (1)	Small (26-50%) (2)	Moderate (51-75%) (3)	Large (76-99%) (4)	All (100%) (5)	Mean (Range=1-5)
What percentage of your practice do you estimate is based on clinical research evidence (i.e. evidence from clinical trials)?	2.7%	21.2%	21.0%	32.3%	21.0%	1.8%	2.5
PART D Items	**0 times (0)**	**1-5 times (1)**	**6-10 times (2)**	**11-15 times (3)**	**16+ times (4)**		**Mean (Range=0-4)**
*I have read/reviewed professional literature (i.e. professional journals & textbooks) related to my practice	3.4%	41.9%	22.6%	8.7%	23.4%		2.1
*I have used an online search engine to search for practice related literature or research	7.9%	39.0%	23.5%	9.9%	19.7%		1.9
*I have read/reviewed clinical research findings related to my practice	7.8%	48.3%	17.4%	7.5%	19.0%		1.8
*I have used professional literature or research findings to assist my clinical decision making	11.0%	52.1%	14.8%	6.3%	15.8%		1.6
*I have used an online database to search for practice related literature or research	28.6%	36.5%	12.4%	6.4%	16.1%		1.4
*I have used professional literature or research findings to change my clinical Practice	23.2%	48.9%	11.3%	4.3%	12.3%		1.3
I have consulted a colleague or industry expert to assist my clinical decision making	22.5%	51.8%	13.5%	4.7%	7.5%		1.2
I have referred to magazines, layperson/ self-help books, or non-government/ non-education institution websites to assist my clinical decision making	35.6%	43.8%	11.1%	4.2%	5.3%		1.0

*The sum of the 6 items with asterisks comprises the "Use" sub-score, which ranges from 0-24. See Figure 3 for frequency distribution graph of the "use" sub-scores. These are responses to the question "Indicate how often you have performed the following activities over the last month".

Table 6 Response frequency and means of Barriers to EBP uptake items (Part E of E-BASE)

PART E Items	Not a barrier (1)	Minor barrier (2)	Moderate barrier (3)	Major barrier (4)	Mean (Range = 1-4)
Lack of time	19.2%	33.0%	34.1%	13.7%	2.4
Lack of clinical evidence in complementary and alternative medicine	18.9%	37.2%	32.2%	11.7%	2.4
Lack of industry support for EBP	31.4%	31.6%	26.3%	10.7%	2.2
Lack of incentive to participate in EBP	34.6%	29.2%	26.2%	10.0%	2.1
Insufficient skills for interpreting research	34.3%	38.7%	19.9%	7.1%	2.0
Insufficient skills for locating research	39.7%	37.3%	16.8%	6.2%	1.9
Insufficient skills to critically appraise/evaluate the literature	35.8%	39.8%	18.8%	5.6%	1.9
Lack of colleague support for EBP	44.1%	32.7%	17.0%	6.2%	1.9
Insufficient skills to apply research findings to clinical practice	39.9%	41.5%	15.8%	2.8%	1.8
Lack of relevance to chiropractic practice	47.1%	29.1%	17.8%	6.0%	1.8
Patient preference for treatment	41.5%	38.0%	16.8%	3.7%	1.8
Lack of interest in EBP	52.5%	30.5%	12.6%	4.4%	1.7
Lack of resources (i.e. access to a computer, the internet or online databases)	60.0%	26.8%	10.4%	2.8%	1.6

These are responses to the question "On a scale ranging from 'not a barrier' to 'major barrier', to what extent do the following factors prevent you from participating in EBP"?

likely that many of our participants never received what would now be considered foundational training in EBP.

Additionally, our results suggest that educational emphasis should be focused on improving the skills of appraising and applying research evidence in clinical practice. This needs to be done in a way that provides clinicians with 'real life' clinical examples, in order to overcome the barriers of lack of interest or clinical relevance to chiropractic practice. This issue was addressed in the second phase of our project, which explores the effectiveness of online EBP educational modules and "booster exercises" that incorporate clinical examples

Table 7 Response frequency and means of Facilitators of EBP uptake items (Part F of E-BASE)

PART F Items	Not useful (1)	Slightly useful (2)	Moderately useful (3)	Very useful (4)	Mean (Range = 1-4)
Access to the Internet in your workplace	3.4%	5.2%	13.5%	77.9%	3.7
Access to free online databases in the workplace, such as Cochrane and PubMed	2.0%	8.9%	18.9%	70.2%	3.6
Ability to download full-text / full-length journal articles	2.1%	11.5%	20.9%	65.5%	3.5
Access to online education materials related to evidence based practice	1.4%	9.3%	23.7%	65.6%	3.5
Access to critical reviews of research evidence relevant to your field (these are critical reviews of multiple research papers addressing a single topic)	1.8%	11.3%	31.4%	55.5%	3.4
Free access to online databases that usually require license fees, such as DynaMed and CINAHL	6.9%	15.1%	19.7%	58.3%	3.3
Access to critically appraised topics relevant to your field (these are critical appraisals of single research papers)	2.2%	15.6%	35.2%	47.0%	3.3
Access to tools used to assist the critical appraisal/evaluation of research evidence	3.4%	17.6%	36.7%	42.3%	3.2
Access to research rating tools that facilitate critical appraisal of single research papers	4.3%	21.9%	35.5%	38.3%	3.1
Access to online tools that assist you to conduct your own critical appraisals of multiple research papers related to a single topic	6.8%	22.9%	30.4%	39.9%	3.0

These are responses to the question "On a scale ranging from 'not useful' to 'very useful', to what extent would the following strategies assist you in participating in EBP"?

relevant to chiropractors. Results of the second phase of this project will be reported in a future publication.

The results of this survey also indicate that there are serious gaps in the uptake of research evidence into chiropractic practice, with nearly half reporting only a very small proportion of what they do in their clinical practice is based on research evidence. DCs appear to have challenges with performing online searches of the literature and interpreting the results of systematic reviews. Although most DCs in our sample reported they had above average skills in locating literature online, they also indicated that they did not engage in the uptake of EBP on a frequent basis (> six times a month). This apparent contradiction may be associated with the issues of time and lack of evidence, as discussed in the next paragraph. However, almost 90% of our sample indicated that they were interested in learning or improving the skills necessary to incorporate EBP into their practices (Table 3). Educational interventions and strategies are more likely to be successful if they are informed by known barriers and facilitators [36-39].

On the whole, most DCs indicated there were few barriers to their uptake of EBP, which is consistent with their generally positive attitudes toward EBP. It is worth noting however, that almost half of DCs indicated that the two biggest barriers to EBP uptake were 'lack of time' and 'lack of clinical evidence in CAM'. A sizeable proportion (a quarter to one third) also cited: 'lack of industry support'; 'lack of incentive'; 'insufficient skills for interpreting research'; 'locating and critically appraising research'; 'lack of colleague support for EBP'; and 'lack of relevance to chiropractic practice'. Many of the barriers identified in this study are similar to those found for chiropractors in Australia [19], Canada [20] and Great Britain [21] as well as a sub-specialty of chiropractic orthopedists in the US [22]. Interestingly, many of the same barriers are encountered in the medical and nursing professions [5,6], leading us to conclude that the challenges facing the chiropractic profession in implementing EBP are not unique.

Interestingly, very few DCs indicated that computer, internet, or database access were barriers to their uptake of EBP. Coupled with our sample's perceived usefulness of all of the listed facilitator items, these findings underscore the importance of providing clinicians with training in EBP skills, particularly through online resources. Our findings also suggest a need for greater support from professional organizations to facilitate collegial support of EBP, as well as better collaboration between scientists and practitioners in the design of clinically applicable research. Indeed, while educational strategies are an important part of narrowing the gap between science and practice for chiropractic and other health disciplines, they will likely be insufficient on their own to accomplish true change. Comprehensive and multi-faceted approaches that take into account all the relevant levels affecting EBP, including professional, managerial, organizational and health systems, will likely be needed to integrate research into practice [41].

There were several limitations to this study. The first is inherent to any type of survey design, which is reliance on self-reporting. For example, the 'skills' sub-score was based upon the participants' self-perceived level of skill; we did not directly test a participant's knowledge or skills in EBP. It would be useful in future studies to correlate an actual "grade" from tests or quizzes of EBP knowledge with the self-reported survey data. Another inherent limitation is selection bias; it is possible that the 'attitudes' sub-scores were skewed toward higher values because participants were already in favor of an evidence-based practice paradigm prior to commencing the survey.

Although we had a relatively large number of survey responders (n = 1,314), this number represents only a small proportion of the approximately 60,000 licensed chiropractors in the US. We made some minor modifications in the original EBASE questionnaire, chiefly to use the word "chiropractic" in certain questions. We do not believe these minor changes altered the intrinsic properties of the EBASE, however we did not formally conduct a psychometric evaluation of this modified version.

Conclusion

The results of this survey have provided new insights into the attitudes, skills and use of EBP among US chiropractors. The information gained from this survey will be most helpful in informing the design of future educational interventions for chiropractors to improve their level of EBP literacy and use of evidence in clinical practice. Overall, American chiropractors appear very similar to chiropractors in other countries, as well as other health professionals in terms of their favorable attitudes towards EBP, while expressing limitations and barriers related to EBP skills, research relevance, and lack of time. This suggests that the design of future EBP interventions for chiropractic should capitalize on the growing body of EBP implementation research evidence developing in other health disciplines. This will likely include broadening the approach beyond a sole focus on EBP education, and taking a multilevel approach that also targets professional, organizational and health policy domains.

Additional file

Additional file 1: EBASE Questionnaire and Scoring Rubric.

Abbreviations

ACA: American Chiropractic Association; CAM: Complementary and Alternative Medicine; DELIVER: Distance Education Online Intervention for

Evidence-Based Practice Literacy; DC: Doctor of Chiropractic; EBP: Evidence-Based Practice; EBASE: Evidence-Based Practice Attitude and Utilization Survey; UPitt: University of Pittsburgh; NCCAM: National Center for Complementary and Alternative Medicine.

Competing interests

The authors declare that they have no competing interests.

Authors' contributions

MS was the principal investigator of the DELIVER study and was responsible for securing the funding and administration of the research grant. He was responsible for data collection, analysis, and a majority of the manuscript preparation. RE contributed to the conceptualization, design and funding acquisition of this work; she participated in data collection implementation and monitoring as well as decisions regarding data analysis and interpretation of results. She worked with the primary author to prepare the manuscript for publication and contributed content to the background and discussion sections. MH was responsible for assisting in designing the study, and interpretation of findings, as well as drafting and editing the manuscript. GC contributed to the initial concept and design of the study, was involved in meetings assessing progress, and critically reviewed the drafts of the manuscript, including data analyses. CH contributed to the initial concept and design of the study, interpretation of findings, as well as editing the manuscript. ML was involved in the design and funding of the study, development of the outcome measure, drafting of the methods, and editing of the draft and final manuscript. CL contributed to the initial concept and design of the study, was involved in meetings assessing progress, and critically reviewed the drafts of the manuscript, including data analyses. CV worked with the primary author and co-authors to prepare the manuscript. She also participated in the implementation of Phase II of the DELIVER study. OW made significant contributions to the conception and design, acquisition and analysis of data; he was involved in drafting/revising the manuscript and gave final approval of the version to be published. LT performed the statistical analyses of the data and assisted with the interpretations of the results. She prepared the tables and worked with the primary author to write the methods, statistical analyses, and results sections of the manuscript. All authors read and approved the final manuscript.

Acknowledgements

This research was made possible by Grant Number R21AT007547 from the National Center for Complementary and Integrative Health (NCCIH; formerly NCCAM) at the National Institutes of Health (NIH). The views expressed in this article are solely those of the authors and do not necessarily represent the official views of the NCCIH, NCCAM or NIH.

The authors would like to acknowledge the hard work and assistance of our senior research associate Kris Gongaware and our research coordinator Christine McFarland. We would also like to acknowledge the important contributions of our database and information technology consultant Jack Doman.

Author details

[1]Department of Physical Therapy, School of Health and Rehabilitation Sciences, Clinical and Translational Science Institute, University of Pittsburgh, Pittsburgh, PA, USA. [2]Center for Spirituality and Healing, Integrative Health and Wellbeing Research Program, University of Minnesota, Minneapolis, MN, USA. [3]University of Western States, Portland, OR, USA. [4]School of Nursing and Midwifery, University of South Australia, Adelaide, SA, Australia. [5]Logan College of Chiropractic, Chesterfield, MO, USA. [6]Palmer Center for Chiropractic Research, Palmer College of Chiropractic, Davenport, IA, USA. [7]National University of Health Sciences, Lombard, IL, USA. [8]The Commonwealth Medical College, Scranton, PA, USA. [9]Department of Occupational Therapy, School of Health and Rehabilitation Sciences, University of Pittsburgh, Pittsburgh, PA, USA.

References

1. Sackett DL, Rosenberg WM, Gray JA, Haynes RB, Richardson WS. Evidence based medicine: what it is and what it isn't. BMJ. 1996;312:71–2.
2. Claridge JA, Fabian TC. History and development of evidence-based medicine. World J Surg. 2005;29:547–53.
3. Balakas K, Potter P, Pratt E, Rea G, Williams J. Evidence equals excellence: the application of an evidence-based practice model in an academic medical center. Nurs Clin North Am. 2009;44:1–10.
4. Glasziou P, Ogrinc G, Goodman S. Can evidence-based medicine and clinical quality improvement learn from each other? BMJ Qual Saf. 2011;20:13–7.
5. Ubbink DT, Guyatt GH, Vermeulen H. Framework of policy recommendations for implementation of evidence-based practice: a systematic scoping review. BMJ Open. 2013; doi:10.1136/bmjopen-2012-001881.
6. Cabana MD, Rand C, Powe N, Wu A, Wilson M, Abboud P, et al. Why don't physicians follow clinical practice guidelines? A framework for improvement. JAMA. 1999;282(15):1458–65.
7. Academic Consortium for Complementary & Alternative Health Care, Competencies for Optimal Practice in Integrated Environments. 2011. http://accahc.org/images/stories/accahc_competencies_optimal_february2012.pdf. Accessed 3 February 2015.
8. Evans R, Maiers M, Delagran L, Kreitzer MJ, Sierpina V. Evidence informed practice as the catalyst for culture change in CAM. Explore. 2012;8(1):68–72.
9. Haas M, Leo M, Peterson D, Lefebvre R, Vavrek D. Evaluation of the effects of an evidence-based practice curriculum on knowledge, attitudes, and self-assessed skills and behaviors in chiropractic students. J Manipulative Physiol Ther. 2012;35(9):701–9.
10. Sullivan BM, Furner SE, Cramer GD. Development of a Student Mentored Research Program between a Complementary and Alternative Medicine University and a Traditional, Research Intensive University. Acad Med. 2014;89(9):1220–6.
11. Cramer GD, Guiltinan J, Maiers M, Laird S, Goertz C, Furner SE, et al. Benefits, Challenges And Culture Change Related To Collaborations Between Complementary And Alternative Medicine And Traditional Research-Intensive Institutions. Med Sci Educator. 2014. doi:10.1007/s40670-014-0077-3.
12. Shaw L, Descarreaux M, Bryans R, Duranleau M, Marcoux H, Potter B, et al. A systematic review of chiropractic management of adults with Whiplash-Associated Disorders: recommendations for advancing evidence-based practice and research. Work. 2010;35(3):369–94.
13. Bussieres A, Stuber K. The Clinical Practice Guideline Initiative: A joint collaboration designed to improve the quality of care delivered by doctors of chiropractic. J Can Chiropr Assoc. 2013;57(4):279–84.
14. Hawk C, Schneider M, Evans Jr MW, Redwood D. Consensus Process to Develop a Best-Practice Document on the Role of Chiropractic Care in Health Promotion, Disease Prevention, and Wellness. J Manipulative Physiol Ther. 2012;35(7):556–67.
15. Hawk C, Schneider M, Dougherty P, Gleberzon B, Killinger L. Best practices recommendations for chiropractic care for older adults: results of a consensus process. J Manipulative Physiol Ther. 2010;33(6):464–73.
16. Hawk C, Schneider M, Ferrance R, Hewitt E, Van Loon M, Tanis L. Best practices recommendations for chiropractic care for infants, children, and adolescents: results of a consensus process. J Manipulative Physiol Ther. 2009;32(8):639–47.
17. Institute of Medicine Committee on Quality of Health Care in America. Crossing the quality chasm: a new health system for the 21st century. Washington, DC: National Academies Press; 2001.
18. Schillinger D. An Introduction to Effectiveness, Dissemination and Implementation Research. P. Fleisher and E. Goldstein, eds. From the Series: UCSF Clinical and Translational Science Institute (CTSI) Resource Manuals and Guides to Community-Engaged Research, P. Fleisher, editor. Published by Clinical Translational Science Institute Community Engagement Program, University of California San Francisco; 2010.
19. Walker BF, Stomski N, Hebert J, French S. A survey of Australian chiropractors' attitudes and beliefs about evidence-based practice and their use of research literature and clinical practice guidelines. Chiropr Man Therap. 2013;21(1):44.
20. Suter E, Vanderheyden L, Trojan L, Verhoef M, Armitage G. How important is research-based practice to chiropractors and massage therapists? J Manipulative Physiol Ther. 2007;30(2):109–15.
21. Hall G. Attitudes of chiropractors to evidence-based practice and how this compares to other healthcare professionals: a qualitative study. Clin Chiropractic. 2011;14:106–11.
22. Roecker CB, Long C, Vining R, Lawrence D. Attitudes toward evidence-based clinical practice among doctors of chiropractic with diplomate-level training in orthopedics. Chiropr Man Therap. 2013;21(1):43.

23. Putting evidence into practice: Dr. Michael Schneider talks about the DELIVER study. Dynamic Chiropractic. Feb 1, 2013. http://www.dynamicchiropractic.com/mpacms/dc/article.php?id=56343. Accessed 13 Feb 2015.
24. Your Opinion Counts. J Amer Chiropr Assoc. 2012;49(6):33. http://www.acatoday.org/content_css.cfm?CID=5060.
25. Leach MJ, Gillham D. Evaluation of the Evidence-Based practice Attitude and utilization SurvEy for complementary and alternative medicine practitioners. J Eval Clin Pract. 2008;14(5):792–8.
26. Leach MJ, Gillham D. Are complementary medicine practitioners implementing evidence based practice? Complement Ther Med. 2011;19(3):128–36.
27. Christensen MG, Kerkhoff D, Kollash M. Job Analysis of Chiropractic. Greeley, CO: National Board of Chiropractic Examiners; 2000.
28. Christensen MG. Kollash M, Ward R, Webb K, Day M. zum Brunnen J. Job Analysis of Chiropractic. Greeley, CO: National Board of Chiropractic Examiners; 2005.
29. Christensen MG, Kollash M, Hyland J. Job Analysis of Chiropractic. Greeley, CO: National Board of Chiropractic Examiners; 2010.
30. Gaglio B, Phillips SM, Heurtin-Roberts S, Sanchez MA, Glasgow RE. How pragmatic is it? Lessons learned using PRECIS and RE-AIM for determining pragmatic characteristics of research. Implement Sci. 2014;9:96.
31. Slawson DC, Shaughnessy A. Teaching evidence-based medicine: Should we be teaching information management instead? Acad Med. 2005;80:685–9.
32. Murthy L, Shepperd S, Clarke MJ, Garner SE, Lavis JN, Perrier L, Roberts NW, Straus SE. Interventions to improve the use of systematic reviews in decision-making by health system managers, policy makers and clinicians. Cochrane Database Syst Rev. 2012;Issue 9. Art. No.: CD009401. doi:10.1002/14651858.CD009401.pub2.
33. Zwickey H, Schiffke H, Fleishman S, Haas M, Cruser D, LeFebvre R, et al. Teaching Evidence-Based Medicine at Complementary and Alternative Medicine Institutions: Strategies, Competencies, and Evaluation. J Altern Complement Med. 2014;20(12):925–31.
34. Long CR, Ackerman D, Hammerschlag R, Delagran L, Peterson D, Berlin M, et al. Faculty development initiatives to advance research literacy and evidence-based practice at CAM academic institutions. J Altern Complement Med. 2014;20(7):563–70.
35. Clar C, Tsertsvadze A, Court R, Hundt GL, Clarke A, Sutcliffe P. Clinical effectiveness of manual therapy for the management of musculoskeletal and non-musculoskeletal conditions; systematic review and update of UK evidence report. Chiropr Man Therap. 2014;28(22):1.
36. Bartholomew LK, Parcel GS, Kok G, Gottlieb NH. Planning Health Promotion Program: An Intervention Mapping Approach. San Francisco, California: Jossey-Bass; 2006.
37. French SD, Green SE, O'Connor DA, McKenzie JE, Francis JJ, Michie S, et al. Developing theory-informed behaviour change interventions to implement evidence into practice: a systematic approach using the Theoretical Domains Framework. Implement Sci. 2012;7:38.
38. QUERI Implementation Guide Quality Enhancement Research Initiative. US Department of Veterans Affairs; 2014. http://www.queri.research.va.gov/implementation/default.cfm Accessed 4 December 2014.
39. Kawchuk G, Newton G, Srbely J, Passmore S, Bussières A, Busse J, et al. Knowledge transfer within the Canadian Chiropractic Community. Part 2: Narrowing the evidence-practice gap. J Can Chiropr Assoc. 2014;58(3):206–14.

18

The simulated early learning of cervical spine manipulation technique utilising mannequins

Peter D Chapman[1], Norman J Stomski[2], Barrett Losco[3] and Bruce F Walker[3*]

Abstract

Background: Trivial pain or minor soreness commonly follows neck manipulation and has been estimated at one in three treatments. In addition, rare catastrophic events can occur. Some of these incidents have been ascribed to poor technique where the neck is rotated too far. The aims of this study were to design an instrument to measure competency of neck manipulation in beginning students when using a simulation mannequin, and then examine the suitability of using a simulation mannequin to teach the early psychomotor skills for neck chiropractic manipulative therapy.

Methods: We developed an initial set of questionnaire items and then used an expert panel to assess an instrument for neck manipulation competency among chiropractic students. The study sample comprised all 41 fourth year 2014 chiropractic students at Murdoch University. Students were randomly allocated into either a usual learning or mannequin group. All participants crossed over to undertake the alternative learning method after four weeks. A chi-square test was used to examine differences between groups in the proportion of students achieving an overall pass mark at baseline, four weeks, and eight weeks.

Results: This study was conducted between January and March 2014. We successfully developed an instrument of measurement to assess neck manipulation competency in chiropractic students. We then randomised 41 participants to first undertake either "usual learning" (n = 19) or "mannequin learning" (n = 22) for early neck manipulation training. There were no significant differences between groups in the overall pass rate at baseline ($\chi^2 = 0.10$, $p = 0.75$), four weeks ($\chi^2 = 0.40$, $p = 0.53$), and eight weeks ($\chi^2 = 0.07$, $p = 0.79$).

Conclusions: This study demonstrates that the use of a mannequin does not affect the manipulation competency grades of early learning students at short term follow up. Our findings have potentially important safety implications as the results indicate that students could initially gain competence in neck manipulation by using mannequins before proceeding to perform neck manipulation on each other.

Keywords: Chiropractic, Education, Neck manipulation, Randomised trial, Mannequin, Simulated learning

Background

Neck manipulation is a commonly used manual therapy for pain and stiffness and is likely to have been practised for centuries [1]. In more modern times it has become even more popular as a technique used by chiropractors and others; however it has been a source of controversy as to its risk/benefit ratio [2, 3]. Complications associated with neck manipulation have been estimated at a rate of one in three treatments but these adverse events are usually negligible causing minor soreness [4]. However, rare catastrophic events can occur. Over the past 30 years there has been a growing awareness of complications arising from the use of neck manipulation, in particular, stroke has become a prominent and worrying concern for practitioners of manual therapy and patients [5–10]. This adverse event may result in permanent impairment or more rarely death. Estimates of vertebral artery stroke (VAS) incidence following neck manipulation are likely to be between 1 in 400,000 cervical manipulations [11] and 1 in 100,000 patients receiving cervical spinal manipulative therapy (SMT) [5].

Some of these serious incidents have been ascribed to poor manipulative technique where the neck is excessively

* Correspondence: bruce.walker@murdoch.edu.au
[3]Discipline of Chiropractic, School of Health Professions, Murdoch University, 90 South St, Murdoch 6150, WA, Australia
Full list of author information is available at the end of the article

rotated. In a University setting where inexperienced students are learning manipulation it may be logical to speculate that these un-skilled operators may deliver a technique that contributes towards a greater complication risk.

The current method of teaching students the psychomotor skills of manipulation is to have students practice on each other. This is problematic for several reasons; a) the necessary skills (speed and accuracy) are not yet present in the student; b) a force that is not fully controlled is being put through the joints of fellow students and c) joints that do not need manipulation are being manipulated. In total this may lead to over stretching of the joint tissues with resulting soreness. To become proficient at the skill of neck manipulation a great amount of practice is needed and to obtain mastery a student has to practice many repetitive movements [12]. This usually means that over the course of an undergraduate chiropractic program the students may perform hundreds of manipulations on each other, with consequent increases in the risk of adverse reactions of varying severities. We found no evidence that stroke has occurred during neck manipulation training however it is intuitive that adverse events are more likely during this first phase of skills training. For example an epidemiological survey of chiropractic students enrolled in the chiropractic program offered at Parker College of Chiropractic in Dallas, Texas, USA revealed that 25 % (143/572) of respondents reported an injury as a result of manipulation being performed on them by other students during their studies [13]. These results are lower than those reported by an earlier study where 55 % of study participants experienced an injury as a result of learning to perform spinal manipulation [14].

Ndetan et al. (2009) reported that the most frequently injured region of the body as a result of students receiving spinal manipulation as part of their training was the neck and shoulder region [13]. However, Macanuel et al. (2005) differ slightly and suggest that this region is the second most commonly injured region, with the lumbopelvic region being the most commonly injured region, amongst chiropractic students when learning to perform spinal manipulative therapy [14].

It has been suggested that chiropractic students may be exposed to injuries to the cervical spine as a result of receiving "amateurish adjustments" or manipulations that deliver a substantial rotatory effect upon the cervical spine from other students [13].

It is therefore important in the early phases of training to search for innovative methods such as simulation to assist chiropractic students achieve a level of mastery of the manipulation techniques but with a low risk of adverse events. To this end we hypothesise that it may be useful to have students reach a level of proficiency by practicing on a mannequin with a flexible neck that approximates the resistance of a human cervical spine. To date very little research has been published on cervical manipulation mannequins and whether they assist the student with skill mastery or the effect upon student safety.

The teaching of spinal manipulative techniques at Murdoch University is consistent with that described by Harvey et al. [15]. Students are first introduced to the theoretical aspects of spinal manipulation by attending didactic lectures in areas such as anatomy, biomechanics and spinal manipulative technique, they then combine this knowledge with the subjective assessment of observing an instructor/expert perform spinal manipulative techniques. The students then progress to copy the demonstrated movements, which usually involves one student acting as a simulated patient while another student attempts to replicate the instructor's execution of the technique. This includes correct hand positions, patient pre-positioning, as well as the direction and magnitude of force required to perform the manipulative technique. Instructors then provide qualitative verbal feedback.

The aims of this study were first to design an instrument to measure competency of neck manipulation technique, and then to use this instrument to measure the suitability of using a simulation mannequin to teach the necessary psychomotor skills for chiropractic manipulative therapy of the neck.

Methods

Questionnaire development

We developed an initial set of questionnaire items in consultation with Murdoch staff members who taught cervical manipulation technique. An expert panel was then formed, who used a Content Validity Index (CVI) to ensure that the questionnaire was relevant to assess neck manipulation competency among chiropractic students [16, 17]. The expert panel consisted of seven chiropractors who teach neck manipulation at several Australian universities and one international university. The composition and size of this expert panel was congruent with guidelines that propose that the panel members' professional backgrounds reflect that of the target population, and that the ideal number is between six to twelve members [16, 17]. Every panel member evaluated each item using four categories: not relevant, unable to assess relevance without major revision, relevant but needs minor alteration, and very relevant. A value of one was assigned to the "very relevant" and "relevant but needs minor alteration" categories, whereas a value of zero was assigned to the other categories. The I-CVI for each item was derived by summing the values for each rater and then dividing by the number of raters. Items were retained if the CVI exceeded 0.79 [16, 17]. After the initial expert panel evaluation and feedback, the pilot version of the questionnaire was expanded considerably in the domains of rating expertise. In the second round of evaluation, the I-CVI for individual items ranged from 0.86-1.0 and all items were retained. The S-CVI, which is the proportion of items rated as either "relevant but needs minor alteration" or "very relevant" by all raters, was 0.94.

The final questionnaire comprised five assessment criteria, of which three contained several sub-criteria. The five assessment criteria were:

1) Patient and practitioner positioning
   - Is the patient positioned correctly?
   - Is the headrest in the correct position?
   - Is the practitioner positioned correctly?
2) Joint pre-tension
   - Has the joint been placed into the pre-manipulative tension position correctly?
3) Contact points
   - Is the contact point on the patient correct?
   - Has the correct side of the patient been contacted?
   - Is the contact on the practitioner's hand correct?
   - Is the practitioner's indifferent/stabilising hand correctly positioned?
4) Vector of correction/line of drive
   - Is the vector of correction correctly aligned with the presentation of the facet joints at the level manipulated?
5) Procedure
   - Is the amplitude of the thrust applied sufficient to address the fixation?
   - Is the speed of the thrust applied sufficient to address the fixation?
   - Was the demonstrated manipulation/adjustment executed safely?

Sample

All students enrolled in the fourth of the five year chiropractic program at Murdoch University during 2014 (N = 41) were invited to participate. Paper copy information notices were distributed in the first lecture of 2014, and a non-teaching staff member delivered an information session and provided an opportunity for students to raise questions about the study to inform the consent process. Students were informed that participation was entirely voluntary, and electing to participate or not participate, would not affect their relationship with University staff in any way. The Murdoch University Human Research Ethics Committee approval number was 2013/200. All 41 students initially invited to participate provided consent to have their results included in the final analysis.

Randomisation and blinding procedure

A staff member, not involved with group allocation, used a random number generator to generate a randomisation list. The group assignment was placed in sequentially numbered, opaque, sealed envelopes. After obtaining informed consent, staff not assessing neck manipulation competency opened the envelope and allocated students to one of two groups: usual learning or mannequin learning. Staff assessing neck manipulation competency, and undertaking data entry and analysis were blinded to group allocation.

Due to the nature of the study it was not possible to blind students to their group allocation, however at all times the assessor remained unaware of the group randomisation. Students are aware that under Australian Law, unless they are a registered practitioner with the Australian Health Professions Regulatory Authority, performing cervical spine manipulation outside of a recognised training program is prohibited [18]. Thus it is unlikely that students practised cervical spine manipulation outside of their usual teaching times.

The mannequin

The cervical mannequin is known as "Flexi-man" and is shown in Figs. 1 & 2. Fleximan has been developed and manufactured by Dr. Timothy Young, Chiropractor [19]. The mannequin consists of a flexible imitation of shoulders, neck and head made of a pliant "rubberised" material. The weight of the mannequin is 4.8 kgs with the specific head weight unknown, however a proxy head weight was 3.2 kgs. This proxy weight was established by laying the mannequin prone with the head recumbent on weight scales. The mannequin was designed to allow students to set up, place contacts and deliver a thrust in a line of drive of their choosing. It does not however allow for pre-manipulative tension. The mannequin is a stylised human facsimile and is not designed to mimic a human specimen. It does not have the variability of human subjects receiving manipulation, for example height, weight, and tissue compliance. The makers state that the mannequin is best used in the introductory phases of training [20].

Educational interventions

The usual learning group practised neck manipulation techniques on each other under supervision consistent with the description provided in the introduction to this article. This learning approach has been used since the inception of the Murdoch University chiropractic program in 2002. The mannequin learning group practiced the neck manipulation techniques on a mannequin with a flexible neck, once again under supervision. The mannequin learning approach was a novel method not previously used at Murdoch University. Each group received

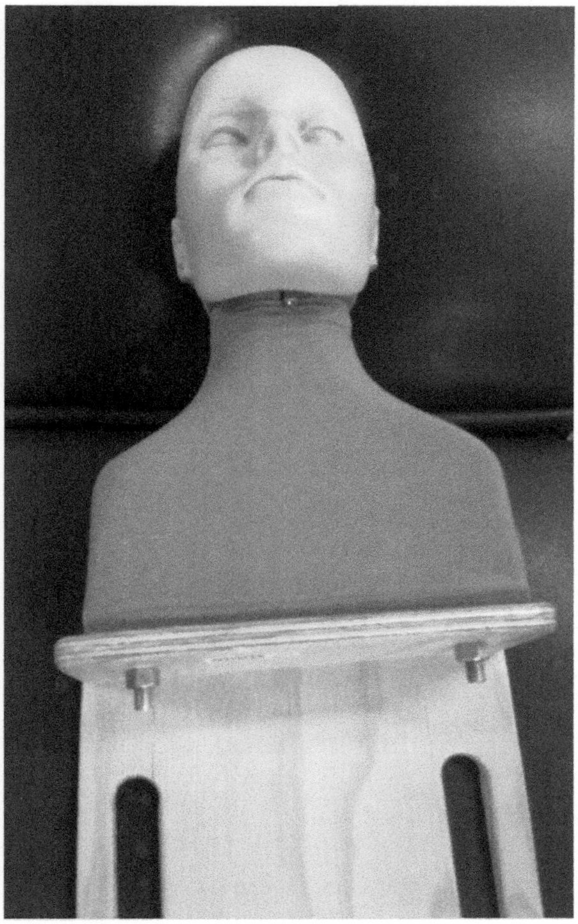

Fig. 1 The mannequin

three, two hour weekly training sessions in the performance of a commonly used cervical spine manipulation technique referred to as the index pillar push [21]. During the weekly training sessions and to ensure that the assessor remained blinded to group allocation students were supervised by academics not involved in the assessment of the students. The supervising academics provided each student with regular personalised feedback relating to their performance of the required technique during the weekly training sessions. After the third weekly training session, all members of each group crossed over and undertook three additional training sessions using the alternate method. The flow of the study is displayed in Fig. 3.

All fourth year students who participated in the study had already received training in neck manipulation in the third year of the program but there is a long summer break between third and fourth year so skills usually diminish. On the first week back at University, a staff member experienced in manipulation assessment who was blinded to group randomisation, assessed the student's performance of the index pillar push procedure at baseline on the mannequin (immediately before the first training session) and then again at four weeks, and eight weeks, by using the validated instrument of measurement.

Assessing student performance of the index pillar push technique involved the assessor requesting the student to perform the technique on both the left and the right hand side of the mannequin. Each student was allowed to perform the technique once on both sides, while the assessor graded their performance.

The maximum total score on the validated questionnaire is 100 %. In order to pass the assessment a student must achieve a minimum score of 69 % overall.

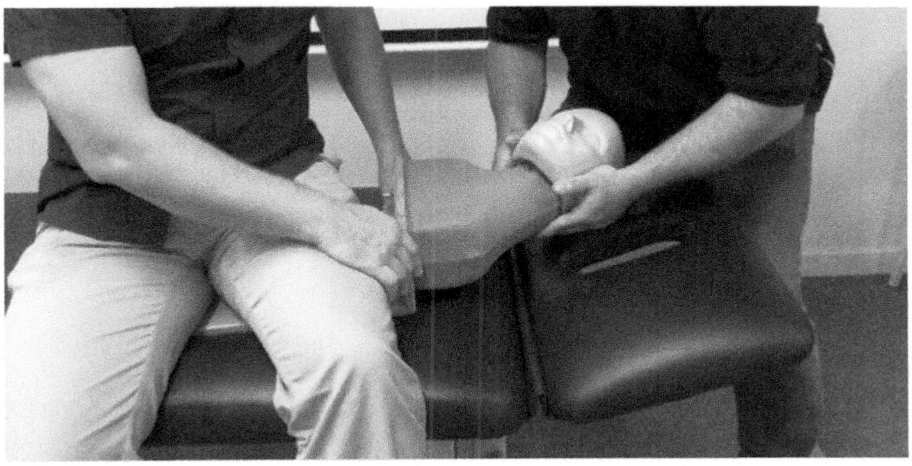

Fig. 2 Technique demonstration on the mannequin

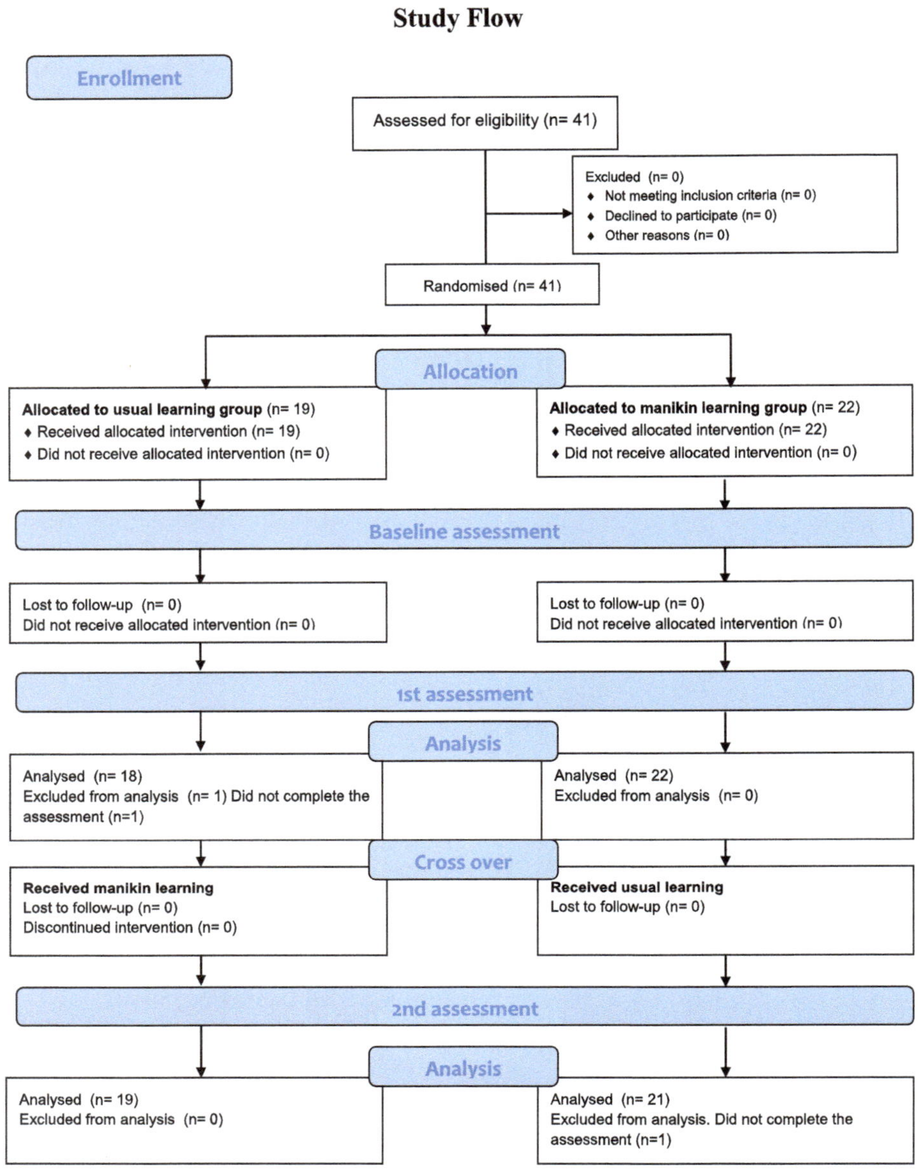

Fig. 3 Flow chart of study

Each of the five identified assessment criteria are considered critical to the successful performance of the required technique. If a student fails to perform one of these five assessment criteria adequately the student is awarded an overall score of 69 %. Should the student fail to perform two of the five assessment criteria adequately they are awarded a score of 49 %. Less than satisfactory performance of three criteria results in a score of 29 %. Inadequate performance of four assessment criteria results in a score of 19 % being awarded to the student. If all five assessment criteria are unsatisfactorily performed or the student is unable to perform the required technique, the student is awarded a score of zero.

Statistical analysis

All data were entered manually into SPSS v.21, cleaned and checked for implausibilities. A chi-square test was used to examine differences between groups for the proportion of students achieving an overall pass mark at baseline, four weeks, and eight weeks.

Results

This study was conducted between January and March 2014. We randomised 41 participants to first undertake either usual learning (n = 19) or mannequin (n = 22). The proportion of female participants was 36.8 % in the usual learning group, and 45.4 % in the mannequin group. The mean age was 23.3 (SD 4.7) years in the usual learning group, and 22.8 (SD 3.4) years in the mannequin group. All participants crossed over to undertake the alternative learning method after four weeks.

There were no significant differences between groups in the overall pass rate at baseline ($\chi^2 = 0.10$, $p = 0.75$), four weeks ($\chi^2 = 0.40$, $p = 0.53$), or at eight weeks ($\chi^2 = 0.07$, $p = 0.79$). The proportion of participants achieving an overall pass in each group at each time point is displayed in Table 1. There were no reported adverse events in the students' group from the therapy administered.

Discussion

Our findings show that mannequins can be used to teach cervical neck manipulation technique without affecting the grades for neck manipulation competency of chiropractic students. This result was consistent with a previous study examining the use of mannequins in teaching cervical manipulation [22]. These findings have important implications for the delivery of chiropractic curricula because the use of mannequins reduces the number of manipulations received by fellow students, which thereby improves the safety of chiropractic training.

In a previous study, differences in learning outcomes were examined by comparing students who undertook either practitioner-positioning training or complete practice training [15]. The practitioner-positioning approach involved students learning the components of spinal manipulation without ever delivering the thrust component. The complete practice approach incorporated the thrust component under instructor supervision and with proprioceptive feedback. This study was administered soon after students' commenced training in the first year of a Master's degree program at Macquarie University in Sydney, New South Wales, Australia which is the equivalent to the 4th year of Murdoch University's program. The study reported that the complete practice approach resulted in significantly higher peak force, and significantly lower time to peak force, both of which are thought to demonstrate higher proficiency in performing spinal manipulation [15]. So, although including the thrust component early in training may enhance the acquisition of manipulation competency, it could also potentially increase the likelihood of students experiencing adverse events. Therefore, by introducing the mannequin into the early stages of students' training, students could experience enhanced learning outcomes without any risk of decreased competency or adverse events.

Several studies have suggested that quantitative assessment of spinal manipulation is superior to qualitative assessment for the acquisition of psychomotor skills [23–25]. Traditionally, students were provided qualitative spinal manipulation feedback by instructors who evaluated parameters such as thrust vector, preload force, amplitude, velocity, and body position. Indeed, these parameters comprised the assessment criteria we derived for the instrument used in this study. Qualitative assessment may be prone to feedback inconsistency due to instructor experience, differing opinions between instructors, and observational oversights, which all may impede the acquisition of psychomotor skills. However, these inconsistencies can be addressed by the use of quantitative feedback devices that measure peak force or force time histories [25–27]. Quantitative feedback has an immediate positive impact upon all parameters relating to the performance of lumbar spine manipulation including subjective patient ratings of task performance [28], and has been shown to be superior to qualitative feedback [29]. Timely quantitative feedback allows the student to make rapid changes to their performance of the required technique [28]. Given this, we recommend that as a next step further research examine how apparatus capable of producing quantitative feedback could be most effectively incorporated with the use of cervical mannequins.

A strength of this study was the use of an expert panel to evaluate the content validity of the neck manipulation competency questionnaire. This resulted in the development of a questionnaire that is appropriate to assess the skills of chiropractic students learning neck manipulation. However, we did not assess the test-retest reliability of the questionnaire, and its reliability should be further determined in other studies. Another limitation of this study was not evaluating intra-rater examiner reliability, so the extent to which this may have influenced the findings remains unclear. Finally, we used a convenience sample so the study may have been underpowered however the results for a reasonable class size allowed us to conclude equivalence between the methods of teaching.

Table 1 Overall pass rate for cervical manipulation

	Number of participants achieving overall pass at baseline	Number of participants achieving overall pass at four weeks	Number of participants achieving overall pass at eight weeks
Participants first undertaking usual learning (n = 19)	22.2 % (4/18)	44.4 % (8/18)	84.2 % (16/19)
Participants first undertaking mannequin training (n = 22)	18.2 % (4/22)	54.5 % (12/22)	81.0 % (17/21)

Conclusions

This study consolidates previous research concerning the use of mannequins to teach neck manipulation skills and confirms that the use of mannequins does not affect the manipulation competency grades of students. Our findings have potentially important safety implications as the results indicate that students could initially gain competence in neck spinal manipulation by using mannequins before proceeding to perform neck manipulation on each other, which is likely to lessen the risk of students experiencing adverse events.

Competing interests

The corresponding author (Walker) is the Editor-in-Chief of *Chiropractic & Manual Therapies*. Walker was blinded to all reviewers' identities and did not select the managing Associate Editor. No other authors had competing interests to declare.

Authors' contributions

PC was responsible for the concept development, design, data collection, literature search, writing of the article and the critical review. NS was responsible for design, literature search, data analysis, writing of the article and the critical review. BL was responsible for design, data collection, writing of the article and the critical review. BW was responsible for design, supervision, writing of the article and the critical review. All authors read and approved the final manuscript.

Authors' information

PC is in private practice but was a lecturer in clinical chiropractic at Murdoch University who taught chiropractic manipulative techniques.

BL is a senior lecturer in clinical chiropractic at Murdoch University and teaches chiropractic manipulative techniques.

NS is a senior health research officer in the School of Health Professions at Murdoch University.

BW is Head of Discipline for Chiropractic at Murdoch University.

Acknowledgments

This study was funded by a grant from the Clinical Simulation Support Unit, Health Department, Government of Western Australia.

Author details

[1]6 Claredon Court, Alexander Heights 6064, WA, Australia. [2]School of Health Professions, Murdoch University, 90 South St, Murdoch 6150, WA, Australia. [3]Discipline of Chiropractic, School of Health Professions, Murdoch University, 90 South St, Murdoch 6150, WA, Australia.

References

1. Burke GL. Backache: From Occiput to Coccyx. Richmond, Canada: Macdonald Publishing; 2008.
2. Gross A, Miller J, D'Sylva J, Burnie SJ, Goldsmith CH, Graham N, et al. Manipulation or mobilisation for neck pain: a Cochrane Review. Man Ther. 2010;15(4):315–33.
3. Hebert JJ, Stomski NJ, French SD, Rubinstein SM: Serious Adverse Events and Spinal Manipulative Therapy of the Low Back Region: A Systematic Review of Cases. *J Manipulative Physiol Ther* 2013.
4. Hurwitz EL, Morgenstern H, Harber P, Kominski GF, Yu F, Adams AH. A randomized trial of chiropractic manipulation and mobilization for patients with neck pain: clinical outcomes from the UCLA neck-pain study. Am J Public Health. 2002;92(10):1634–41.
5. Rothwell DM, Bondy SJ, Williams JI. Chiropractic manipulation and stroke: a population-based case-control study. Stroke. 2001;32(5):1054–60.
6. Smith WS, Johnston SC, Skalabrin EJ, Weaver M, Azari P, Albers GW, et al. Spinal manipulative therapy is an independent risk factor for vertebral artery dissection. Neurology. 2003;60(9):1424–8.
7. Dittrich R, Rohsbach D, Heidbreder A, Heuschmann P, Nassenstein I, Bachmann R, et al. Mild mechanical traumas are possible risk factors for cervical artery dissection. Cerebrovasc Dis. 2007;23(4):275–81.
8. Walker BF, Losco B, Clarke BR, Hebert J, French S, Stomski NJ. Outcomes of usual chiropractic, harm & efficacy, the ouch study: study protocol for a randomized controlled trial. Trials. 2011;12:235.
9. Cassidy JD, Boyle E, Cote P, He Y, Hogg-Johnson S, Silver FL, et al. Risk of vertebrobasilar stroke and chiropractic care: results of a population-based case-control and case-crossover study. Spine (Phila Pa 1976). 2008;33(4 Suppl):S176–183.
10. Walker BF, Hebert JJ, Stomski NJ, Clarke BR, Bowden RS, Losco B, French SD: Outcomes of usual chiropractic. The OUCH randomized controlled trial of adverse events. *Spine (Phila Pa 1976)* 2013, 38(20):1723-1729.
11. Klougart N, Leboeuf-Yde C, Rasmussen LR. Safety in chiropractic practice, Part I; The occurrence of cerebrovascular accidents after manipulation to the neck in Denmark from 1978-1988. J Manipulative Physiol Ther. 1996;19(6):371–7.
12. Kovacs G. Procedural skills in medicine: linking theory to practice. J Emerg Med. 1997;15(3):387–91.
13. Ndetan HT, Rupert RL, Bae S, Singh KP. Prevalence of musculoskeletal injuries sustained by students while attending a chiropractic college. J Manipulative Physiol Ther. 2009;32(2):140–8.
14. Macanuel K, Deconinck A, Sloma K, Ledoux M, Gleberzon BJ. Characterization of side effects sustained by chiropractic students during their undergraduate training in technique class at a chiropractic college: a preliminary retrospective study. J Can Chiropr Assoc. 2005;49(1):46–55.
15. Harvey MP, Wynd S, Richardson L, Dugas C, Descarreaux M. Learning spinal manipulation: a comparison of two teaching models. J Chiropr Educ. 2011;25(2):125–31.
16. Lynn MR. Determination and quantification of content validity. Nurs Res. 1986;35(6):382–5.
17. Polit DF, Beck CT. The content validity index: are you sure you know what's being reported? Critique and recommendations. Res Nurs Health. 2006;29(5):489–97.
18. Anon: Health Practitioner Regulation National Law (WA) Act 2010. URL: http://www.slp.wa.gov.au/legislation/statutes.nsf/main_mrtitle_12107_homepage.html
19. Young T: FLEXI-MAN. Cervical Manikin Version 4. Pacific Paradise, Queensland.: T&S Young; 2003.
20. Young T: Flexi-Man. Practice makes perfect. Pacific Paradise, Queensland.: T&S Young; 2003.
21. Bergmann T, Peterson D. Chiropractic Technique: Principles and Procedures. Missouri: Elsevier; 2011.
22. Young TJ, Hayek R, Philipson SA. A cervical manikin procedure for chiropractic skills development. J Manipulative Physiol Ther. 1998;21(4):241–5.
23. Triano JJ, Rogers CM, Combs S, Potts D, Sorrels K. Quantitative feedback versus standard training for cervical and thoracic manipulation. J Manipulative Physiol Ther. 2003;26(3):131–8.
24. Descarreaux M, Dugas C, Lalanne K, Vincelette M, Normand MC. Learning spinal manipulation: the importance of augmented feedback relating to various kinetic parameters. Spine J. 2006;6(2):138–45.
25. Descarreaux M, Dugas C. Learning spinal manipulation skills: assessment of biomechanical parameters in a 5-year longitudinal study. J Manipulative Physiol Ther. 2010;33(3):226–30.
26. Scaringe JG, Chen D, Ross D. The effects of augmented sensory feedback precision on the acquisition and retention of a simulated chiropractic task. J Manipulative Physiol Ther. 2002;25(1):34–41.
27. Rogers CM, Triano JJ. Biomechanical measure validation for spinal manipulation in clinical settings. J Manipulative Physiol Ther. 2003;26(9):539–48.
28. Triano JJ, Scaringe J, Bougie J, Rogers C. Effects of visual feedback on manipulation performance and patient ratings. J Manipulative Physiol Ther. 2006;29(5):378–85.
29. Downie AS, Vemulpad S, Bull PW. Quantifying the high-velocity, low-amplitude spinal manipulative thrust: a systematic review. J Manipulative Physiol Ther. 2010;33(7):542–53.

The effect of spinal manipulation on deep experimental muscle pain in healthy volunteers

Søren O'Neill[2,1*], Øystein Ødegaard-Olsen[1] and Beate Søvde[3]

Abstract

Background: High-velocity low-amplitude (HVLA) spinal manipulation is commonly used in the treatment of spinal pain syndromes. The mechanisms by which HVLA-manipulation might reduce spinal pain are not well understood, but often assumed to relate to the reduction of biomechanical dysfunction. It is also possible however, that HVLA-manipulation involves a segmental or generalized inhibitory effect on nociception, irrespective of biomechanical function. In the current study it was investigated whether a local analgesic effect of HVLA-manipulation on deep muscle pain could be detected, in healthy individuals.

Methods and materials: Local, para-spinal muscle pain was induced by injection of 0.5 ml sterile, hyper-tonic saline on two separate occasions 1 week apart. Immediately following the injection, treatment was administered as either a) HVLA-manipulation or b) placebo treatment, in a randomized cross-over design. Both interventions were conducted by an experienced chiropractor with minimum 6 years of clinical experience. Participants and the researcher collecting data were blinded to the treatment allocation. Pain scores following saline injection were measured by computerized visual analogue pain scale (VAS) (0-100 VAS, 1 Hz) and summarized as a) Pain duration, b) Maximum VAS, c) Time to maximum VAS and d) Summarized VAS (area under the curve). Data analysis was performed as two-way analysis of variance with treatment allocation and session number as explanatory variables.

Results: Twenty-nine healthy adults (mean age 24.5 years) participated, 13 women and 16 men. Complete data was available for 28 participants. Analysis of variance revealed no statistically significant difference between active and placebo manipulation on any of the four pain measures.

Conclusion: The current findings do not support the theory that HVLA-manipulation has a non-specific, reflex-mediated local or generalized analgesic effect on experimentally induced deep muscle pain. This in turn suggests, that any clinical analgesic effect of HVLA-manipulation is likely related to the amelioration of a pre-existing painful problem, such as reduction of biomechanical dysfunction.

Background

Spinal manipulation is commonly used in an effort to alleviate musculoskeletal pain, but the exact mechanisms by which such treatments can reduce pain are not well understood. It is commonly assumed however, that when pain arises from biomechanical dysfunction, spinal manipulation may affect pain relief through the reduction of such dysfunction. Pain relief following spinal manipulation is thus assumed to indicate curative treatment of painful biomechanical dysfunction.

A number of clinical studies now indicate, that spinal manipulation may be a prudent choice for patients with musculoskeletal pain, not least spinal pain syndromes [1]. It is difficult however, to reliably identify those patients who are most likely to benefit from spinal manipulation and it is also a challenge to demonstrate the presence of biomechanical dysfunction in a valid and reliable manner [2, 3].

*Correspondence: soren@oneill.dk
[2] Institute of Regional Health Research, University of Southern Denmark, Campusvej 55, 5230 Odense, DK, Denmark
[1] Spine Centre of Southern Denmark, Lillebælt Hospital, Østre Hougvej 55, 5500 Middelfart, DK, Denmark
Full list of author information is available at the end of the article

A pragmatic solution which has been suggested, is a trial of a few treatments to assess the potential benefit of further spinal manipulation for a given patient [4, 5]. This is perfectly sensible, assuming that pain relief with 2–4 such treatments indicates reduction of some underlying painful mechanical lesion or dysfunction. However, if spinal manipulation has non-specific, reflex-mediated pain-inhibitory effects irrespective of the underlying cause of nociception, such pain relief may in fact simply mask the symptoms of other painful disorders, which are not appropriately treated with *high-velocity, low-amplitude* (HVLA) manipulation. In other words: If spinal manipulation has substantial local or regional, non-specific analgesic effects irrespective of the cause of pain, such treatment could potentially obfuscate serious pathology.

Any such non-specific, reflex-mediated pain-inhibitory effect is likely to be neurophysiological in nature and neural mechanisms have played a central role in many of the theoretical models of spinal manipulation. By the same token, the first detailed theoretical model of a central reflex-mediated nociceptive modulatory mechanism focused specifically on the impact of mechano-sensory input on nociceptive processing (the pain-gate theory proposed by Melzack and Wall [6]). In more recent years several studies have demonstrated that mechanical stimulation such as joint manipulation/mobilization can inhibit pain: In laboratory animal models of inflammatory joint pain Sluka and Wright [7] and Skyba et al. [8] demonstrated a hypoalgesic effect with joint mobilization, and showed that this effect is mediated by serotonin and noradrenaline sensitive pathways. Extra-cellular thalamic recordings of nociceptive specific and wide-dynamic-range neurons (which are known to be involved in pain processing in states of central pain hypersensitivity) in rats has demonstrated that HVLA manipulation raises the mechanical response threshold, and furthermore that variations in the manipulation amplitude, but not duration affects the resulting hypoalgesia [9, 10]. Song et al. [11] demonstrated an effect of daily manipulations over a week (by Activator®) on pain from nerve-root inflammation, assessed by both behavioral pain measures and intracellular recordings in rats. These findings and other like them provide objective evidence of a central nociceptive inhibitory effect of mechanical stimuli in laboratory animals, which appear to be reliant on serotonin and noradrenaline sensitive pathways, thus hinting at a descending pain control mechanism from the periaquaductal gray matter and rostro-ventral medial medulla of the brain stem (see Lewis et al. [12] for a recent review of conditioned pain modulation in chronic pain).

Obviously, the translational value of animal models in pain research can be questioned [13, 14] but human research supports the presence of hypoalgesic effects of manipulation which are not mediated by (segmental) opioid sensitive pathways [15] and the findings of hypoalgesia, sympathetic facilitation and changes in motor-control by Vicenzino et al. [16, 17] and Sterling et al. [18] support a mechanism of descending inhibitory control from the brain stem. The later study by Bishop et al. [19] which demonstrated changes in thermal summation pain both segmentally and caudal to the manipulation also support descending inhibition as a likely mechanism of HVLA induced hypoalgesia.

It seems plausible then, that HVLA manipulation could exert a diffuse hypoalgesic effect on the basis of descending inhibitory control from the brain stem. A number of factors may have influenced previous findings, including (but not limited to) the study population, the time scale within which the effect of HVLA-manipulation is sought and the method with which pain sensitivity has been examined.

Whereas the specific cause and nature of pain in clinical spinal pain states is often undetermined, experimental pain can be induced in a manner which is controlled and well understood – researchers inducing experimental pain know the precise nature and tissue site of the pain they have induced and research indicates that spinal manipulation has a significant analgesic effect on such experimental pain whether induced by pressure, mechanical stretching, capsaicin or electrical stimulation [20, 21]. Most studies however, have examined and demonstrated that the effect is evident at the same spinal level or in the neighboring region of the experimental pain stimulus and HVLA manipulation.

The literature summarized by the reviews by Millan et al. [20] and Coronado et al. [21] examines the effects of spinal manipulation on *experimental* pain. Some of the reviewed literature is on healthy volunteers [19, 22–29], but most [16–18, 30–44] of the studies actually examine populations of patients with *clinical* pain conditions ranging from mechanical neck pain and low back pain to tender-points and latent trigger points. It is therefor possible, that any observed local hypoalgesic effect of spinal manipulation in those studies, is due to an effect on the underlying painful clinical condition itself or changes in central pain modulation specifically related to those clinical conditions.

In order to gain a better understanding of the mechanisms by which spinal manipulation may afford such hypoalgesic effects, it is necessary to distinguish between effects inherent to the manipulation itself, and effects mediated by the potential influence on an underlying clinical pain condition – is any observed difference in pain sensitivity caused by a diffuse anti-nociceptive effect of manipulation, or by reduction of some underlying (mechanical) painful condition, such as latent trigger points?

Furthermore, the manner in which experimental pain sensitivity is tested may prove important. Research suggests that different aspects of the pain experience are not simple correlates [45–50]; deep and superficial pain sensitivity may vary, as may sensitivity to different pain modalities (thermal, chemical, mechanical, etc) and the choice of pain indicators (thresholds, distribution, duration, modulation, quality, etc) may also be important.

The purpose of this study was examine the immediate, local, deep-tissue hypoalgesic effect of spinal manipulation in healthy volunteers with no assumption of underlying painful clinical or sub-clinical conditions.

Method and materials

Design

A randomized, controlled, crossover study.

Recruitment

Participants were recruited from the student population of the chiropractic degree program at the University of Southern Denmark. Only healthy volunteers without known contraindications to spinal manipulation were invited to participate.

As part of the university degree program, all chiropractic students are evaluated by a certified chiropractor during their 3rd semester, in order to detect possible contradictions for HVLA manipulations. Four study participants were recruited from the 2nd semester and prior to study participation these were interviewed and examined for contraindications for HVLA manipulation by a senior chiropractor at The Spinecentre of Southern Denmark, Lillebaelt Hospital, Denmark.

Participants with chronic pain, previous back surgery, current back problems, somatic or psychological conditions were excluded.

Study participants were recruited through verbal information in the classroom and written information was sent electronically to those who expressed an interest in participating.

The Regional Scientific Ethical Committee for Southern Denmark approved the study (S-0080137) and written consent was obtained from all participants.

Experimental procedure

The experiment was carried out at the Spinecentre of Southern Denmark, Lillebaelt Hospital. Two assistants (graduate students) and two senior chiropractors from the department conducted the study.

Participants were informed that they would receive two effective, but different treatments and that the aim of the study was to compare any difference in effectiveness between them. All participants were treated on two separate occasions at least 1 week apart and treatment sessions were identical apart from the actual manual treatment performed: a) active HVLA-manipulation treatment, and b) placebo treatment with an Activator instrument. Participants were not informed that one of the treatments was a placebo.

Treatments at both the first and second session were directed at the 6th thoracic level. Allocation of treatment was done randomly according to a pre-hoc computer generated list in which treatment and session was randomized, but balanced.

On each occasion, in preparation of the test procedure, assistant 1 (BS) identified the spinous process of the 6th thoracic segment through palpation (counting down from the bony landmark of the C7 spinous process). The T6 segment was marked with a pen and anesthetic cream (EMLA cream, Astra Zeneca – an eutectic mixture of the local anesthetics Lidocain and Prilocain) was applied para-spinally on the right side of the T6 spinous process and covered by a patch with self-adhesive borders (Tegaderm, 5 × 7 cm) to keep the cream in place. The anesthetic cream was applied to ensure that experimental pain was induced primarily from deep tissues and not from needle-puncture of superficial structures.

After 20 min, assistant 2 (ØØO) removed the patch, wiped off the anesthetic cream and instructed the participant in the use of the computerized visual analogue pain scale, before asking the participant to lie prone on a chiropractic treatment table.

The injection point was the same for all participants; para-spinally at T6 (center of the anesthetized area) which was wiped down twice with alcohol swaps, as per standard aseptic injection technique. Assistant 2 proceeded to aspirate and gradually (over approx 2 s) inject 0.5 ml sterile hyper-tonic saline solution (Sodium SAD 1 mmol/ml) at room temperature, into the right T6 paraspinal musculature at approximately 2 cm depth. Immediately thereafter, assistant 2 left the room and one of the two senior chiropractors delivered the allocated treatment.

Placebo treatment was performed immediately next to the injection site. The chiropractor stabilized the chosen segment with the left hand, while holding the activator in the right hand, placing it on the anesthetized skin on the right side of the transverse process. The participant was asked to take a deep breath. Upon exhalation the Activator was pressed twice, releasing two 'click' sounds, while giving no mechanical impulse (amplitude = 0 mm).

HVLA-manipulation was performed with bilateral thenar contact (Carver bridge) on both transverse processes on the T6 segment. The participant was asked to take a deep breath and upon exhalation the HVLA manipulation was administered over the segment resulting in a mechanical impulse, in most instances with an accompanying articular cavitation.

Immediately after administering the treatment, the chiropractor left the room and (the blinded) assistant 2 returned. Assistant 2 ensured, that the participant indicated the intensity of pain from the saline injection as it developed over time (computerized VAS). The computerized VAS consisted of a scale marked 'No pain' at one end and 'Worst possible pain' at the other, corresponding to a value between 0 and 100 respectively. The VAS was sampled with a frequency of 1 Hz and data was stored electronically, allowing for a time-series of VAS measurements (see Fig. 1 for an illustration). During the recording, there was complete silence and no activity in the treatment room.

Data recording was considered complete when the patient indicated that the pain declined to near 0 – typically within 3–5 min.

The participants were all chiropractic students with personal knowledge of spinal manipulative procedures, which challenges the validity of the chosen placebo treatment. For that reason, upon completion of the experimental part of the study, 14 participants were randomly selected for a phone interview and questioned if they had, at any point been aware that one of the treatments was a placebo treatment.

Data

The VAS data was summarized as four outcome variables: a) duration of pain, b) max VAS value, c) time from pain onset to max VAS value and d) accumulated area under the curve (VAS over time). See Fig. 1 for an illustration.

Statistical analysis

Data are presented as median values with minimum, maximum and 1st and 3rd quartiles. The results are analyzed with two-way Anova with treatment allocation and session number as explanatory variables. Homogeneity of variance was analyzed with Fligner-Killeen test. An alpha level of 5 % was considered statistically significant. Analysis was performed using R version 3.0.2 (2013-09-25) for Linux [51].

Results

A total of 29 participants took part in the study; 13 women and 16 men (mean age 24.5 years).

No complications or side effects were reported by any of the participants and there were no dropouts. Due to technical computer problems however, raw data for 1 participant (male) was lost, leaving complete data for both sessions for 28 subjects.

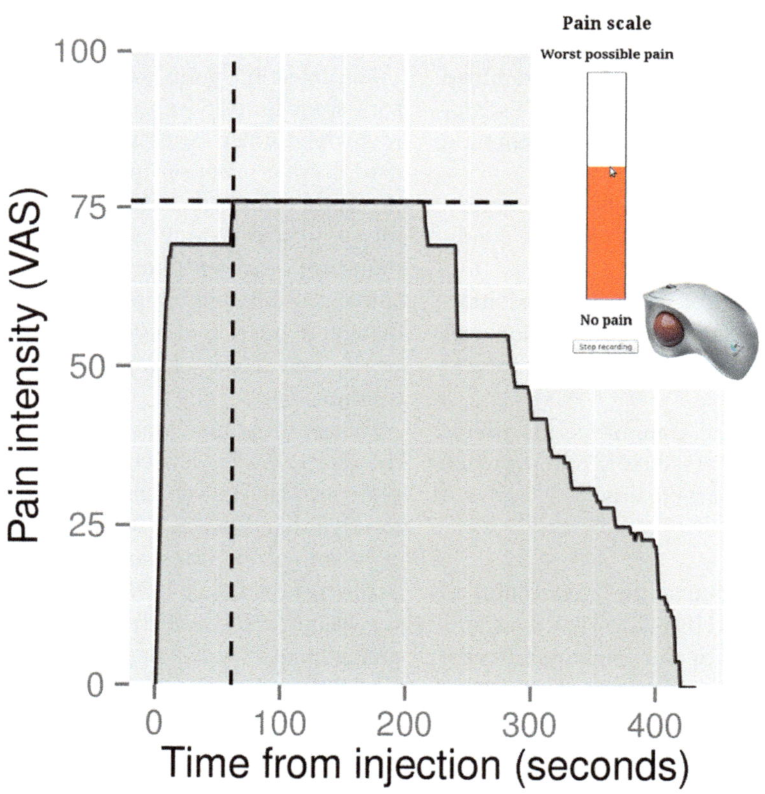

Fig. 1 Illustration of computerized VAS data. Pain intensity was measured using an on-screen visual analogue pain scale (insert in figure) controlled by the participant with a common computer trackball. The pain intensity was sampled with a frequency of 1 Hz and the resulting time-series data is illustred in the graph

Fourteen (14) participants received the active treatment on the first session (and placebo on the second), and vice versa.

The median duration of saline induced pain was 219 s (min = 101, 1. quartile = 178, 3. quartile = 274, max = 433), the median maximum VAS was 48 VAS (min = 7, 1.quartile = 35, 3.quartile = 66, max = 98), the median time from pain onset to max VAS was 44.5 s (min = 1, 1.quartile = 27, 3.quartile = 90.25, max = 143) and the median area-under-the-curve was 6117 VAS×seconds (min = 1019, 1.quartile = 3572, 3.quartile = 9182, max = 25010).

Fligner-Killeen test of homogeneity of variance for each of the four outcome variables, by each of the two explanatory variables yielded P values between 0.26 and 0.92, i.e. no heteroscedasticity of variance was observed.

Two-way analysis of variance revealed no significant differences in the 4 outcome variables by either explanatory variable, with one exception: A significant effect ($p =$ 0.005) of session number on duration of pain was found, with longer duration of pain on the first session (mean = 256 s, 95 % QI [227;285]) compared to the second session (mean = 202 s, 95 % QI [178;226]).

A post-hoc power-calculation (based on paired t-test) revealed, that with $n = 28$, alpha = 0.05 and beta = 0.8, a moderate effect size (0.55) would have been detected if present.

None of the 14 randomly selected participants interviewed following the experiment indicated that they had any suspicion that the Activator treatment had been a placebo treatment.

Discussion

If the effects of HVLA-manipulation was due primarily to an immediate, non-specific and reflex-mediated inhibition of nociception, we would have expected to observe a difference in saline induced pain in the current study between active and placebo treatment, but no such difference was observed.

Current findings in relation to previous publications

At first, the present findings appear to be in contrast to most of the published literature on HVLA-manipulation and experimentally induced pain, as summarized in the two recent reviews by Millan et al. and Coronado et al. [20, 21]. The authors reported significant pain inhibitory effects of HVLA-manipulation on experimentally induced pain.

However, the published literature was mostly based on populations with clinical or sub-clinical conditions [16–18, 30–44], i.e. patients with clinical pain states such as neck and low back pain, or non-clinical populations in which HVLA-manipulation was directed at tissues identified as pain hypersensitive (tender-points, trigger points). In those instances, it is unclear whether any effect of HVLA-manipulation should be ascribed to a non-specific reflex-mediated pain-inhibitory effect of the manual procedure itself, or a specific effect on the (sub-)clinical condition. In the present study, manipulation was not directed at any such clinical or sub-clinical condition and all participants were tested (arbitrarily) at the T6 segment. Any effect of HVLA-manipulation, had it been observed in the present study could thus have been ascribed to such non-specific, reflex-mediated pain inhibition.

Of the previous studies investigating healthy, pain free participants [19, 22–29] reviewed by Millan et al. and Coronado et al., the majority relied on pressure-pain thresholds and reported contradictory findings: Fernández-de-las-Penãs et al. [22, 23] used placebo-controlled designs and demonstrated an increase in pressure pain thresholds following cervical manipulation. This is in contrast to the controlled studies by Hamilton [25] and Soon [27], who reported no effect of manipulation on pressure pain thresholds. The study by Bishop et al. [19] which also involved a control group found a difference in thermal sensory summation between groups, but no difference in pressure pain or thermal pain thresholds.

The studies by Krouwel et al. [26] and Willet et al. [29] are harder to interpret as they did not involve clear-cut control groups: There is a tendency for experimental pain sensitivity to be higher on the first test, compared to subsequent tests which was also the finding in several of the papers discussed here – this underlines the importance of a control group in paired *before/after* pain sensitivity studies. In any case, the studies by Krouwel et al. [26] and Willet et al. [29] are similar in several respects, and while they both include a treatment group receiving simple sustained (*quasi-static*) pressure which could be interpreted as a minimalist intervention control group, this is not clearly stated. In any case, no group differences in pain thresholds are reported in either study.

Finally, the studies by George et al. [24] and Terrett and Vernon [28] both employed superficial pain stimuli (thermal and electrical, respectively). Whereas Terrett and Vernon reported a 140 % increase in superficial pain tolerance thresholds following manipulation, George et al. reported only few differences between those receiving manipulation, performing extension exercises or simply riding a stationary bicycle. Clearly, the literature on manipulation induced hypoalgesia in *healthy, pain-free subjects* is not concordant.

Care should be exercised when comparing animal and human pain research, but as described in the *Background* section, animal research indicates the presence of a non-specific anti-nociceptive effect of manipulation, possibly based on descending inhibitory control. The current findings did not demonstrate such an effect.

Differences between the present methodology and previous publications

The present study differs from the previously published literature on HVLA manipulation in the choice of pain stimulus: intra-muscular injection of hyper-tonic saline. Most of the previously published studies have used either pressure pain thresholds or superficial (skin) stimuli [20, 21]. Injection of hyper-tonic saline is a common experimental model of muscle pain [52], albeit less common than the ubiquitous pressure algometer. Slater et al. [53] also induced experimental pain by injection of hypertonic saline, albeit in adjunct to *delayed onset muscle soreness (DOMS)* of the extensor carpi radialis muscle and reported no difference in saline pain intensity, nor in pressure pain sensitivity following *mobilization-with-movement* manual therapy compared to placebo. In this respect, the present study is in alignment with the methodology and findings of Slater et al.

Although the specific seat and nature of most clinical spinal pain states for which spinal manipulation is used is unknown, it is rarely thought to originate in superficial structures, such as skin, subcutaneous connective tissues, etc. Furthermore, spinal manipulation is typically administered in an attempt to affect deep tissues such as facet joints, intervertebral disks and segmental musculature, but obviously also affects superficial tissues. The use of intra-muscular injection of hyper-tonic saline and a superficial anesthetic cream in the present study was chosen to ensure that the pain stimulus was indeed primarily delivered to deep spinal tissues.

The anesthetic cream was applied to reduced the superficial pain of the needle puncture and thus ensure that the induced experimental pain stemmed primarily from the deep intra-muscular saline. Whereas the cream will not have affected the deep experimental pain to any appreciable degree, it could arguably have affected the *profile* of sensory input in relation to the manipulation. The current study was not designed to cast light on any (potential) effect of superficial sensation or anesthesia on the effects of spinal manipulation, but this might be worth investigating in future research.

Conversely, the clinical pain for which HVLA spinal manual therapy is delivered, is of longer duration than the experimental pain induced in the current study – typically 2–4 min. This is a potential limitation of the current design and if, as some animal research indicates HVLA manipulation exerts anti-nociceptive effects through descending inhibitory control, a much longer time-frame is likely necessary to demonstrate such effects.

As there is no consensus on which experimental pain stimulus best simulate clinical pain or which tests most reliably reveals changes in pain sensitivity, a selection of diverse pain stimuli and measures are often recommended. In the present study only a single pain stimuli was used, however it could be argued that deep muscle pain more closely resembles clinical back pain than mechanical pressure or superficial thermal or electrical stimuli. The outcome measures used in the present study were related to several aspects of the pain experience: pain onset, intensity and duration. Other aspects such as pain detection- and tolerance threshold, spatial distribution, qualitative pain description, conditioned pain modulation and others could equally have been relevant, but as always a balance had to be struck between feasibility and methodological rigor.

Several studies in the pain literature conclude that pain sensitivity is complex and multi-modal, and that adequate assessment requires a battery of different quantitative sensory tests of pain sensitivity [45–50, 54]. The only study published on the *generalizability* of quantitative sensory testing of experimental pain [54], suggests that composite pain scores, such as those affected by e.g. both pain intensity and duration, offer greater generalizability than single scores such as e.g. pain threshold. We can not exclude however, that group differences could have been revealed by other quantitative sensory pain tests.

As an incidental finding, significantly longer pain duration on the first session, compared to the second session, was observed. This is not unusual in experimental pain research and is likely due to a degree of anxiety and unfamiliarity with the pain stimulus in the first session. For this reason some researchers employ an 'introductory'-session to familiarize study participants with the stimulus, some time well in advance of the actual study. This was not the case in the present study; instead the effect was countered by random allocation of treatments to session 1 and 2.

Study population

A potential limitation of the current study was the study population: students recruited from the chiropractic program at the University of Southern Denmark. This represents a potential bias, as the study population has prior knowledge of manipulative techniques and therefor might be in a position to recognize the placebo treatment as such. The study population was chosen for practicality, availability and economy, despite the potential sources of bias. According to Vernon et al. [55] it is difficult, but possible to construct a valid placebo treatment for manual procedures if it meets the following criteria; 1) the intervention should have no significant treatment effect and 2) the subject should be unable to determine whether they have received a sham treatment. All participants in the current study were unaware of the order of treatment and the existence of a placebo intervention, and none of the 14 participants, randomly chosen for interview after the study were aware of the use of a placebo treatment. We would thus argue that the inactivated Activator treatment represents a true placebo treatment in the current study.

Interpretation of findings

The current findings should not be over-interpreted. They indicate however, that HVLA-manipulation does not affect an immediate non-specific, reflex-mediated inhibition of deep-tissue segmental pain. Indirectly the findings thus lend support to the assumption that pain relief from HVLA-manipulation is likely to represent reduction of pain from some underlying painful condition, e.g. biomechanical dysfunction. This, in turn, suggests that the approach recommended by Leboeuf-Yde et al. and Axén et al. [4, 5], with a trial of 2–4 treatments to assess the effect of HVLA-manipulation is indeed a pragmatic and safe one. As stated above however, necessary choices regarding pain stimulus, pain measures, time frame etc should temper the conclusions based on a single study.

Future studies should take into consideration both the study population, the test- and treatment-sites and the chosen outcome measures. When quantifying experimentally induced pain in participants with painful clinical conditions, it becomes difficult to separate the intrinsic effects of HVLA manipulation from those of a clinical effect on the underlying cause of pain. Furthermore, if the intent is to disentangle the underlying neurological mechanisms of HVLA-manipulation induced hypoalgesia, test sites should be chosen which are appropriate for the hypothesis; local, segmental or generalized effects. And finally, the choice of pain measures is important and a battery of tests covering both different pain modalities and response domains is to be preferred.

Conclusion

The current study indicates, that HVLA-manipulation does not have an immediate non-specific, reflex-mediated local hypoalgesic effect on experimentally induced deep para-spinal muscle pain in healthy volunteers after skin anesthesia.

Competing interests

The authors declare that they have no competing interests.

Author's contributions

All authors contributed to the study design. ØØO and BS contributed to data collection and analysis. ØØO and SON contributed to manuscript preparation. All authors read and approved the final manuscript.

Author details

[1]Spine Centre of Southern Denmark, Lillebælt Hospital, Østre Hougvej 55, 5500 Middelfart, DK, Denmark. [2]Institute of Regional Health Research, University of Southern Denmark, Campusvej 55, 5230 Odense, DK, Denmark. [3]Stathelle Healthcentre, Brugata 10, 3960 Stathelle, Norway.

References

1. Clar C, Tsertsvadze A, Court R, Hundt GL, Clarke A, Sutcliffe P. Clinical effectiveness of manual therapy for the management of musculoskeletal and non-musculoskeletal conditions: systematic review and update of UK evidence report. Chiropr man ther. 2014;22(1):12. Accessed 2014-10-09.
2. Hestœk L, Leboeuf-Yde C. Are chiropractic tests for the lumbo-pelvic spine reliable and valid? a systematic critical literature review. J Manipulative Physiol Ther. 2000;23(4):258–75. Accessed 2014-10-17.
3. Huijbregts PA. Spinal motion palpation: A review of reliability studies. J Man Manip Ther. 2002;10(1):24–39. Accessed 2014-10-17.
4. Leboeuf-Yde C, Grønstvedt A, Borge JA, Lothe J, Magnesen E, Nilsson Ø, et al. The nordic back pain subpopulation program: demographic and clinical predictors for outcome in patients receiving chiropractic treatment for persistent low back pain. J Manipulative Physiol Ther. 2004;27(8):493–502.
5. Axén I, Jones JJ, Rosenbaum A, Lövgren PW, Halasz L, Larsen K, et al. The nordic back pain subpopulation program: validation and improvement of a predictive model for treatment outcome in patients with low back pain receiving chiropractic treatment. J Manipulative Physiol Ther. 2005;28(6):381–5.
6. Melzack R, Wall PD. Pain mechanisms: a new theory. Science (New York, N Y). 1965;150(3699):971–9.
7. Sluka KA, Wright A. Knee joint mobilization reduces secondary mechanical hyperalgesia induced by capsaicin injection into the ankle joint. Eur J Pain. 2001;5(1):81–7. doi:10.1053/eujp.2000.0223. Accessed 2015-05-19.
8. Skyba DA, Radhakrishnan R, Rohlwing JJ, Wright A, Sluka KA. Joint manipulation reduces hyperalgesia by activation of monoamine receptors but not opioid or GABA receptors in the spinal cord. Pain. 2003;106(1–2):159–68.
9. Reed WR, Pickar JG, Sozio RS, Long CR. Effect of spinal manipulation thrust magnitude on trunk mechanical activation thresholds of lateral thalamic neurons. J Manip Physiol Ther. 2014;37(5):277–86. doi:10.1016/j.jmpt.2014.04.001.
10. Reed WR, Sozio R, Pickar JG, Onifer SM. Effect of spinal manipulation thrust duration on trunk mechanical activation thresholds of nociceptive-specific lateral thalamic neurons. J Manipulative Physiol Ther. 2014;37(8):552–60. doi:10.1016/j.jmpt.2014.08.006.
11. Song XJ, Gan Q, Cao JL, Wang ZB, Rupert RL. Spinal manipulation reduces pain and hyperalgesia after lumbar intervertebral foramen inflammation in the rat. J Manip Physiol Ther. 2006;29(1):5–13. doi:10.1016/j.jmpt.2005.10.001.
12. Lewis GN, Rice DA, McNair PJ. Conditioned pain modulation in populations with chronic pain: a systematic review and meta-analysis. J Pain. 2012;13(10):936–44.
13. Mogil JS. Animal models of pain: progress and challenges. Nat Rev Neurosci. 2009;10(4):283–94. doi:10.1038/nrn2606. Accessed 2015-05-26.
14. Olesen AE, Andresen T, Staahl C, Drewes AM. Human experimental pain models for assessing the therapeutic efficacy of analgesic drugs. Pharmacol Rev. 2012;64(3):722–79. doi:10.1124/pr.111.005447. Accessed 2015-05-26.
15. Paungmali A, O'Leary S, Souvlis T, Vicenzino B. Naloxone fails to antagonize initial hypoalgesic effect of a manual therapy treatment for lateral epicondylalgia. J Manip Physiol Ther. 2004;27(3):180–5. doi:10.1016/j.jmpt.2003.12.022.
16. Vicenzino B, Collins D, Wright A. The initial effects of a cervical spine manipulative physiotherapy treatment on the pain and dysfunction of lateral epicondylalgia. Pain. 1996;68(1):69–74.
17. Vicenzino B, Collins D, Benson H, Wright A. An investigation of the interrelationship between manipulative therapy-induced hypoalgesia and sympathoexcitation. J Manipulative Physiol Ther. 1998;21(7):448–53.
18. Sterling M, Jull G, Wright A. Cervical mobilisation: concurrent effects on pain, sympathetic nervous system activity and motor activity. Man Ther. 2001;6(2). doi:10.1054/math.2000.0378.
19. Bishop MD, Beneciuk JM, George SZ. Immediate reduction in temporal sensory summation after thoracic spinal manipulation. Spine J. 2011;11(5):440–6. doi:10.1016/j.spinee.2011.03.001.

20. Millan M, Leboeuf-Yde C, Budgell B, Amorim M-A. The effect of spinal manipulative therapy on experimentally induced pain: a systematic literature review. Chiropr Man Therap. 2012;20(1):26.
21. Coronado RA, Gay CW, Bialosky JE, Carnaby GD, Bishop MD, George SZ. Changes in pain sensitivity following spinal manipulation: A systematic review and meta-analysis. J Electromyogr Kinesiol. 2012;22(5):752–67. Accessed 2014-10-09.
22. Fernandez-de-Las-Penas C, Alonso-Blanco C, Cleland JA, Rodriguez-Blanco C, Alburquerque-Sendin F. Changes in pressure pain thresholds over C5-C6 zygapophyseal joint after a cervicothoracic junction manipulation in healthy subjects. J Manipulative Physiol Ther. 2008;31(5):332–7. doi:10.1016/j.jmpt.2008.04.006.
23. Fernandez-de-las-Penas C, Perez-de-Heredia M, Brea-Rivero M, Miangolarra-Page JC. Immediate effects on pressure pain threshold following a single cervical spine manipulation in healthy subjects. J Orthop Sports Phys Ther. 2007;37(6):325–9. doi:10.2519/jospt.2007.2542.
24. George SZ, Bishop MD, Bialosky JE, Zeppieri GJ, Robinson ME. Immediate effects of spinal manipulation on thermal pain sensitivity: an experimental study. BMC Musculoskelet Disord. 2006;7:68. doi:10.1186/1471-2474-7-68.
25. Hamilton L, Boswell C, Fryer G. The effects of high-velocity, low-amplitude manipulation and muscle energy technique on suboccipital tenderness. Int J Osteopathic Med. 2007;10(2–3):42–9. doi:10.1016/j.ijosm.2007.08.002. Accessed 2015-04-29.
26. Krouwel O, Hebron C, Willett E. An investigation into the potential hypoalgesic effects of different amplitudes of PA mobilisations on the lumbar spine as measured by pressure pain thresholds (PPT). Man Ther. 2010;15(1):7–12. doi:10.1016/j.math.2009.05.013.
27. Soon BTC, Schmid AB, Fridriksson EJ, Gresslos E, Cheong P, Wright A. A crossover study on the effect of cervical mobilization on motor function and pressure pain threshold in pain-free individuals. J Manipulative Physiol Ther. 2010;33(9):652–8. doi:10.1016/j.jmpt.2010.08.014.
28. Terrett AC, Vernon H. Manipulation and pain tolerance. A controlled study of the effect of spinal manipulation on paraspinal cutaneous pain tolerance levels. Am J Phys Med. 1984;63(5):217–25.
29. Willett E, Hebron C, Krouwel O. The initial effects of different rates of lumbar mobilisations on pressure pain thresholds in asymptomatic subjects. Man Ther. 2010;15(2):173–8. doi:10.1016/j.math.2009.10.005.
30. Bialosky JE, Bishop MD, Robinson ME, Zeppieri GJ, George SZ. Spinal manipulative therapy has an immediate effect on thermal pain sensitivity in people with low back pain: a randomized controlled trial. Phys Ther. 2009;89(12):1292–1303. doi:10.2522/ptj.20090058.
31. Côté P, Mior SA, Vernon H. The short-term effect of a spinal manipulation on pain/pressure threshold in patients with chronic mechanical low back pain. J Manipulative Physiol Ther. 1994;17(6):364–8.
32. de Camargo VM, Alburquerque-Sendin F, Berzin F, Stefanelli VC, de Souza DPR, Fernandez-de-las-Penas C. Immediate effects on electromyographic activity and pressure pain thresholds after a cervical manipulation in mechanical neck pain: a randomized controlled trial. J Manipulative Physiol Ther. 2011;34(4):211–20. doi:10.1016/j.jmpt.2011.02.002.
33. Fernandez-Carnero J, Cleland JA, Arbizu RLT. Examination of motor and hypoalgesic effects of cervical vs thoracic spine manipulation in patients with lateral epicondylalgia: a clinical trial. J Manipulative Physiol Ther. 2011;34(7):432–40. doi:10.1016/j.jmpt.2011.05.019.
34. Fernandez-Carnero J, Fernandez-de-las-Penas C, Cleland JA. Immediate hypoalgesic and motor effects after a single cervical spine manipulation in subjects with lateral epicondylalgia. J Manipulative Physiol Ther. 2008;31(9):675–81. doi:10.1016/j.jmpt.2008.10.005.
35. Fryer G, Carub J, McIver S. The effect of manipulation and mobilisation on pressure pain thresholds in the thoracic spine. J Osteopathic Med. 2004;7(1):8–14. doi:10.1016/S1443-8461(04)80003-0.
36. Mansilla-Ferragut P, Fernandez-de-Las Penas C, Alburquerque-Sendin F, Cleland JA, Bosca-Gandia JJ. Immediate effects of atlanto-occipital joint manipulation on active mouth opening and pressure pain sensitivity in women with mechanical neck pain. J Manipulative Physiol Ther. 2009;32(2):101–6. doi:10.1016/j.jmpt.2008.12.003.
37. Mohammadian P, Gonsalves A, Tsai C, Hummel T, Carpenter T. Areas of capsaicin-induced secondary hyperalgesia and allodynia are reduced by a single chiropractic adjustment: a preliminary study. J Manipulative Physiol Ther. 2004;27(6):381–7. doi:10.1016/j.jmpt.2004.05.002.
38. Oliveira-Campelo NM, Rubens-Rebelatto J, Marti N-Vallejo FJ, Alburquerque-Sendi N F, Fernandez-de-Las-Penas C. The immediate effects of atlanto-occipital joint manipulation and suboccipital muscle inhibition technique on active mouth opening and pressure pain sensitivity over latent myofascial trigger points in the masticatory muscles. J Orthop Sports Phys Ther. 2010;40(5):310–7. doi:10.2519/jospt.2010.3257.
39. Parkin-Smith GF, Penter CS. A clinical trial investigating the effect of two manipulative approaches in the treatment of mechanical neck pain: a pilot study. J Neuromusculoskeletal Syst. 1998;1998(6):6–16.
40. Ruiz-Saez M, Fernandez-de-las-Penas C, Blanco CR, Martinez-Segura R, Garcia-Leon R. Changes in pressure pain sensitivity in latent myofascial trigger points in the upper trapezius muscle after a cervical spine manipulation in pain-free subjects. J Manipulative Physiol Ther. 2007;30(8):578–83. doi:10.1016/j.jmpt.2007.07.014.
41. Shearar KA, Colloca CJ, White HL. A randomized clinical trial of manual versus mechanical force manipulation in the treatment of sacroiliac joint syndrome. J Manipulative Physiol Ther. 2005;28(7):493–501. doi:10.1016/j.jmpt.2005.07.006.
42. Thomson O, Haig L, Mansfield H. The effects of high-velocity low-amplitude thrust manipulation and mobilisation techniques on pressure pain threshold in the lumbar spine. Int J of Osteopath Med. 2009;12(2):56–62. doi:10.1016/j.ijosm.2008.07.003. Accessed 2015-04-29.
43. van Schalkwyk R, Parkin-Smith GF. A clinical trial investigating the possible effect of the supine cervical rotatory manipulation and the supine lateral break manipulation in the treatment of mechanical neck pain: a pilot study. J Manipulative Physiol Ther. 2000;23(5):324–31.
44. Vernon HT, Aker P, Burns S, Viljakaanen S, Short L. Pressure pain threshold evaluation of the effect of spinal manipulation in the treatment of chronic neck pain: a pilot study. J Manipulative Physiol Ther. 1990;13(1):13–16.
45. Janal MN, Glusman M, Kuhl JP, Clark WC. On the absence of correlation between responses to noxious heat, cold, electrical and ischemic stimulation. Pain. 1994;58(3):403–11.
46. Lautenbacher S, Rollman GB, McCain GA. Multi-method assessment of experimental and clinical pain in patients with fibromyalgia. Pain. 1994;59(1):45–53.
47. Hastie BA, Riley JL, Robinson ME, Glover T, Campbell CM, Staud R, et al. Cluster analysis of multiple experimental pain modalities. Pain. 2005;116(3):227–37.
48. Greenspan JD, Slade GD, Bair E, Dubner R, Fillingim RB, Ohrbach R, et al. Pain sensitivity risk factors for chronic TMD: Descriptive data and empirically identified domains from the OPPERA case control study. J Pain. 2011;12(11):61–74.
49. Neziri AY, Curatolo M, NÃijesch E, Scaramozzino P, Andersen OK, Arendt-Nielsen L, et al. Factor analysis of responses to thermal, electrical, and mechanical painful stimuli supports the importance of multi-modal pain assessment. Pain. 2011;152(5):1146–55.
50. O'Neill S, Manniche C, Graven-Nielsen T, Arendt-Nielsen L. Association between a composite score of pain sensitivity and clinical parameters in low-back pain. Clin J Pain. 2014;30(10):831–8.
51. R Core Team. R: a language and environment for statistical computing. Vienna, Austria: R Foundation for Statistical Computing; 2013. http://www.R-project.org/.
52. Graven-Nielsen T, Arendt-Nielsen L. Assessment of mechanisms in localized and widespread musculoskeletal pain. Nat Rev Rheumatol. 2010;6(10):599–606. doi:10.1038/nrrheum.2010.107. Accessed 2015-05-16.
53. Slater H, Arendt-Nielsen L, Wright A, Graven-Nielsen T. Effects of a manual therapy technique in experimental lateral epicondylalgia. Man Ther. 2006;11(2):107–17. doi:10.1016/j.math.2005.04.005. Accessed 2015-07-09.
54. O'Neill S, O'Neill L. Improving QST reliability – more raters, tests, or occasions? a multivariate generalizability study. J Pain. 2015;16(5):454–62. doi:10.1016/j.jpain.2015.01.476.
55. Vernon H, MacAdam K, Marshall V, Pion M, Sadowska M. Validation of a sham manipulative procedure for the cervical spine for use in clinical trials. J Manipulative Physiol Ther. 2005;28(9):662–6.

Change in lumbar lordosis during prone lying knee flexion test in subjects with and without low back pain

Amir M Arab[1*], Ailin Talimkhani[2], Noureddin Karimi[2] and Fetemeh Ehsani[2]

Abstract

Background: Prone lying knee flexion (PLKF) is one of the clinical tests used for assessment of the lumbo-pelvic movement pattern. Considerable increase in lumbar lordosis during this test has been considered as impairment of movement patterns in lumbar-pelvic region. However, no study has directly evaluated the change in lordosis during active PLKF test in subjects with low back pain (LBP). The purpose of this study was to investigate the change of lumbar lordosis in PLKF test in subjects with and without LBP.

Methods: A convenience sample of 80 subjects participated in the study. Subjects were categorized into two groups: those with chronic non-specific LBP (N = 40, mean age: 40.84 ± 17.59) and with no history of LBP (N = 40, mean age: 23.57 ± 10.61). Lumbar lordosis was measured with flexible ruler, first in prone position and then on active PKF test in both subjects with and without LBP. Data was analyzed by using statistical methods such as, independent t-test and paired t-test.

Results: There were statistically significant differences in lumbar lordosis between prone position and after active PLKF in both subjects with and without LBP ($P < 0.0001$). The amount of change in lordosis during PLKF test was not significant between the two groups ($P = 0.65$). However these changes were greater among patients with LBP.

Conclusion: Increase in lumbar lordosis during this test may be due to excessive flexibility of movement of the lumbar spine in the direction of extension and abnormal movement patterns in the individuals with LBP.

Keywords: Low back pain, Lumbar lordosis, Movement pattern, Prone knee flexion, Flexible ruler

Background

Low back pain (LBP) is a world-wide health problem and the most common and costly musculoskeletal disorder in the today's societies [1,2]. The prevalence of LBP is estimated to be between 10% and 80% depending on the population [3,4]. Despite its high prevalence and detrimental effects on subjects' activities, the exact causes of mechanical LBP have not yet been fully understood. However, during the past decades the approach in evaluation and management of LBP has been changed from strengthening or stretching of the lumbo-pelvic muscles toward modification of the motor system and movement pattern [5].

A balanced motor system is obtained from coordinated activity of synergist and antagonist muscles. Normal functioning of the trunk depends not only on passive joint mobility, but also on normal muscular activity and central nervous system regulation. Muscles produce and control the movement and stabilize the spine, protecting if from excessive load during functional activities [6,7].

With regard to this point of view, repetitive movements and long-term faulty postures and movements can change muscle tissue characteristics and can lead to muscle dysfunction, altered movement pattern, pain and finally movement disorders [5]. Hence, the main emphasis has been recently placed on assessment of the altered movement pattern in patients with musculoskeletal pain and disorders such as LBP and on the important of achieving normal pattern of the movement for the prevention and treatment of LBP [6-11].

* Correspondence: arabloo_masoud@hotmail.com
[1]Department of Physical Therapy, University of Social Welfare and Rehabilitation Sciences, Velenjak, Tehran, Iran
Full list of author information is available at the end of the article

Several studies have demonstrated that LBP is associated with muscle imbalance and altered activation pattern of the lumbo-pelvic muscles during different tasks [12-15]. Some clinical tests have been used to assess the altered movement pattern in subjects with musculoskeletal disorders. Prone lying knee flexion (PLKF) is an accepted test for assessment and treatment of the lumbo-pelvic movement patterns [5]. In this test, a patient lays prone and actively flexes his or her dominant knee as far as possible. Muscle imbalance and altered activation of the lumbo-pelvic muscles has been reported during PLKF test in patients with chronic LBP [5]. Excessive anterior pelvic tilt, lumbar rotation, lumbar hyperextension, increased lumbar lordosis and decreased knee flexion during the PLKF has been considered as abnormal movement patterns during PLKF [5]. Coordination between muscles in the lumbo-pelvic region is thought to balance the position of the pelvis in normal posture and during the lower limb or trunk movement. It has been assumed that during PLKF, lack of sufficient stiffness in the abdominal and anterior supporting structures of the lumbar spine produces anterior tilt in the pelvic and increased lumbar lordosis specially in person with lower cross syndrome [5].

However, to our knowledge, no study has investigated the change in lumbar lordosis during PLKF in patients with chronic LBP. The purpose of this study was to investigate the change in the degree of lumbar lordosis during PLKF in subjects with and without chronic LBP and to determine if this change varies between two groups.

Methods

Subjects

The quasi-experimental study design with repeated measurements was used to investigate the lumbar lordosis changes during PLKF in two groups: subjects with chronic non-specific LBP (N = 40, average age: 40.84 [SD = 17.59] years old, average height: 165.0 [SD = 9.0] cm, average weight: 70.31 [SD = 16.06] kg, body mass index (BMI): 25.55 [SD = 3.99] kg/m^2) and subjects with no history of LBP (N = 40, average age: 23.57 [SD = 10.61] years old, average height: 162.0 [SD = 7.0] cm, average weight: 55.62 [SD = 6.55] kg, BMI: 21.05 [SD = 2.26] kg/m^2).

Power analysis was used to determine the sample size for test. Type I error (α) was set at 0.05 and power of the test was 0.80. Considering this, the calculated sample size showed that sample size in this study was appropriate to test the hypothesis and the results derived from the study are meaningful.

The subject population in this study was a sample of convenience. The LBP patients were referred by orthopedic specialist and physiotherapy clinics. The patients were included if they had a history of non-specific LBP for more than six weeks duration before the study date. They were also included if had intermittent (on and off) LBP with at least three previous episodes each lasting more than one week, during the year before the study [16].

The control group was evaluated and found to have no complaint of any pain or dysfunction in their low back, pelvis, thoracic and lower extremities. The healthy subjects were recruited from the university students.

The exclusion criteria in both groups were pregnancy, history of dyspnea, history of hip pain, dislocation or fracture, history of lumbar spine surgeries, history of anterior knee ligament injury or rupture, history of anterior knee pain, inability to perform active PLKF without pain, history of lower extremity injury in the past 3 months, shortness of hip flexors, positive neurological symptoms and cardiopulmonary disorders. Each eligible subject was enrolled after signing an informed consent form approved by the human subjects committee at the University of Social Welfare and Rehabilitation Sciences. Ethical approval for this study was granted from the internal ethics committee at the University of Social Welfare and Rehabilitation Sciences (Date: 2013.03.09).

Procedures

The subject was on the examining table in the prone position. The lumbar lordosis was measured first in prone position. Then the subject was asked to perform knee flexion (PLKF) and then the lumbar lordosis was measured after PLKF test in both subjects with and without LBP. The dominant leg was chosen for investigation.

Measuring lumbar lordosis

A standard flexible ruler was used to measure the degree of lumbar lordosis in prone position before and after active knee flexion (Figure 1). For this purpose, the subject's position was prone lying on a treatment table with the arms along the sides and head face was down. The base of sacrum and spinous process of L1 was located by palpation and marked with removable stickers.

A standard flexible ruler was fitted on subject's lumbar curve, over the lumbar spinous processes of L1 – S1. The curve of the flexible ruler, resembling the size of subject's lumbar curvature, was graphed on a paper, noting where the two reference points for L1 and S1 were located. The method explained by others was used to quantify the degree of lumbar lordosis [16-20].

Two points on the curve, representing L1 and S1, were connected by a line (L). A perpendicular line (H), representing the height of the lumbar curve, bisected line L. The length of each line was calculated in millimeters, and the values were used in the following formula to calculate the degree of lumbar lordosis.

$$\theta = 4\,[\text{Arc tan}\,(2H/L)]$$

A very high correlation (r = 0.92) has been found between degrees of lumbar lordosis measured by a flexible

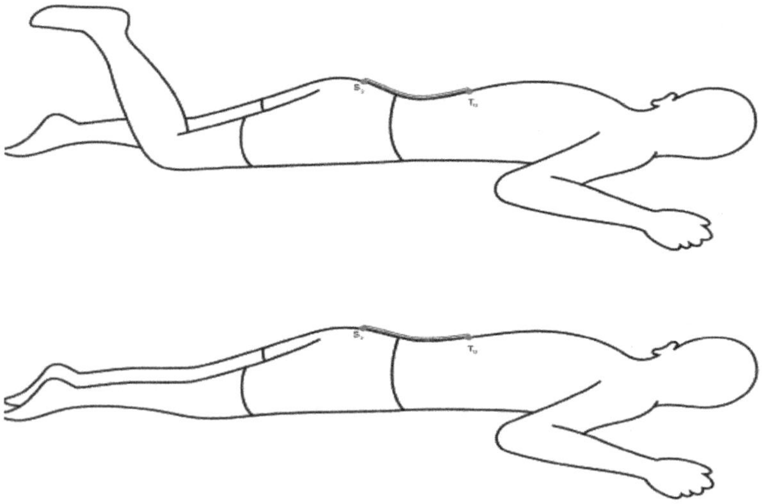

Figure 1 Measurement of lumbar lordosis with flexible ruler in prone position and active PLKF.

ruler and from lumbar X-rays [21-23]. The reliability of flexible curve for measurement of lumbar lordosis has been previously established [24].

Data analysis

Statistical analysis was performed using SPSS version 16.0.

A paired *t*-test was used to demonstrate changes in lumbar lordosis before and after PLKF test in both subjects with and without LBP.

An independent *t*-test was used to compare changes in lumbar lordosis during PLKF between subjects with and without LBP and also to compare demographic data between subjects with and without LBP. Statistical significance was attributed to P value less than 0.05.

Ethical approval

This research was reviewed and was approved by the Human Subject Committee at University of Social Welfare and Rehabilitation Sciences.

Results

The demographic data for the subjects are presented in Table 1. No statistical significance was found in the height between groups. However, there was a statistically significant difference in subjects' age, weight and BMI between the two groups (P = 0.000).

There was no significant difference in lumbar lordosis at the baseline in prone relaxed position between two groups (P = 0.21, %95 CI: 1.77-7.44). There was a statistically significant difference in lumbar lordosis between prone position and after PLKF in subjects without LBP (P = 0.000) and subjects with LBP (P = 0.000) (Table 2, Figure 2). Overall, the lumbar lordosis was significantly greater in the PLKF compared to prone-relaxed position in both subjects with and without LBP. The mean difference in lumbar lordosis between positions was 6.47 and 5.65 for subjects with LBP and without LBP respectively.

There was no statistically significant difference in the changes of lumbar lordosis after performing PLKF between subjects with and without LBP (P = 0.65) (Table 3). However, the changes in lumbar lordosis were greater among patients with LBP compared to those without LBP.

Discussion

The current study shows changes in lumbar lordosis during active PLKF test in subjects with and without LBP. The results of this study demonstrated that there were statistically significant differences in lumbar lordosis between prone position and after PLKF in both subjects with and without LBP ($P < 0.0001$). But the amount of changes in lordosis during PLKF test was not significant between two

Table 1 Demographic data of the subjects in each group

Variables	With no LBP (n = 40)	With LBP (n = 40)
Age (years)	23.57 (10.61)	40.84 (17.59)
Weight (kg)	55.62 (6.55)	70.31 (16.06)
Height (cm)	162.0 (7.0)	165.0 (9.0)
BMI (kg/m^2)	21.05 (2.26)	25.55 (3.99)

Continuous data: Mean (Standard Deviation).
LBP = Low Back Pain, BMI = Body Mass Index.

Table 2 Lumbar lordosis in both groups

Variables	Before PLKF	After PLKF	P-value
With no LBP	35.02 (9.25)	40.67 (13.09)	**0.000**
With LBP	32.35 (12.43)	38.82 (14.43)	**0.000**

Continuous data: Mean (Standard Deviation). Bold p-values indicate statistical significance.
LBP = Low Back Pain, PLKF = Prone Lying Knee Flexion.

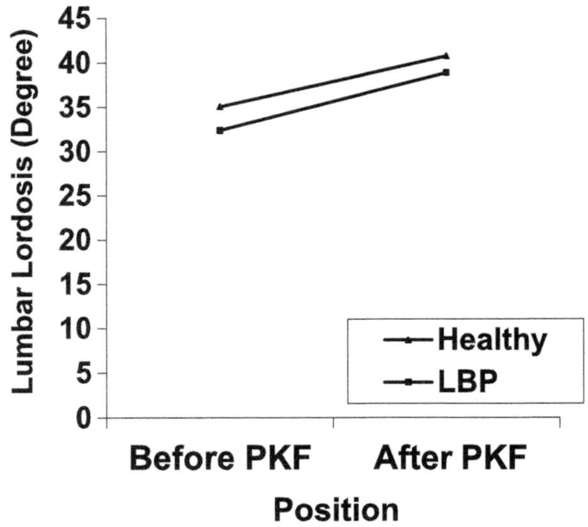

Figure 2 Lumbar lordosis during PLKF in subjects with and without LBP.

groups (P = 0.65). These changes were greater among patients with LBP compared to subjects without LBP.

In this study, the subjects had no pain during the test and none of the subjects reported that pain was a limiting factor to perform PLKF test, so, direct effects of pain on the measurement can be minimized.

Lumbar extension and anterior rotation of the pelvis are often observed during the PLKF test. Increase in the degree of lumbar lordosis during PLKF test found in both groups can be attributed to the accompanied lumbar extension during flexion of the knee. In theory, it is proposed that excessive anterior pelvic tilt, lumbar hyperextension and increased lumbar lordosis during the PLKF are commonly seen as abnormal movement patterns in patients with chronic LBP [5]. Investigators attributed these to muscle imbalance and altered activation of the lumbo-pelvic muscles [5].

Previous investigators attributed excessive lumbar extension and hyper lordosis during PLKF to a deficiency in controlling anterior pelvic rotation during PLKF because of muscular dysfunction in the lumbo-pelvic region [5,25]. Sahrmann [5] proposed the concept of "relative flexibility or stiffness" that has been linked to uncontrolled movement, pain and pathology by causing direction related stress and strain during various functional movements in the patients with LBP. Sahrmann [5] suggested that increased stiffness of the anterior supporting structures of the thigh, hip, knee and lumbar spine can result in compensatory exaggerated anterior pelvic tilt with lumbar extension motion during prone knee flexion or hip extension. In this study, stiffness in thigh and anterior supporting structures of the lumbar spine was not measured, just measured the change in lumbar lordosis during PLKF.

Table 3 Changes in lumbar lordosis between two groups

Variable	With no LBP (n = 40)	With LBP (n = 40)	P-value
Changes in lumbar lordosis during PLKF	5.65 (10.13)	6.47 (6.67)	0.65

Continuous data: Mean (Standard Deviation).
LBP = Low Back Pain, PLKF = Prone Lying Knee Flexion.

Scholtes et al. [26] found that during knee flexion and hip lateral rotation in prone lying, subjects with LBP demonstrated a greater maximal lumbar-pelvic rotation angle compared to those without LBP, as the lumbar-pelvic region may move more frequently during the early ranges of lower limb movement in daily activities.

In this study, lumbar lordosis was significantly higher during PLKF compared to prone relaxed position in both subjects with and without LBP. However, this change in lumbar lordosis during PLKF was not significant between two groups. The reason for this may be due to the healthy subjects being recruited from university students and staff used to performing sustained postures and repeated movements in their daily activities.

It has been thought that, if the lumbar-pelvic motion occurs more during a limb movement, then the frequency of lumbar-pelvic motion may be increased through the day. The increased frequency of the movements in lumbar-pelvic region can contribute to increased mechanical stress and strain on lumbar-pelvic region. This can also change the characteristics of muscular tissue, in turn, leading to abnormal movement patterns in lumbar-pelvic region [26,27]. Previous studies supported increased mobility of the lumbar-pelvic region in LBP patients which can be associated with degeneration of lumbar-pelvic region tissues [28,29].

In this study, compensatory lumbar extension motion during active PLKF test may be due to instability in lumbar-pelvic region and also, excessive flexibility of movement of the lumbar spine in the direction of extension. This hypothesis has been supported by findings which suggest active limb movements which contribute to accumulation of tissue stress can affect decrease in spinal stability in patients with LBP [30]. However, more studies are needed to resolve the existing ambiguities in this field.

Limitations

We acknowledge some limitations. In this study the patients with chronic non-specific LBP were examined and other LBP patients (acute or specific LBP) were not examined. Another limitation of this study was that LBP subjects were not categorized based on movement system impairment-based categories for LBP as described by Sahrmann [5].

It has been suggested investigating the lumbar lordosis change in LBP patients with different movement system impairment-based categories. Again in this study, we did not measure lumbar -pelvic kinematics and electromyography (EMG) activity of the stabilizing and prime mover muscles during PLKF to find the pattern of muscles recruitment.

The fact that the healthy subjects were recruited from university students and staff performing sustained postures and repeated movements in their daily activities may be used to question the results showing no significant difference in lumbar lordosis change during PLKF between two groups.

Considering the non statistically different but measurable changes in lumbar lodosis during PLKF between subjects with and without LBP, we suggest that PLKF can be used as an evaluation tool of lumbar-pelvic movement patterns in the individuals with LBP and even healthy individuals with poor postural alignment and poor movement habits.

Conclusion

This study investigated the chansge in lumbar lordosis during PLKF test between subjects with and without LBP. The results of this study indicate an increase in the degree of lumbar lordosis during PLKF compared to prone-relaxed position in subjects with and without LBP. However, greater change in lumbar lordosis was found in the subjects with LBP compared to healthy subjects. More studies are needed to resolve the existing ambiguities in this field.

Competing interests

The authors declare that they have no competing interests.

Authors' contributions

AMA contributed to conception, design, analysis, interpretation of data and drafting the manuscript. AT carried out the data collection and drafting the manuscript. NK participated in design and interpretation of data. FE participated in analysis and helped to draft the manuscript. All authors read and approved the final manuscript.

Author details

[1]Department of Physical Therapy, University of Social Welfare and Rehabilitation Sciences, Velenjak, Tehran, Iran. [2]University of Social Welfare and Rehabilitation Sciences, Velenjak, Tehran, Iran.

References

1. Marras WS, Allread WG, Burr DL, Fathallah FA. Prospective validation of a low-back disorder risk model and an assessment of ergonomic interventions associated with manual materials handling tasks. Ergonomics. 2000;43:1866–86.
2. Lahiri S, Markkanen P, Levenstein C. The cost-effectiveness of occupational health interventions: preventing occupational back pain. Am J Ind Med. 2005;48(6):515–29.
3. Verhaak PF, Kerssens JJ, Dekker J, Sorbi MJ, Bensing JM. Prevalence of chronic benign pain disorder among adults: a review of the literature. Pain. 1998;77(3):231–9.
4. Gilgil E, Kacar C, Butun B, Tuncer T, Urhan S, Yildirim C, et al. Prevalence of low back pain in a developing urban setting. Spine. 2005;30:1093–8.
5. Sahrmann S. Diagnosis and treatment of movement impairment syndromes. 1. Missouri: Mosby. Inc; 2002. p. 121–92.
6. Jull GA, Janda V. Muscles and motor control in low back pain: Assessment and management. In: Twomey LT, Taylor JR, editors. Physical Therapy of the Low Back. Chuchill Livingstone: New York; 1987. p. 253–78.
7. Norris CM. Spinal stabilisation: an exercise programme to enhance lumbar stabilistion. Phys Ther. 1995;81(3):13–39.
8. Cholewicki J, Van Dieen JH, Arsenault AB. Muscle function and dysfunction in the spine. J Electromyoger Kinesiol. 2003;13(4):303–4.
9. Janda V. On the concept of postural muscles and posture in man. Aust J Physiother. 1983;29:83–4.
10. Janda V. Pain in the locomotor system-A broad approach. Aspects of manipulative therapy. Melbourne: Churchill Livingstone; 1985. p. 148–51.
11. O'Sullivan P, Phyty D, Twomey L, Allison GT. Evaluation of specific stabilizing exercise in the treatment of chronic low back pain with radiologic diagnosis of spondylolysis or spondylolisthesis. Spine. 1997;22(24):2959–67.
12. Hodges P, Moseley G. Pain and motor control of the lumbopelvic region: effect and possible mechanisms. J Electromyogr Kinesiol. 2003;13:361–70.
13. Hungerford B, Gilleard W, Hodges P. Evidence of altered lumbopelvic muscle recruitment in the presence of sacroiliac joint pain. Spine. 2003;28:1593–600.
14. Leinonen V, Kankaanpaa M, Airaksinen O, Hanninen O. Back and hip extensor activities during trunk flexion/extension: Effects of low back pain and rehabilitation. Arch Phys Med Rehabil. 2000;81:32–7.
15. Newcomer K, Jacobson T, Gabriel D, Larson DR, Brey RH, An KN. Muscle activation patterns in subjects with and without low back pain. Arch Phys Med Rehabil. 2002;83:816–21.
16. Nourbakhsh MR, Arab AM. Relationship between mechanical factors and incidence of low back pain. J Orthop Sports PhysTher. 2002;32:447–60.
17. Link CN, Nicholson GG, Shaddeau SA, Birch R, Gossman MR. Lumbar curvature in standing and sitting in two types of chairs: relationship of hamstring and hip flexor muscle length. PhysTher. 1990;70:611–8.
18. Nourbakhsh MR, Arab AM, Salavati M. The relationship between pelvic cross syndrome and chronic low back pain. J Back Musculoskeletal Rehabil. 2006;19:119–28.
19. Youdas JW, Garrett TR, Harmsen SS. Lumbar lordosis and pelvic inclination of asymptomatic adults. Phys Ther. 1996;76:1066–81.
20. Youdas JW, Garrett TR, Egan KS, Therneau TM. Lumbar lordosis and pelvic inclination in adults with chronic low back pain. Phys Ther. 2000;80:261–75.
21. Seidi F, Rajabi R, Ebrahimi TJ, Tavanai AR, Moussavi SJ. The Iranian flexible ruler reliability and validity in lumbar lordosis measurments. Sport Sci. 2009;2(2):95–9.
22. Hart DL, Rose SJ. Reliability of a noninvasive method for measuring the lumbar curve. Orthop Sports Phys Ther. 1986;8(4):180–4.
23. Youdas JW, Vj S, Garrett TR. Reliability of measurments of lumbar spine sagittal mobility obtained with the flexible curve. Orthop Sports Phys Ther. 1995;21(1):13–20.
24. Nourbakhsh MR, Moussavi SJ, Salavati M. Effects of lifestyle and work-related physical activity on the degree of lumbar lordosis and chronic low back pain in a Middle East population. Spinal Disord. 2001;14:283–92.
25. Jae-Seop O. Effects of Peforming an abdominal drwing-in maneuver during prone hip extension exercises on hip and back extensormuscle activity and amount of anterior pelvic tilt. J OrthopSports Phys Ther. 2007;37(6):320–4.
26. Scholtes SA, Gombatto SP, Van Dillen LR. Differences in lumbopelvic motion between people with and people without low back pain during two lower limb movement tests. Clin Biomech. 2009;24(1):7–12.
27. Van Dillen LR, Sahrmann SA, Norton BJ, Caldwell CA, Fleming D, McDonnell MK, et al. Effect of active limb movements on symptoms in patients with low back pain. J Orthop Sports Phys Ther. 2001;31:402–18.
28. Leone A, Guglielmi G, Cassar-Pullicino VN, Bonomo L. Lumbar intervertebral instability: a review. Radiology. 2007;245(1):62–77.
29. Singer KP, Fitzgerald D, Milne N. Neck retraction exercises and cervical disk disease. In: Singer KP, editor. Proceeding of the Biennial manipulative physiotherapist conference. Australia: Perth; 1993. p. 88–93.
30. Scholtes SA, Van Dillen LR. Gender-related differences in prevalence of lumbopelvic region movement impairments in people with low back pain. J Orthop Sports Phys Ther. 2007;37:744–53.

21

The establishment of a primary spine care practitioner and its benefits to health care reform in the United States

Donald R Murphy[1,2*], Brian D Justice[3], Ian C Paskowski[4], Stephen M Perle[5] and Michael J Schneider[6]

Abstract

It is widely recognized that the dramatic increase in health care costs in the United States has not led to a corresponding improvement in the health care experience of patients or the clinical outcomes of medical care. In no area of medicine is this more true than in the area of spine related disorders (SRDs). Costs of medical care for SRDs have skyrocketed in recent years. Despite this, there is no evidence of improvement in the quality of this care. In fact, disability related to SRDs is on the rise. We argue that one of the key solutions to this is for the health care system to have a group of practitioners who are trained to function as primary care practitioners for the spine. We explain the reasons we think a primary spine care practitioner would be beneficial to patients, the health care system and society, some of the obstacles that will need to be overcome in establishing a primary spine care specialty and the ways in which these obstacles can be overcome.

Keywords: Low Back Pain, Neck Pain, Health Care Reform, Primary Care, Health Policy

Introduction

One of the most talked about issues in the United States (US) is health care reform. In other countries as well, discussion commonly revolves around the issue of how health care services can be improved while containing costs. Many in the US have described the current health care situation as a "crisis" [1-4]. In March 2010, the US Congress passed and the President signed into law the Affordable Care Act, which puts in place comprehensive health care reform measures [5]. While various models for providing care to patients have been considered, such as accountable care organizations [6], it is recognized that any meaningful approach to health care reform will require three goals to be achieved: 1. improved patient health; 2. improved patient experience; 3. decreased per capita costs [7].

Spine-related disorders (SRDs) are among the most common, costly and disabling problems in Western society. For the purpose of this commentary, we define SRDs as the group of conditions that include back pain, neck pain, many types of headache, radiculopathy, and other symptoms directly related to the spine. Virtually 100% of the population is affected by this group of disorders at some time in life. Low back pain (LBP) in the adult population is estimated to have a point prevalence of 28%-37%, a 1-year prevalence of 76% and a lifetime prevalence of 85% [8,9]. Up to 85% of these individuals seek care from some type of health professional [10,11]. Two-thirds of adults will experience neck pain some time in their lives, with 22% having neck pain at any given point in time [12].

The burden of SRDs on individuals and society is huge [13]. Direct costs in the United States (US) are US$102 billion annually [14] and $14 billion in lost wages were estimated for the years 2002-4 [13]. Other indirect costs are substantially higher than this. As far back as 1996 it was estimated that in The Netherlands total costs for neck pain was US$686 million, with half of that cost arising from disability [15]. And the problem appears to be worsening. In the years between 1997 and 2005, expenditures for back and neck pain rose 65%, adjusted for inflation [14]. During this time measures of mental health, physical functioning and work, school and social activity among patients with SRDs declined [14]. With regard to

* Correspondence: rispine@aol.com
[1]Clinical Director, Rhode Island Spine Center, 600 Pawtucket Avenue, Pawtucket, RI 02860 USA
Full list of author information is available at the end of the article

work-related LBP, this is the most common disorder that leads to lost work days [16] and while it comprises up to 25% of injuries in the workplace it accounts for up to 1/3 of all workers' compensation costs [17,18].

A variety of physicians and other providers have traditionally been involved with the diagnosis and treatment of these patients. This includes primary care physicians, chiropractic physicians, orthopedic surgeons, neurosurgeons, physiatrists, osteopathic physicians, physical therapists, psychologists, massage therapists, kinesiologists, naprapaths and acupuncturists. This has resulted in what has been termed the "supermarket approach" to the management of SRDs [19]. That is, the SRD patient is faced with an environment in which there is a large number of practitioners, each offering a solution to SRDs, with the patient left to sort out which of these disparate approaches is best for his or her particular problem. Oftentimes this determination is based more on salesmanship and marketing than on science, clinical benefit and cost-effectiveness [19].

Treatment for SRDs has become increasingly specialist-focused, imaging-oriented, invasive and expensive. According to Deyo, et al [20] between 1994 and 2004 LBP related Medicare expenditures in the US increased 629% for epidural steroid injections, 423% for opioid medications, 307% for magnetic resonance imaging and 220% for lumbar fusion surgeries. This dramatic rise in medical costs was not shown to have resulted in improved outcomes for SRD patients. In fact, despite the tremendous amount of time and money spent on the diagnosis and treatment of patients with SRDs, chronicity and disability related to these disorders appears to be steadily on the rise [14,20,21]. We are not aware of any other health condition in which a similar level of worsening outcomes has occurred despite significant increase in health care expenditures.

One approach to health care reform would designate primary care physicians (PCPs) or groups of PCPs as "patient homes", responsible for the comprehensive care and management of a designated patient population under a risk-sharing agreement. However, there is a projected gap between the availability of traditional PCPs and societal needs in the near future, especially if a national health care program is implemented [22]. Currently, LBP is the second most common reason for symptomatic physician visits [23-25] and increasing the number of SRD patients seeing PCPs will serve to further exacerbate the problem of under-availability of traditional PCPs. Thus, in the area of SRDs, a different approach to primary care is needed.

In their book Redefining Health Care [26], Porter and Teisberg state that for health care reform to be successful, it must incentivize competition based on *value*, i.e., outcome per dollar spent. To maximize value in health care, they recommend physicians and other health care providers organize themselves around conditions in which they have maximal expertise and experience (chronic kidney disease, diabetes, SRDs) rather than around medical specialties (orthopedics, internal medicine, neurology, etc.) and compete on the level of providing the best health outcomes for these conditions at the best possible cost (i.e., providing value). Having groups organized based on their medical specialty rather than their focused expertise is inefficient because different health conditions require different diagnostic strategies, treatment approaches, outcome measurements and monitoring [26].

SRDs have specific features that differentiate them from other types of health conditions. For example, diagnosis is challenging because, unlike conditions such as heart disease and diabetes, there usually is no well-defined lesion that can be clearly detected via imaging studies or other special tests [27]. In addition, many, and perhaps most, cases of SRDs are multifactorial, involving somatic, neurophysiological and psychological processes that interact to produce the suffering experienced by the patient [28,29]. Thus, management of patients with SRDs requires a level of expertise that can respond to these challenges.

In our view, a fundamental problem lies at the heart of the "supermarket approach" to SRDs; the lack of a "general practitioner" who has advanced training in spine care, who understands the multifactorial nature of SRDs and who can sort out the most appropriate clinical choices for the patient with low back or neck pain. Essentially, we think that the health care system needs an appropriately trained and skilled clinician who can fill the role of a primary care provider for the diagnosis and non-surgical management of SRDs; a "primary care physician for the spine".

Primary Care for the Spine

"Primary care" is defined by the American Academy of Family Physicians (AAFP) as "that care provided by physicians specifically trained for and skilled in comprehensive first contact and continuing care for persons with any undiagnosed sign, symptom, or health concern (the "undifferentiated" patient) not limited by problem origin (biological, behavioral, or social), organ system, or diagnosis" [30]. The role of the traditional PCP is to apply comprehensive knowledge about the differential diagnosis of conditions that might arise in *any* bodily system, including the spine and musculoskeletal system. However, recent studies have shown that traditional PCPs are not well trained in the differential diagnosis and management of musculoskeletal disorders [31-33], probably due to the heavy emphasis on internal diseases in medical school education and in primary care residency programs. Even those traditional PCPs who profess to have a special interest in SRDs tend to have anachronistic beliefs about best practices for managing these disorders [34]. And guidelines do little to change practitioners' beliefs and practice

[35]. The traditional PCP is not likely to be the best choice in the primary care of SRDs [36].

We are not using the term *primary care* in the context of a generalist who provides medical care for any condition involving virtually any organ system. We are using the term *primary spine care* in the context of a focused practitioner who provides medical care for all patients with problems related to a specific organ system - the spine. This model is analogous to the general dentist, who provides "primary care" for oral health. To paraphrase the AAFP definition for our purpose, "primary spine care" can be defined as "that care provided by practitioners specifically trained for and skilled in comprehensive first contact and continuing care for persons with any undiagnosed sign, symptom, or health concern (the "undifferentiated" patient) not limited by problem origin (biological, behavioral, or social), *involving the spine*".

Primary spine care would be provided by practitioners who are specifically trained to diagnose and manage the majority of patients with SRDs with the most evidence-based methods. They would also coordinate the referral and follow up of the minority of SRD patients who might require special tests (e.g. radiographs, MRI or electrodiagnostic testing) or more intensive (e.g. multidisciplinary rehabilitation) or invasive (e.g. injection and surgery) procedures.

The primary spine care practitioner would function as the first contact for patients with SRDs, i.e. the first practitioner that a patient consults when he or she develops a spine problem. The primary spine care practitioner could also function as a resource for traditional PCPs (family practice physicians, general internal medicine physicians, pediatric, obstetrical/ gynecological physicians, primary care nurse practitioners or physician's assistants) to refer patients who present with SRDs.

The Necessary Skill Set of the Primary Spine Care Practitioner

The primary spine care practitioner would require several important characteristics in order to provide maximum value to society. Some of these characteristics include:

1. *Skills in Differential Diagnosis*: Serious pathology as a cause of spinal pain occurs in only 1% of patients [37]. However this means that the busy primary spine care practitioner could potentially see at least one case every couple of months. Thus, skill in the recognition of serious pathology is essential, as many of these disorders require immediate investigation or treatment. This includes an understanding of what diagnostic tests to order when certain "red flags" are present. Also essential in this regard is an understanding of when diagnostic testing is *not* necessary [38] as efficiency and cost-effectiveness would be an essential aspect of primary spine care.
2. *Skills in the management of the majority of patients with spine pain*: Any primary level practitioner should ideally be able to manage the majority of patients he or she sees without the need for referral. The first-line treatments that the primary spine care practitioner would employ would include those methods shown to be evidence-based, minimally invasive and cost-effective. There is a variety of such treatment methods that have been found to be effective and have broad application which include manual therapies, particularly manipulation and mobilization [39,40], the McKenzie method [41], neural mobilization techniques [42-44], various forms of exercise [45-47], patient-specific, evidence-based education [47,48], non-steroidal anti-inflammatory and non-opioid analgesics [27] (most of which are available over-the-counter) and nutritional approaches [49,50]. The primary spine care practitioner would be required to be knowledgeable and skilled in the application of these strategies without the need for referral.
3. *A wide ranging understanding of spinal pain*: SRDs are currently understood to be a complex mixture of biopsychosocial phenomena [29,51,52]. It is increasingly being recognized that the experience of spinal pain and its related disability involves a combination of biological and psychological processes that occur within a certain social context. The primary spine care practitioner would require a keen understanding of these disparate but interrelated processes. Patient satisfaction in spine care is closely tied to the clinician providing a clear explanation of the problem [53,54]. Therefore, the primary spine care practitioner would be required to clearly articulate the complexities of spine pain to patients in simple terms. The ability to recognize the many facets of some complex SRDs [28], educate the patient about his or her condition, its natural history and the patient's role in recovery [55], and then motivate the patient to actively participate in care [56] are all necessary, but quite refined, skills that the competent spine provider must have.
4. *The ability to detect and manage psychological factors:* It is increasing recognized the psychological factors play an important, and in many cases the most important, role in the perpetuation of pain, suffering and disability in patients with SRDs [57-60]. The primary spine care practitioner would have to be knowledgeable and skilled in the detection of processes such as fear-avoidance, catastrophizing, passive coping, poor self-efficacy, cognitive fusion and depression and to be able to address these as part of the overall management strategy [61]. As a purely psychological approach may not be effective [62] it is essential that management of

these factors is incorporated by the primary spine care practitioner into the management of the somatic factors [63,64].

5. *An appreciation of minimalism in spine care*: The primary spine care practitioner would have to understand that often in spine care "less is more". That is, an approach that focuses on education regarding the natural history of SRDs, maximizes patient empowerment and minimizes practitioner-driven intervention is likely to be most beneficial [65,66]. This would allow the practitioner to focus on the *value* of care (i.e. outcome per unit cost [67]) which would not only benefit patients with SRDs but also the health care system and society as a whole by helping control costs while expediting early return to a productive life. This approach would also minimize the growing problem in spine care of patient dependency, whether on pharmaceuticals, interventional procedures, passive modalities or other practitioner-provided services [56].

6. *An understanding of the methods, techniques and indications of intensive rehabilitation, interventional treatments and surgical procedures*: It would be the responsibility of the primary spine care practitioner to coordinate the referral and follow up for the minority of patients who need secondary and tertiary level treatment. This would require knowledge and experience regarding the appropriate indications for these interventions, an ability to explain them to patients and an ability to follow up with these patients after the intervention to monitor the progress and outcome [68].

7. *An understanding of the unique features of work-related SRDs:* SRDs that begin in the workplace have particular features that differentiate them from those that are not perceived as work-related [69-71]. Many physicians, particularly traditional PCPs, are uncomfortable with work-related back pain and have misperceptions about the important role that early return to work and return to other normal activities plays in recovery [72-74]. The primary spine care practitioner would be required to understand the nuances of work-related SRDs and the unique aspects of management that are required to effectively care for this patient population [75].

8. *An understanding of the unique features of SRDs related to motor vehicle collisions:* Similar to work-related SRDs, those related to motor vehicle collisions (particularly whiplash associated disorders) have particular features that require specialized knowledge. The primary spine care practitioner would require an understanding of issues that are unique to this type of patient such as injury mechanisms [76,77], patterns of injury [78-80], risk factors for chronicity [81], medicolegal reporting and the delicate balance between the need for early, aggressive treatment [82] and the potential role this can play in chronicity [65,66].

9. *Public Health Perspective*: The primary spine care practitioner would require a broad perspective regarding how spine problems and spine care fits in the grander scheme of public health. For example, many of the health conditions that are the focus of public health education and promotion campaigns are associated with SRDs as complicating factors. These include: smoking, obesity, type II diabetes, lack of physical exercise, and mental health disorders. Public health campaigns regarding SRDs are in the early stages [83,84] and it can be expected that further public health efforts regarding this widespread set of problems will be undertaken [85] and will require input from primary-level practitioners with expertise in this area.

10. *The ability to coordinate the efforts of a variety of practitioners*: As we stated earlier, a high-quality primary spine care practitioner should be able to manage the majority of patients with SRDs without the need for referral. However, in those patients who require specialized services, the primary spine care practitioner would have to be skilled in the coordination of these services and in follow up to ensure that maximum benefit is derived.

11. *The ability to follow patients over the long term*: As SRDs typically take on a recurrent course [86,87] that is life-long [88] the primary spine care practitioner would have to be skilled in the long term follow up of patients to monitor recurrences, teach patients how to effectively interpret and self-manage the majority of these recurrences, and provide management of those recurrences for which self-management is not effective.

The primary spine care practitioner: potential benefits for patients

Any patient benefits that may result from a focused management strategy with a well trained primary spine care practitioner would have to be investigated through a rigorous research effort. However, based on the current understanding of SRDs we would anticipate a number of such benefits. Some examples include:

1. *Faster recovery:* By providing targeted, evidence-based care the well-trained primary spine care practitioner would avoid unnecessary treatment, promote active care plans and patient empowerment and appropriately triage when necessary [89]. This can be expected to facilitate maximal outcomes in the shortest time.

2. *Cost savings:* The primary spine care practitioner could save patients considerable time and money both at the point of encounter and in the future by ordering diagnostic tests only when necessary, applying evidence-based treatments, avoiding unnecessary treatment and taking a "less is more" approach through education and motivation in self-directed care [27].
3. *Avoiding iatrogenic disability:* Judicious use of imaging and appropriate communication of findings may also help avoid the iatrogenic disability that can arise as a result of the medicalization of imaging findings that are of questionable clinical significance, such as "disc degeneration" [90]. Inappropriate communication of diagnostic test results can lead to unnecessary catastrophizing of benign spine pain that may result in prolonged disability [91] and unnecessary invasive procedures [92]. Having a primary spine care practitioner who understands when advanced imaging is necessary and when it is not necessary, and who can put into the proper perspective the findings of these tests, can help to reverse the costly imaging- and specialist-dominated culture that has developed in the area of SRDs.
4. *Increased productivity:* Encouragement to remain active, particularly with work-related SRDs and engaging in a targeted stay at work/ return to work strategy [93,94] would lessen the likelihood of work loss and its resultant economic hardship [95].
5. *Decreased likelihood of becoming a "chronic pain sufferer":* Appropriate care plans that focus on active care and patient empowerment are likely to help the patient avoid becoming a chronic pain sufferer [96]. The recognition of "yellow flags" of psychosocial involvement can lead to early intervention, before these factors lead patients down the path of prolonged disability [58,61].
6. *High patient satisfaction:* In the age of consumer-driven health care, the importance of the patient's overall experience of health care is of great importance [97]. Cost effective and clinically effective care provided by a practitioner who has good communication skills to educate, motivate and empower the patient will likely lead to high levels of satisfaction [54,98].
7. *Shared decision making:* The primary spine care practitioner would have a wide-ranging understanding of the various diagnostic and management strategies available to patients with SRDs and thus could provide information, resources and support in making decisions regarding their care.
8. *Focus on prevention:* While no program of prevention of future SRDs has been shown to be completely successful, it has been demonstrated that taking a preventative approach can help limit disability related to SRDs [82,99,100] and well as reduce the frequency of future episodes [101,102].

The primary spine care practitioner: potential benefits to society

As with patient benefits, research would be required to determine any societal benefits that may result from the institution of a primary spine care practitioner. However we anticipate that there are many potential benefits to society of having a practitioner who is charged with providing primary care for patients with SRDs. Some examples include:

1. *Knowledgeable care coordinator:* A wide variety of practitioners is currently involved in the management of SRDs with little coordination of their efforts [19]. This leads to inefficiency and compromises value [26]. In our view it would be much more efficient and valuable to create teams of professionals with expertise in SRDs working together to provide efficient and effective patient care [26]. The primary spine care practitioner could play the role of "team captain" by organizing and supervising the work of the various disciplines that may be contributing to the management of any particular patient. This could be expected to improve outcomes by turning what is oftentimes a disjointed effort into a coordinated effort. It would also be likely to help control costs by having a single person in charge of monitoring a particular treatment to determine if it is bringing about meaningful improvement and should continue or is not bringing about meaningful improvement and should be altered or stopped.
2. *SRDs as a public health initiative:* Increased recognition is being given to the potential of a public health approach to SRDs [84,85]. The primary spine care practitioner can spearhead efforts in this area to facilitate and implement such public health campaigns as well as reinforce public health messages on an individual level with patients. Community-wide approaches to back pain have been successful in the past [84]. These programs involve a consistent evidence-based approach by primary contact providers coupled with community-wide education programs to inform the public on how to prevent disability related to SRDs and what to do if spine pain occurs. The success of these programs requires an understanding on the part of the primary spine care practitioner of the essential public health messages regarding SRDs. A community-wide public health initiative regarding SRDs has the potential to save millions of dollars and to prevent needless human suffering [84].
3. *Improved worker productivity:* SRDs trigger significant amounts of absenteeism [103] and "presenteeism" (the worker being present at the workplace but with significant losses in work productivity) [104,105]. The

economic impact of these losses to a community is substantial. The establishment of a primary spine care practitioner could potentially lead to significant community-wide savings in both direct [14] and indirect [106] costs of SRDs.

4. *Less long term disability:* A significant portion of health care costs related to SRDs goes toward the management of chronic and recurrent conditions [17,107]. Appropriate initial evaluation and treatment can significantly reduce the number of acute pain patients who become chronic [82], and to reduce the cost of medical care, lost productivity and disability. A "culture of disability" can spread through a family or business or community, creating emotional and financial hardship for society [108]. Having a primary spine care practitioner who is skilled in disability management could potentially help reduce the risk of long term disability by acting at the early stages of a SRD episode [109,110].

The primary spine care practitioner: potential benefits for the health care system

At present the delivery of health care to patients with SRDs follows the inefficient and expensive "supermarket approach" [19]. Having a primary spine care provider to manage patients with SRDs may benefit the health care system in a number of ways, including:

1. *Controlling costs:* The health care system in Western Society has been burdened with runaway costs. In no area is this more an issue than with SRDs [20]. By having a primary spine care practitioner who has the skills to manage the majority of patients with SRDs without the need for special tests or referral to specialists or other practitioners, a dramatic decrease in the cost of SRDs could be realized.

2. *Unburdening traditional PCPs:* The traditional PCP has the responsibility of managing the overall health needs of his or her patients. This includes, in many cases, multiple co-morbidities. The primary spine care practitioner would handle a significant portion of the traditional PCP's current case load, increasing the PCP's availability to the numerous other responsibilities of these practitioners. Thus, traditional PCPs would benefit by being relieved of the burden of caring for a large group of patient complaints for which they have little training [31-33]. This could also potentially result in a decrease in the projected PCP shortfall [22]. Having a primary spine care practitioner to whom traditional PCPs can refer patients with SRDs, or whom these patients can consult directly without having to see their PCP (a more efficient pathway), would remove from the already-overbooked schedule of traditional PCPs those conditions (SRDs) for which they have minimal training in diagnosis and management. This will allow them to focus on what they do best.

3. *More strategic specialist referrals:* Specialists who care for patients with SRDs would benefit for a similar reason as would traditional PCPs. Many patients with SRDs who see specialists such as orthopedic surgeons, neurosurgeons, interventional physiatrists or pain management physicians have no indications for surgery, injections or other invasive procedures. In addition, it has been found that in many cases these specialists do not have a keen understanding of the management of non-surgical SRDs [111]. This is likely because the bulk of the training of these specialists is focused on the application of interventional and surgical procedures in complex cases. By having all SRD patients see the primary spine care practitioner, who is trained to recognize those who require more invasive procedures, only those patients who need such procedures would be channeled to the surgical or interventional specialist. This would allow these specialist practitioners to focus their practice on doing what they do best - applying skilled surgical or interventional procedures.

4. *Disruptive innovation:* The establishment of clinicians who can provide primary spine care would represent a significant "disruptive innovation" [112] in health care. According to Christensen, et al [112] disruptive innovation is the process in which complex, expensive products and services are transformed into simple, affordable ones. Disruptive innovation in any industry occurs when a company, a group of individuals, or a profession comes along with new ideas and a new approach that leads to the transformation of the industry so that products and services become dramatically more affordable and accessible. This happened in the 1970s when Toyota disrupted the auto industry and in the early 1980s when Apple disrupted the computer industry [112]. We suggest that the introduction of the primary spine care practitioner can serve as a disruption in the delivery of spine care services that could potentially lead to dramatic improvements in the delivery, accessibility, cost and outcomes of this care. This viewpoint is supported by the example of the Spine Care Program at Jordan Hospital in Plymouth, Massachusetts where the primary spine care practitioner model has been implemented in an ACO-style environment. Preliminary evidence indicates that this program has been successful in the areas of outcomes, patient satisfaction and cost efficiency [113]. In addition, 80% of the patients in this program are referred by traditional PCPs supporting our viewpoint that the primary

spine care practitioner model would be helpful in reducing the burden on these practitioners.

5. *Standardization of care:* Inconsistent clinical decision-making, unnecessary ordering of imaging studies, overutilization of invasive procedures, over-prescription of pharmaceuticals and excessive reliance on passive care approaches all trigger huge health care losses both in money and time [20]. A standardized, evidence based patient care pathway followed by knowledgeable practitioners has the potential to greatly minimize these costs.

6. *New evidence and technologies:* Currently, new treatment approaches or technologies regarding SRDs are often driven into the health care system more by marketing efforts than by good science [19]. With the introduction of a single group of primary spine care practitioners throughout the health care system, quality, evidence-based technologies and procedures could more quickly and efficiently be introduced.

Obstacles to the implementation of the primary care for the spine model

There are a number of hurdles to overcome for the successful implementation of a primary care of spine model. These obstacles include:

1. *Educational changes:* Currently, none of the major health care educational institutions are consistently graduating providers who meet all the criteria necessary to be successful primary spine care practitioners. However with some basic fundamental changes, and a commitment from state and federal governments, trade organizations and school administrators and faculty, this obstacle can be overcome. Institutions of chiropractic medicine, for example, provide training that is focused primarily on the spine. Many of the skills required of the primary spine care practitioner are already taught at these schools. By instituting some specific changes, that are already being discussed within this health care profession [114,115], these institutions can become at least one source of appropriately trained primary spine care practitioners. Other disciplines that include some level of spine care training within their respective curricula are institutions of osteopathic medicine and physical therapy. The primary focus of most osteopathic programs in the US is the diagnosis and treatment of internal disorders with a majority of osteopathic physicians working in the field of family medicine. Physical therapy education does contain some spine related coursework, but is more broadly focused on musculoskeletal, neuromuscular, cardiopulmonary, and wound care. Thus, significant changes in these curricula would be required if they are to successfully train primary spine care practitioners.

2. *Incentivizing value:* Traditionally, in the area of SRDs and as in other areas of health care, providers have typically been paid by the procedure, thus incentivizing more procedures. This would have to change for successful implementation of primary spine care services into the health care system. Primary spine care practitioners would have to be adequately paid for activities such as patient education, coordination of care and stay at work/ return to work strategies. In addition, they would have to be financially incentivized to take a "less is more" approach. There are signs that this is starting to occur, however. As the health care system moves from fee for service toward a shared risk management model, providers and care pathways that add value to the system will be the leaders, thus increasing the support of their programs and services [67,97]. The concept of the primary spine care practitioner fits well into this model, allowing a "less is more" approach that involves fewer procedures and greater patient empowerment to replace the present "supermarket" approach [19] to SRDs.

3. *Overcoming prejudice:* It is likely that the best candidates to be groomed to become primary care spine providers may not come from the allopathic medical profession. This may be resisted in some aspects of the medical community. It would be important that a competent, appropriately trained provider be accepted regardless of the degree after his or her name. The institution of new models of health care in general, including primary spine care, will require non-traditional ways of thinking about which provider will become the "team captain" for any particular medical condition.

4. *The detrimental effect on those invested in the "supermarket approach":* For health care practitioners who currently see a large volume of patients with SRDs and who remain invested in the current incentive system in which more procedures are emphasized without regard for outcome or value, the institution of a primary spine care practitioner could be detrimental. If a system in which value rather than volume is rewarded, some practitioners will be negatively impacted and some may even go out of business [26]. Thus, the disruption of the health care system that the institution of a primary spine care practitioner will be a part of will undoubtedly be resisted by some individuals or groups who are unable or unwilling to embrace this change. However, such resistance has occurred in response to major disruptions of other industries [112] and we would anticipate that the benefits of the disruption we are suggesting will overcome any opposition that will inevitably arise.

5. *Resistance from within the profession(s) that could potentially be the source of primary spine care practitioners:* For whatever profession or professions that respond to the need for a primary spine care practitioner, this will be a significant disruption to the traditional practice patterns or self-image of these professions. As a result, the role that we are introducing here will be actively resisted [115]. However, given the fact that SRDs affect virtually 100% of the population it can be expected that whatever profession accepts the role of primary spine care practitioner will likely dramatically increase the volume of patients that seeks its services.

6. *Implementation:* The implementation of primary spine care services will require support from several areas of the health care system, including the profession(s) from which the non-surgical spine care practitioner will arise, third party payors, who will have to provide the financial incentive to bring value to spine care, regulatory and legislative bodies that may have to institute changes in allowing this area of health care to fully realize its societal benefits and other members of the health care system who will have to support and accept the implementation of primary spine care services. Again, disruptive innovations in other industries have required such changes and we would anticipate that the same can occur in response to the primary spine care innovation.

7. *Sustainability:* Any disruptive innovation has to be sustained in order for society to fully realize its benefits. Because of the great need we have presented here for high-quality, low cost (i.e., valuable) spine care, we feel that this need, and the benefits realized as a result of the institution of primary spine care services, will drive the sustainability of these services. However, this sustainability will also be dependent on the consistent supply of practitioners who are appropriately skilled in providing primary spine care. As we indicated earlier, this will require commitment on the part of whatever health care profession(s) elects to supply the system with appropriately trained practitioners.

Conclusion

The need for some type of reform in our health care system is recognized by the public, industry and providers. The exact form that health care reform will take is not known but it is widely held that primary care services will have a significant clinical and administrative role and that shared risk among all stakeholders will be beneficial. Any meaningful approach to health care reform will require that three goals be achieved: 1. improved patient health, 2. improved patient experience 3. decreased per capita costs. That is, emphasis must be placed on value in health care. To achieve these goals, health care services in general must be redesigned away from the traditional fee-for-service model to a model based on value that is accessible, practical and sustainable.

It is our view that the addition of a primary spine care provider who is responsible for front-line diagnosis, management and triage would help achieve these goals, bringing greater value in the care of patients with SRDs. Moreover, the addition of this practitioner would be aligned with developing models of health care such as the patient-centered medical home and the accountable care organization. The establishment of such a practitioner is not unprecedented; primary oral health care is currently provided by the general dentist, who manages the majority of society's oral health needs him- or herself, with referral to specialist practitioners in those relatively few circumstances in which it is warranted. We think that the same model can be applied to SRDs.

The primary spine care practitioner will require a particular skill set that includes the ability to apply evidence-based procedures, appropriately educate and motivate patients and effectively prevent and manage disability related to SRDs. The benefits in terms of improved outcomes of care for SRDs, improved patient satisfaction, and reduced costs (i.e., the value of care for SRDs) would be well worth the effort of grooming practitioners toward filling this role.

Disclosures

The authors declare that they have no competing interests.

Author details

[1]Clinical Director, Rhode Island Spine Center, 600 Pawtucket Avenue, Pawtucket, RI 02860 USA. [2]Clinical Assistant Professor, Alpert Medical School of Brown University, Box G-A, Providence, RI 02912 USA. [3]Private Practice of Chiropractic, Rochester Chiropractic Group, 1687 English RoadRochester, NY 14616 USA. [4]Medical Director, Medical Back Pain Program at Jordan Hospital, 10 Cordage Park Circle, Suite 225, Plymouth, MA 02360 USA. [5]Professor of Clinical Sciences, University of Bridgeport, Bridgeport, CT 06604 USA. [6]Assistant Professor, School of Health and Rehabilitative Sciences, University of Pittsburgh, 4028 Forbes Tower, Pittsburgh, PA 15260 USA.

Authors' contributions

DRM originally conceived of the conceptual basis of the paper and wrote the initial manuscript. BDJ, ICP, SMP and MJS then made individual contributions to various sections of the manuscript. All authors took part in editing and revising the manuscript on multiple occasions. All authors reviewed the final manuscript prior to submission.

References

1. Rushton FE: **US health-care crisis.** *Pediatr Int* 2009, **51(5)**:603-605.
2. Diamond GA, Kaul S, Boden WE: **A 300-year-old solution to the health care crisis.** *Arch Intern Med* 2009, **169(11)**:1019-1021.
3. Tumulty K: **The health care crisis hits home.** *Time* 2009, **173(10)**:26-31.
4. Clark RM: **America's health care crisis: a family doctor's perspective.** *J Med Assoc Ga* 2008, **97(3)**:16-17.

5. **Understanding the Affordable Care Act.** [http://www.healthcare.gov/law/about/index.html].
6. McClellan M, McKethan AN, Lewis JL, Roski J, Fisher ES: **A national strategy to put accountable care into practice.** *Health Aff (Millwood)* 2010, **29(5)**:982-990.
7. **National Committee for Quality Assurance Accountable Care Organization Criteria.** [http://www.ncqa.org/tabid/1266/Default.aspx].
8. Schmidt CO, Raspe H, Pfingsten M, Hasenbring M, Basler HD, Eich W, Kohlmann T: **Back pain in the German adult population: prevalence, severity, and sociodemographic correlates in a multiregional survey.** *Spine (Phila Pa 1976)* 2007, **32(18)**:2005-2011.
9. Cassidy JD, Carroll LJ, Cote P: **The Saskatchewan health and back pain survey. The prevalence of low back pain and related disability in Saskatchewan adults.** *Spine (Phila Pa 1976)* 1998, **23(17)**:1860-1866, discussion 1867.
10. Carey TS, Evans AT, Hadler NM, Lieberman G, Kalsbeek WD, Jackman AM, Fryer JG, McNutt RA: **Acute severe low back pain. A population-based study of prevalence and care-seeking.** *Spine (Phila Pa 1976)* 1996, **21(3)**:339-344.
11. Carey TS, Evans A, Hadler N, Kalsbeek W, McLaughlin C, Fryer J: **Care-seeking among individuals with chronic low back pain.** *Spine (Phila Pa 1976)* 1995, **20(3)**:312-317.
12. Cote P, Cassidy JD, Carroll L: **The Saskatchewan Health and Back Pain Survey. The prevalence of neck pain and related disability in Saskatchewan adults.** *Spine (Phila Pa 1976)* 1998, **23(15)**:1689-1698.
13. *United States Bone and Joint Decade. The Burden of Musculoskeletal Diseases in the United States* Rosemont, IL: American Academy of Orthopaedic Surgeons; 2008.
14. Martin BI, Turner JA, Mirza SK, Lee MJ, Comstock BA, Deyo RA: **Trends in health care expenditures, utilization, and health status among US adults with spine problems, 1997-2006.** *Spine (Phila Pa 1976)* 2009, **34(19)**:2077-2084.
15. Borghouts JA, Koes BW, Vondeling H, Bouter LM: **Cost-of-illness of neck pain in The Netherlands in 1996.** *Pain* 1999, **80(3)**:629-636.
16. Hashemi L, Webster BS, Clancy EA, Volinn E: **Length of disability and cost of workers' compensation low back pain claims.** *J Occup Environ Med* 1997, **39(10)**:937-945.
17. Webster BS, Snook SH: **The cost of 1989 workers' compensation low back pain claims.** *Spine* 1994, **19(10)**:1111-1115, discussion 1116.
18. Atlas SJ, Chang Y, Keller RB, Singer DE, Wu YA, Deyo RA: **The impact of disability compensation on long-term treatment outcomes of patients with sciatica due to a lumbar disc herniation.** *Spine* 2006, **31(26)**:3061-3069.
19. Haldeman S, Dagenais S: **A supermarket approach to the evidence-informed management of chronic low back pain.** *Spine J* 2008, **8(1)**:1-7.
20. Deyo RA, Mirza SK, Turner JA, Martin BI: **Overtreating chronic back pain: time to back off?** *J Am Board Fam Med* 2009, **22(1)**:62-68.
21. Martin BI, Deyo RA, Mirza SK, Turner JA, Comstock BA, Hollingworth W, Sullivan SD: **Expenditures and health status among adults with back and neck problems.** *Jama* 2008, **299(6)**:656-664.
22. Phillips RL Jr, Bazemore AW: **Primary care and why it matters for U.S. health system reform.** *Health Aff (Millwood)* 2010, **29(5)**:806-810.
23. Wolsko PM, Eisenberg DM, Davis RB, Kessler R, Phillips RS: **Patterns and perceptions of care for treatment of back and neck pain: results of a national survey.** *Spine (Phila Pa 1976)* 2003, **28(3)**:292-297, discussion 298.
24. Hart LG, Deyo RA, Cherkin DC: **Physician office visits for low back pain. Frequency, clinical evaluation, and treatment patterns from a U.S. national survey.** *Spine (Phila Pa 1976)* 1995, **20(1)**:11-19.
25. Deyo RA, Mirza SK, Martin BI: **Back pain prevalence and visit rates: estimates from U.S. national surveys, 2002.** *Spine (Phila Pa 1976)* 2006, **31(23)**:2724-2727.
26. Porter ME, Teisberg EO: *Redefining Health Care: Creating Value-Based Competition on Results* Boston, MA: Harvard Business School Press; 2006.
27. Chou R, Qaseem A, Snow V, Casey D, Cross JT Jr, Shekelle P, Owens DK: **Diagnosis and treatment of low back pain: a joint clinical practice guideline from the American College of Physicians and the American Pain Society.** *Ann Intern Med* 2007, **147(7)**:478-491.
28. Langevin HM, Sherman KJ: **Pathophysiological model for chronic low back pain integrating connective tissue and nervous system mechanisms.** *Med Hypotheses* 2007, **68(1)**:74-80.
29. Peters ML, Vlaeyen JWS, Weber WEJ: **The joint contribution of physical pathology, pain-related fear and catastophizing to chronic back pain disability.** *Pain* 2005, **113(1-2)**:45-50.
30. **American Academy of Family Practitioners.** http://www.aafp.org/online/en/home/policy/policies/p/primarycare.html(accessed 23 February 2011) http://www.aafp.org/online/en/home/policy/policies/p/primarycare.html.
31. Matheny JM, Brinker MR, Elliott MN, Blake R, Rowane MP: **Confidence of graduating family practice residents in their management of musculoskeletal conditions.** *Am J Orthop (Belle Mead NJ)* 2000, **29(12)**:945-952.
32. Matzkin E, Smith EL, Freccero D, Richardson AB: **Adequacy of education in musculoskeletal medicine.** *Journal of Bone & Joint Surgery* 2005, **87-A(2)**:310-314.
33. Freedman KB, Bernstein J: **Educational deficiencies in musculoskeletal medicine.** *J Bone Joint Surg* 2002, **84(4)**:604-608.
34. Buchbinder R, Staples M, Jolley D: **Doctors with a special interest in back pain have poorer knowledge about how to treat back pain.** *Spine (Phila Pa 1976)* 2009, **34(11)**:1218-1226, discussion 1227.
35. Bishop A, Foster NE: **The implementation of guidelines for the management of patients with low back pain: the role of practitioners' attitudes and perceptions.** *Internat Muscluskel Med* 2010, **32(4)**:151-156.
36. Williams CM, Maher CG, Hancock MJ, McAuley JH, McLachlan AJ, Britt H, Fahridin S, Harrison C, Latimer J: **Low back pain and best practice care: A survey of general practice physicians.** *Arch Intern Med* 2010, **170(3)**:271-277.
37. Henschke N, Maher CG, Refshauge KM, Herbert RD, Cumming RG, Bleasel J, York J, Das A, McAuley JH: **Prevalence of and screening for serious spinal pathology in patients presenting to primary care settings with acute low back pain.** *Arthritis Rheum* 2009, **60(10)**:3072-3080.
38. Chou R, Fu R, Carrino JA, Deyo RA: **Imaging strategies for low-back pain: systematic review and meta-analysis.** *Lancet* 2009, **373(9662)**:463-472.
39. Bronfort G, Haas M, Evans RL: **Efficacy of spinal manipulation and mobilization for low back pain and neck pain: a systematic review and best evidence synthesis.** *Spine J* 2004, **4(3)**:335-356.
40. Gross AR, Hoving JL, Haines TA, Goldsmith CH, Kay T, Aker P, Bronfort G: **A Cochrance review of manipulation and mobilization for mechanical neck disorders.** *Spine* 2004, **29(1)**:1541-1548.
41. Clare HA, Adams R, Maher CG: **A systematic review of efficacy of McKenzie therapy for spinal pain.** *Aust J Physiother* 2004, **50**:209-216.
42. Murphy DR, Hurwitz EL, Gregory AA, Clary R: **A nonsurgical approach to the management of patients with cervical radiculopathy: A prospective observational cohort study.** *J Manipulative Physiol Ther* 2006, **29(4)**:279-287.
43. Murphy DR, Hurwitz EL, Gregory AA, Clary R: **A non-surgical approach to the management of lumbar spinal stenosis: a prospective observational cohort study.** *BMC Musculoskelet Disord* 2006, **7**:16.
44. Murphy DR, Hurwitz EL, McGovern EE: **A non-surgical approach to the management of patients with lumbar radiculopathy secondary to herniated disc: A prospective observational cohort study with follow up.** *J Manipulative Physiol Ther* 2009, **32(9)**:723-733.
45. Mayer J, Mooney V, Dagenais S: **Evidence-informed management of chronic low back pain with lumbar extensor strengthening exercises.** *Spine J* 2008, **8(1)**:96-113.
46. Standaert CJ, Weinstein SM, Rumpeltes J: **Evidence-informed management of chronic low back pain with lumbar stabilization exercises.** *Spine J* 2008, **8(1)**:114-120.
47. Hurwitz EL, Carragee EJ, van der Velde G, Carroll LJ, Nordin M, Guzman J, Peloso PM, Holm LW, Cote P, Hogg-Johnson S, *et al*: **Treatment of neck pain: noninvasive interventions: results of the Bone and Joint Decade 2000-2010 Task Force on Neck Pain and Its Associated Disorders.** *Spine* 2008, **33(4 Suppl)**:S123-152.
48. Brox JI, Storheim K, Grotle M, Tveito TH, Indahl A, Eriksen HR: **Evidence-informed management of chronic low back pain with back schools, brief education, and fear-avoidance training.** *Spine J* 2008, **8(1)**:28-39.
49. Seaman DR: **The diet-induced proinflammatory state a cause of chronic pain and other degenerative diseases.** *J Manipulative Physiol Ther* 2002, **25(3)**:168-179.
50. Giannetti BM, Staiger C, Bulitta M, Predel HG: **Efficacy and safety of comfrey root extract ointment in the treatment of acute upper or lower back pain: results of a double-blind, randomised, placebo controlled, multicentre trial.** *Br J Sports Med* 2010, **44(9)**:637-641.

51. Waddell G: *The Back Pain Revolution.* 2 edition. Edinburgh: Churchill Livingstone; 2004.
52. Burton AK: **Back injury and work loss: biomechanical and psychosocial influences.** *Spine* 1997, **22(21)**:2575-2580.
53. Wallace AS, Freburger JK, Darter JD, Jackman AM, Carey TS: **Comfortably numb? Exploring satisfaction with chronic back pain visits.** *Spine J* 2009, **9(9)**:721-728.
54. Laerum E, Indahl A, Skouen JS: **What is "the good back consultation?" a combined qualitative and quantitative study of chronic low back pain patients' interaction with and perceptions of consultations with specialists.** *J Rehabil Med* 2006, **38(4)**:255-262.
55. Henrotin Y, Cedraschi C, Duplan B, Bazin T, Duquesnoy B: **Information and low back pain management: a systematic review.** *Spine* 2006, **31(11)**:E326-E334.
56. Haldeman S, Carroll LJ, Cassidy JD: **The empowerment of people with neck pain: introduction: the Bone and Joint Decade 2000-2010 Task Force on Neck Pain and Its Associated Disorders.** *Spine (Phila Pa 1976)* 2008, **33(4 Suppl)**:S8-S13.
57. Verhagen AP, Karels CH, Schellingerhout JM, Willemsen SP, Koes BW, Bierma-Zeinstra SM: **Pain severity and catastrophising modify treatment success in neck pain patients in primary care.** *Man Ther* 2010, **15(3)**:267-272.
58. Main CJ, Foster N, Buchbinder R: **How important are back pain beliefs and expectations for satisfactory recovery from back pain?** *Best Pract Res Clin Rheumatol* 2010, **24(2)**:205-217.
59. Vlaeyen JWS, Kole-Snijders AMJ, Boeren RGB, van Eek H: **Fear of movement/reinjury in chronic low back pain and its relation to behavioral performance.** *Pain* 1995, **62**:363-372.
60. Crombez G, Vlaeyen JWS, Heuts PHTG, Lysens R: **Pain-related fear is more disabling than pain itself: evidence on the role of pain-related fear in chronic back pain disability.** *Pain* 1999, **80(1-2)**:329-339.
61. Main CJ, Buchbinder R, Porcheret M, Foster N: **Addressing patient beliefs and expectations in the consultation.** *Best Pract Res Clin Rheumatol* 2010, **24(2)**:219-225.
62. Jellema P, Windt van der, Windt van der, van der Horst HE, Blankenstein AH, Bouter LM, Stalman WAB: **Why is a treatment aimed at psychosocial factors not effective in patients with (sub)acute low back pain?** *Pain* 2005, **118**:350-359.
63. Klaber Moffett JA, Carr J, Howarth E: **High fear-avoiders of physical activity benefit from an exercise program for patients with back pain.** *Spine* 2004, **29(11)**:1167-1172.
64. Smeets R, Vlaeyen J, Kester A, Knottnerus J: **Reduction of pain catastrophizing mediates the outcome of both physical and cognitive-behavioral treatment in chronic low back pain.** *J Pain* 2006, **7(4)**:261-271.
65. Cote P, Hogg-Johnson S, Cassidy D, Carroll L, Frank JW, Bombardier C: **Initial patterns of clinical care and recovery from whiplash injuries.** *Arch Intern Med* 2005, **165**:2257-2263.
66. Cote P, Hogg-Johnson S, Cassidy JD, Carroll L, Frank JW, Bombardier C: **Early aggressive care and delayed recovery from whiplash: Isolated finding or reproducible result?** *Arthritis Rheum* 2007, **57(5)**:861-868.
67. Porter ME, Teisberg EO: **How physicians can change the future of health care.** *Jama* 2007, **297(10)**:1103-1111.
68. Chou R, Loeser JD, Owens DK, Rosenquist RW, Atlas SJ, Baisden J, Carragee EJ, Grabois M, Murphy DR, Resnick DK, *et al*: **Interventional therapies, surgery, and interdisciplinary rehabilitation for low back pain: an evidence-based clinical practice guideline from the American Pain Society.** *Spine (Phila Pa 1976)* 2009, **34(10)**:1066-1077.
69. Harris I, Mulford J, Solomon M, van Gelder JM, Young J: **Association between compensation status and outcome after surgery: a meta-analysis.** *Jama* 2005, **293(13)**:1644-1652.
70. Rainville J, Pransky G, Indahl A, Mayer E: **The physician as disability advisor for patients with musculoskeletal complaints.** *Spine* 2005, **30(22)**:2579-2584.
71. Atlas SJ, Tosteson TD, Blood EA, Skinner JS, Pransky GS, Weinstein JN: **The impact of workers' compensation on outcomes of surgical and nonoperative therapy for patients with a lumbar disc herniation: SPORT.** *Spine (Phila Pa 1976)* 2010, **35(1)**:89-97.
72. Linton SJ, Vlaeyen J, Ostelo R: **The back pain beliefs of health care providers are we fear-avoidant?** *J Occup Rehab* 2002, **12(4)**:223-232.
73. Pransky G, Katz JN, Benjamin K, Himmelstein J: **Improving the physician role in evaluating work ability and managing disability: a survey of primary care practitioners.** *Disabil Rehabil* 2002, **24(16)**:867-874.
74. Zinn W, Furutani N: **Physician perspectives on the ethical aspects of disability determination.** *J Gen Intern Med* 1996, **11(9)**:525-532.
75. von Korff M, Barlow W, Cherkin D, Deyo RA: **Effects of practice style in managing back pain.** *Ann Intern Med* 1994, **121**:187-195.
76. Kaneoka K, Ono K, Inami S, Hayashi K: **Motion analysis of cervical vertebrae during whiplash loading.** *Spine* 1999, **24(8)**:763-769.
77. Stemper BD, Yoganandan N, Pintar FA: **Gender- and region-dependant local facet joint kinematics in rear impact: implications in whiplash injury.** *Spine* 2004, **29(16)**:1764-1771.
78. Ivancic PC, Ito S, Tominaga Y, Rubin W, Coe MP, Ndu AB, Carlson EJ, Panjabi MM: **Whiplash causes increased laxity of cervical capsular ligament.** *Clin Biomech (Bristol, Avon)* 2008, **23(2)**:159-165.
79. Ettlin T, Schuster C, Stoffel R, Bruderlin A, Kischka U: **A distinct pattern of myofascial findings in patients after whiplash injury.** *Arch Phys Med Rehabil* 2008, **89(7)**:1290-1293.
80. Kaale BR, Krakenes J, Albrektsen G, Wester K: **Clinical assessment techniques for detecting ligament and membrane injuries in the upper cervical spine region–a comparison with MRI results.** *Man Ther* 2008, **13(5)**:397-403.
81. Carroll LJ, Holm LW, Hogg-Johnson S, Cote P, Cassidy JD, Haldeman S, Nordin M, Hurwitz EL, Carragee EJ, van der Velde G, *et al*: **Course and prognostic factors for neck pain in whiplash-associated disorders (WAD): results of the Bone and Joint Decade 2000-2010 Task Force on Neck Pain and Its Associated Disorders.** *Spine* 2008, **33(4 Suppl)**:S83-92.
82. Rosenfeld M, Seferiadis A, Carlsson J, Gunnarsson R: **Active intervention in patients with whiplash-associated disorders improves long-term prognosis a randomized controlled clinical trial.** *Spine* 2003, **28(22)**:2491-2498.
83. Waddell G, O'Connor M, Boorman S, Torsney B: **Working Backs Scotland: a public and professional health education campaign for back pain.** *Spine* 2007, **32(19)**:2139-2143.
84. Buchbinder R, Jolley D, Wyatt M: **Population based intervention to change back pain beliefs and disability: three part evaluation.** *BMJ* 2001, **322(7301)**:1516-1520.
85. Cassidy JD, Cote P: **Is it time for a population health approach to neck pain?** *J Manipulative Physiol Ther* 2008, **31(6)**:442-446.
86. Cote P, Cassidy JD, Carroll LJ, Kristman V: **The annual incidence and course of neck pain in the general population: a population-based cohort study.** *Pain* 2004, **112(3)**:267-273.
87. Cassidy JD, Cote P, Carroll LJ, Kristman V: **Incidence and course of low back pain episodes in the general population.** *Spine* 2005, **30(24)**:2817-2823.
88. Hartvigsen J, Christensen K: **Pain in the back and neck are with us until the end: a nationwide interview-based survey of Danish 100-year-olds.** *Spine* 2008, **33(8)**:909-913.
89. Haldeman S, Dagenais S: **What have we learned about the evidence-informed management of chronic low back pain?** *Spine J* 2008, **8(1)**:266-277.
90. Jarvik JJ, Hollingworth W, Heagerty P, Haynor DR, Deyo RA: **The longitudinal assessment of imaging and disability of the back (LAIDback) study Baseline Data.** *Spine* 2001, **29(10)**:1158-1166.
91. Crook J, Milner R, Schultz IZ, Stringer B: **Determinants of occupational disability following a low back injury a critical review of the literature.** *J Occup Rehabil* 2002, **12(4)**:277-295.
92. Lurie JD, Birkmeyer NJ, Weinstein JN: **Rates of advanced spinal imaging and spine surgery.** *Spine (Phila Pa 1976)* 2003, **28(6)**:616-620.
93. Murphy DR: **Motivating patients to return to work. Part 1.** *Occup Med Clin Care Update* 2008, **15(2)**:1-2.
94. Murphy DR: **Motivating patients to return to work. Part 2.** *Occup Med Clin Care Update* 2008, **15(3)**:1-2.
95. Zampolini M, Bernardinello M, Tesio L: **RTW in back conditions.** *Disabil Rehabil* 2007, **29(17)**:1377-1385.
96. Whitfill T, Haggard R, Bierner SM, Pransky G, Hassett RG, Gatchel RJ: **Early intervention options for acute low back pain patients: a randomized clinical trial with one-year follow-up outcomes.** *J Occup Rehabil* 2010, **20(2)**:256-263.
97. Porter ME: **A strategy for health care reform–toward a value-based system.** *N Engl J Med* 2009, **361(2)**:109-112.
98. Staiger TO, Jarvik JG, Deyo RA, Martin B, Braddock CH 3: **BRIEF REPORT: Patient-physician agreement as a predictor of outcomes in patients with back pain.** *J Gen Intern Med* 2005, **20(10)**:935-937.

99. Rutten GM, Degen S, Hendriks EJ, Braspenning JC, Harting J, Oostendorp RA: **Adherence to clinical practice guidelines for low back pain in physical therapy: do patients benefit?** *Phys Ther* 2010, **90(8)**:1111-1122.
100. Team UBT: **United Kingdom back pain exercise and manipulation (UK BEAM) randomised trial: effectiveness of physical treatments for back pain in primary care.** *BMJ* 2004, **329**:1377-1381.
101. Hides JA, Jull GA, Richardson CA: **Long-term effects of specific stabilizing exercises for first-episode low back pain.** *Spine* 2001, **26(11)**:e243-e248.
102. Larsen K, Weidick F, Leboeuf-Yde C: **Can passive prone extensions of the back prevent back problems? A randomized, controlled intervention trial of 314 military conscripts.** *Spine* 2002, **27(24)**:2747-2752.
103. Guo HR, Tanaka S, Halperin WE, Cameron LL: **Back pain prevalence in US industry and estimates of lost workdays.** *Am J Public Health* 1999, **89(7)**:1029-1035.
104. Maniadakis NM, Gray A: **The economic burden of back pain in the UK.** *Pain* 2000, **84(1)**:95-104.
105. van den Heuvel SG, Ijmker S, Blatter BM, de Korte EM: **Loss of productivity due to neck/shoulder symptoms and hand/arm symptoms: results from the PROMO-study.** *J Occup Rehabil* 2007, **17(3)**:370-382.
106. Nimgade A, McNeely E, Milton D, Celona J: **Increased expenditures for other health conditions after an incident of low back pain.** *Spine (Phila Pa 1976)* 2010, **35(7)**:769-777.
107. Wasiak R, Kim J, Pransky G: **Work disability and costs caused by recurrence of low back pain: longer and more costly than in first episodes.** *Spine* 2006, **31(2)**:219-225.
108. Raspe H, Hueppe A, Neuhauser H: **Back pain, a communicable disease?** *Int J Epidemiol* 2008, **37(1)**:69-74.
109. Bonde J, Rasmussen MS, Hjollund H, Svendsen SW, Kolstad HA, Jenson LD, Wieclaw J: **Occupational disorders and return to work: a randomized controlled study.** *J Rehabil Med* 2005, **37(4)**:230-235.
110. Stephens B, Gross DP: **The influence of a continuum of care model on the rehabilitation of compensation claimants with soft tissue disorders.** *Spine* 2007, **32(25)**:2898-2904.
111. Finestone AS, Raveh A, Mirovsky Y, Lahad A, Milgrom C: **Orthopaedists' and family practitioners' knowledge of simple low back pain management.** *Spine (Phila Pa 1976)* 2009, **34(15)**:1600-1603.
112. Christensen CM, Grossman JH, Hwang J: *The Innovator's Prescription: A Disruptive Solution for Health Care* New York: McGraw-Hill; 2009.
113. Paskowski I, Schneider M, Stevans J, Ventura JM, Justice BD: **A hospital-based standardized spine care pathway: report of a multidisciplinary, evidence-based process.** *J Manipulative Physiol Ther* 2010, **34(2)**:98-106.
114. Wyatt LH, Perle SM, Murphy DR, Hyde TE: **The necessary future of chiropractic education: a North American perspective.** *Chiropractic & Osteopathy* 2005, **13(10)**:1-15.
115. Murphy DR, Schneider MJ, Seaman DR, Perle SM, Nelson CF: **How can chiropractic become a respected mainstream profession? The example of podiatry.** *Chiropr Osteop* 2008, **16**:10.

A method for quantitative measurement of lumbar intervertebral disc structures: an intra- and inter-rater agreement and reliability study

Andreas Tunset[1], Per Kjaer[1,2*], Shadi Samir Chreiteh[3] and Tue Secher Jensen[2]

Abstract

Background: There is a shortage of agreement studies relevant for measuring changes over time in lumbar intervertebral disc structures. The objectives of this study were: 1) to develop a method for measurement of intervertebral disc height, anterior and posterior disc material and dural sac diameter using MRI, 2) to evaluate intra- and inter-rater agreement and reliability for the measurements included, and 3) to identify factors compromising agreement.

Methods: Measurements were performed on MRIs from 16 people with and 16 without lumbar disc herniation, purposefully chosen to represent all possible disc contours among participants in a general population study cohort. Using the new method, MRIs were measured twice by one rater and once by a second rater. Agreement on the sagittal start- and end-slice was evaluated using weighted Kappa. Length and volume measurements were conducted on available slices between intervertebral foramens, and cross-sectional areas (CSA) were calculated from length measurements and slice thickness. Results were reported as Bland and Altman's limits of agreement (LOA) and intraclass correlation coefficients (ICC).

Results: Weighted Kappa (K_w (95% CI)) for start- and end-slice were: intra-: 0.82(0.60;0.97) & 0.71(0.43;0.93); inter-rater: 0.56 (0.29;0.78) & 0.60(0.35;0.81). For length measurements, LOA ranged from [−1.0;1.0] mm to [−2.0;2.3] mm for intra-; and from [−1.1; 1.4] mm to [−2.6;2.0] mm for inter-rater. For volume measurements, LOA ranged from [−293;199] mm^3 to [−582;382] mm^3 for intra-, and from [−17;801] mm^3 to [−450;713] mm^3 for inter-rater. For CSAs, LOA ranged between [−21.3; 18.8] mm^2 and [−31.2; 43.7] mm^2 for intra-, and between [−10.8; 16.4] mm^2 and [−64.6; 27.1] mm^2 for inter-rater. In general, LOA as a proportion of mean values gradually decreased with increasing size of the measured structures. Agreement was compromised by difficulties in identifying the vertebral corners, the anterior and posterior boundaries of the intervertebral disc and the dural sac posterior boundary. With two exceptions, ICCs were above 0.81.

Conclusions: Length measurements and calculated CSAs of disc morphology and dural sac diameter from MRIs showed acceptable intra- and inter-rater agreement and reliability. However, caution should be taken when measuring very small structures and defining anatomical landmarks.

Keywords: Magnetic resonance imaging, Intervertebral disc, Disc herniations, Measurement, Spinal canal, Dural sac, Agreement, Reliability, Limits of agreement, Intraclass correlation coefficient

* Correspondence: pkjaer@health.sdu.dk
[1]Department of Sports Science and Clinical Biomechanics, University of Southern Denmark, Campusvej 55, Odense M DK-5230, Denmark
[2]Research Department, Spine Centre of Southern Denmark, Lillebaelt Hospital, Oestre Hougvej 55, Middelfart DK-5500, Denmark
Full list of author information is available at the end of the article

Background

In 1934, Mixter and Barr introduced the concept of lumbar disc herniations (LDH) as an explanation for radiating pain to the lower extremities [1,2]. Since then, extensive effort has been put into investigating the pathogenesis, clinical presentation, treatment and morphological changes involved in LDH [2]. LDH is generally regarded as a potential source of low back pain (LBP) and/or pain radiating to the leg, often below the knee [3]. In patients with clinical signs of nerve root compromise, about nine out of ten patients have disc-related findings on magnetic resonance imaging (MRI) [4]. On the other hand, LDH may be present without any pain or other clinical symptoms [5].

Dural sac size and intervertebral disc height have previously been found to be related to LDH, either clinically or biologically. The dural sac has a direct anatomical relationship with the intervertebral disc [6], and a direct mechanical influence is therefore possible due to an LDH taking up space in the spinal canal [7]. In addition, a correlation between a narrowed spinal canal and LBP and/or leg pain has been reported in cross-sectional studies [8-10]. Intervertebral disc height is possibly affected by LDH as material migrates posteriorly from the disc herniation. A study has shown a correlation between the classification of extended disc contour and disc height [11]. As there is evidence that disc height reduction is associated with LDHs and thus of potential clinical relevance, it was included in the current study.

Anterior disc material is similarly relevant, since it has been proposed that anterior LDHs may cause pain and symptoms [12,13]. Though this condition is rare, this imaging finding was also included in the current study, in order to be comprehensive.

Good long-term prognosis over a follow-up period of 6 months has been reported for a majority of people with LDH [14-17], and forms the current understanding of LDH among health care professionals [18,19]. In the context of clinical prognosis, it is relevant to know how LDHs change in size over time. Previous studies evaluating the change in size of LDHs over time have focused mainly on symptoms in clinical study populations [16,20-24]. Some studies have investigated the quantitative change in size of LDHs over time based on diagnostic imaging [25-29]. Three of these studies have reported the quantitative change in size over time of disc material relative to the spinal canal at multiple follow-ups [27-29], where measurements were based on a method developed by Kato et al. [27]. However, this method is described in insufficient detail to be replicated, due to the absence of definitions of anatomical boundaries.

For evaluation of disc changes over time, the ideal method is to use measurements from multiple image slices. The value of a multi-slice approach is that multiple length and area measurements can be combined into cross-sectional areas (CSA) or volumes, respectively, thereby increasing the chance of capturing changes that might otherwise be missed from single-slice methods. This multi-slice approach has been used in several studies [30-34]. It is also desirable that the method be described in sufficient detail to allow replication. Studies have provided method descriptions in varying detail [30,35-38] and in some cases, this detail is inadequate for replication.

Bland and Altman´s Limits of Agreement (LOA) is the most popular [39], and recommended statistical method for evaluation of agreement [40-44]. The standard error of measurement (SEM) is similarly regarded as a suitable parameter of agreement [45], but is, however, sensitive to variability in the population [46]. Although a recent study reported use of LOA for evaluating agreement of measurements on intervertebral disc morphology [47], it is rarely used when evaluating agreement in the measurement of intervertebral discs, LDH, or the spinal canal [48].

No method for quantitatively measuring intervertebral discs, LDH, and the dural sac was found in the literature that described in adequate detail a multi-slice technique and used LOA (Additional file 1). For a series of planned studies, we required a method to evaluate the changes in size over time of LDHs and their influence over time on dural sac size and intervertebral disc height, and their relationship with LBP. Therefore, we had need of a multi-slice technique for evaluating size of structures that was described in adequate detail and that used LOA to evaluate agreement.

The objectives of this study were:

1) to develop methods for quantitative measurement of anterior and posterior disc heights, extension of anterior and posterior lumbar disc material and dural sac diameter on MRI,
2) to evaluate the intra- and inter-rater agreement and reliability of the measurements included in these methods, and
3) to identify sources of measurement error in the measurement procedures.

Materials and methods

Design

The study is an intra- and inter-rater reliability study using repeated measurements of individual MRIs.

Study population

The sample of MRIs was selected from the longitudinal cohort-study entitled 'Backs on Funen, Denmark', which investigated potential risk factors for LBP. The Office of Civil Registrations sampled a cohort of 40-year old Danes in 2000. All subjects were from the general population living in the county of Funen, Denmark. One out of nine people in this age group was selected (625 individuals) and invited to participate by postal mail. People were excluded if they were severely disabled, had ferromagnetic implants, suffered from claustrophobia, or were not able to communicate in Danish [49]. From this cohort, 412 participated in 2001 at baseline and were re-invited to take part in 2005. At the second measurement of the cohort in 2005, 348 participated and were re-invited to take part in 2009. At the last measurement in 2009, 293 participated. At every measurement of the cohort, all participants had a lumbar MRI and filled in a questionnaire about their LBP. Permission for the original cohort study was granted by the local ethics committee (ref. no. 20000042) and the Danish Data Protection Agency (ref. no. 2000-53-0037) [49].

Sixteen participants assessed as having a disc herniation were purposefully selected by one of the co-authors not involved in the actual measurements (PK) to represent cases with all available types of disc herniations based on previous readings of the MRIs (see below). In the upper lumbar spine, LDH was found to be almost non-existent; therefore, we chose only the three lowest levels. A list of identification numbers, levels, types of herniation, and time of examination was generated and the sample was selected to be truly representative of all types of LDH. Sixteen other participants assessed as not having a disc herniation were randomly selected to participate in the agreement analysis as controls for comparison. Only one MRI per patient was selected among the three MRIs taken at the three available time-points.

MRI

MRI scans were performed with an open, low field 0.2 T magnetic resonance unit (Magnetom Open Viva, Siemens AG, Erlangen, Germany). The lumbar spine was scanned with participants in the supine position, using a combined body/surface coil. Sagittal T1- and T2-weighted and axial T2-weighted MRIs were performed with axial images placed in the plane of the five lower discs. The following sequences were performed at all three time-points:

- A localiser sequence of five images, 40/10/40 degrees (TR/TE/flip angle) consisting of two coronal and three sagittal images in orthogonal planes.
- Sagittal T1-weighted spin echo, 621/26 (TR/TE), 144 × 256 matrix, 300 mm. FOV, 11 slices of 4 mm. thickness, interslice gap of 0.8 mm., 2 acquisitions, 6 min. 1 sec. scan time.
- Sagittal T2-weighted turbo spin echo 4609/134 (TR/effective TE), 210 × 256 matrix, 300 mm. FOV, 11 slices of 4 mm. thickness, interslice gap of 0.8 mm., 2 acquisitions, 8 min. 42 sec. scan time.
- Axial T2-weighted turbo spin echo 6415/134 (TR/effective TE), 180 × 256 matrix, 250 mm. FOV, 3 slices of 5 mm. thickness, interslice gap of 1.0 mm., 2 acquisitions, 7 min. 49 sec. scan time. Slices were placed in the plane of the five lower discs.

To account for scoliosis and vertebral rotation, the radiographers were instructed to align the sagittal images in the best way possible in all three planes. This meant that more than one sagittal series might have been performed in cases of serious scoliosis or vertebral rotation. For the purpose of this study, only the sagittal series that had the best alignment was used for measurement.

An experienced musculoskeletal radiologist evaluated the MRI scans of the lumbar spine from all three time-points using a standardised evaluation protocol [50].

Raters

Inter-rater agreement was tested between two raters: one of whom was a student enrolled in a Master degree in clinical biomechanics (AT) who had no prior training in the interpretation of MRIs (Rater 1); the other was an experienced back pain researcher (TSJ) with extensive experience in interpreting MRIs for research purposes (Rater 2). These raters were purposely chosen to represent an inexperienced, and an experienced, interpreter of MRI. The intra-rater agreement was tested between measures performed by Rater 1.

Development of measurement method

Various methods for measuring the anatomical structures from MRI investigated in the current study have been reported previously [7-10,30-38,48,51-72] (Additional file 1). None of these articles described an ideal method for detecting the longitudinal change in size of LDH. A new method was therefore developed based on knowledge from the literature and the experience of the authors (AT, PK & TSJ).

Sagittal T2-weigthed MRIs were chosen for the measurements. We chose to use sagittal images because only three axial slices were available for each disc level in this study. The T2- rather than the T1-weighted sequence was chosen because of the increased contrast between the cerebrospinal fluid and the posterior part of the intervertebral disc and dural sac. Measures of length, cross-sectional area and volume were taken at the disc levels L3-L4, L4-L5 and L5-S1.

The following length measurements were defined: anterior and posterior intervertebral height (AIVH, PIVH), and the horizontal dimensions of the intervertebral disc (IVDL), anterior and posterior disc material extending beyond the corners of the vertebra (ADML, PDML) and dural sac. From these measures it was possible to calculate cross-sectional areas (CSAs): CSA of the anterior intervertebral height (CAIH), CSA of the posterior intervertebral height (CPIH), CSA of the intervertebral disc

(CIVD), CSA of the anterior disc material (CADM), CSA of the posterior disc material (CPDM)s, and CSA of the dural sac (CDS). Furthermore, volume measurements were also defined for the anterior and posterior disc material that extended beyond the vertebral rim. The definitions of measurement parameters and descriptions of their mode of application are shown in Figure 1 and Table 1.

Training of raters

For the training sessions, 10 participants from the final data collection period, who were judged by the radiologist to have LDH only at this time point, were randomly selected for training. Prior to the actual agreement study, each rater reviewed the 10 cases independently, after which the cases were collectively reviewed and consensus reached on the measurement procedures.

Measurements

All measurements were evaluated for the appropriate disco-vertebral segments on each sagittal T2-image from the first left image with a visible pedicle (start slice) to the last right image with a visible pedicle (end slice), delineating the bottom and top of an intervertebral foramina (Figure 1). All images were magnified between 1100%-1200% during measurements, showing the relevant intervertebral disc horizontally on the screen. For brightness and contrast, default settings of images were used. Length measurements were conducted using the OsiriX 'length-tool`. Length measurements taken from all included sagittal MRIs from every structure were used for calculating the CSAs of those structures (Figures 1 and 2). Volume measurements were calculated by means of OsiriX measurement software using the 'pencil-tool' for manually tracing regions of interest (ROIs) from all slices on each sagittal image, and the 'Compute volume...' tool (Figures 2 and 3).

Insertion positions on the corners of the vertebrae were defined as the most anterior point for anterior corners, and the most posterior point for posterior corners. Possible osteophytes were regarded as part of the vertebral body, as delineation of these was challenging. Insertion positions on the boundaries between structures were defined by the point showing the most contrast between structures (Figure 1). The tracing of disc material areas, used for calculating volumes, was defined as the dark visual material located anteriorly or posteriorly to the already inserted line for disc height (Figure 3). Disc material protruding inferiorly or superiorly was included until visual delineation became indistinct, because alternative ways of distinguishing outlines of disc material and its segregation from adjacent longitudinal ligaments were all more challenging. A three-dimensional illustration of the approach for measuring and calculating structures is shown in Figure 2.

To avoid potential bias due to differences of equipment and software both raters used Apple 13" MacBooks with integrated touchpads. The free open-source measurement software OsiriX (version 4.1.2) was used by both raters. This version of OsiriX is designed for scientific use [73].

Data generated from length and volume measurements were stored as comma-separated values (CSV) files, using the OsiriX ROI plugin-tool 'export ROI'. CSV files were named with identification number, segment number, and the first and last section numbers of the MRI scan. In scans containing sections with fewer measurements of dural sac length, additional naming information was included. This naming added brackets following the initial

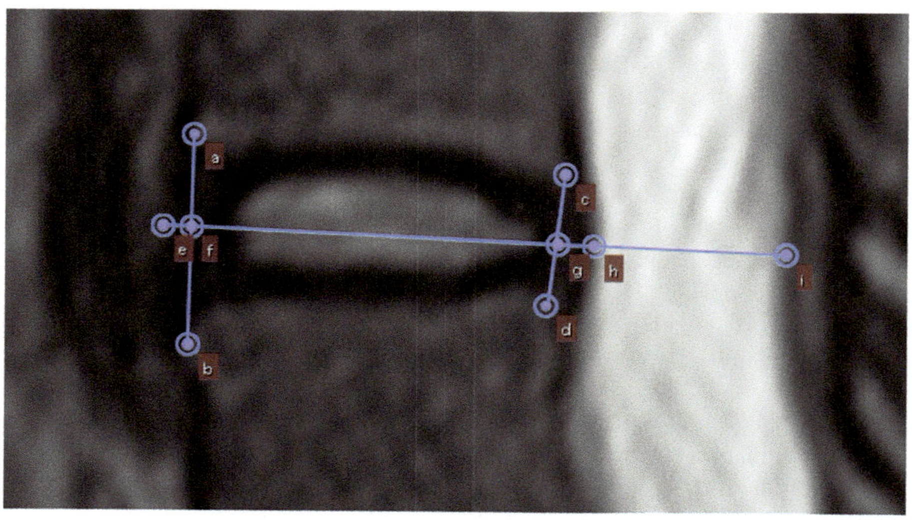

Figure 1 Positioning of measured structures (a-i); (a-b) Anterior intervertebral height; (c-d) Posterior intervertebral height; (e-f) Anterior disc material; (f-g) Intervertebral disc; (g-h) Posterior disc material; (h-i) Dural sac.

Table 1 Abbreviations and definitions for measurement parameters

Measurements & calculations	Definitions of measurement parameters	Details of measurement execution
Length measurements		
Anterior intervertebral height (AIVH)	Distance between anterior-superior and anterior-inferior corners at vertebrae located at relevant intervertebral disc	OsiriX 'length-tool' between most anterior point at superior corner and most anterior corner at inferior corner (Figure 1: a-b)
Posterior intervertebral height (PIVH)	Distance between posterior-superior and posterior-inferior corners at vertebrae located at relevant intervertebral disc	OsiriX 'length-tool' between most posterior point at superior corner and most posterior corner at inferior corner (Figure 1: c-d)
Intervertebral disc length (IVDL)	Distance between anterior and posterior boundaries of intervertebral disc	OsiriX 'length-tool' between midway of AIVH and midway of PIVH (Figure 1: f-g)
Anterior disc material length (ADML)	Distance between anterior and posterior boundaries of anterior herniated disc material	OsiriX 'length-tool' between most anterior located boundary of anterior disc material and midway of AIVH. Linear continuation of IVDL (Figure 1: e-f)
Posterior disc material length (PDML)	Distance between anterior and posterior boundaries of posterior herniated disc material	OsiriX 'length-tool' between midway of PIVH and most posterior located boundary of posterior disc material. Linear continuation of IVDL (Figure 1: g-h)
Antero-posterior dural sac length (ADSL)	Distance between anterior and posterior boundaries of dural sac	OsiriX 'length-tool' between most posterior located boundary of posterior disc material and most posterior located boundary of dural sac. Linear continuation of PDML (Figure 1: h-i)
Cross-sectional area (CSA) calculations		
CSA of anterior intervertebral height (CAIH)	Sum of areas estimated by the product of length measurements of anterior intervertebral height, slice thickness, and inter-slice gap distance (Figure 2a)	Calculation of CSA using all slices for AIVH length measurements. (Additional file 2: Calculating software)
CSA of posterior intervertebral height (CPIH)	Sum of areas estimated by product of length measurements of posterior intervertebral height, slice thickness, and interslice gap distance (Figure 2c)	Calculation of CSA using all slices for PIVH length measurements. (Additional file 2: Calculating software)
CSA of intervertebral disc (CIVD)	Sum of areas estimated by product of length measurements of intervertebral disc, slice thickness, and interslice gap distance (Figure 2b)	Calculation of CSA using all slices for IVDL length measurements. (Additional file 2: Calculating software)
CSA of anterior disc material (CADM)	Sum of areas estimated by product of length measurements of anterior disc material, slice thickness, and interslice gap distance	Calculation of CSA using all slices for ADML length measurements. (Additional file 2: Calculating software)
CSA of posterior disc material (CPDM)s	Sum of areas estimated by product of length measurements of posterior disc material, slice thickness, and interslice gap distance (Figure 2d)	Calculation of CSA using all slices for PDML length measurements. (Additional file 2: Calculating software)
CSA of dural sac (CDS)	Sum of areas estimated by product of length measurements of dural sac, slice thickness, and interslice gap distance	Calculation of CSA using all slices for ADSL length measurements. (Additional file 2: Calculating software)
Volume measurements		
Volume of anterior disc material (VADM)s	Calculated volume of anterior disc material, from tracing of sagittal areas in all slices	OsiriX 'pencil-tool' tracing area of anterior disc material anterior of AIVH at all chosen slices. Osirix 'Compute volume…' tool for volume read-out (Figure 3: a)
Volume of posterior disc material (VPDM)s	Calculated volume of posterior disc material, from tracing of sagittal areas in all slices	OsiriX'pencil-tool' tracing area of posterior disc material posterior of PIVH at all chosen slices. Osirix 'Compute volume…' tool for volume read-out (Figure 3: b)

Abbreviations used throughout the study, detailed definition of all measurement parameters, and details of measurement execution listed in sequence applied.

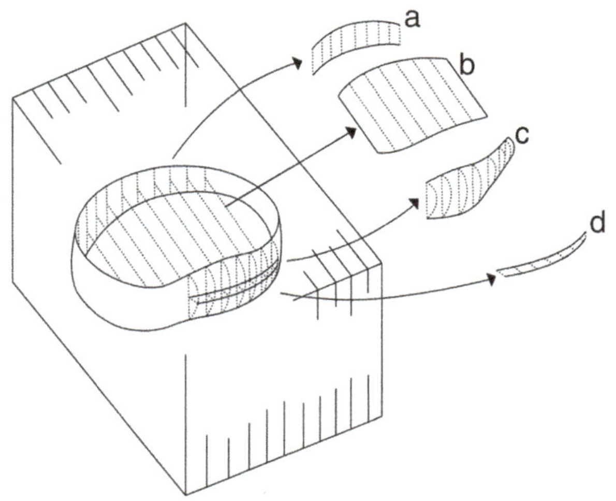

Figure 2 Schematic drawing of 3D cross-sectional areas (CSA) and volume of disc measures from sagittal image slices. a) CSA of anterior intervertebral height (AIVH), **b)** CSA of intervertebral disc (CIVD), **c)** Volume of posterior disc material (VPDM) and **d)** CSA of posterior disc material (CPDM).

section's numbers containing missing dural sac identifiers. CSV files were further converted into XLSX files and converted into spread-sheets by customised software (Additional file 2) designed specifically for this study by an engineer (SSC) at the Institute of Sports Science and Clinical Biomechanics at the University of Southern Denmark, Odense, Denmark. The customised software calculated the length from the X, Y coordinates from the measurements. Calculation of CSA included the number of slices measured slice thickness, as well as the interslice gap. The CSA of the anterior intervertebral height (CAIH) and the CSA of the posterior intervertebral height (CPIH) showed the CSA in the frontal plane and the remaining CSA in the axial plane (Figure 2).

Measurement data extracted by the custom-made software and stored in Excel were checked for consistency against the original ROI files supplied by OsiriX. All calculated results were screened for obvious errors by comparing them with the ROI files (Figure 4). Errors due to any altered order of measurements were manually corrected.

Blinding

To enhance the quality and applicability of the study, the raters were blinded in several ways [74]. Each rater was blinded to the findings of the other rater during measurements in the inter-rater analysis. In the intra-rater analysis, the rater was blinded to his own prior measurements. This was achieved by storing the data from the first measurement on a portable flash memory stick, which was stored by another project colleague. The order of participants was randomly changed between the two intra-rater measurement sessions. There was an 11-day interval between the first and second measurement sessions to lessen the likelihood of recognition of participants. All participants were anonymised for name, birth date, project ID, MRI access number, examination date, gender, and scan location.

Data analysis

An important issue when comparing measures is whether they are performed on the same slices. Therefore, we recorded all slice numbers and compared the raters' selections. The intra- and inter-rater agreement about the

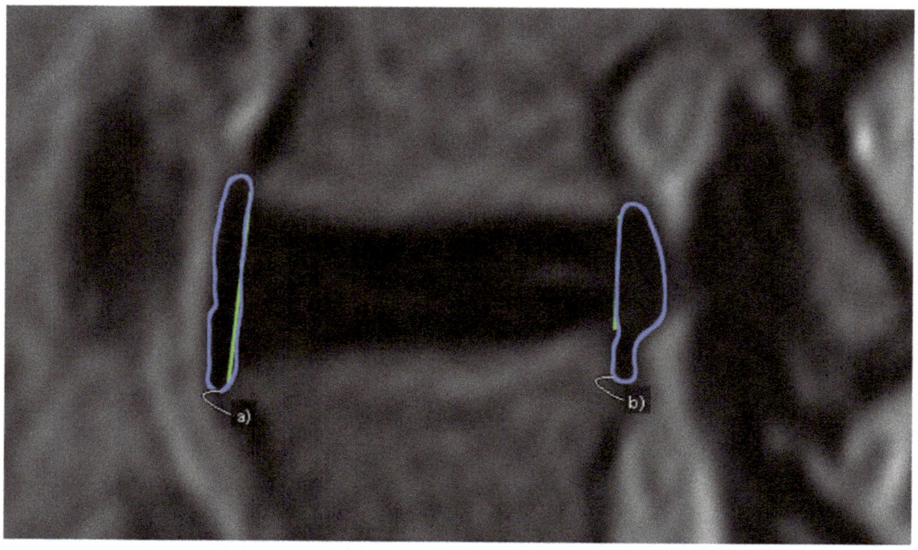

Figure 3 Illustration of outlining used for volume measurements. Outlining regions of interest in sagittal areas of **a)** anterior and **b)** posterior disc material. Volume calculated from combined areas from all slices, slice thickness, and interslice gaps. The pre-set boundary between the vertebral corners and visual boundaries completes the outlining.

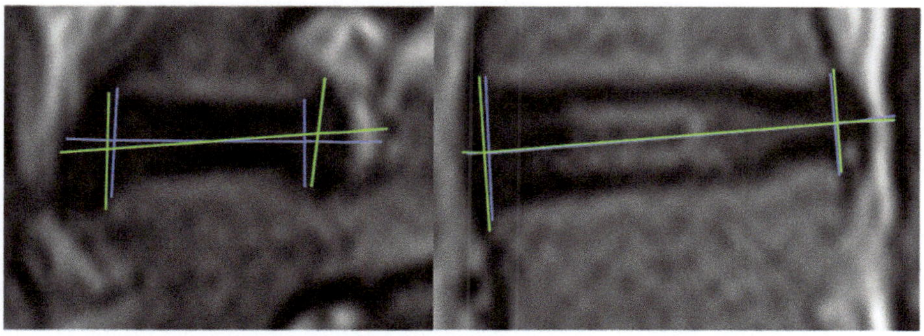

Figure 4 Examples of stored measurement images, used in data validation. Measurements stored as regions of interest during measurements were used for data validation. Single measurements were localised if needed and were checked against each other to ensure correct results. Images show a set of measurements with somewhat poor agreement between two measurements, and one with almost perfect agreement.

selection of the first (1, 2, 3 or 4) and last slice (6, 7, 8 or 9) for measuring sagittal images (disc parameters and dural sac), were analysed using weighted Kappa statistics and reported as weighted Kappa coefficients (K_w) with 95% CI. Since our focus was on the between-rater agreement of the measurements, we only compared measures that we performed on the same slice. For volume measurements and CSA calculations, the sets of data from all subjects where the start and end slice were not the same were excluded from the analysis.

The intra- and inter-rater agreement of the length and volume measurements, as well as the CSA calculations, were analysed using Bland & Altman's [41] LOA. LOA is based on graphical techniques and simple calculations, and provides a plot of differences between the means of the measures, a bias shown as the mean difference, as well as the SD of the differences. This enables the calculation of 95% LOA to define ranges within which most differences between measures will lie (Figure 5). The 95% CI was reported to describe the precision of the mean difference (bias). Bias was considered present if the 95% CI did not include zero. Examples of good and poor results are given in Figures 6 and 7.

Furthermore, LOA were presented as a proportion of mean values for each structure. The proportion was calculated as follows: ((upper LOA +(−1*(lower LOA))/the mean)*100. To the best of our knowledge, no reference standard for an acceptable cut-off proportion exists. Therefore, we arbitrarily considered percentages lower than 50% as an indicator of acceptable precision.

Intra- and inter-rater reliability was evaluated with ICC type 2.1 [75]. These statistical analyses were conducted with STATA statistical software package Version 12.1 [76].

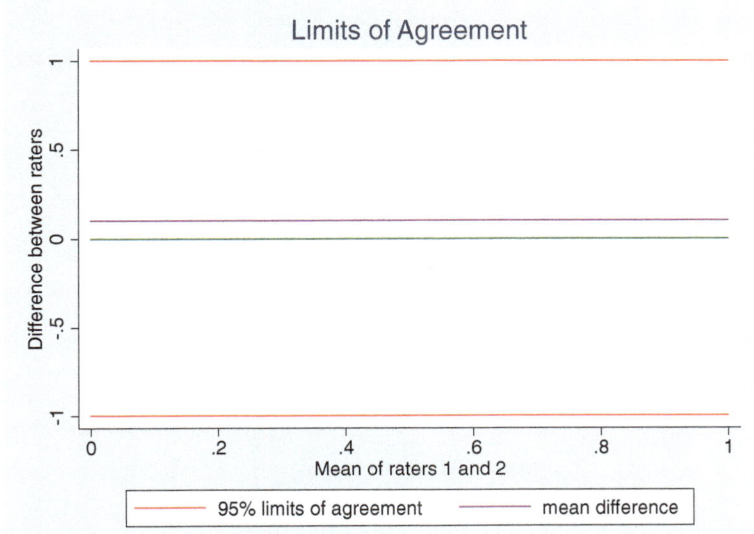

Figure 5 The Bland and Altman's plot. The y-axis shows the difference between raters' measurements, and the x-axis shows the mean value of both raters' measurements. The purple line shows the mean difference between measurements. Red lines show the 95% Limits of Agreement, between which 95% of all measurement differences are located.

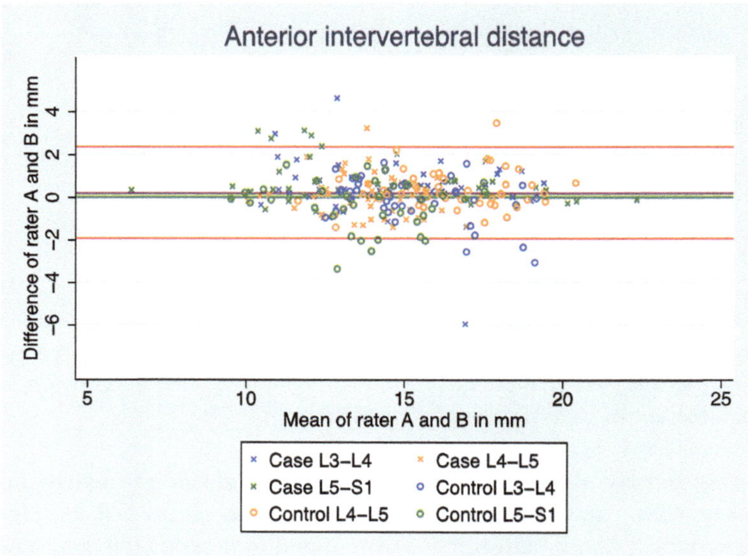

Figure 6 Bland and Altman's plot. Example of a good result for length of anterior intervertebral distance.

Sample size considerations

A Kappa power calculation using the formula $n=2k^2$ from Haas et al. [77] for four response option categories estimated a required sample size of 32 participants. For each participant, approximately eight measurements were made for each structure.

A post hoc estimation of the precision of the LOA was also performed based on the formula suggested by Bland and Altman [41,78] and the standard deviations from the current study. Based on this, the 95% CI for LOA was 0.21 times the standard deviation (SD) for the 257 length measurements (all < 0.26 mm), 0.69 times the SD for the 24 intra-rater CSA calculations (all < 13.2 mm^2), and 0.88 times the SD for the 15 inter-rater volume measurements (all < 262 mm^3). These figures indicate the sample size to be sufficient for acceptable precision of LOA for the length measures and the CSA measures but not the volume measures.

According to Bonett, an approximate sample of 15 is needed for estimating ICC with an expected coefficient of 0.9, an alpha level of 5%, a width of 0.2, and two categories [79]. The number of participants and measures exceeded that which was needed for satisfactory accuracy for evaluating reliability.

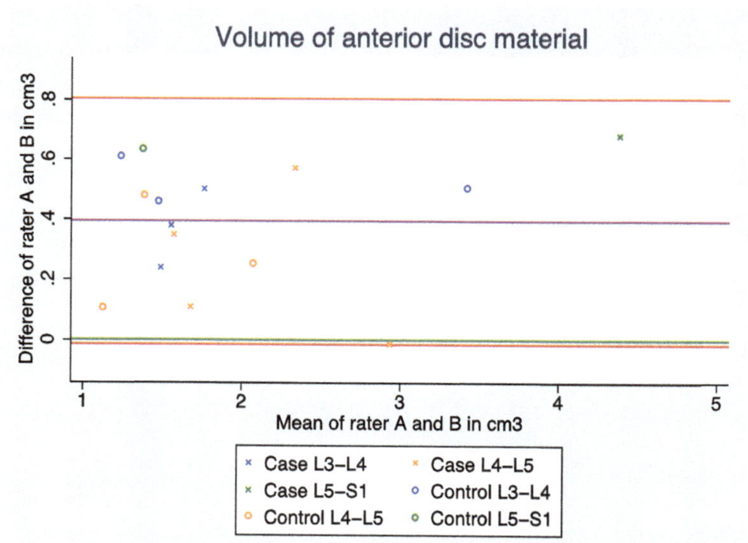

Figure 7 Bland and Altman's plot. Example of a poor result for volume of anterior disc material.

Factors that compromise agreement

After analysis, the graphs depicting LOA were examined and outliers identified by visually distinguishing measurement differences that were far above or below the LOA on the graphs. These measurements were compared with the ROI files to identify possible reasons for 'out of range' measurements and reported in a narrative form. An example of comparison is given in Figure 4.

Post hoc analysis

Due to poor inter-rater agreement on the start- and end-slices in the original analysis, a post-hoc re-analysis was undertaken. The definitions of the start- and end-slices were revised to include the requirement of visualisation of a full pedicle. This second inter-rater evaluation and weighted Kappa analysis of start- and end-slice for all structures, excluding the dural sac, were performed using the new criterion. Length and volume measurements were not repeated.

Results

Description of all measured parameters

In total, the lumbar MRIs from 32 participants were included in this study for evaluation of both intra- and inter-rater agreement and reliability. There were 17 females and 15 males, all aged between 40 and 49 years. Of all the measurements conducted, 10 were on segment level L3-L4, 12 on segment level L4-L5 and 10 on segment level L5-S1. Of all the available posteriorly located disc materials, 12 were classified as normal, 4 as bulged 5 as focal protrusions, 5 as broad-based protrusions, 5 as extrusions and 1 as sequestration.

Intra-rater agreement

Description of measured parameters

For length measurements, 258 slices were included in the analysis for each parameter. For CSA calculations and volume measurements, 24 participants were included in the analysis for each parameter and eight participants were excluded due to differing numbers of slices. The exception was for CSA calculation for ADSL, which included 25 participants in the analysis and similarly excluded seven participants due to differing numbers of slices.

Start- and end-slice on measurements

Weighted Kappa for the choice of start-slice on dural sac length measurements was (K_w (95% CI)): 0.84 (0.65 - 0.97) and on remaining structures (K_w (95% CI)): 0.82 (0.60 - 0.97)). Weighted Kappa for the end-slice on dural sac length measurements was (K_w (95% CI): 0.87 (0.71 - 0.97) and on all remaining structures was (K_w (95% CI): 0.71 (0.43 - 0.93)). Cross tabulations are available in Additional file 3.

Measurements of length

The mean difference of all length measurements ranged between −0.1 mm and 0.2 mm, with 95% CI ranging between −0.2 mm and 0.3 mm. LOA ranged between [−1.0; 1.0] mm and [−2.0; 2.3] mm, and between 6.8% and 62.9% of mean values (Table 2 and Additional file 4).

Estimation of cross-sectional area

The mean difference of all CSA calculations ranged between −3.8 mm^2 and 6.2 mm^2, with 95% CI ranging between −11.5 mm^2 and 14.3 mm^2. LOA ranged between [−21.3; 18.8] mm^2 and [−31.2; 43.7] mm^2, and between 3.6% and 40.1% of mean values (Table 2 and Additional file 4).

Measurements of volume

Mean differences for both volume measurements were −100 mm^3 and −47 mm^3, with 95% CI ranging between −204 mm^3 and 6 mm^3. LOA ranged between [293; 199] mm^3 and [−582; 382] mm^3, and between 37.3% and 45.1% of mean values (Table 2 and Additional file 4).

Intra-rater reliability

ICCs ranged from 0.90 (95% CI 0.88-0.92) to 0.99 (0.99-1.00) for length measurements and from 0.95 (0.89-0.98) to 1.00 (1.00-1.00) for CSAs. ICCs for measurement of volume were 0.95 (0.88-0.98) for anterior disc material and 0.95 (0.89-0.98) for posterior disc material (Table 3).

Inter-rater agreement

Description of measured parameters

For length measurements, 257 slices were included in the analysis for each parameter. For CSA calculations and volume measurements, 15 participants were included in the analysis for each parameter and 17 participants were excluded due to differing numbers of slices. The exception was the CSA calculation for ADSL, which included eight participants in the analysis and excluded 24 participants due to differing numbers of slices.

Start- and end-slice for measurements

Weighted Kappa for the choice of start-slice on dural sac length measurements was (K_w (95% CI): 0.22 (0.08 - 0.42) and on remaining structures was (K_w (95% CI): 0.35 (0.17 - 0.56)). Weighted Kappa for the choice of end-slice on dural sac length measurements was (K_w (95% CI): 0.22 (0.05 - 0.43) and on all remaining structures (K_w (95% CI): 0.37 (0.08 - 0.66)). *Post hoc* analysis for start- and end-slice on all structures except dural sac showed weighted Kappa for start- (K_w (95% CI): 0.56 (0.29 - 0.78)) and for end-slice (K_w (95% CI): 0.60 (0.35 - 0.81)). Cross tabulations are available in Additional file 3.

Table 2 Intra-rater measures agreement results

Measurement	n (slices)	Mean (mm)	Standard deviation (mm)	Mean difference (bias) [95% CI] (mm)	95% LOA (mm)	LOA as proportion of mean values (%)
Length - AIVH	258	14.7	1.1	0.2 [0.0; 0.3]	−2.0; 2.3	29.3
Length - PIVH	258	9.5	0.8	0.1 [0.0; 0.2]	−1.5; 1.6	32.6
Length - IVDL	258	31.1	0.5	−0.1 [−0.1; 0.0]	−1.1; 1.0	6.8
Length - ADML	258	3.5	0.6	0 [−0.1; 0.1]	−1.1; 1,1	62.9
Length - PDML	258	3.6	0.5	0 [−0.1; 0.1]	−1.0; 1.0	55.6
Length - ADSL	227	8.5	0.8	−0.1 [−0.2; 0.0]	−1.6; 1.4	35.3
	n (participants)	**(mm^2)**	**(mm^2)**	**(mm^2)**	**(mm^2)**	**(%)**
Area - CAIH	24	512.6	19.1	6.2 [−1.8; 14.3]	−31.2; 43.7	14.6
Area - CPIH	24	327.6	11.7	4.5 [−0.4; 9.4]	−18.4; 27.4	14.0
Area - CIVD	24	1101.3	10.2	−1.2 [−5.5; 3.1]	−21.3; 18.8	3.6
Area - CADM	24	118.8	10.2	1 [−3.3; 5.3]	−19.0; 21.1	33.8
Area - CPDM	24	121.8	12.5	−1.6 [−6.9; 3.7]	−26.0; 22.8	40.1
Area - CDS	25	267.9	18.6	−3.8 [−11.5; 3.9]	−40.3; 32.7	27.2
		(mm^3)	**(mm^3)**	**(mm^3)**	**(mm^3)**	**(%)**
Volume - VADM	24	2136.7	246	−100 [−204; 4]	−582; 382	45.1
Volume - VPDM	24	1314.8	126	−47 [−100; 6]	−293; 199	37.4

Number of slices measured for length, and participants measured for cross-sectional area and volume measurements, overall mean values, standard deviation, mean difference between measurements with 95% confidence intervals (CI), 95% limits of agreement (LOA), and LOA as a proportion of mean values. Due to absence of dural sac at certain otherwise measured slices, a lower number of slices were measured. Participants with unequal start- and end-slices were excluded from the analyses, leading to varying numbers of included participants.

Table 3 Intra-rater measures reliability results

Measurement	n (slices)	ICC [95% CI]
Length - AIVH	258	0.91 [0.88, 0.93]
Length - PIVH	258	0.90 [0.88, 0.92]
Length - IVDL	258	0.99 [0.99, 1.00]
Length - ADML	258	0.95 [0.94, 0.96]
Length - PDML	258	0.94 [0.92, 0.95]
Length - ADSL	227	0.98 [0.98, 0.99]
	n (participants)	
Area – CAIH	24	0.99 [0.98, 1.00]
Area – CPIH	24	0.98 [0.96, 0.99]
Area - CIVD	24	1.00 [1.00, 1.00]
Area - CADM	24	0.97 [0.94, 0.99]
Area - CPDM	24	0.95 [0.89, 0.98]
Area - CDS	25	0.97 [0.93, 0.99]
Volume - VADM	24	0.95 [0.89, 0.98]
Volume - VPDM	24	0.95 [0.88, 0.98]

Number of slices measured for length and participants measured for cross-sectional area and volume measurements, intraclass correlation coefficient (ICC), and accompanying 95% confidence intervals (CI). Due to absence of dural sac at certain otherwise measured slices, a lower number of slices were measured. Participants with unequal start- and end-slices were excluded from the analyses, leading to varying numbers of included participants.

Measurements of length

The mean difference of all length measurements ranged between −0.7 mm and 0.3 mm, with 95% CI ranging between −0.8 mm and 0.4 mm. LOA ranged between [−1.1; 1.4] mm and [−2.6; 2.0] mm, and between 9.7% and 105.9% of mean values (Table 4 and Additional file 4).

Estimation of cross-sectional area

The mean difference for all CSA calculations ranged between −19.5 mm^2 and 6.4 mm^2, with 95% CI ranging between −31.7 mm^2 and 19.7 mm^2. LOA ranged between [−10.8; 16.4] mm^2 and [−64.6; 27.1] mm^2, and between 4.5% and 48.4% of mean values (Table 4 and Additional file 4).

Measurements of volume

Mean differences were 131 mm^3 and 392 mm^3, with 95% CI ranging between −33 mm^3 and 508 mm^3. LOA ranged between [−17; 801] mm^3 and [−450; 713] mm^3, and between 44.7% and 104.1% of mean values (Table 4 and Additional file 4).

Inter-rater reliability

ICCs ranged from 0.73 (0.69-0.79) to 0.98 (0.90-0.99) for length measurements and from 0.88 (0.69-0.96) to 0.99 (0.97-1.00) for CSAs. ICCs for measurement of volume were 0.57 (0.13-0.83) for anterior disc material and 0.90 (0.00-0.98) for posterior disc material (Table 5).

Table 4 Inter-rater measures agreement results

Measurement	n (slices)	Mean (mm)	Standard deviation (mm)	Mean difference (bias) [95% CI] (mm)	95% Limits of agreement (LOA) (mm)	LOA as proportion of mean values (%)
Length - AIVH	257	14.9	1.2	−0.5 [−0.7; −0.4]	−2.8; 1.8	30.9
Length - PIVH	257	9.6	1.2	−0.3 [−0.4; −0.2]	−2.6; 2.0	47.9
Length - IVDL	257	31.2	0.8	−0.7 [−0.8; −0.6]	−2.2; 0.8	9.7
Length - ADML	257	3.4	0.6	0.1 [0.0; 0.2]	−1.1; 1.4	73.6
Length - PDML	257	3.4	0.9	0.3 [−0.2; 0.4]	−1.5; 2.1	105.9
Length - ADSL	229	8	1.1	0.2 [0.0; 0.3]	−2.0; 2.3	53.8
	n (participants)	**(mm2)**	**(mm^2)**	**(mm^2)**	**(mm^2)**	**(%)**
Area - CAIH	15	568.2	23.4	−18.7 [−31.7; −5.7]	−64.6; 27.1	16.2
Area - CPIH	15	362.8	17.3	−13.3 [−22.9; −3.7]	−47.3; 20.7	18.7
Area - CIVD	15	1190.4	13.7	−19.5 [−27.1; −11.9]	−46.4; 7.4	4.5
Area - CADM	15	126.2	7	2.8 [−1.1; 6.7]	−10.8; 16.4	21.6
Area - CPDM	15	121.7	15	6.4 [−2.0; 14.7]	−23.1; 35.8	48.4
Area - CDS	8	286	17.8	4.8 [−10.1; 19.7]	−30.1; 39.8	24.4
		(mm^3)	**(mm^3)**	**(mm^3)**	**(mm^3)**	**(%)**
Volume - VADM	15	1830.3	209	392 [277; 508]	−17; 801	44.7
Volume - VPDM	15	1117.6	297	131 [−33; 296]	−450; 713	104.1

Number of slices measured for length and participants measured for cross-sectional area and volume measurements, overall mean values, standard deviation, mean difference between measurements (bias) with 95% confidence intervals (CI), 95% limits of agreement (LOA), and LOA as a proportion of mean values. Due to absence of dural sac at certain otherwise measured slices, a lower number of slices were measured. Participants with unequal start- and end-slices were excluded from the analyses, leading to varying numbers of included participants.

Bias estimates

The 95% CI for mean differences suggested no statistically significant bias for intra-rater measures, and suggested a possible significant bias in a negative direction for seven out of 14 inter-rater parameters.

Factors that compromise agreement

A total of 27 outliers consisting of single intra-rater measurements and 20 outliers consisting of single inter-rater measurements were seen from the LOA plots. Three reasons were identified:

1) A different interpretation of vertebral corners at both the anterior and posterior locations, as well as superior and inferior locations was the reason for seven AIVH and PIVH outliers, nine IVDL outliers, one ADML outlier, and three PDML outliers. This may have been the reason for the IVDL and PDML outliers due to their dependence on AIVH and PIVH measurements.
2) Inconsistent distinction between structural boundaries due to lack of contrast was identified as inherent in three separate causes for outliers. The first was that five outliers were caused by a different interpretation of the anterior boundary of ADML. The second was that six outliers were caused by a different interpretation of the boundary between PDML and ADSL. The third was that fifteen outliers

Table 5 Inter-rater measures reliability results

Measurement	n (slices)	ICC [95% CI]
Length - AIVH	257	0.88 [0.82 – 0.92]
Length - PIVH	257	0.81 [0.76 – 0.85]
Length - IVDL	257	0.98 [0.90 – 0.99]
Length - ADML	257	0.93 [0.91 – 0.95]
Length - PDML	257	0.73 [0.64 – 0.79]
Length - ADSL	229	0.96 [0.95 – 0.97]
	n (participants)	
Area - CAIH	15	0.96 [0.81 – 0.99]
Area - CPIH	15	0.93 [0.68 – 0.98]
Area - CIVD	15	0.99 [0.78 – 1.00]
Area - CADM	15	0.99 [0.97 – 1.00]
Area - CPDM	15	0.88 [0.69 – 0.96]
Area - CDS	8	0.95 [0.79 – 0.99]
Volume - VADM	15	0.90 [0.00 – 0.98]
Volume - VPDM	15	0.57 [0.13 – 0.83]

Number of slices measured for length and participants measured for cross-sectional area and volume measurements, intraclass correlation coefficient (ICC), and accompanying 95% confidence intervals (CI). Due to absence of dural sac at certain otherwise measured slices, a lower number of slices were measured. Participants with unequal start- and end-slices were excluded from the analyses, leading to varying numbers of included participants.

were caused by a different interpretation of the posterior boundary of ADSL.
3) A single outlier for each of IVDL, ADML, PDML and ADSL was identified as an error in measurement execution. These errors were included in the CSAs and therefore influenced their results.

Discussion

This study reports a new method for measuring lumbar disc-related structures for use in research and in clinical practice. Intra-rater reliability in selecting start- and end-slice was substantial and inter-rater reliability changed from poor to moderate after revision of the method [80]. The Bland and Altman's LOA showed very little bias (mean difference) and a small range for all intra-rater measurements and calculations. Reliability was high with most ICCs > 0.90. For inter-rater measurements and calculations the Bland and Altman's LOA showed slightly higher bias and slightly higher ranges, with the exception of volume measurements, which had considerably larger bias and ranges. Reliability was slightly lower but most ICCs were > 0.73. The uncertainty around volume measures was considerable. In general, LOA as a percentage of the mean values gradually decreased with increased size of the measured structures.

The results indicate that when measuring very small structures (e.g. ADML and PDML) on MRI, the changes over time have to be relatively large in order to detect changes. Combining length measures into volume measures reduces the LOA as a proportion of the mean. The measurement of volume by manual tracing seems to be dependent on the observer and the VPDM seems to be particularly problematic to agree upon.

The intra-rater measurements and calculations showed better agreement than inter-rater measurements, although the differences were not large. This indicates a good consensus regarding the anatomical delineation between length measurements by the same rater, but also acceptable consensus between the two raters. The same does not apply with volume measurements, where the inter-rater agreement was not acceptable. It seems the cumulative error in the marking of multiple anatomical structures was not accurate enough between multiple raters, resulting in differences that were unacceptably high. The same applies for start- and end-slice, where it seems agreement between raters is poor unless sufficient consensus on measurements is made beforehand. This appears to be due to difficulty in determining the slice delineating the boundary of the foramina, when using the criterion of visualisation of a fully visible pedicle, a criterion previously described in the literature [81].

Outliers found during the validation of the results could generally be traced to two main reasons: one being inexact positioning of vertebral corners; the other being difficulties in distinguishing between the anterior or posterior boundaries between structures. As for positioning of vertebral corners, a possible interfering factor could be the presence of osteophytes, by their modifying the visual appearance of the vertebra. For future use of this method, specification in advance of measurements, and persistent implementation of detailed definitions for aforementioned positionings, should be conducted by all raters. We were not able to find articles that definitively discussed any of these factors regarding similar problems with positioning or boundary distinction. Videman et al. [82] previously used a more thorough method for defining 'theoretical' vertebral corners. However, such an approach is likely to be more complicated and time-consuming.

A similar method of measuring the spinal canal was performed by Dora et al. [8]. They used sagittal MRIs and ICC and reported good inter-rater reliability (ICC>0.95). Other studies have used similar methods for measuring the spinal canal or the dural sac, but have not documented any kind of reproducibility [9,28,63,68,69]. A similar method is also used for measuring disc herniations and the spinal canal in some studies [27-29], but the method is described inadequately, and there is no reporting of analysis of agreement or reliability. One study performed similar quantitative measurements of similar structures on MRIs using LOA for determining agreement [48]. In this study, one finding on intervertebral disc length is comparable with the current study and indicates similar LOA. That study sample consisted of children and therefore their population was not directly comparable with ours. A study that compared results of MRIs in different positions showed anteriorly and posteriorly herniated disc material length measurements with almost exactly the same values [83]. A direct comparison with other studies is difficult, as this is the first study, to our knowledge, with the current statistical approach and such a detailed description of the method.

Agreement, together with reliability, is generally embedded in the expression reproducibility. In the literature, agreement and reliability are often used interchangeably, although their foci are different. Agreement focuses on measurement error when the focus is change in health status over time, while reliability is concerned with measurement error plus the variability between study objects and the focus is distinction between persons [45]. deVet et al. recommend reporting agreement parameters such as LOA, and further, when reporting reliability using ICC, they should be reported together with error estimates such as SEM [45]. This study uses both agreement and reliability, but the clear distinction between their use and meaning has been preserved.

Our review of the available literature (Additional file 1) showed a common pattern in methodological limitations through the use of inappropriate methods for longitudinal measurements, inadequate descriptions of methods, as well as unsatisfying statistical analyses of agreement. Out of 34 studies, only 17 reported reproducibility, and only one of these studies [48] used an appropriate statistical method – in that case, LOA. Eight of the remaining studies [8,33,34,38,48,52,55,57] used ICC, which is a measure of reliability, not agreement [45]. Furthermore, only one out of these eight studies reported an error estimate [55].

We interpret our results as indicating that the measurement method used in this study is suitable for further use, with the exception of volume measurements. The method also makes it possible to validate data regarding errors made during measurements and those made during calculations, as well as indications for how to correct relevant errors in advance of the analysis. This data validation method may also be used for localising the reasons for outliers. As seen in the post-hoc analysis, a focus on consensus between raters is important for obtaining agreement about start- and end-slices. Our study is likely to be useful for future research because the method is appropriate for longitudinal measurements it contains a full and detailed description of the method and includes adequately conducted agreement and reliability analyses. In future studies and in clinical practice, this method can be used to detect changes larger than the LOA in disc morphology over time in individuals and between groups of patients. However, the size of the measure of interest has to be considered, since the relative precision increases with the size of the measurement (LOA as a percentage of the mean, Tables 2 and 4). In our research group, this method will form the basis for a series of research projects with the aims of investigating the changes in disc morphology over time and their association with clinical outcomes.

There could be a number of reasons for the observed poor agreement of inter-rater volume measurements. A possible explanation is a lack of certainty when manually tracing the anterior and posterior herniated disc material – an issue reported in earlier studies addressing volume measurements using MRIs [84,85]. Another explanation is a possible difficulty in separating herniated disc material from the longitudinal ligament, as these structures appear with almost the same signal intensity on MRI.

One limitation of this study may be the low resolution of the MRIs and the high magnification levels used. With a 144×256 matrix, 300 mm field of view and 4 mm slice thickness [49], the DICOM reader software digitally reconstructed the high detail of anatomical structures visible on the MRIs. This, in addition to the high magnification levels, increases the measurement precision but may reduce the accuracy of the image's representativeness of the actual anatomy. Any length measurement below the size of one voxel (1.2(height) × 1.4(width) × 4.0(depth) mm) could therefore be considered relatively inaccurate. As for the length measurements of the anterior and posterior herniated disc material, there is a possibility that most of the anterior or posterior position is above or below the measured level, leading to possible underestimation of disc material sizes. Furthermore, as this study is not a test-retest study, it does not take into account the measurement errors that would be associated with repositioning patients, diurnal variations and the effect of activities within its estimates of intra- and inter-rater reliability.

The original study cohort was representative of the general population but the selection of a sample of cases and controls for the current study may affect the generalisability of the results. The reported means of measurements will not reflect those of the original cohort since only 22-25% in it had LDH. Although the prevalence of LDH, especially the more severe types, is likely to be higher in a clinical population, we believe that the measurement method will work in clinical populations. Our aim was to establish reproducibility and reliability, not to report prevalence or reference values for either a general or a clinical population.

It is possible that the ICCs and weighted Kappa values are inflated in this study, due to the large variability in the measures when purposefully selecting a sample representative of all types of LDH and of controls without LDH. The results may also be inflated by excluding a number of the more lateral MRI slices, when there was disagreement on start- and end-slice. The reason for this is that the LOA were relatively smaller for the larger structures. Another factor that may have increased the reproducibility and reliability is that only two raters were performing the measurements. However, when comparing ICCs in our study with those in other studies using the same measure of reliability, the results were very similar [8,34,38].

In this study, we have performed several statistical analyses with an alpha level of 5% which by definition increases the risk of at least one chance finding in every twenty tests. However, the trends for the LOA and the ICCs are all in the same direction for the included measures. The variability in lumbar levels, LDH and normal discs in the study sample could lead to a suspicion that the LOA would be different for certain subgroups. However, in the Bland and Altman's LOA plots (Additional file 4), colours indicate the different levels as well as cases and controls. And when looking carefully at these, there are no obvious differences.

The strengths of this study are the high number of single length measurements, the carefully planned execution, the extensive review of the available literature as well as the well-described method. The high number of length measurements is also the basis for the CSAs. This study also followed a structured protocol from the beginning and adhered throughout to guidelines for studies of agreement [44,74]. Finally a comprehensive description of the method is available, as is the freeware measurement software [73]. This method also only takes 5 to 20 minutes per MRI to measure and interpret, depending on equipment, software preparation, and experience. In a clinical setting, a selection of relevant parameters such as CPDM, CPIH, and CDS may reduce the time consumption considerably.

Conclusion

This new method of quantifying length measurements of disc morphology and dural sac diameter from MRIs showed good intra- and inter-rater agreement as well as reliability. Quantitative volume measurements showed unacceptable agreement and reliability. However, caution should be taken when selecting start- and end-slice, measuring very small structures, and when defining anatomical landmarks. This method for quantitative measurement of lumbar intervertebral discs and related structures is suitable for testing in broader contexts, including in more diverse clinical samples, and in quantitative research that involves serial measurement of anatomical structures over multiple follow-up time periods.

Additional files

Additional file 1: Literature review.

Additional file 2: Description of calculating software (computer program available from the authors on request).

Additional file 3: Cross tabulations for start- and end-slices.

Additional file 4: Graphs of limits of agreement.

Abbreviations

ADML: Anterior disc material length; ADSL: Antero-posterior dural sac length; AIVH: Anterior intervertebral height; AT: Andreas Tunset; BSc: Bachelor of Science; CADM: Cross-sectional area of anterior disc material; CAIH: Cross-sectional area of anterior intervertebral height; CDS: Cross-sectional area of dural sac; CI: Confidence interval; CIVD: Cross-sectional area of intervertebral disc; CPDM: Cross-sectional area of posterior disc material; CPIH: Cross-sectional area of posterior intervertebral height; CSA: Cross-sectional area; CSV: Comma separated values; DICOM: Digital imaging and communities in medicine; ICC: Intra-class correlation coefficient; ID: Identification; IVDL: Intervertebral disc length; K_w: Weighted Kappa; LBP: Low back pain; LDH: Lumbar Disc Herniation; LOA: Limits of agreement; MRI: Magnetic resonance imaging; MSc: Master of Science; PDML: Posterior disc material length; PhD: Doctor of Philosophy; PIVH: Posterior intervertebral height; PK: Per Kjaer; ROI: Region of interest; SSC: Shadi Samir Chreiteh; T: Tesla; TSJ: Tue Secher Jensen; VADM: Volume of anterior disc material; VPDM: Volume of posterior disc material.

Competing interests

There are no competing interests among authors.

Authors' contributions

AT, PK and TSJ developed the concept and design and administered the study, developed the method used in the study, performed the analysis and drafted the manuscript. AT and TSJ conducted all intra- and inter-rater measurements. SSC developed the software for calculating the data. AT drafted the manuscript. PK and TSJ reviewed the manuscript several times. All authors approved the manuscript in its final form.

Authors' information

An additional list of each author's qualifications and affiliations is available at the start of the article. This study is part of the undergraduate research education of a Master program in Clinical Biomechanics being undertaken by AT.

Acknowledgements

The Faculty of Health Sciences at The University of Southern Denmark granted a scholarship for execution of the undergraduate research education for AT. The Chiropractic Fund for Research and Postgraduate Education financially supported this study. The authors wish to thank Professor Tom Bendix for his role in designing the original study and securing primary funding from the Industrial Insurance Company, now Topdanmark. We also thank Professor Claus Manniche and The Spine Centre of Southern Denmark for hosting the entire project and, in particular, for making the third data collection possible by supplying secretarial support and providing imaging of the participants. Finally, we thank Annette Wille for completing the artwork for Figure 2.

Author details

[1]Department of Sports Science and Clinical Biomechanics, University of Southern Denmark, Campusvej 55, Odense M DK-5230, Denmark. [2]Research Department, Spine Centre of Southern Denmark, Lillebaelt Hospital, Oestre Hougvej 55, Middelfart DK-5500, Denmark. [3]DELTA, Venlighedsvej 4, Hørsholm DK-2970, Denmark.

References

1. Mixter WJ, Barr JS: **Rupture of the Intervertebral Disc with Involvement of the Spinal Canal.** *N Engl J Med* 1934, **211**(5):210–215.
2. Casey E: **Natural history of radiculopathy.** *Phys Med Rehabil Clin N Am* 2011, **22**(1):1–5.
3. Konstantinou KDK: **Sciatica – Review of epidemiological studies and prevalence estimates.** *Spine* 2008, **33**(22):2464–2472.
4. Jensen TS, Albert HB, Soerensen JS, Manniche C, Leboeuf-Yde C: **Natural course of disc morphology in patients with sciatica - An MRI study using a standardized qualitative classification system.** *Spine* 2006, **31**(24):1605–1612.
5. Endean APK, Coggon D: **Potential of magnetic resonance imaging findings to refine case definition for mechanical low back pain in epidemiological studies: a systematic review.** *Spine* 2011, **36**(2):160–169.
6. Renowden SA: **Normal anatomy of the spinal cord.** *Pract Neurol* 2012, **12**(6):367–370.
7. Carragee EJ, Kim DH: **A prospective analysis of magnetic resonance imaging findings in patients with sciatica and lumbar disc herniation. Correlation of outcomes with disc fragment and canal morphology.** *Spine (Phila Pa 1976)* 1997, **22**(14):1650–1660.
8. Dora C, Walchli B, Elfering A, Gal I, Weishaupt D, Boos N: **The significance of spinal canal dimensions in discriminating symptomatic from asymptomatic disc herniations.** *Eur Spine J* 2002, **11**(6):575–581.
9. Visuri T, Ulaska J, Eskelin M, Pulkkinen P: **Narrowing of lumbar spinal canal predicts chronic low back pain more accurately than intervertebral disc degeneration: a magnetic resonance imaging study in young Finnish male conscripts.** *Mil Med* 2005, **170**(11):926–930.
10. Pneumaticos SG, Hipp JA, Esses SI: **Sensitivity and specificity of dural sac and herniated disc dimensions in patients with low back-related leg pain.** *J Magn Reson Imaging* 2000, **12**(3):439–443.
11. O'Neill C, Kurgansky M, Kaiser J, Lau W: **Accuracy of MRI for diagnosis of discogenic pain.** *Pain physician* 2008, **11**(3):311–326.
12. Luoma K, Riihimaki H, Luukkonen R, Raininko R, Viikari-Juntura E, Lamminen A: **Low back pain in relation to lumbar disc degeneration.** *Spine (Phila Pa 1976)* 2000, **25**(4):487–492.
13. Wong-Chung JK, Naseeb SA, Kaneker SG, Aradi AJ: **Anterior disc protrusion as a cause for abdominal symptoms in childhood discitis. A case report.** *Spine (Phila Pa 1976)* 1999, **24**(9):918–920.
14. Weber H, Holme I, Amlie E: **The natural course of acute sciatica with nerve root symptoms in a double-blind placebo-controlled trial evaluating the effect of piroxicam.** *Spine (Phila Pa 1976)* 1993, **18**(11):1433–1438.
15. Saal JA, Saal JS: **Nonoperative treatment of herniated lumbar intervertebral disc with radiculopathy. An outcome study.** *Spine (Phila Pa 1976)* 1989, **14**(4):431–437.

16. Weber H: **Lumbar disc herniation. A controlled, prospective study with ten years of observation.** *Spine (Phila Pa 1976)* 1983, **8**(2):131–140.
17. Hakelius A: **Prognosis in sciatica. A clinical follow-up of surgical and non-surgical treatment.** *Acta orthopaedica Scandinavica Supplementum* 1970, **129:**1–76.
18. Jacobs WC, van Tulder M, Arts M, Rubinstein SM, van Middelkoop M, Ostelo R, Verhagen A, Koes B, Peul WC: **Surgery versus conservative management of sciatica due to a lumbar herniated disc: a systematic review.** *Eur Spine J* 2011, **20**(4):513–522.
19. van Tulder M, Peul W, Koes B: **Sciatica: what the rheumatologist needs to know.** *Nat Rev Rheumatol* 2010, **6**(3):139–145.
20. Suri P, Hunter DJ, Jouve C, Hartigan C, Limke J, Pena E, Li L, Luz J, Rainville J: **Nonsurgical treatment of lumbar disk herniation: are outcomes different in older adults?** *J Am Geriatr Soc* 2011, **59**(3):423–429.
21. Weinstein JN, Lurie JD, Tosteson TD, Tosteson AN, Blood EA, Abdu WA, Herkowitz H, Hilibrand A, Albert T, Fischgrund J: **Surgical versus nonoperative treatment for lumbar disc herniation: four-year results for the Spine Patient Outcomes Research Trial (SPORT).** *Spine* 2008, **33**(25):2789–2800.
22. Kohlboeck G, Greimel KV, Piotrowski WP, Leibetseder M, Krombholz-Reindl M, Neuhofer R, Schmid A, Klinger R: **Prognosis of multifactorial outcome in lumbar discectomy: a prospective longitudinal study investigating patients with disc prolapse.** *Clin J Pain* 2004, **20**(6):455–461.
23. Azimi P, Mohammadi HR, Montazeri A: **An outcome measure of functionality and pain in patients with lumbar disc herniation: a validation study of the Japanese Orthopedic Association (JOA) score.** *J Orthop Sci* 2012, **17**(4):341–345.
24. Ng LC, Sell P: **Outcomes of a prospective cohort study on peri-radicular infiltration for radicular pain in patients with lumbar disc herniation and spinal stenosis.** *Eur Spine J* 2004, **13**(4):325–329.
25. Saal JA, Saal JS, Herzog RJ: **The natural history of lumbar intervertebral disc extrusions treated nonoperatively.** *Spine* 1990, **15**(7):683–686.
26. Modic MT, Obuchowski NA, Ross JS, Brant-Zawadzki MN, Grooff PN, Mazanec DJ, Benzel EC: **Acute low back pain and radiculopathy: MR imaging findings and their prognostic role and effect on outcome.** *Radiology* 2005, **237**(2):597–604.
27. Kato F, Mimatsu K, Kawakami N, Iwata H, Miura T: **Serial changes observed by magnetic resonance imaging in the intervertebral disc after chemonucleolysis. A consideration of the mechanism of chemonucleolysis.** *Spine* 1992, **17**(8):934–939.
28. Yukawa Y, Kato F, Matsubara Y, Kajino G, Nakamura S, Nitta H: **Serial magnetic resonance imaging follow-up study of lumbar disc herniation conservatively treated for average 30 months: relation between reduction of herniation and degeneration of disc.** *J Spinal Disord* 1996, **9**(3):251–256.
29. Masui T, Yukawa Y, Nakamura S, Kajino G, Matsubara Y, Kato F, Ishiguro N: **Natural history of patients with lumbar disc herniation observed by magnetic resonance imaging for minimum 7 years.** *J Spinal Disord Tech* 2005, **18**(2):121–126.
30. Malko JA, Hutton WC, Fajman WA: **An in vivo magnetic resonance imaging study of changes in the volume (and fluid content) of the lumbar intervertebral discs during a simulated diurnal load cycle.** *Spine* 1999, **24**(10):1015–1022.
31. Holodny AI, Kisza PS, Contractor S, Liu WC: **Does a herniated nucleus pulposus contribute significantly to a decrease in height of the intervertebral disc? Quantitative volumetric MRI.** *Neuroradiology* 2000, **42**(6):451–454.
32. Violas P, Estivalèzes E, Pédrono A, Sales De Gauzy J, Sévely A, Swider P: **A method to investigate intervertebral disc morphology from MRI in early idiopathic scoliosis: a preliminary evaluation in a group of 14 patients.** *Magn Reson Imaging* 2005, **23**(3):475–479.
33. Autio RA, Karppinen J, Niinimäki J, Ojala R, Kurunlahti M, Haapea M, Vanharanta H, Tervonen O: **Determinants of spontaneous resorption of intervertebral disc herniations.** *Spine* 2006, **31**(11):1247–1252.
34. Hamanishi C, Matukura N, Fujita M, Tomihara M, Tanaka S: **Cross-sectional area of the stenotic lumbar dural tube measured from the transverse views of magnetic resonance imaging.** *J Spinal Disord* 1994, **7**(5):388–393.
35. Carlisle E, Luna M, Tsou PM, Wang JC: **Percent spinal canal compromise on MRI utilized for predicting the need for surgical treatment in single-level lumbar intervertebral disc herniation.** *Spine J* 2005, **5**(6):608–614.
36. Zaaroor M, Kosa G, Peri-Eran A, Maharil I, Shoham M, Goldsher D: **Morphological study of the spinal canal content for subarachnoid endoscopy.** *Minim Invasive Neurosurg* 2006, **49**(4):220–226.
37. Grams AE, Gempt J, Forschler A: **Comparison of spinal anatomy between 3-Tesla MRI and CT-myelography under healthy and pathological conditions.** *Surg Radiol Anat* 2010, **32**(6):581–585.
38. Ogura H, Miyamoto K, Fukuta S, Naganawa T, Shimizu K: **Comparison of magnetic resonance imaging and computed tomography-myelography for quantitative evaluation of lumbar intracanalar cross-section.** *Yonsei Med J* 2011, **52**(1):137–144.
39. Zaki R, Bulgiba A, Ismail R, Ismail NA: **Statistical methods used to test for agreement of medical instruments measuring continuous variables in method comparison studies: a systematic review.** *PloS one* 2012, **7**(5):e37908.
40. Hanneman SK: **Design, analysis, and interpretation of method-comparison studies.** *AACN Adv Crit Care* 2008, **19**(2):223–234.
41. Bland JM, Altman DG: **Statistical methods for assessing agreement between two methods of clinical measurement.** *Lancet* 1986, **1**(8476):307–310.
42. McAlinden C, Khadka J, Pesudovs K: **Statistical methods for conducting agreement (comparison of clinical tests) and precision (repeatability or reproducibility) studies in optometry and ophthalmology.** *Ophthalmic Physiol Opt* 2011, **31**(4):330–338.
43. Chatburn RL: **Evaluation of instrument error and method agreement.** *AANA J* 1996, **64**(3):261–268.
44. Kottner J, Audige L, Brorson S, Donner A, Gajewski BJ, Hrobjartsson A, Roberts C, Shoukri M, Streiner DL: **Guidelines for Reporting Reliability and Agreement Studies (GRRAS) were proposed.** *Int J Nurs Stud* 2011, **48**(6):661–671.
45. de Vet HC, Terwee CB, Knol DL, Bouter LM: **When to use agreement versus reliability measures.** *J Clin Epidemiol* 2006, **59**(10):1033–1039.
46. Atkinson G, Nevill AM: **Statistical methods for assessing measurement error (reliability) in variables relevant to sports medicine.** *Sports Med* 1998, **26**(4):217–238.
47. Belavy DL, Armbrecht G, Felsenberg D: **Evaluation of lumbar disc and spine morphology: long-term repeatability and comparison of methods.** *Physiol Meas* 2012, **33**(8):1313–1321.
48. Masharawi Y, Kjaer P, Bendix T, Manniche C, Wedderkopp N, Sorensen JS, Peled N, Jensen TS: **The reproducibility of quantitative measurements in lumbar magnetic resonance imaging of children from the general population.** *Spine* 2008, **33**(19):2094–2100.
49. Kjaer P, Leboeuf-Yde C, Korsholm L, Sorensen JS, Bendix T: **Magnetic resonance imaging and low back pain in adults: a diagnostic imaging study of 40-year-old men and women.** *Spine* 2005, **30**(10):1173–1180.
50. Solgaard Sorensen J, Kjaer P, Jensen ST, Andersen P: **Low-field magnetic resonance imaging of the lumbar spine: reliability of qualitative evaluation of disc and muscle parameters.** *Acta Radiol* 2006, **47**(9):947–953.
51. Zhao L, Qu DB, Jin DD: **Lumbar MRI measurement in normal adults and its clinical relevance.** *Chin J Clin Rehabil* 2004, **8**(20):4112–4113.
52. Cooley JR, Danielson CD, Schultz GD, Hall TA: **Posterior disk displacement: morphologic assessment and measurement reliability-lumbar spine.** *J Manipulative Physiol Ther* 2001, **24**(5):317–326.
53. Alomari RS, Corso JJ, Chaudhary V: **Labeling of lumbar discs using both pixel- and object-level features with a two-level probabilistic model.** *IEEE Trans Med Imaging* 2011, **30**(1):1–10.
54. Malko JA, Hutton WC, Fajman WA: **An in vivo MRI study of the changes in volume (and fluid content) of the lumbar intervertebral disc after overnight bed rest and during an 8-hour walking protocol.** *J Spinal Disord Tech* 2002, **15**(2):157–163.
55. Lurie JD, Tosteson AN, Tosteson TD, Carragee E, Carrino JA, Kaiser J, Sequeiros RT, Lecomte AR, Grove MR, Blood EA: **Reliability of magnetic resonance imaging readings for lumbar disc herniation in the Spine Patient Outcomes Research Trial (SPORT).** *Spine* 2008, **33**(9):991–998.
56. Violas P, Estivalezes E, Briot J, Sales de Gauzy J, Swider P: **Objective quantification of intervertebral disc volume properties using MRI in idiopathic scoliosis surgery.** *Magn Reson Imaging* 2007, **25**(3):386–391.
57. Dora C, Schmid MR, Elfering A, Zanetti M, Hodler J, Boos N: **Lumbar disk herniation: do MR imaging findings predict recurrence after surgical diskectomy?** *Radiology* 2005, **235**(2):562–567.
58. Zou J, Yang H, Miyazaki M, Wei F, Hong SW, Yoon SH, Morishita Y, Wang JC: **Missed lumbar disc herniations diagnosed with kinetic magnetic resonance imaging.** *Spine* 2008, **33**(5):E140–144.
59. Puigdellivol-Sanchez A, Prats-Galino A, Reina MA, Maches F, Hernandez JM, De Andres J, van Zundert A: **Three-dimensional magnetic resonance**

image of structures enclosed in the spinal canal relevant to anesthetists and estimation of the lumbosacral CSF volume. *Acta anaesthesiologica Belgica* 2011, **62**(1):37–45.
60. Pneumaticos SG, Chatziioannou AN, Hipp J, Chatziioannou SN: **Prediction of successful discectomy using MRI quantitation of dural sac and herniated disc dimensions.** *Int J Clin Pract* 2010, **64**(1):13–18.
61. Chung SS, Lee CS, Kim SH, Chung MW, Ahn JM: **Effect of low back posture on the morphology of the spinal canal.** *Skelet Radiol* 2000, **29**(4):217–223.
62. Lee GY, Lee JW, Choi HS, Oh KJ, Kang HS: **A new grading system of lumbar central canal stenosis on MRI: an easy and reliable method.** *Skelet Radiol* 2011, **40**(8):1033–1039.
63. Hirasawa Y, Bashir WA, Smith FW, Magnusson ML, Pope MH, Takahashi K: **Postural changes of the dural sac in the lumbar spines of asymptomatic individuals using positional stand-up magnetic resonance imaging.** *Spine* 2007, **32**(4):E136–140.
64. Grenier N, Kressel HY, Schiebler ML, Grossman RI, Dalinka MK: **Normal and degenerative posterior spinal structures: MR imaging.** *Radiology* 1987, **165**(2):517–525.
65. Speciale AC, Pietrobon R, Urban CW, Richardson WJ, Helms CA, Major N, Enterline D, Hey L, Haglund M, Turner DA: **Observer variability in assessing lumbar spinal stenosis severity on magnetic resonance imaging and its relation to cross-sectional spinal canal area.** *Spine* 2002, **27**(10):1082–1086.
66. Schizas C, Theumann N, Burn A, Tansey R, Wardlaw D, Smith FW, Kulik G: **Qualitative grading of severity of lumbar spinal stenosis based on the morphology of the dural sac on magnetic resonance images.** *Spine* 2010, **35**(21):1919–1924.
67. Madsen R, Jensen TS, Pope M, Sorensen JS, Bendix T: **The effect of body position and axial load on spinal canal morphology: an MRI study of central spinal stenosis.** *Spine* 2008, **33**(1):61–67.
68. Knirsch W, Kurtz C, Haffner N, Langer M, Kececioglu D: **Normal values of the sagittal diameter of the lumbar spine (vertebral body and dural sac) in children measured by MRI.** *Pediatr Radiol* 2005, **35**(4):419–424.
69. Jeong ST, Song HR, Keny SM, Telang SS, Suh SW, Hong SJ: **MRI study of the lumbar spine in achondroplasia. A morphometric analysis for the evaluation of stenosis of the canal.** *J Bone Joint Surg Br Vol* 2006, **88**(9):1192–1196.
70. Jeffrey JE, Campbell DM, Golden MH, Smith FW, Porter RW: **Antenatal factors in the development of the lumbar vertebral canal: a magnetic resonance imaging study.** *Spine* 2003, **28**(13):1418–1423.
71. Haig AJ, Weiner JB, Tew J, Quint D, Yamakawa K: **The relation among spinal geometry on MRI, paraspinal electromyographic abnormalities, and age in persons referred for electrodiagnostic testing of low back symptoms.** *Spine* 2002, **27**(17):1918–1925. discussion 1924–1915.
72. Ahn TJ, Lee SH, Choi G, Ahn Y, Liu WC, Kim HJ, Lee HY: **Effect of intervertebral disk degeneration on spinal stenosis during magnetic resonance imaging with axial loading.** *Neurologia medico-chirurgica* 2009, **49**(6):242–247. discussion 247.
73. *Osirix Imaging Software.* http://www.osirix-viewer.com/license.pdf.
74. Lucas NP, Macaskill P, Irwig L, Bogduk N: **The development of a quality appraisal tool for studies of diagnostic reliability (QAREL).** *J Clin Epidemiol* 2010, **63**(8):854–861.
75. Krebs DE: **Declare your ICC type.** *Phys Ther* 1986, **66**(9):1431.
76. StataCorp: **Stata Statistical Software.** In *Version 12 edn.* Texas, USA: College Station; 2011.
77. Haas M: **Statistical methodology for reliability studies.** *J Manipulative Physiol Ther* 1991, **14**(2):119–132.
78. *How can I decide the sample size for a study of agreement between two methods of measurement?.* http://www-users.york.ac.uk/~mb55/meas/sizemeth.htm.
79. Bonett DG: **Sample size requirements for estimating intraclass correlations with desired precision.** *Stat Med* 2002, **21**(9):1331–1335.
80. Landis JR, Koch GG: **The measurement of observer agreement for categorical data.** *Biometrics* 1977, **33**(1):159–174.
81. Attias N, Hayman A, Hipp JA, Noble P, Esses SI: **Assessment of magnetic resonance imaging in the diagnosis of lumbar spine foraminal stenosis–a surgeon's perspective.** *J Spinal Disord Tech* 2006, **19**(4):249–256.
82. Videman T, Battie MC, Parent E, Gibbons LE, Vainio P, Kaprio J: **Progression and determinants of quantitative magnetic resonance imaging measures of lumbar disc degeneration: a five-year follow-up of adult male monozygotic twins.** *Spine* 2008, **33**(13):1484–1490.
83. Parent EC, Videman T, Battie MC: **The effect of lumbar flexion and extension on disc contour abnormality measured quantitatively on magnetic resonance imaging.** *Spine* 2006, **31**(24):2836–2842.
84. Prodhomme O, Seguret F, Martrille L, Pidoux O, Cambonie G, Couture A, Rouleau C: **Organ volume measurements: comparison between MRI and autopsy findings in infants following sudden unexpected death.** *Arch Dis Child Fetal Neonatal Ed* 2012, **97**(6):F434–F438.
85. Shimada YJ, Shiota T: **Underestimation of left atrial volume by three-dimensional echocardiography validated by magnetic resonance imaging: a meta-analysis and investigation of the source of bias.** *Echocardiography* 2012, **29**(4):385–390.

23

Reliability and validity of a simple and clinically applicable pain stimulus: sustained mechanical pressure with a spring-clamp

Søren O'Neill[1,2,3*], Thomas Graven-Nielsen[1], Claus Manniche[2,3] and Lars Arendt-Nielsen[1]

Abstract

Background: Generalized hyperalgesia, a widespread increased sensitivity to painful stimuli, has been demonstrated in a range of chronic pain conditions including low-back pain. The evidence suggests, that generalized hyperalgesia may be an important factor in the development of chronicity, but it is not commonly assessed in clinical practice. Whereas a range of tools and procedures for the quantitative sensory testing of pain sensitivity is available for laboratory pain research, most experimental pain stimuli are not well suited for clinical practice. In the current study, a simple and inexpensive mechanical spring-clamp was tested as a potential experimental pain stimulus.

Methods: Ten seconds of mechanical pressure was applied to the thumb of 242 study participants: Healthy volunteers and low-back-pain patients (hospital and primary care). Pain intensity was measured by visual analogue scale before and after conditioned pain modulation by cold-pressor test (CPT). Correlation to pressure pain threshold (PPT) of the infraspinatus muscle and cold-pressor test pain intensity, time to pain onset and time to non-tolerance, was examined. Test/re-test reliability of clamp pain was also assessed and the stimulus–response relationship was examined with a set of 6 different clamps.

Conclusions: Clamp pain was sensitive to changes in pain sensitivity provoked by conditioned pain modulation (CPM). Test/re-test reliability of the spring-clamp pain was better for healthy volunteers over a period of days, than for hospital patients over a period of weeks. A strong correlation ($\rho = 0.73$, $P > 0.0001$) was found between clamp force and evoked pain intensity. Correlation to other pain stimuli varied, with a strong correlation between pre and post-CPM clamp pain intensity ($\rho = 0.81$, $P > 0.0001$), moderate correlation between clamp pain and PPT ($\rho = -0.43$, $P > 0.0001$), as well as CPT pain intensity ($\rho = 0.32$, $P > 0.0001$) and a weak correlation with time to onset of CPT pain ($\rho = -0.14$, $P < 0.05$).

The application of mechanical pressure is commonly employed to assess general pain sensitivity, and a simple spring-clamp seems a potentially useful instrument for quantitative sensory testing in a clinical setting.

Keywords: Experimental pain, Quantitative sensory testing, Low-back pain, Central sensitization, Generalized hyperaglesia, Pain sensitivity

* Correspondence: soeren.oneill@rsyd.dk

[1]SMI Laboratory for Human Experimental Pain Research, Center for Sensory- motor Interaction, Department of Health Science and Technology, University of Aalborg, Fredrik Bajers Vej 7, Bld. D3, 9220 Aalborg, Denmark

[2]RCF Spine Center of Southern Denmark, Lillebælt Hospital, Østre Hougvej 55, 5500 Middelfart, Denmark

Full list of author information is available at the end of the article

Background

Assessing general pain sensitivity is clinically relevant, as generalised hyperalgesia appears to be an important factor in the chronification of many pain conditions, including e.g. low back pain (LBP) [1-5]. However standardized assessment of pain sensitivity and central modulation of pain sensitivity is probably used only rarely in clinical practice. Chiropractors and other healthcare providers who deal with musculoskeletal pain routinely assess mobility, muscular function, neurological integrity and similar aspects of the patient presentation in *semi-standardized* ways as taught in pre-graduate training and described in common textbooks. In contrast, no corresponding standardized method of quantifying pain sensitivity and modulation locally, segmentally or generally have been described for musculoskeletal problems and we suspect such examination procedures are not in common clinical use. Subjective patient reports of widespread pain, abnormal pain descriptions and disproportionate exacerbations with physical activity, may alert the clinican to potential abnormal pain sensitivity and modulation, and such suspicions should arguable be documented by quantitative sensory testing (QST).

Like clinical tests of e.g. spinal mobility and deep tendon reflexes, QST should be safe, easy and fast to perform and ideally should not rely on expensive specialist equipment. Otherwise it is unlikely they will be used in busy clinical practice. Unfortunately, the range of experimental pain stimuli which are available in the laboratory, are generally prohibitively expensive and/or difficult to use in a clinical setting. Such laboratory procedures include deep and superficial electrical stimulation, injection or topical application of noxious substances, controlled mechanical or thermal stimuli and many others. For the most part these require considerable training and experience to perform and interpret, and furthermore they often require expensive equipment such as constant current stimulators or peltier thermodes.

Different QST procedures measure different aspects of pain sensitivity, whilst others overlap to some degree [6-8]. The pressure algometer is often used to assess pain detection thresholds of deep-tissue structures [9], but quantifying the effects of temporal summation or conditioned pain modulation (CPM), require a more complicated set-up [10]. In any case, a single pain test is most likely insufficient to get an adequate picture of pain sensitivity in a complex clinical context, where different pathways and mechanisms are involved. Rather, it is a question of choosing the right *selection* and *combination* of QST procedures [6-8]. Obviously, the more QST procedures in such a selection of tests, the more expensive, time-consuming and difficult it becomes and therefore less likely to be adopted in clinical practice.

Mechanical pressure pain sensitivity of the thumb has been advocated as a good choice of a *'neutral'* site for testing general pain sensitivity – i.e. a site at which general pain sensitivity can be assessed, unaffected by any localized tissue pain such as e.g. low-back pain [3,11]. Clauw et al. [4] reported a moderate correlation ($\rho = 0.38\text{-}0.52$) between pressure pain detection and tolerance thresholds of the thumb and physical function and pain in LBP sufferers. Pain sensitivity of the thumb and thenar muscles have also been used as an indicator of general pain sensitivity in reports of hyperalgesia in relation to vulvodynia [12], the peri-menstrual period [13] and myofacial jaw pain [14]. Giesecke et al. [3] used mechanical pressure of the thumb in a study of chronic LBP and fibromyalgia to demonstrate increased pain sensitivity compared to pain-free controls.

To adequately assess pain sensitivity, the clinician would most likely need a *battery* of carefully selected pain tests. In this study, we examined the reliability of an in-expensive spring-clamp, which could potentially be useful as one such test in a battery of clinically applicable standardized QST in the assessment of general pain sensitivity.

Methods

Subjects and materials

It was our deliberate intention to include a heterogeneous group of participants with or without low-back pain, of different characteristics (chronic/acute, with/without leg pain, etc.). For that reason, participants were recruited from three different populations: Hospital LBP outpatients, LBP patients in primary sector chiropractic clinics, and healthy volunteers.

By virtue of the free access to chiropractic care in the primary sector and the restrictive referral criteria which apply to hospital referral, hospital patients tend to be more chronic and severely affected. This was confirmed by the current data (details published elsewhere [2]).

Patients were recruited consecutively on pre-defined, pseudo-random days in both the primary care and hospital settings. No particular inclusion criteria were applied apart from low-back pain being the primary complaint.

A total of 242 participants were recruited. 127 woman and 115 men, 119 hospital patients, 79 patients from primary care and 44 healthy volunteers. Mean age was 45.4 years (95% CI 43.8-47.0).

Hospital patients, primary chiropractic care patients and healthy volunteers are collectively referred to as *QST participants* hereafter. In addition to QST participants, 20 (healthy, pain free) experimenters were recruited to perform reliability and dose–response measurements of the spring-clamp.

The current study was concerned mainly with the reliability and validity of the spring clamp as an experimental pain stimulus with potential clinical applicability. Parts of the data has also been analysed and published in another manuscript focused on differences in pain sensitivity between clinical subgroups [2].

The experiment was conducted in accordance with the Helsinki Declaration and IASP guidelines for human pain research [15]. Approval was granted by The Regional Committees on Health Research Ethics for Southern Denmark (ref. S-20090003).

Clinical data

Hospital patients and primary care patients were asked to indicate *average*, *current* and *worst* LBP intensity (with or without radicular pain) on 100 mm paper VAS (0–100) and healthy volunteers were asked to confirm, that they did not suffer any pain complaints, after which QST was performed. Furthermore low-back pain patients (hospital and private practice) completed the Roland-Morris disability questionnaire [16] and EQ5D forms [17] for descriptive purposes.

Experimental QST protocol

QST consisted of pressure pain detection threshold (PPT) of the left infraspinatus muscle, spring-clamp pain intensity with 10 seconds sustained pressure over the left thumb nail-bed, conditioned pain modulation (CPM) with cold-pressor test (CPT) as the conditioning stimulus and (repeat) spring-clamp pain intensity as the test stimulus. Spring-clamp pain was re-tested at the first subsequent consultation for hospital patients.

QST data was collected by SON or one of two research assistants. Prior to data collection both assistants (senior clinical interns) were instructed in the correct QST procedure and all three examiners practised the procedures together until confident they were performed as uniformly as could reasonably be expected. No formal testing of variation between testers was performed.

Pressure pain threshold

Pressure was applied manually with an algometer (Somedic pressure algometer with a 1 cm^2 probe, model 2, Hørby, Sweden) on the left Infraspinatus muscle, with a near-constant velocity of 50 kPa/s until the subject indicated the pressure as becoming painful by pressing an indicator button connected to the algometer.

PPT measurements were repeated 3 times with 5–10 seconds interval and the average was used for further analysis. The probe of the algometer was placed such that repeat applications overlapped partly. If no pain had been elicited by 1000 kPa, this was recorded as the PPT. If the first and second measurement was 1000 kPa, a third was not performed.

Clamp – sustained mechanical pressure

The spring-clamp (Millarco 100 mm with two 14×13 mm^2 pressure pads, Prod.Nr. 72644, Millarco, Lystrup, Denmark – see Figure 1) was placed on the left thumbnail for 10 seconds, after which participants were asked to score the pain intensity on a 100 mm paper VAS, marked *'No pain'* and *'Worst pain imaginable'* at either end (scored as 0–100 VAS).

Care was taken to ensure that the upper pad of the clamp was placed as far proximal on the nail as possible, but not overlapping the eponychium (cuticula) and the lower pad proximal enough to prevent the clamp sliding forward. In a few instances when participants had a particularly short or curved nail, it was necessary to manually prevent the clamp from sliding forward.

Conditioned pain modulation

A 25 litre water-tub (Dometic Waeco Mobicool C40, Dubai, United Arab Emirates) was kept refrigerated at 0–2 degrees Celsius and temperature was confirmed by means of a thermometer immediately before each cold-pressor test.

Participants were instructed to immerse their right, non-clenched hand to the wrist in the circulating water (Reich submersible water pump, 15 l/min, 0.5 bar, Reich, Arnhem, Netherlands) and keep it there for 1 minute or until pain became unbearable. Participants were asked to verbally indicate onset of pain and time from immersion to pain-onset was noted. Similarly, time from submersion to withdrawal was recorded when participants could not tolerate the full 1 minutes cold-pressor test.

Participants were informed when 30 and 50 seconds had passed and immediately after withdrawal participants indicated cold-pressor pain intensity on a 100 mm VAS, marked *'No pain'* and *'Worst pain imaginable'* at either end (scored as 0–100 VAS).

Mechanical pressure on the left thumb nail with the spring-clamp, as described above, was repeated 5–15

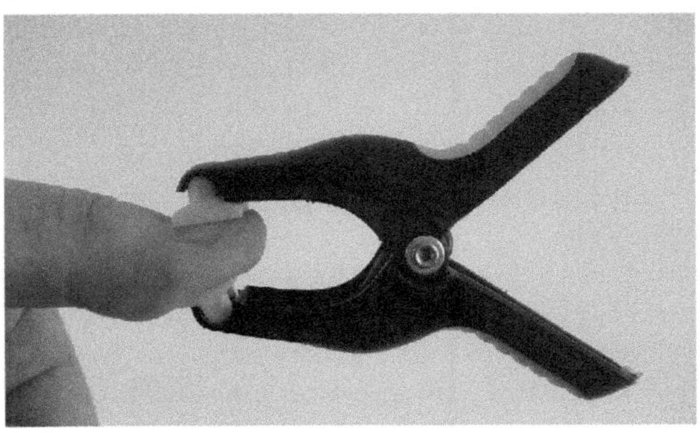

Figure 1 Mechanical spring clamp. Generic, inexpensive wood-working spring-clamp.

seconds after CPT, thus serving as test-stimulus in assessment of conditioned pain modulation (CPM), with CPT as conditioning stimulus. The same clamp was used for all QST participants, for both these tests.

Test/re-test – hospital patients

On the first subsequent visit following the initial examination, hospital patients were re-tested with a spring-clamp, by the attending clinician. Logistically, there was a need for several clamps for the re-test, and therefore a random clamp was selected for each patient – I.e. test and re-test were performed with two different clamps (of the same type).

No re-test was possible for primary care patients.

Test/re-test and stimulus–response by experimenters

Ten pairs of senior clinical interns were recruited as experimenters (*examiner* and *test-subject*) and instructed how to test a selection of six clamps of different types. Clamps were of different makes and models, with different sizes/forces, but all with 14×13 mm^2 pads – the same 6 clamps were used for test and re-test.

The clamps being used were shielded from view of the *(blinded)* test-subject. The examiner applied the 6 clamps in a pre-determined random order, with a pause of approximately 10 seconds between tests.

After 10 seconds of pressure application, the test-subject rated the pressure on a 100 mm plastic VAS. The VAS was denoted *'No sensation'*, *'Pain threshold'* and *'Worst pain imaginable'* corresponding to a score of 0, 50 and 100, respectively. A written instruction was supplied, explaining that any non-painful sensation should be rated between *'No sensation'* and *'Pain threshold'*, and similarly any painful sensation between *'Pain threshold'* and *'Worst pain imaginable'*.

Finally, the examiner measured the mechanical force generated by each of the six clamps, using a scale (Kern HDB 10 K10, Kern & Sohn Gmbh, Balingen, Germany) in a custom made aluminium frame, with the jaws of the clamp opened to 7 mm.

The same six clamps were re-tested, in a new random order, a few days later, by the same examiner and test-subject pairs.

Variation in clamp force, including temperature and degree of opening

To assess inter-clamp variability, the force generation of all sixty-two available, similar spring-clamps were tested once (by SON). To assess intra-clamp variability a random selection of ten clamps were tested ten times each, using the Kern scale.

Five other clamps were selected at random and submerged in 40 degree Celsius warm water. As the water cooled, the clamp force was measured at 40, 35, 30, 25 and 20 degrees Celsius.

Finally ten clamps were randomly selected and, using a set of 1.5 mm thick washers and the Kern scale, the clamp force was measured with the jaws of the clamps opened to 7, 8.5, 10, 11.5 and 13 mm.

Statistical analysis

Data was analysed using R version 2.13.1 (R Foundation for Statistical Computing, Vienna, Austria) for Linux and an P-level of 0.05 was accepted as significant. P-values are reported numerically or by star-annotation, where * is $P < 0.05$, ** is $P < 0.01$, *** is $P < 0.001$ and **** is $P < 0.0001$.

Non-parametric analysis was employed: Summary statistics are reported as *median* value (95% CI) [inter-quartile range], except where otherwise stated. Correlations were calculated as Spearmans ρ and reliability of repeat measurements were analysed with Limits of Agreement.

Results

Summary of clinical data

The distribution of VAS scores for average, current and worst low-back pain is illustrated in Figure 2.

Eighteen low-back pain patients (and 44 healthy volunteers) did not report duration of low back pain. Of the remaining, 58 reported LBP for 3 months or less and 122 reported LBP for more than 3 months. 67 participants reported LBP for more than a year.

Of 198 low-back pain patients, 22 did not complete the Roland-Morris disability questionnaire, nor the Quality of Life (EQ5D). The median EQ5D score (adjusted to the Danish population norm) was 0.723 (IQR [0.59;0.82]) and the median Roland-Morris score was 10 (IQR [4;15]).

Quantitative sensory testing

The results of QST are illustrated in Figure 3. Median pressure pain threshold was 447 kPa (IQR [341;588]) (in 8 participants PPT was right-censored as 1000kPa), median VAS score with clamp before CPT was 21 (IQR [7;41]), median clamp VAS after CPT was 13 (IQR [4;30]), median time to onset of pain with CPT was 12 seconds (IQR [8;19]), median CPT VAS score was 73 (IQR [59;85]) and median time to discontinuation of CPT was 60 seconds (IQR [34;60]).

Clamp pain correlation to other pain modalities

Bi-plots of correlation between clamp pain (before CPM) and other QST are illustrated in Figure 4. A moderate correlation was found between clamp pain intensity and PPT ($\rho = -0.43$, $P < 0.0001$) and CPT pain ($\rho = 0.32$, $P < 0.0001$). A weak correlation was found between clamp pain and time from start of CPT until CPT pain ($\rho = -0.14$, $P < 0.05$) and a strong correlation was found between

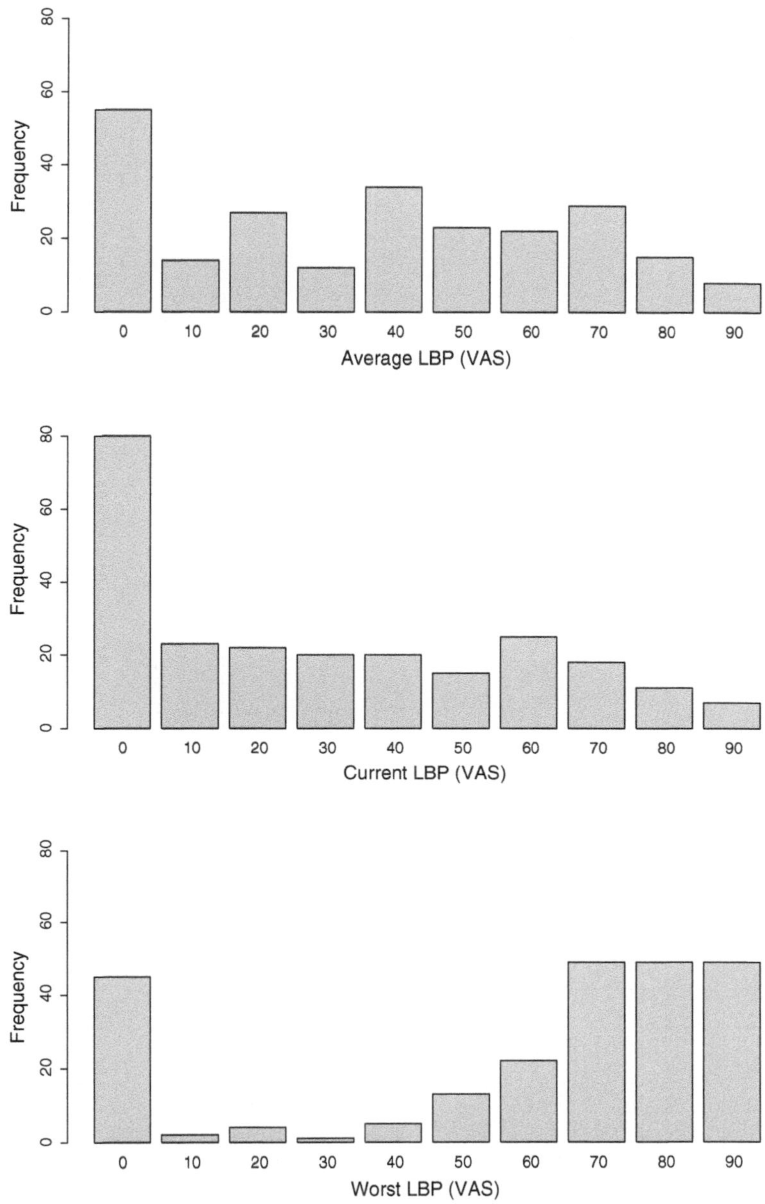

Figure 2 Low back pain intensity. Distribution of average, current and worst low-back pain intensity.

clamp pain intensity before and after CPT ($\rho = 0.81$, $P < 0.0001$).

Conditioned pain modulation

Spring-clamp pain dropped significantly after conditioned pain modulation (Wilcoxon signed rank test, $p < 0.0001$). The median change in absolute VAS score was only 3 (IQR [0.0;13.8]), but the median relative change in VAS score was 27.2% (IQR [0.0;62.8]).

Test/re-test

The experimenters (*examiners* and *test-subjects*) re-tested the set of 6 clamps 1–21 days (mean 6.5) after the first test. The Limits of agreement plot illustrates a mean difference in test/re-test VAS scores of 1.84 (SD = 13.81). See upper-left panel of Figure 5.

Similarly, re-test clamp VAS scores were obtained for 81 hospital patients. Re-test was performed 5–154 days (mean 35) after the first test. Mean difference was 1.54 (SD = 24.45). See upper-right panel of Figure 5.

Stimulus/response

A stimulus–response plot of the mechanical pressure of the 6 different clamps and the corresponding VAS scores is illustrated in the lower right-hand frame of Figure 5. A strong and highly significant correlation was found ($\rho = 0.73$, $P < 0.0001$).

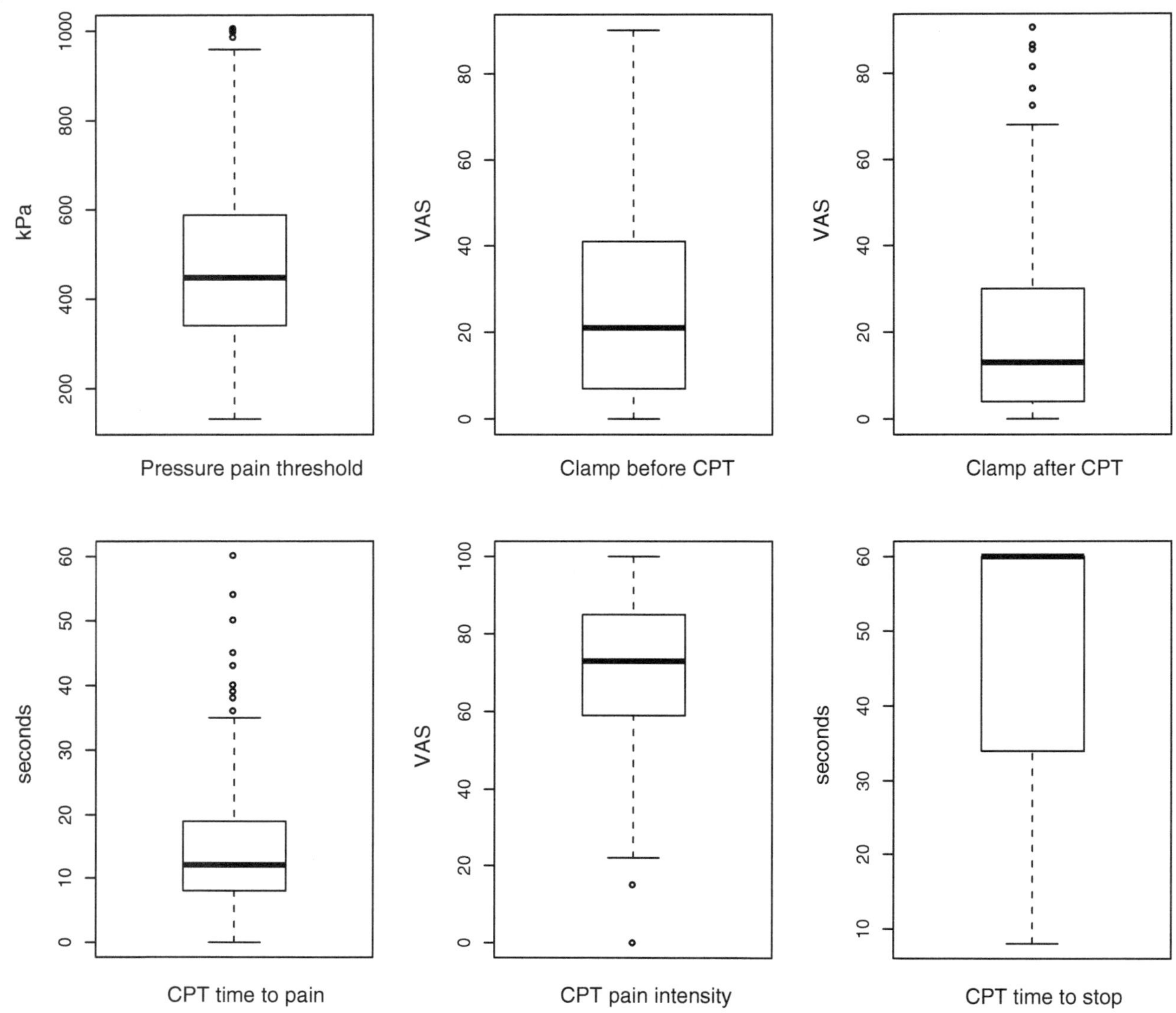

Figure 3 Quantitative sensory testing. Box plots of QST. Box plots illustrate median value and inter-quartile range. Whiskers represents nearest value to 1.5 · IQR. Outliers are plotted separately.

Variation between and within clamps

The force generated by the 62 available clamps of similar design, is illustrated in Figure 6. The median clamp force was 5.8 kg (4.8-6) [3.5;6.4].

On repeated testing of 10 random clamps 10 times, the standard deviation (normalized relative to each clamp) was 0.04 kg.

Variation with temperature and degree of clamp opening

A strong linear relationship between degree of clamp jaw opening (7–13 mm) and generated clamp force was found. Conversely, temperature and clamp force did not correlate. See Figure 7.

Discussion

Mechanical properties

Individual clamps reliably re-produced a consistent force on re-test with an SD of only 0.04 kg. By contrast there was considerable variation between apparently identical clamps of the same model and the distribution was not normally distributed, as illustrated in Figure 6.

The clamp force was not affected notably by temperature variations, but was affected by the degree of clamp jaw opening (as would be expected). With the clamps used in the present study, a difference of 4 mm in clamp jaw opening translated into a change in clamp force of approximately 1 kg, which suggests that variations in clamp jaw opening should be either

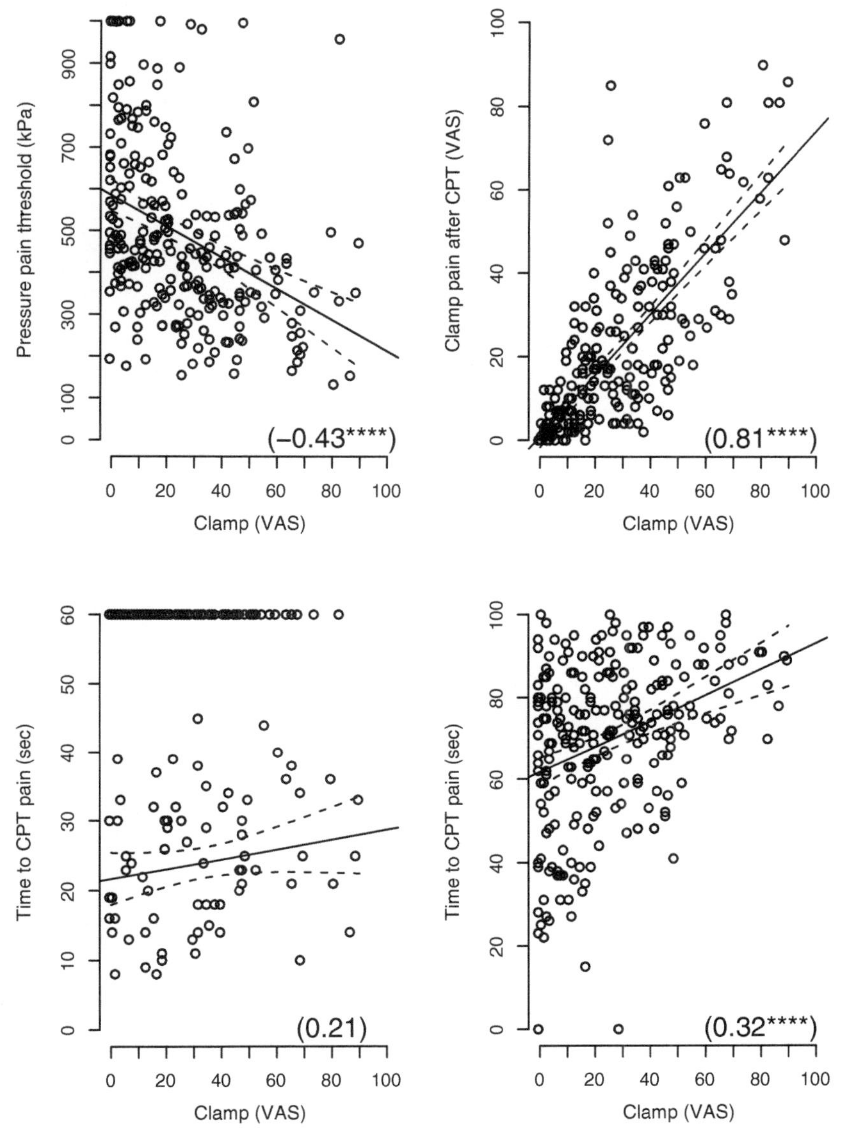

Figure 4 Spring clamp pain and other QST. Linear regression of spring-clamp VAS score and other pain stimuli (with 95%CI). Data was obtained from all participants (n = 242). Numbers in lower-right corner of plot area are Spearmans ρ with statistical significance level (star-annotation). For the *CPT time to discontinued*, all data have been plotted, but only observations <60 seconds have been included in regression and correlation analysis.

controlled or reported in future studies employing a spring-clamp.

Properties as a pain stimulus

Stability

Clamp pain was more stable over a period of days in healthy volunteers, compared to chronic hospital patients over a period of weeks: Arguably because of greater inherent variability in chronic pain patients and potentially also because of the greater time lapse between tests. Furthermore the use of two different clamps at test and re-test in hospital patients is likely to induce greater variation – As the current data demonstrate, there is notable variation in clamp force between individual clamps of the same make and model. This suggests that the force should be recorded if spring clamps are to be used in a clinical setting or for further research.

Correlation

The clamp pain was correlated in varying degrees to other QST: clamp pain score after CPM, PPT, CPT pain score and time from CPT start until CPT pain onset. No correlation was found to CPT tolerance. In other words, clamp pain intensity correlated to other QST to varying degrees, which is in line with the literature which suggests, that

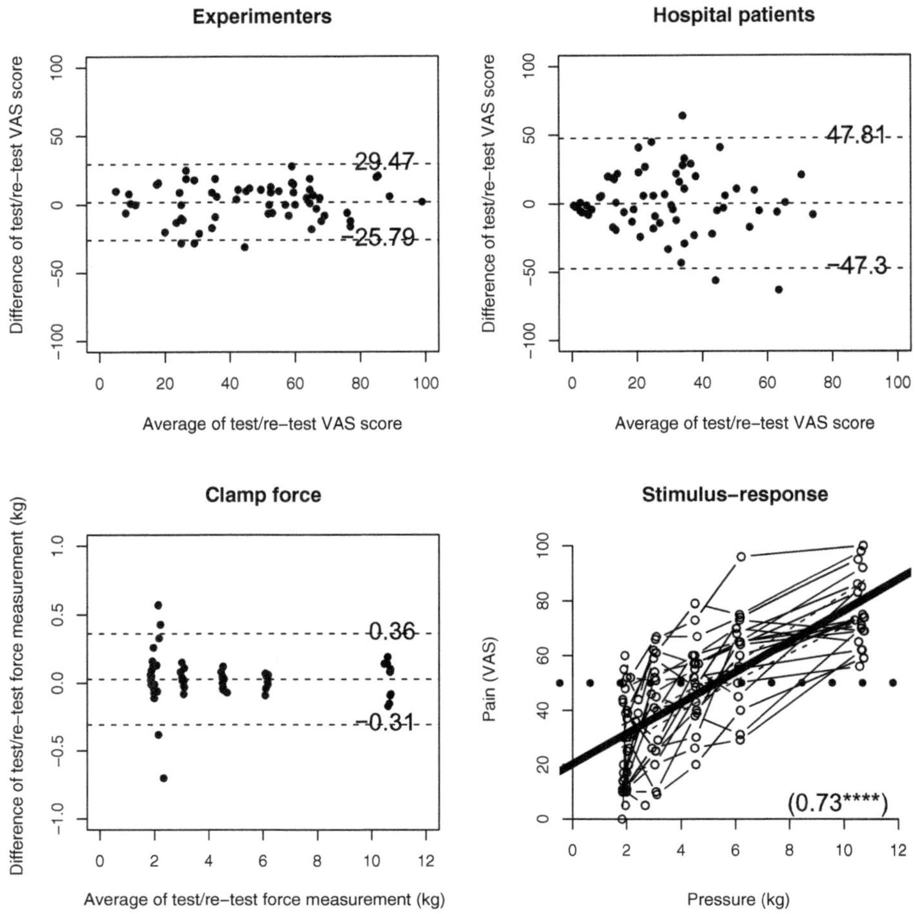

Figure 5 Test-retest and Stimulus-response relationship. Test/re-test limits of agreement (95%) and dose-response relationship. The panels *'Experimenters'* and *'Clamp force'* represents repeat measurements with the same 6 clamps (of different types and forces). The panel *'Hospital patients'* represent repeat measurements with two different clamps of the same type. *'Stimulus-response'* illustrates linear regression and lists Spearmans ρ with statistical significance level.

different methods of QST measure different aspects of pain sensitivity and modulation [6,7,18,19].

Applicability

Unlike the algometer, the spring-clamp can only be used to apply a fixed, sustained pressure but as spring-clamps are commercially available in a large variety of sizes, it should be possible to prepare a set of clamps of gradually increasing force for clinical use. By applying 6 different clamps in what is essentially a *multiple random staircase* model [20], we observed a clear dose–response relationship between pain scores and clamps-forces.

If only a single clamp is used, that particular clamp should be of sufficient calibre/strength to actually induce pain in the majority of study subjects – a pressure in the range of 5–10 kg with an application pad area of 1–2 cm^2 seems a good candidate when applied to the thumb.

A further consideration is the tissues to which the spring-clamp can be applied, which is limited by the degree of opening permitted by the spring-clamp jaws. It is feasible to apply a spring-clamp to skin-folds, fingers, toes, ear-lobes etc. and probably also small, peripheral muscle groups such as the thenar and hypo-thenar muscles – this has not been investigated in the current study however and the validity of the spring clamp as a pain stimulus may differ between test sites.

Conditioned modulation of clamp pain

The spring-clamp was sensitive to changes in pain sensitivity as a result of conditioned pain modulation. A significant change in spring-clamp pain intensity were observed, with the majority of participants reporting less clamp pain after conditioned pain modulation. This suggests that pain induced by the spring clamp is sensitive to changes in central pain modulation. Futhermore, the spring clamp has previously been used to examine differences in pain sensitivity between clinical subgroups (acute and chronic LBP patients and healthy controls) [2].

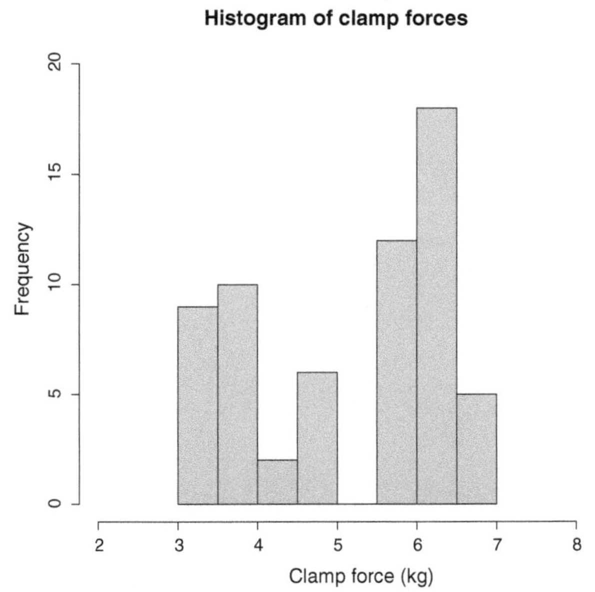

Figure 6 Clamp forces. Histogram of forces generated by the 62 available spring-clamps.

Previous studies

During data collection of the present study, Egloff et al. [21] published a similar study employing a clothes peg as the pain stimulus. The authors examined differences in pain response between two different clinical sub-groups (orthopaedic versus medical/psychosomatic pain), reported good correlation to pressure pain detection and tolerance thresholds and good test/re-test stability. The correlations between clothes-peg pain intensity and pressure pain thresholds, using a standard algometer, were reported as Spearmans ρ between -0.38 and -0.62 – i.e. of similar magnitude to the current findings ($\rho = -0.43$). All-in-all, the findings of the current study and those of Egloff et al. align.

Two other LBP studies have been published in which mechanical pain sensitivity of the thumb has been used as an indicator of general pain sensitivity [3,4], but these have used a traditional algometer to measure PPTs and a custom made apparatus with hydraulic valves and calibrated weights. To our knowledge, the study by Egloff et al. is the only other work using a simple clamp/peg technique.

Perspectives for future use

The association between chronic pain and generalized hyperalgesia is well supported in the literature and may play an important part in clinical management of painful disorders. However, establishing a reliable *diagnosis* of altered central pain modulation in e.g. specific LBP cases, is not yet possible [22]. If such a diagnosis is to have clinical benefits, it should be made early in the course of pain. Chiropractors in primary practice are in a position to examine such patients, early in the course of pain.

If a diagnosis is to be made based on an individuals changes in pain sensitivity over time, as opposed to population reference values, this underlines the need for quick, reliable and simple pain tests early in the clinical course of pain. The spring clamp tested in the current study could serve as one such a pain stimulus, possibly as part of a larger test battery.

Conclusions

No single QST provides a complete picture of pain sensitivity or mechanisms of central nociceptive modulation and the spring-clamp has obvious limitations, but it does offer a simple, reliable and clinically applicable pain stimulus for assessing pain patients in clinical practice. The clinical assessment and implications of such testing is still unclear.

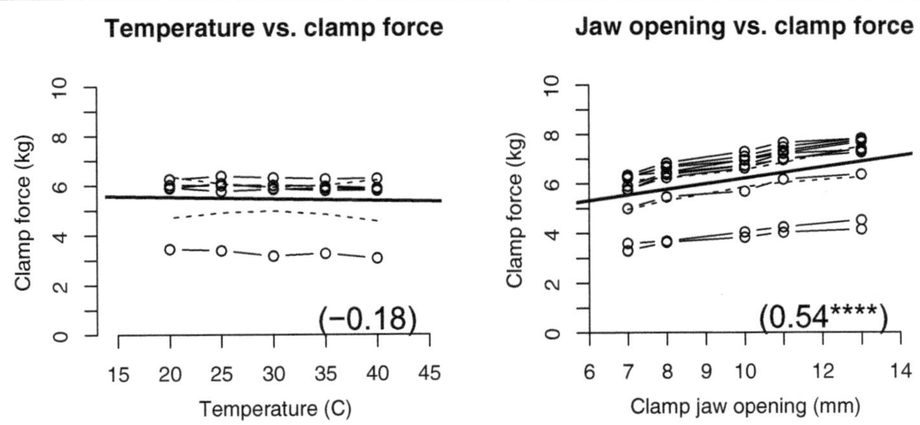

Figure 7 Effect of temperature and degree of clamp opening. Correlation of clamp force with temperature and degree of clamp jaw opening. Numbers in lower-right corner of plot area is Spearmans ρ with statistical significance level (star-annotation). Five random clamps tested for sensitivity to temperature changes and 10 random clamps tested for degree of jaw opening.

Abbreviations
CPM: Conditioned Pain Modulation; LBP: Low-back pain; PPT: Pressure Pain Detection Threshold; QST: Quantitative Sensory Testing.

Competing interests
We the authors declare no conflicts of interest or competing interests in the preparation of the present manuscript.

Authors' contributions
Author SO'N: Contributed significantly to the design of the project, manuscript authoring, data collection and analysis. Author TG-N: Contributed significantly to the design of the project and manuscript authoring. Author CM: Contributed significantly to the design of the project and manuscript authoring. Author LA-N: Contributed significantly to the design of the project and manuscript authoring. The manuscript has been approved by all 4 authors.

Acknowledgements
Contributions which do not justify authorship: none.
Technical help: none.
Financial and material support: none.
Conflicts of interest: none.
The authors state *no conflicts of interest* in the preparation of this manuscript and the research on which it is based.

Author details
[1]SMI Laboratory for Human Experimental Pain Research, Center for Sensory- motor Interaction, Department of Health Science and Technology, University of Aalborg, Fredrik Bajers Vej 7, Bld. D3, 9220 Aalborg, Denmark. [2]RCF Spine Center of Southern Denmark, Lillebælt Hospital, Østre Hougvej 55, 5500 Middelfart, Denmark. [3]SDU Institute of Regional Health Research, University of Southern Denmark, Campusvej 55, 5230 Odense, Denmark.

References
1. O'Neill S, Kjær P, Graven-Nielsen T, Manniche C, Arendt-Nielsen L: **Low pressure pain thresholds are associated with, but does not predispose for, low back pain.** *Eur Spine J* 2011, **20:**2120–2125.
2. O'Neill S, Manniche C, Graven-Nielsen T, Arendt-Nielsen L: **Association between a composite score of pain sensitivity and clinical parameters in Low-back pain.** *Clin J Pain* 2013. Epub Ahead of Print (doi:10.1097/AJP.0000000000000042).
3. Giesecke T, Gracely RH, Grant MA, Nachemson A, Petzke F, Williams DA, Clauw DJ: **Evidence of augmented central pain processing in idiopathic chronic low back pain.** *Arthritis Rheum* 2004, **50:**613–623.
4. Clauw DJ, Williams D, Lauerman W, Dahlman M, Aslami A, Nachemson AL, Kobrine AI, Wiesel SW: **Pain sensitivity as a correlate of clinical status in individuals with chronic low back pain.** *Spine* 1999, **24:**2035–2041.
5. Puta C, Schulz B, Schoeler S, Magerl W, Gabriel B, Gabriel HHW, Miltner WHR, Weiss T: **Enhanced sensitivity to punctate painful stimuli in female patients with chronic low back pain.** *BMC Neurol* 2012, **12:**98.
6. Greenspan JD, Slade GD, Bair E, Dubner R, Fillingim RB, Ohrbach R, Knott C, Mulkey F, Rothwell R, Maixner W: **Pain sensitivity risk factors for chronic TMD: descriptive data and empirically identified domains from the OPPERA case control study.** *J Pain* 2011, **12:**T61–T74.
7. Hastie BA, Riley JL, Robinson ME, Glover T, Campbell CM, Staud R, Fillingim RB: **Cluster analysis of multiple experimental pain modalities.** *Pain* 2005, **116:**227–237.
8. Neziri AY, Curatolo M, Nüesch E, Scaramozzino P, Andersen OK, Arendt-Nielsen L, Jüni P: **Factor analysis of responses to thermal, electrical, and mechanical painful stimuli supports the importance of multi-modal pain assessment.** *Pain* 2011, **152:**1146–1155.
9. Finocchietti S, Takahashi K, Okada K, Watanabe Y, Graven-Nielsen T, Mizumura K: **Deformation and pressure propagation in deep tissue during mechanical painful pressure stimulation.** *Med Biol Eng Comput* 2013, **51:**113–122.
10. Yarnitsky D: **Conditioned pain modulation (the diffuse noxious inhibitory control-like effect): its relevance for acute and chronic pain states.** *Curr Opin Anaesthesiol* 2010, **23:**611–615.
11. Petzke F, Khine A, Williams D, Groner K, Clauw DJ, Gracely RH: **Dolorimetry performed at 3 paired tender points highly predicts overall tenderness.** *J Rheumatol* 2001, **28:**2568–2569.
12. Giesecke J, Reed BD, Haefner HK, Giesecke T, Clauw DJ, Gracely RH: **Quantitative sensory testing in vulvodynia patients and increased peripheral pressure pain sensitivity.** *Obstet Gynecol* 2004, **104:**126–133.
13. Isselée H, Laat AD, Bogaerts K, Lysens R: **Long-term fluctuations of pressure pain thresholds in healthy men, normally menstruating women and oral contraceptive users.** *Eur J Pain* 2001, **5:**27–37.
14. Michelotti A, Farella M, Stellato A, Martina R, Laat AD: **Tactile and pain thresholds in patients with myofascial pain of the jaw muscles: a case–control study.** *J Orofac Pain* 2008, **22:**139–145.
15. Charlton E: **Ethical guidelines for pain research in humans. Committee on ethical issues of the international association for the study of pain.** *Pain* 1995, **63:**277–278.
16. Albert HB, Jensen A-M, Dahl D, Rasmussen MN: **Criteria validation of the Roland Morris questionnaire. A Danish translation of the international scale for the assessment of functional level in patients with low back pain and sciatica.** *Ugeskr Laeger* 2003, **165:**1875–1880.
17. Sørensen J, Davidsen M, Gudex C, Pedersen KM, Brønnum-Hansen H: **Danish EQ-5D population norms.** *Scand J Public Health* 2009, **37:**467–474.
18. Janal MN, Glusman M, Kuhl JP, Clark WC: **On the absence of correlation between responses to noxious heat, cold, electrical and ischemic stimulation.** *Pain* 1994, **58:**403–411.
19. Lautenbacher S, Rollman GB, McCain GA: **Multi-method assessment of experimental and clinical pain in patients with fibromyalgia.** *Pain* 1994, **59:**45–53.
20. Gracely RH, Lota L, Walter DJ, Dubner R: **A multiple random staircase method of psychophysical pain assessment.** *Pain* 1988, **32:**55–63.
21. Egloff N, Klingler N, von Känel R, Cámara RJA, Curatolo M, Wegmann B, Marti E, Ferrari M-LG: **Algometry with a clothes peg compared to an electronic pressure algometer: a randomized cross-sectional study in pain patients.** *BMC Musculoskelet Disord* 2011, **12:**174.
22. Curatolo M: **Diagnosis of altered central pain processing.** *Spine Phila Pa 1976* 2011, **36**(25 Suppl):S200–S204.

The role of information search in seeking alternative treatment for back pain: a qualitative analysis

Hoda McClymont[1*], Jeff Gow[2,3] and Chad Perry[1]

Abstract

Background: Health consumers have moved away from a reliance on medical practitioner advice to more independent decision processes and so their information search processes have subsequently widened. This study examined how persons with back pain searched for alternative treatment types and service providers. That is, what information do they seek and how; what sources do they use and why; and by what means do they search for it?

Methods: 12 persons with back pain were interviewed. The method used was convergent interviewing. This involved a series of semi-structured questions to obtain open-ended answers. The interviewer analysed the responses and refined the questions after each interview, to converge on the dominant factors influencing decisions about treatment patterns.

Results: Persons with back pain mainly search their memories and use word of mouth (their doctor and friends) for information about potential treatments and service providers. Their search is generally limited due to personal, provider-related and information-supply reasons. However, they did want in-depth information about the alternative treatments and providers in an attempt to establish apriori their efficacy in treating their specific back problems. They searched different sources depending on the type of information they required.

Conclusions: The findings differ from previous studies about the types of information health consumers require when searching for information about alternative or mainstream healthcare services. The results have identified for the first time that limited information availability was only one of three categories of reasons identified about why persons with back pain do not search for more information particularly from external non-personal sources.

Keywords: Back pain, Information search, Search effort, Complementary and alternative treatments, Australia

Background

Health consumers are moving away from a heavy reliance on medical practitioner advice to more independent decision processes [1,2]. In countries such as Australia, the United Kingdom and the United States shared decision making and patient self-management are key components of health policy [3]. There are five steps to the consumer health decision making process: need recognition; information search; evaluation of alternatives; purchase decision and post-purchase behavior [4]. In this paper a qualitative examination of the second step, information search, in managing chronic back pain is undertaken.

Information search is particularly relevant to consumers with chronic diseases where doctors cannot recommend one best treatment that will solve the problem [2,5]. One such chronic condition is back pain caused by musculoskeletal disease. Traditionally, information about solutions to back pain and the available treatments has been provided by mainstream health providers such as physiotherapists and, in more serious cases, by surgeons. However, more recent trends indicate that an increasing number of persons with back pain are turning to alternative or complementary treatments such as chiropractic treatments, homeopathy, naturopathy, Bowen therapy, kinesiology and reflexology [5]. This change in treatment direction combined with the multitude of treatment solutions necessitates factual and effective information in order to guide consumer's choices.

* Correspondence: hoda@usq.edu.au
[1]School of Management and Enterprise, University of Southern Queensland, 4350 Toowoomba, QLD, Australia
Full list of author information is available at the end of the article

This area of research is particularly important because back pain is a significant problem affecting people globally [6]. In industrialised countries, more than 80 per cent of people will experience back pain sometime in their life and up to half of the workforce will suffer at least one episode of back pain each year resulting in work absences, lower productivity and increased costs to businesses [6]. For example, half of all working Americans experience back pain each year and it is one of the most common reasons for missing work [7]. In the United Kingdom, there are approximately three million persons with back pain and of the 131 million working days lost to sickness, 34.4 million are due to musculoskeletal conditions such as back pain, neck pain and limb problems [8]. In turn, musculoskeletal disorders are the leading cause of disability in Australia; they accounted for more disability than any other medical condition with 14% (2.8 million people) experiencing back pain and disc disorders [9].

Despite this significance of back pain problems and a trend towards alternative information sources and treatment options, little is known about the information search processes used by persons with back pain to select appropriate treatment types and service providers in particular. This gap is important because persons with back pain search behavior are the *start* of any treatment chain. Other research has addressed search behavior by patients and/or patients' families searching for information about areas like hospitals, physicians and healers [10-12], aged care homes [11], mental health services [13] and cancer [14,15]. Recent research has covered search behavior on the internet for health related issues that did not include back pain [16,17]. But persons with back pain overall information search behavior has not been researched [18] and so requires some qualitative investigation to uncover.

This study aims to extend previous research on information search in healthcare by using the convergent interviewing methodology to investigate how persons with back pain apply three essential elements of the search process to acquire information about treatment types and service providers: what sources do they use and why; what information content do they seek and how; and how do they search for it?

The next section briefly reviews literature on information search in the health care context. Then data collection and analysis methods of convergent interviewing used in this research are described. Analysis of the research data to develop schemas of information search behaviour by persons with back pain, and their implications, follow.

Prior theory - information search

This research extends prior theory to back pain situations and so that theory needs to be established first. Accessing the right information efficiently reduces uncertainty and anxiety [2] and guides the decision making of health consumers. To undertake this information search, a typical consumer has to decide on three key issues that became the three research questions about back pain that drove the data collection and analysis phases of this research: where to search for it [19], what information content to look for [20], and how much search effort to expend when looking for information [21].

Information sources

Firstly, consider sources of information. The literature on information search identifies two main sources: internal and external sources. Internal search comprises searching one's memory to access information about solutions to an existing problem [19,22,23]. This information is basically stored knowledge and experiences gathered over time [24]. Thus prior knowledge is a key to undertaking any effective search for it provides the basis for evaluating new information in later, external search. Furthermore, prior knowledge has been shown to influence both the amount and type of information sought. However, this influence appears to be context specific [25] with certain contexts leading to more information search with greater knowledge while others lead to less information search with greater knowledge [26]. Despite its contextual nature, no studies were found on the use of internal information search within a health care context. Thus, the question arises about how much consumers with back pain rely on their memories (internal sources) for treatment type and service provider information and how does this internal search impact the amount and type of external information search?

In turn, if internal information is deficient, external information sources are usually used. External information search constitutes seeking information from the outside environment [24]. In contrast to the scant research about internal sources, some research findings are available about external information sources used to make health treatment and service provider selections [10,27-29]. For example, [30] suggested that information about mainstream health care services is effectively distributed through external sources such as pamphlets, health professionals and formal educational programs. However, other studies indicate that information search by patients does not rely on these sources and instead uses more "personal" external sources; for example, information about general health matters could be sought from family members, friends, work colleagues and doctors [1,31]. For back pain, studies show booklets and physical-related cues might be effective but other sources like video are not [32,33]. Other external sources about back pain are online [34,35]. But are these *all* the sources for back pain information? This was the first research question.

Information content

The second issue raised in the information search literature is the nature of the content of the information patients look for or indeed avoid looking for [12,36]. The information content sought by health consumers is context specific [20]. For example, [37] found that women going through menopause searched for information to work out which symptoms were 'normal' for their age group; which symptoms they experienced were related to menopause; to get information to prepare for their visit to the doctor, and to later confirm the doctor's diagnosis and expand their knowledge of issues raised by the doctor. As another example, parents of children often have concerns and require specific information to combat misconceptions, and address their doubts about the safety/efficacy of treatments [38]. A final example relates to female cancer patients' whereby women search for information topics relating to therapies available, how to manage a recurrence of cancer if a treatment stops working, types of surgery that can be undertaken for the cancer and pain issues [39]. What context-specific information do persons with back pain seek? This was the second research question.

Search effort

The third element of information search behavior is the search effort expended by consumers. While the search effort construct [40,41] is well recognized and accepted in the marketing literature, there does not appear to be an accepted way to measure it. For example [42], measured this construct using two items: the amount of time and the amount of effort used to locate information [43] also measured search effort for home shoppers using the single item of the number of advertisements referred to in catalogues [21] defined search effort based on the number of sources consulted and the amount of effort required to gather and comprehend information. In health care research [44], measured internet search effort based on a single scale of measuring the extent of agreement/disagreement with the statement: "it took a lot of effort to get the information you needed". Other health care research investigating information search behaviours appear to ignore this issue totally [45]. In brief, search effort has been measured using time, number of sources, effort level or a combination thereof. But what defines search effort by persons with back pain? This was the third and final research question.

Methods

Qualitative research methods are appropriate for the investigation of how and/or why a social phenomenon occurs, and are therefore appropriate for this study's research problems [46,47]. That is, "the aim of qualitative research is to develop concepts that can help us understand social phenomena in natural settings, giving emphasis on the meanings, experiences and views of the participants" [48], p.11. The qualitative method of convergent interviewing was selected. It involved a series of long, initially rather unstructured interviews [49-51]. The interviewer analysed the data and refined the interview questions after each interview, to converge on the emerging issues in the topic area. In brief, flexible exploration of this complex and sensitive topic was possible through the convergent interviewing technique.

This convergent interviewing methodology is *justified* for this research in four ways [50]. Firstly, it converges quickly on important issues. The required number of interviewees in convergent interviewing should be less than traditional interviewing's because any points of convergence or divergence among interviewees are examined after each interview to develop the questions and probes for the next interview; that is, the methodology is a thorough one. Moreover, this efficiency is important when interviewees are time-limited, like many of the busy interviewees in this research project. Secondly, convergent interviewing has a mechanism for knowing when to stop collecting data – the "stability" described below. Finally, it sets a sound stage for further research methodologies such as case research.

However, there are limitations related to convergent interviewing as a research methodology. Firstly, convergent interviews are time consuming and require many consecutive interviews with many different people [46]. But the analysis after each interview allowed a convergence on key issues, and the use of the prior theory permitted a focus on important issues. Secondly, there is a risk of bias because the researcher, as the interviewer, is a participant in the data collection process. This risk was mitigated by the researcher's understanding and experience of the methodology and her use of appropriate interview techniques [52]. Moreover, the methodology's analysis after each interview reduces bias that may exist in traditional interviewing's one-off data analysis process that starts after the final interview. Indeed, the methodology could perhaps be called 'convergent and divergent interviewing' because explanations for any differences of opinion are probed for in each interview. Next, convergent interviewing is an exploratory technique and therefore should be used in conjunction with later research, and this limitation is acknowledged in the 'further research' section below. Finally the lack of interviewee validation could result in misinterpretation of the results by the researcher, but asking interviewees to decide the validity of the social-scientific rendering of interpretations of the interviews would be unreasonable because of their lack of discipline-specific knowledge [53].

Interviews were conducted with adult persons with back pain who had sought either one or more types of treatment for their problem. Study participants were recruited in Australia through notices in physiotherapy practices, government offices and one university. The twelve interviewees were purposively selected to ensure gender, age and educational balance in the sample, as shown in Table 1.

A key question is, "How many interviews should have been conducted?" The answer to this question about convergent interviewing revolves around the concept of "stabilty" or "saturation" when no new information or patterns in the data emerge from the interviews [54]. This stabilty depends on the skill of the interviewer, the type of research problem, the cases themselves, and the depth of data analysis [55], p.245 summarises this difficulty of deciding how many interviews are needed: "The validity, meaningfulness and insights generated from qualitative inquiry have more to do with the information-richness of the cases selected and the observational/analytical capabilities of the researcher than with sample size." The interviewer was an experienced qualitative researcher who had previous interviewing experience and who had a working knowledge of the subject matter.

Estimates of the required number of interviews vary. That minimum can be about six [54,55], 10 [56] or 15 [57]. The maximum can be about 50 [56,58]. Stability is often reached after only five or so convergent interviews [50]. The final convergent interview occurs when interview data analysis of that interview shows there is stability through a consistent pattern of agreements and disagreements in the last two interviews [46,50,51]. In this study, this stability appeared after the eleventh interview. To ensure that stability had been reached, an additional interview was conducted but no new information emerged.

At each interview, the researcher clarified a number of administrative issues including ethical clearance and whether the interview could be taped. The opening question was broad [46] and then detail-oriented probes, elaboration probes, and clarification probes were used within the interview [59]. Incidentally, "back pain" is defined in this report in general terms: "a pain in the lumbar, lumbosacral, or cervical regions of the back, varying in sharpness and intensity. Causes may include muscle strain or pressure on the root of a nerve" [60]. Each interview ran for approximately 60 minutes and was taped and then transcribed before analysis. Each interview was transcribed within a day of the interview and the transcript was triangulated with the notes taken by the researcher during the interview. The interviewer undertook preliminary analysis of each of the interview transcripts and accessed literature about issues that emerged as a result of the interview in order to better understand the subject matter. These steps allowed the researcher to modify the interviewer's guide as necessary (in line with the convergent interviewing methodology) to obtain more detailed and relevant information in the following interviews.

Table 1 Sample characteristics of convergent interview interviewees (n = 12)

	Frequency		Frequency
Gender		**Highest education level**	
Females	5	Secondary	5
Males	7	Post secondary	2
		Tertiary	5
Age			
Less than 25 years		**Occupation**	
25 – less than 40 years	2	Professional	6
40 – less than 60 years	3	Semi-professional	2
	7	Trades	1
		Student	2
		Disability pension	1

Data reduction was undertaken to condense data to assist in the development of a conceptual framework. Thus, transcripts were coded into themes and sub-themes according to the issues identified during the literature review. The three themes were information sources, information content and search effort although each of these were further divided into sub-themes such as internal information sources, external personal sources and external non-personal sources under the information sources theme. Where new and contrary information was found in the data, these were coded to new categories and discussed later. Next, the data from the various coded themes and sub-themes were linked together to find regularities and make sense of the data [61]. These regularities were tallied in a table next to each theme or sub-themes and the interviewee number and quote recorded alongside them.

In order to validate findings and their interpretations, one researcher undertook the analysis and discussed the findings with the other researchers. Next, the analysis was put aside for some time and then returned to by the researcher and re-analysed. This action resulted in some minor errors in the initial interpretations. These were rectified by revisiting the interview transcripts to clarify what the interviewees had said and assessing the logic with which ideas were categorized into a theme or sub-theme based on prior literature and data reduction techniques.

Ethical approval was obtained from the University of Southern Queensland's Human Research Ethics Committee (Ethical Approval number: H05REA495).

Results and discussion

Research question 1: what sources of information do persons with back pain use, and why?

Persons with back pain use a variety of internal, external personal (subjective) and external non-personal (objective) information sources during decision making, as summarized in Table 2, where the relative importance of each item is estimated.

Table 2 Information sources used to select treatment types/service providers

Information sources	Interviewees	No. of interviewees using each source	Rank of frequency of sources used
Internal source – memory of past knowledge and experiences	1, 2, 3, 4, 5, 7, 8, 9, 10, 11, 12	6	2
External personal sources			
Word of mouth – friends	1, 2, 4, 5, 7, 9, 11	7	1
Doctor/other therapists' referrals	1, 4, 5, 7, 9, 11	6	2
Word of mouth – family	1, 5, 8, 9	4	3
Word of mouth – work colleagues	1, 2, 6, 12	4	3
Speaking with a provider prior to appointment	2, 10	2	5
Word of mouth - other (for example, teacher, receptionist at my doctor's practice)	3, 10	2	5
External non-personal sources			
Yellow/white pages	1, 2, 3, 8	4	3
Promotional sign at provider's office	2, 3, 11	3	4
Internet	5, 7	2	5
Books	5	1	6
Radio talk back show	7	1	6

One of the two most important sources of information is *internal.* Almost all interviewees (11 of 12 interviewees) stated using internal sources in one or more of their decision making situations for back pain treatment selection This frequent use of internal information sources (including past knowledge and/or personal experiences) reflects other consumer research about services that require experience to evaluate [4] and indicates that persons with back pain tend to rely on their own memories. But how comprehensive and accurate is their internal information?

In order to ascertain how accurate and comprehensive interviewee's knowledge and experiences were, they were asked to explain why they chose the treatment type that they had. The majority (66%, or interviewees 2, 3, 4, 5, 7, 8, 9, 12) of interviewees explained that they had made their choices based on their perceptions of their back problem, their perception of what each treatment type could offer and thus which would be most suitable for their problem. For example, interviewee 9 said:

> *'I thought my muscles were tight from sitting at the computer every day at work so the masseuse would relax my muscles. I didn't think I had a medical problem to be sorted out by a chiropractor or physiotherapist'.*

Misconceptions and biases about chiropractors and physiotherapists

An interesting finding was that most interviewees had misconceptions of the nature of their problem and workings of chiropractic and physiotherapy treatments even though these treatments were the ones most used by interviewees. Some misconceptions were:

- That they perceived their bones were 'out' of their spine' and that they needed to be 'put back in'

> *Chiropractors manipulate the bones and put them in so they loosen the muscles but they don't retighten them. Physiotherapists don't actually put the bones in but they make the muscles work so that the bones go in by themselves. I know this from my suppositions mainly and from talking to physiotherapists* (Interviewee 3).

> *But, I knew chiropractors put bones back into place and so in my first accident when I popped a vertebra out I knew a chiropractor would put the bones back into place ... I picked [Bowen Therapy] because I thought that chiropractors put people's bones into place but I also knew that muscles keep your bones in place and so there is no point getting your bones put into place if they (your muscles) are not working right. So I wanted to go to Bowen therapy* (Interviewee 5).

> *I chose a chiropractor because I knew it was something structural – something was 'out' and it had to be put back in. And my perception is the physiotherapists work more with muscles and give massage and exercise things. But I felt like something had gone out so I just felt like I needed to have it pushed back in* (Interviewee 9).

- That physiotherapists have nothing to do with treating pain and muscle spasm:

When people think of physiotherapists, they don't think of them as people who could help heal muscle spasm and pain. And people think of chiropractors as aligning the back which has little to do with muscle pain and spasm (Interviewee 2).

- That physiotherapists and chiropractors only deal with injuries and rehabilitation

I liked the notion that chiropractors could deal with the manipulation ....like the operation of a chiropractic move. Like, they are realigning what you have. So if your back is causing you grief due to the tension that you may be carrying around then they can realign the neck and fix your headache. Whereas other treatments, I am not sure how they work but I don't like the idea of taking a tablet for a headache. I would rather deal with the cause. I always associate physiotherapists with sports injury and rehabilitation (for example, people who have their arm in a cast and they build the muscle up.' (Interviewee 10).

- That chiropractors are only helpful for non-specific back pain

Chiropractors are good for general back pain which I initially had. The treatments allowed me to wake up in the mornings without feeling stiff. They straightened my back which was crooked and I will go back for my general back pain to them but not for the spondylolisthesis. *I try to stretch my treatments to 4–5 weeks now* (Interviewee 7).

- That physiotherapists are better than chiropractors or vice versa

'I thought of seeing a chiropractor but what I had learnt about physiotherapists and chiropractors was the physiotherapists were better' (Interviewee 4).

Knowledge and experience void relating to alternative treatments

Unlike the multitude of opinions provided about physiotherapy and chiropractic care, some interviewees appeared not to know as much or express strong opinions about other treatment types (interviewees 5, 6, 7, 10, 11). Therefore, they relied mainly on their emotions and memories of vicarious learning and recommendations made by others to select a treatment type. For example, interviewee 7 chose an acupuncturist because of desperation rather than because of his knowledge of the treatment: *'I chose this type of treatment out of desperation and the lack of success with physiotherapists and chiropractors. Also, I was curious about this type of treatment and wondered what benefits it could have.'* Interviewee 10 chose chiropractors because she did not like needles despite the fact that acupuncture needles do not function in the same way that injections do: *' I always associate physiotherapists with sports injury and rehabilitation (for example, people who have their arm in a cast and they build the muscle up. And, I don't like acupuncture because I don't like needles'.* Interviewee 5 said: *'I found out about Reiki from mum and her books'. Respondent 1 used memories of vicarious learning to select a treatment type: 'I didn't really know anything about physiotherapists and chiropractors other than they help with pain. But I knew that my sister had had luck with a chiropractor and so I just chose to go to them'* (Interviewee 1).

However, once interviewees had had back problems for some time and had experienced a treatment, they used various criteria to decide on the treatment type and provider. Therefore, their criteria for selection included their past knowledge as well as their present experience with which to construct their decision.

Biased attitudes towards non-mainstream treatments

Some interviewees revealed biases against non-mainstream treatments. For example, interviewee 11 was biased against non-mainstream treatments because of his rural upbringing: *'The others (acupuncture, osteopath or any treatment outside of physiotherapy and chiropractors) are voodoo. ... well I come from a rural background and family members and people I associate with said to go to a physiotherapist. You wouldn't go to a chiropractor because they could injure you, crack your bones. As far as any alternative things like acupuncture – they are extreme'.*

Similarly, interviewee 4 showed bias toward alternative treatments like chiropractic care based on his experience:

I thought of seeing a chiropractor but what I had learnt about physiotherapists and chiropractors, was the physiotherapists were better. I knew a chiropractor as a friend when I told him my symptoms, he said that I am better off with a physiotherapist who works with musculoskeletal issues rather than spinal issues (which is what a chiropractor does).

External sources

Persons with back pain also rely on *external* personal sources to provide credence about the treatment and service they seek. Two external personal sources are word of mouth by friends, and referrals by doctors and other therapists. Other external personal sources used include word of mouth by family and work colleagues, speaking with a provider prior to booking an appointment, and speaking with others such as teachers and receptionists.

External non-personal sources are not used as much as external personal sources, because they do not have the credence of personal sources [4], as discussed below. These external non-personal sources include the telephone directory, advertising signage outside the provider's office, the internet, books and talk-back shows.

No interviewee relied solely on an internal source, even if they have past experience and knowledge to fall back on – all those using an internal source also used an external personal source, and some of them used an external non-personal source as well. Clearly, for back pain services, credence is required as well as experience [4].

Effectiveness of external personal sources

One question that remains unanswered in the literature is how effective are external personal sources in achieving positive treatment outcomes? To investigate this issue, a summary of all incidents in which interviewees outlined information sources used to select a treatment type and subsequent treatment outcomes was developed (refer Table 3).

Table 3 summarises 26 incidents where interviewees had selected a treatment provider based on word of mouth. Of the 26 incidents, only 12 (46.2%) had positive outcomes. A positive outcome is defined as adequate relief of symptoms for an acceptable period of time as judged by the respondent. The other 14 incidents were 11 (42.3%) who had no symptom relief (a negative outcome) and another 3 (11.5%) who had some symptom relief but were not fully satisfied (a somewhat positive outcome). In brief, we propose that although word of mouth is heavily relied on for decisions about which treatment type and provider to use, it might not be the most effective source to use. Further research is warranted to establish the validity of this finding and to identify any other factors which may be contributing to this outcome.

In brief, the findings of the internal and external information sources indicated that persons with back pain have and obtain little if any accurate information about the nature of their problem and what different treatments can and should be used for. As a result, interviewees' final choice of treatment type is based more on trial and error. This finding is supported by a cancer study in which its noted that many patients do not know how to access credible information and make informed decisions about cancer [62].

One poorly resolved issue in the literature relates to the reasons for the limited use of some information sources and this research makes a contribution about this issue. In particular, why are not more external non-personal sources used? Three categories of reasons for *not* searching more extensively for external information about treatment types or service providers emerged in the interviews. First, many interviewees provided *personal* reasons for not searching for information such as:

- A lack of interest as noted by interviewee 11:

I don't look for much information about what my problems are or treatments because usually you are so busy and flat out that you, sort of, are very reactive in everything you do....

- Not wanting to self- diagnose:

Nowadays I suppose you could look on the internet but I don't reckon I would do that probably because I would rather be led by an expert rather than have a look at a whole lot of stuff and start deciding... (Interviewee 12).

- Being able to self-diagnose as stated by interviewee 9: 'No I didn't look for any other information because being a nurse, you self-diagnose a lot.'

The second category of reasons for limiting search of external non-personal sources can be labeled provider-related. Two reasons were offered:

- Loyalty to the treatment provider. For example, interviewee 3 said that her loyalty stopped her from searching for information: "He [the physiotherapist] was the one I went to 25 years ago after my high jump accident, I had success with him and I was ... loyal."
- The provider provided sufficient information about their treatment relative to other providers.

I didn't look for any other information because on my first consultation with the chiropractor, they took me through what chiropractic care is and how it differs from a doctor, physiotherapist or acupuncturist. So I felt they gave me enough information (Interviewee 10).

Finally, *information-supply reasons* for limited use of external sources included reasons such as patients not knowing what information to look for, where to look for information, or the information not being readily available. For example, interviewees 7 and 12 both believed that information was not readily available. Interviewee 7, who suffers from spondylolisthesis, a rare spinal pressure produced by the forward dislocation of one vertebra over the one beneath it, said that he had only looked for information about this problem on the Internet because it is a very specific condition and information could not be found through general sources such as general interest magazines. Interviewee 2 also found it difficult to find information readily and said:

It was difficult to find information about back pain. The Yellow Pages [telephone directory] just had names

Table 3 External personal sources used to select treatment types/service providers

Interviewee	External source	1st ever treatment	2nd treatment	3rd treatment	Treatment outcome
1	WOM – family		Pain subsided from chiropractor		Positive
1	WOM - friend			Pain subsided from physiotherapy	Positive
2	WOM - colleague		Pain subsided from masseuse		Positive
3	WOM – teacher		Paid subsided from chiropractor		Positive
4	GP - referral	Pain relief but problem progressively worsened with physiotherapy			Negative
4	GP - referral		Some pain relief but got problem got progressively worse with physiotherapy		Negative
4	GP - referral			Some pain relief but got problem got progressively worse with physiotherapy	Negative
5	WOM – friends	Inadequate length of pain relief from chiropractor			Negative
5	WOM – family		No pain relief with colour therapy		Negative
5	WOM – family			Inadequate length of pain relief	Negative
6	WOM - colleague	Unhappy with chiropractor's behaviour			Negative
6	WOM – friends		Inadequate length of pain relief from acupuncture		Somewhat positive
6	WOM – friends			Inadequate length of pain relief from acupuncture	Somewhat positive
7	GP and WOM – friends	Not totally pain free with physiotherapy			Somewhat positive
7	WOM – friends		In adequate relief of symptoms with chiropractor		Negative
7	WOM - friend			No pain relief from acupuncture	Negative
8	WOM - mum	Adequate pain relief with chiropractor			Positive
8	WOM and marketing sources		Adequate pain relief with chiropractor		Positive
9	WOM friends/others	Adequate pain relief with chiropractor			Positive
10	Chiropractor's referral		Adequate pain relief		Positive
10	Chiropractor's referral			Adequate pain relief	Positive
11	WOM –friends	Inadequate pain relief			Negative
11	GP referral		Adequate pain relief		Positive
11	WOM – friend and family			Inadequate pain relief	Negative
12	WOM - friend	Adequate pain relief			Positive
12	WOM - friend		Adequate pain relief		Positive

Table 3 External personal sources used to select treatment types/service providers *(Continued)*

All	Total treatment outcomes	**26**
All	Total 'somewhat positives' outcomes*	**3 (11.5%)**
All	Total 'positive' outcomes	**12 (46.2%)**
All	Total negative outcomes	**11 (42.3%)**

*Note: somewhat positive outcomes frequency was excluded from the final calculation because of the outcomes were not satisfactory enough for the patient to remain loyal to the practitioner.

and contact details of physiotherapists and chiropractors but they didn't have a list of people who could assist with back pain."

In turn, interviewee 1 did not know what information to look for or where to look for it: *"I didn't look for information because I didn't know what to look for or where to look for it ... there wasn't any real information in your face."*

In brief, internal and only external *personal* sources of information are most important for persons with back pain. External non-personal information in not as used because of personal, provider or supply related reasons.

Research question 2: what information content is sought by persons with back pain, and how?

Interviewees sought information about two items: their *treatment options*, and their choice of service providers within a selected treatment option. The content sought about treatment options included information about the types of back problems that exist and their symptoms; the types of treatment options that exist and the specific symptoms they address or benefits they have; how each treatment option works and its origins; the efficacy of each treatment option; and self-help tips.

In addition to information sought about treatment options, interviewees wanted information about *service providers* including:

1. Finding service providers within each treatment type and their area of expertise. For example, interviewee 6 said: *"I ended up talking to friends to find out ... which ones [acupuncturists] were good to go to."*
2. Service providers' reputation. For example, interviewee 10 said:

"I went and saw Dr X and he fixed my neck and I went out and my mum was talking to her [the receptionist] about my prescription and how Dr X realigned my neck and she said "I go to a really good chiropractor if you are looking for one" and then she suggested X Chiropractic."

3. Provider's contact details. For example, interviewee 8 said: *"I found out about him through mum ... Then I jumped on the Internet for the White Pages to find his number..."*
4. Proximity to provider. For example, interviewee 1 looked through the Yellow Pages to locate a chiropractor close to where she lived. In turn, interviewee 2 said that he was in pain and walked by the masseuse therapist's shop and decided to go in for a massage. He made this decision because he was in city Y at the time that he experienced this pain and so could not wait to see his masseuse back home in city X.
5. How speedily an appointment could be obtained with the provider. For example, interviewee 11 said: *"And I needed someone that I could get into straight away..."*
6. Accessibility of the provider to discuss matters before making an appointment. For example, interviewee 2 searched for information about a provider by phoning a masseuse therapist, telling him about his problem and asking him what he could do about it.

The relationship between information content and information source

Another issue, not highlighted in the extant literature, emerged from the interview data: there was a link between some information items sought about treatment options and about service providers, and the types of information sources used to locate such information. Figure 1 shows these linkages, with treatment options and service providers on the left and information sources on the right.

To begin, information about *treatment options* was sourced through internal sources (when it was available), and through several external personal and external non-personal sources, as shown in Figure 1. Next, consider the findings about the linkages about *service provider* information and information sources, as also summarized in Figure 1. These linkages had three patterns. First, information about the availability of providers practicing a treatment type and their reputation and expertise was sourced mainly through internal sources (such as past experience) and external personal sources including word of mouth from friends, family, colleagues, doctors and others. Second, very specific information about a service provider such as the contact details, location of practice, speed of obtaining an appointment and access to the provider before an appointment, was sourced mainly from external sources such as the telephone directory, signage outside the practice and through direct contact with the provider prior to

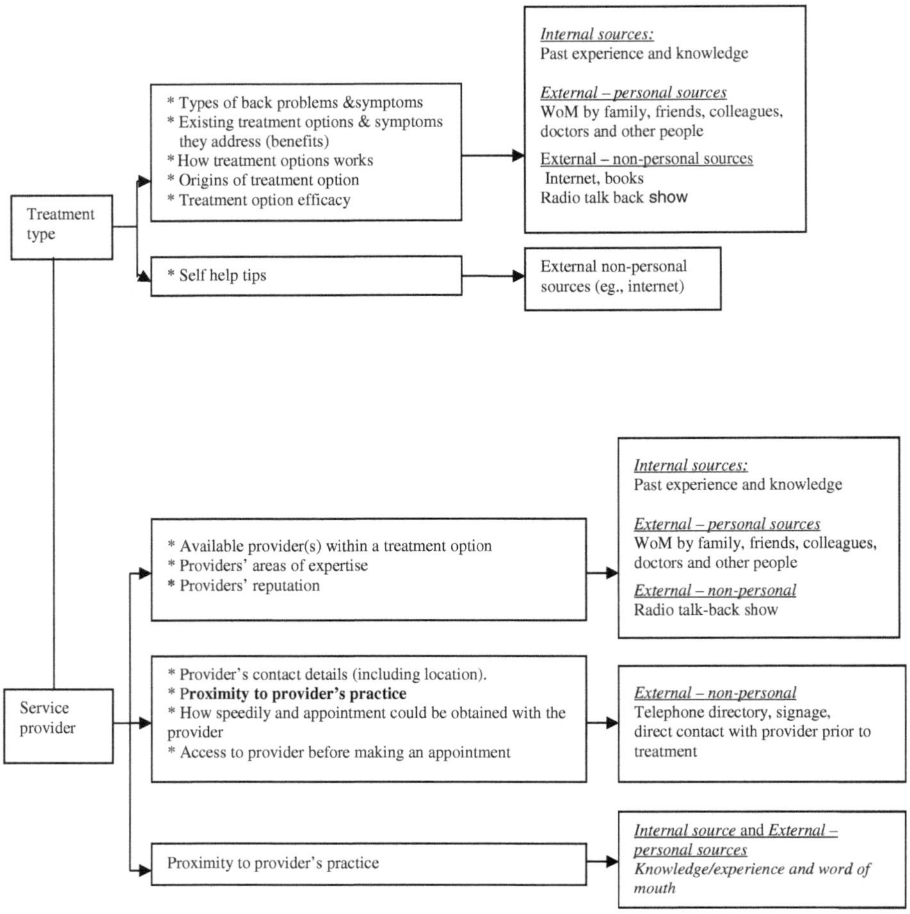

Figure 1 Mapping the relationship between information content and information sources.

treatment bookings. Third, information about the location of a service provider's practice was also sourced through internal sources (that is, past experience and knowledge) and through external personal sources of word of mouth.

In brief, the context-specific items of information sought by persons with back pain were identified for the first time, and the linkages between their sources of information and type of information were identified for the first time for any health care patient.

Research question 3: How do persons with back pain search for information?

The meaning of "search effort" emerged as the number of sources used and whether a patient deliberately or incidentally looked for information prior to making a decision. The term "deliberately" refers to situations where interviewees made a deliberate decision to look for information. By contrast, situations are categorized as "incidentally" when interviewees were exposed to certain information even though they were not deliberately searching for it. This distinction between deliberate and incidental search effort has not been identified before.

First, consider *deliberate* search through the examples provided by interviewees. Naturally, the decision was a deliberate one when the interviewee referred to their memory banks (internal information) to select a suitable treatment type and service provider (for example, interviewees 3, 8 and 9). Similarly, deliberate search was undertaken by interviewees who sought information externally through the Yellow/White Pages, the internet, books, doctors, speaking with service providers before the appointment and, in some cases, speaking with family members (for example, interviewees 1, 2, 4, 5 7, 8 and 10).

Interviewees who deliberately consulted family members about their back problems and sought assistance from them, were dependents living at home. Of the five interviewees (interviewees 1, 3, 5, 8 and 10) who did consult family members, four did so to obtain assistance. For example, the younger, dependent interviewees 3, 5, 8 and 10 had all told their parents about their pain and their parents had then suggested a course of action such as seeing a doctor (interviewees 3, and 10) or seeking treatments from providers such as a reiki healer and a physiotherapist (interviewees 5 and 8). Only interviewee 1 (an adult living independently) did not consult her family for specific back pain assistance, and raised the issue only in conversation with them.

Next, consider *incidental* search. Incidental search occurred when interviewees did not usually deliberately attempt to find information but were exposed to it from external sources such as from colleagues, friends, advertising signs on providers' doors and talkback shows. For example, interviewees 6, 7, 11 and 12 were having a general conversation with a work colleague and the issue of back pain arose as a topic in the conversation. In brief, it became evident from the analysis that search effort is a function of deliberate or incidental search.

Implications

The findings of this research have *implications* for public and private health sectors, and also for marketing management researchers. Persons with back pain rely mainly on internal information and external personal word of mouth by their doctor and friends which does not appear to provide an effective strategy for choosing treatment types and providers. Therefore, the public health system could provide more treatment related information about mainstream *and* complementary and alternative treatments. Furthermore they could provide generic information about how to select a service provider (for example, what steps to take to find a reputable and qualified service provider with the desired area of expertise) through a range of media. As a first option, information can be channeled through GP practices, in preference to the television and radio shows that have been shown to be more effective for the less information savvy, health conscious consumer [28]. However, research indicates that GPs may be unlikely to refer patients to complementary and alternative treatments due to their lack of belief in them [63]. This stance could be due to the fact that many GPs are not familiar with the research advances relating to alternative treatments like chiropractic care and massage. Therefore, an alternative solution is to use social workers who are trained in complementary and alternative treatments [62] and who understand physiology and anatomy. These professionals can assist patients to explore choices, discuss concerns, ask questions to increase understanding and make more informed decisions without judgment or bias.

As well, this information could be channeled through printed pamphlets/booklets in back health professional practices aimed at persons with back pain and their family and friends who are more health conscious and information savvy. Of course, the psychographic and media profiles of all these segments may need to be researched as a precursor to this action.

The findings of this study also have implications for health service providers. Knowledge of the information content required by interviewees can be used to better communicate services so that consumers can make better decisions. Service providers have two options: they can provide information about their service only and/or provide additional information about other competing treatment options available and compare the differences/benefits to their specific treatment offering. Service providers can also target this information through various media. Some of these media include more personal sources like the word of mouth of their own patients (who speak with friends and family) and office staff as well as their websites, pamphlets located in doctor's practices (for more in-depth treatment and service related information), radio advertising, signage and the telephone directory (for contact details and other specific service provider related queries). In order to provide personal ratings of the practice and provider, the websites could host a patient review site where past and present patients can discuss the outcomes of their experiences and even suggest improvements. The website could also provide an appointment availability function whereby patients could book or cancel appointments and find out if appointment slots are available when needed.

Next, the research has implications for market researchers. The convergent interviewing methodology was an efficient and effective way of undertaking inductive research in an under-researched area and so could be used in similar research projects. However, two limitations are evident from this study, each providing grounds for *further research* into this topic. One limitation relates to the sample size, which although adequate for constructing a preliminary model of search behavior, requires statistical generalization (theory testing) through a survey to complement the analytic generalization (theory building) of this research [47]. A final limitation is that we were not able to find any strong deviations in interviewee's answers and this could be because of the sample size. Further *quantitative* research about information search should be undertaken to investigate the presence of deviations in responses and investigate the roles of demographic, psychographic, behavioural and back pain characteristics on response differences.

Conclusions

This study has explored how persons with back pain search for information when trying to choose from a range of treatment options and service providers. Three main issues were researched: where to search for information, what information to search for, and how much effort to expend searching. In terms of where to search for information, persons with back pain rely heavily on their own memories (internal) and external personal sources such as friends and doctors when searching for information about treatment types and service providers. However, more often than not, these perceptions are wrong, biased or too limited to provide a useful guide for decisions.

These findings differ from the findings of previous studies [30] about the types of information health consumers require when searching for information about alternative or mainstream healthcare services. First, internal search was not mentioned in the literature even though it is the source most used and appears to be inaccurate, and interviewees did not rely to any extent on pamphlets. The results have identified for the first time that limited information availability was only one of three categories of reasons identified about why persons with back pain do not search for more information particularly from external non-personal sources.

Next, this study confirms findings from other research [36] that information *content* sought by patients is health context specific. For example, some interviewees required information about self-help techniques for their back problem. Examples of service related information content included the speed with which an appointment with the provider could be obtained, a providers' area of expertise and their reputation. In turn, this research outlined for the first time the exact information items sought by interviewees for both back pain treatment types and service providers, and its linkages to sources. Furthermore, extending previous studies [36], this research showed that the sheer number of treatment options and service providers required interviewees to undertake a more complex search step (combining internal search, and external personal and non-personal search) than in some other health care areas.

Finally, the information sources used by persons with back pain are a function of the information content they seek; this link is a new finding. For example, the use of external non-personal sources such as the telephone directory, contacting the provider directly or using practice signage was reserved for acquiring more detailed service provider information such as the speed of acquiring an appointment; whereas information about the provider's reputation and expertise was obtained from internal and other external personal sources. This situation reflects the information available from each source rather than the information search preferences of these persons with back pain, as evidenced by the reasons given for their low reliance on external non-personal sources.

Competing interests
The authors declare they have no competing interests.

Authors' contributions
HM conceived of the study, conceived the research design, conducted the interviews, undertook data analysis and wrote the first draft of the manuscript and approved the final manuscript. JG assisted in the research design, assisted in the data analysis and wrote additional sections of the second draft of the manuscript as well as writing the final version of the manuscript and approving the final manuscript. CP advised on research design and wrote some sections of the second draft of manuscript and approved the final manuscript.

Acknowledgements
The authors would like to thank the 12 participants who shared their back pain treatment journeys with us.

Author details
[1]School of Management and Enterprise, University of Southern Queensland, 4350 Toowoomba, QLD, Australia. [2]School of Commerce, University of Southern Queensland, Toowoomba, Australia. [3]Research Associate, Health Economics and HIV/AIDS Research Division (HEARD), University of KwaZulu-Natal, Westville Campus, Durban, South Africa.

References
1. Stewart DW, Hickson GB, Pechmann C, Koslow S, Altemeier WA: **Information search and decision making in the selection of family health care.** *J Health Care Market* 1989, **9**(2):29–39.
2. Sepucha KR, Belkora J: **Putting shared decision making to work in breast and prostate cancers: tools for community oncologists.** *Comm Oncol* 2007, **4**(11):685–689.
3. Fullwood C, Kennedy A, Rogers A, Eden M, Gardner C, Protheroe J, Reves D: **Patients' experiences of shared decision making in primary care practices in the United Kingdom.** *Med Decis Making* 2013, **33**(1):26–36.
4. Kotler P, Keller K: *Marketing Management*. New York: Prentice Hall; 2008.
5. Yen L, Jowsey T, McRae S: **Consultation with complementary and alternative medicine by older Australians: Results from a national survey.** *BMC Complement Altern Med* 2013, **13**(73):1–8.
6. Disease Control Priorities Project: *Musculoskeletal Conditions are the Most Common Cause of Chronic Disability*; 2007. Available at: http://www.dcp2.org/file/84/DCPP-Musculoskeletal.pdf (accessed 12 May 2013.
7. American Chiropractic Association: *Back Pain Facts and Statistics*; 2013. Available at: http://www.acatoday.org/level2_css.cfm?T1ID=13&T2ID=68 (accessed 5 September 2013).
8. Office for National Statistics: *31 Million Days Lost to Sickness in 2011 – but it's Falling*; 2012. Available at: ons.gov.uk/ons/rel/mro/news-release/131-million-working-days-lost-to-sickness-in-2011—but-it-s-falling/sanr0512.html, (accessed 21 October 2012).
9. Australian Bureau of Statistics: *Health*. Year Book Australia; 2012. Available at http://www.abs.gov.au/ausstats/abs@.nsf/Lookup/by%20Subject/1301.0~2012~Main%20Features~Health%20status~229. (accessed 21 October 2012).
10. Harris KM: **How do patients choose physicians? Evidence from a national survey of enrolees in employment-related health plans.** *Health Serv Res* 2003, **38**(2):711–732.
11. McClymont H: **Search and evaluation behaviours in hospital selection of rural health consumers.** *Asian J Mark* 2005, **11**(1):81–91.
12. Kind T, Wheeler K, Robinson B, Cahana M: **Do leading children's hospitals have quality websites? A description of children's hospital web sites.** *J Med Internet Res* 2004, **6**(2):e20.
13. Lipscomb T, Root T, Shelley K: **Strategies for seeking mental health services.** *Serv Mark Q* 2004, **25**(4):1–12.
14. Kwon N, Kyunghye K: **Who goes to a library for cancer information in the e-health era? A secondary data analysis of the Health Information National Trends Survey (HINTS).** *Lib Info R* 2009, **31**(3):192–200.
15. Weber K, Solomon D, Meyer B: **A qualitative study of breast cancer treatment decisions: evidence for five decision making styles.** *Health Commun* 2013, **28**(4):408–421.
16. Huh J, DeLorme DE, Reid LN, Kim J: **How Korean and White Americans Evaluate and Use Online Advertising and Non-advertising Sources for Prescription Drug Information.** *Ther Inno Reg Sci* 2013, **47**(1):116–124.
17. Park J, Chung E, Yoo WS: **Is the internet a primary source for consumer information search?: Group comparison for channel choices.** *J Retailing & Consumer Services* 2009, **16**(2):92–99.
18. Mortimer M, Ahlberg G, MUSIC-Norrtalje Study Group: **To seek or not to seek? Care-seeking behaviour among people with low-back pain.** *Scand J Public Healt* 2003, **31**(3):194–203.
19. Moorman C, Diehl K, Brinberg D, Kidwell B: **Subjective knowledge, search, locations and consumer choice.** *J Consum Res* 2004, **31**(3):673–680.

20. Wathen NC, Harris RM: **I try to take care of it myself. How rural women search for health information.** *Qual Health Res* 2007, **17**(5):639–651.
21. Duncan CP, Olshavsky RW: **External search: the role of consumer beliefs.** *J Marketing Res* 1982, **19**(1):32–43.
22. Rijnsoever FJ, Castaldi C, Dijst MJ: **In what sequence are information sources consulted by involved consumers? The case of automobile pre-purchase search.** *J Retail Consum Serv* 2012, **19**(3):343–352.
23. Kitamura S: **The relationship between use of the internet and traditional information sources: an empirical study in Japan.** *SAGE Open* 2013, **3:** doi:10.1177/2158244013489690.
24. Lamb JF, Hair JF, McDaniel C: *Marketing.* Mason: Thompson – South Western; 2009.
25. Rose S, Philip S: **Internal psychological versus external market-driven determinants of the amount of consumer information search amongst online shoppers.** *J Mark Manag* 2009, **25**(1–2):171–190.
26. Johnson EJ, Russo EJ: **Product familiarity and learning new information.** *J Consum Res* 1984, **11**(1):542–550.
27. Diviani N, Camerini A, Reinholz D, Galfetti A, Schulz PJ: **Health literacy, health empowerment and health information search in the field of MMR vaccination: a cross-sectional study protocol.** *BMJ Open* 2012, **19**:2(6).
28. Dutta-Bergman MJ: **Primary sources of health information: comparisons in the domain of health attitudes, health cognitions, and health behaviours.** *Health Commun* 2004, **16**(3):273–289.
29. Flynn M, Smith M, Freese J: **When do older adults turn to the internet for health information? Findings from the Wisconsin longitudinal study.** *J Gen Intern Med* 2006, **21**(12):1295–1301.
30. Ansani NT, Bethany MV, Henderson AF, McKaveney TP, Weber RJ, Smither RB: **Quality of arthritis information on the Internet.** *Am J Health Syst Pharm* 2005, **62**(1):1184–1189.
31. Mahoney C, Heavin C, Sammon D: *A Tool for Analyzing the Information Behavior of Expectant and new Mothers.* Proceedings of the 21st European Conference on Information Systems; 2013. viewed 25 May 2013, < http://www.staff.science.uu.nl/~vlaan107/ecis/files/ECIS2013-0873-paper.pdf.
32. Henrotin YE, Cedraschi C, Duplan B, Bazin T, Duquesnoy B: **Information and low back pain management: a systematic review.** *Spine* 2006, **31**(11):E326–E334.
33. Little P, Roberts L, Blowers H, Garwood J, Cantrell T, Langridge J, Chapman J: **Should we give detailed advice and information booklets to patients with back pain?: a randomized controlled factorial trial of a self-management booklet and doctor advice to take exercise for back pain.** *Spine* 2001, **26**(19):2065–2072.
34. Butler L, Foster N: **Back pain online: a cross-sectional survey of the quality of web-based information on low back pain.** *Spine* 2003, **28**(4):395–401.
35. Li L, Irvin E, Guzmin J, Bombardier C: **Surfing for back pain patients: the nature and quality of back pain information on the Internet.** *Spine* 2001, **26**(5):545–557.
36. Davey HM, Lim J, Butow PN, Barratt A, Houssami N, Higginson R: **Consumer information materials for diagnostic breast tests: women's view on information and their understanding of test results.** *Health Expect* 2003, **4**(6):298–311.
37. Genius SK: **Constructing "sense" from evolving health information: a qualitative investigation of information seeking and sense making across sources.** *J Am Soc Inf Sci Tec* 2012, **63**(8):1553–1566.
38. Kennedy A, LaVail K, Nowak G, Basket M, Landry S: **Confidence about vaccines in the United States: understanding parents' perceptions.** *Health Affair* 2011, **30**(6):1151–1159.
39. Kim SC, Shah DV, Namkoong K, McTavish FM, Gustafson DH: **Predictors of online health information seeking among women with breast cancer: the role of social support perception and emotional well-being.** *J Comput-Mediat Comm* 2013, **18**(2):212–232.
40. Webster FE: **Modeling of industrial buying behavior.** *J Marketing Res* 1965, **2**(4):370–376.
41. Beatty SE, Smith SM: **External search effort: an investigation across several product categories.** *J Consum Res* 1987, **14**(1):83–95.
42. Bunn MD, Butaney GT, Hoffmann NP: **An empirical model of professional buyers' search effort.** *J Bus-Bus Mark* 2001, **8**(4):55–84.
43. Sundaram DS, Taylor RD: **An investigation of external information search effort: replication in in-home shopping situations.** *Advances Consum Res* 1998, **25**:440–445.
44. Geana M, Greiner KA: **Health information and the digital divide.** *J Manag & Mark Healthcare* 2011, **4**(2):108–112.
45. Enwald HPK, Niemelä RM, Keinänen-Kiukaanniemi S, Leppäluoto J, Jämsä J, Herzig K, Oinas-Kukkonen H, Huotari MA: **Human information behaviour and physiological measurements as a basis to tailor health information. An explorative study in a physical activity intervention among prediabetic individuals in Northern Finland.** *Health Info Libr J* 2012, **29**(2):131–140.
46. Carson D, Gilmore A, Gronhaug K, Perry C: *Qualitative Research in Marketing.* London: Sage; 2001.
47. Yin RK: *Case Study Research.* 4th edition. London: Sage; 2009.
48. Al-Busaidi Z: **Qualitative research and its uses in health care.** *Sultan Qaboos University Medical J* 2008, **8**(1):11–19.
49. Driedger SM, Gallois C, Sanders CB, Santesso N: **Finding common ground in team-based qualitative research using the convergent interviewing method.** *Qual Health Res* 2006, **16**(8):1145–1157.
50. Rao S, Perry C: **Convergent interviewing to build a theory in under-researched areas: principles and an example investigation of internet usage in inter-firm relationships.** *Qual Mark Res: An International J* 2003, **6**(4):236–247.
51. Rao S, Perry C: **Convergent interviewing: a starting methodology for an enterprise research program.** In *Innovative Methodologies in Enterprise Research.* Edited by Hine D, Carson D. Northampton: Edward Elgar; 2007.
52. Perry C: *Efficient and Effective Research.* Adelaide: AIB Publications; 2013.
53. Bryman AE: *Member Validation' Accessed: 22 January 2014. Available at:* http://www.referenceworld.com/sage/socialscience/mem_valid.pdf.
54. Guest G, Bunce A, Johnson L: **How many interviews are enough? An experiment with data saturation and variability.** *Field Method* 2006, **18**(1):59–82.
55. Morse JM: **Determining sample size.** *Qual Health Res* 2000, **19**(3):3–5.
56. de Ruyter K, Scholl N: **Positioning qualitative market research: reflections from theory and practice.** *QualMark Res: An International J* 1998, **1**(1):7–14.
57. Betraux D: **From the life-history approach to the transformation of sociological Practice.** In *Biography and Society: The Life History Approach In The Social Sciences.* Edited by Betraux D. London: Sage; 1981:29–45.
58. Mason M: **Sample size and saturation in PhD studies using qualitative interviews.** *Forum: Qualitative Science Research* 2010, **11**(3):8.
59. Patton MQ: *Qualitative Evaluation and Research Methods.* 3rd edition. Newbury Park: Sage; 2002.
60. Medical Dictionary: *Medical Definition of Back Pain*; 2013. The Free Dictionary, viewed 28 May 2013, http://medical-dictionary.thefreedictionary.com/back+pain.
61. Miles MB, Huberman AM: *Qualitative Data Analysis (2nd edition).* Thousand Oaks: Sage; 1994.
62. Runfola J, Levine E, Sherman P: **Helping patients make decisions about complementary and alternative treatments: The social work role.** *J Psychosoc Oncol* 2006, **24**(1):81–106.
63. Charles C, Gafni A, Whelan T: **Self-reported use of shared decision-making among breast cancer specialists and perceived barriers and facilitators to implementing this approach.** *Health Expect* 2004, **7**(4):338–348.

Spinal manipulation under anesthesia: a narrative review of the literature and commentary

Dennis DiGiorgi

Abstract

As exhibited throughout the medical literature over many decades, there is a lack of uniformity in the manner in which spine pain patients have historically qualified for and received manipulation under anesthesia (MUA). Also, for different professions that treat the same types of spinal conditions via the same means, fundamental MUA decision points vary within the published protocols of different professional associations. The more recent chiropractic literature communicates that the evidence to support the efficacy of MUA of the spine remains largely anecdotal. In addition, it has been reported that the types of spinal conditions most suitable for MUA are without clear-cut consensus, with various indications for MUA of the low back resting wholly upon the opinions and experiences of MUA practitioners. This article will provide a narrative review of the MUA literature, followed by a commentary about the current lack of high quality research evidence, the anecdotal and consensus basis of existing clinical protocols, as well as related professional, ethical and legal concerns for the chiropractic practitioner. The limitations of the current medical literature related to MUA via conscious/deep sedation need to be recognized and used as a guide to clinical experience when giving consideration to this procedure. More research, in the form of controlled clinical trials, must be undertaken if this procedure is to remain a potential treatment option for chronic spine pain patients in the chiropractic clinical practice.

Keywords: Manipulation under anesthesia, Spine, Efficacy, Medical evidence, Quality, Ethics

Background

MUA has been reported in the medical literature since the 1930's [1]. Inspection of the literature reveals that medicine assisted manipulation (MAM) [2], across its varied forms- manipulation under general anesthesia or conscious/deep sedation (MUA), manipulation under joint anesthesia (MUJA) or manipulation under epidural anesthesia/epidural steroid injection (MUEA/MUESI)- has been used to treat a host of musculoskeletal conditions [1,3-30]. Table 1 summarizes many of the clinical diagnoses traditionally reported and treated by MAM.

Historically, there has remained a strong theoretical basis for the application of MUA to the axial spine and associated soft tissues. It has been proposed that by disrupting or stretching adhesions [4,12,20,25,31,32] a restoration of articular mechanics can be realized [4,10,12,32,33]. Nevertheless, the most recent review paper on medicine assisted manipulation for chronic low back pain communicates that the theories that MUA more effectively treats adhesions and that adhesion reduction increases flexibility are without the support of experimental research [2]. Of equal inference is the notion that these theories cannot be contested absent such research [2]. Thus, there is a void of medical evidence to either confirm or deny the validity of the principal clinical basis for utilizing spinal MUA.

The addition of anesthesia to the manipulative procedure serves to eliminate pain inhibiting reflexes and to allow for relaxation of muscles so that treatment can be delivered more effectively [10,34]. Essentially, MUA of the spine is intended for use with two general categories of pain conditions [32,35], and when manipulation is the therapeutic procedure of choice [35]:

The acute condition (i.e., acute onset of a recurrent condition)

MUA may be pursued when a patient's pain is so intense and debilitating that medication management and/or the application of standard chiropractic treatment is precluded [35,36]. Immediate relief is desired in an attempt

Correspondence: drdigiorgi@aol.com
DC, CHCQM, CCIC, Consultant Practice- Whitestone, New York, USA

Table 1 Musculoskeletal conditions treated with medicine assisted manipulation (MAM)

Cervical spine		Thoracic spine
Cervical disk herniation/syndrome [4,8]		Intractable intercostal neuritis [10]
Cervical pain [3,5-7]		Thoracic pain [5,7]
Cervical radiculopathy [4,9]		
Cervicogenic headache [3,4]		**Other**
Traumatic torticollis [10]		Acute muscle spasm with subluxation [27]
Lumbar spine/pelvis		Acute osteopathic lesion pathology [17]
Acute low back pain [7]	Lumbar intervertebral disc syndrome [17,25,26]	Acute psoasitis [17]
Arthritic changes of the low back [17]	Lumbarization/sacralization [10]	Chronic muscle contracture [6,27]
Chronic low back pain [5,11-15]	Lumbar nerve root compression syndrome [23,24]	Chronic myositis [27]
Chronic lumbosacral strain [29]	Lumbar post-laminectomy syndrome [22]	Extremity dysesthesias related to cervical or lumbar pain [5]
Chronic sacroiliac strain [1,27]	Lumbar radiculopathy [9]	Fibrosis/(myo)fibrositis [10,17,27,28]
Degenerative lumbar scoliosis [19]	Lumbosacral disc protrusion [11]	Nerve entrapment [27]
Disturbed lumbar disc integrity [10]	Postural defects of the low back [20]	Old compression fractures [10]
Failed back surgery syndrome [12,21]	Recalcitrant synovial joint mediated low back pain [18]	Osteoporosis [10]
Joint stiffness of the low back [17]	Rigidity of the low back [20]	
Low back pain with leg weakness and/or pain [11,12,16]	Spondylolisthesis [17,30]	
Lumbar disc derangement [30]	Spondylosis [30]	

to have the individual return to pre-injury status as soon as possible [35]. In the chiropractic literature it has been reported that MUA is not usually applied in cases of acute trauma [35], but if so, only a single procedure dose would typically be required to return the patient to office-based care [32]. Aside from the single procedure dose approach it has also been reported that the application of intermittent (non-consecutive) MUA procedure doses may be justified in the treatment of acute musculoskeletal conditions [37].

The chronic condition

For the chronic condition MUA is indicated when a patient's pain has proven to be of limited responsiveness in part to trials of traditional office-based manipulative procedures (over a period of weeks [33,35,37]), and when the condition has a measurable detrimental impact upon functionality [5]. Treatment is directed at eliminating the fibrotic adhesions presumed responsible for altering one's ability to engage in routine activities versus pre-injury or pre-condition levels. In qualifying the extent to which physical incapacitation may warrant the use of MUA it has been depicted that condition intensity can render "impossible" patient engagement in therapeutic exercise [38]. The procedure may be most appropriate once other modes of conservative care have been exhausted and the final patient decision scenario of surgery versus MUA is reached [38].

In 1992, Greenman [6] reported that the need for MUA is "not common". Elsewhere, it has been suggested that only a small minority of patients with musculoskeletal disorders/mechanical dysfunctions will require the like, perhaps spanning from 3% to 10% [5,7]). However, these figures on patient candidacy have yet to be validated by way of controlled investigation [2], thereby suggesting lack of substantiating evidence for them.

The MUA procedure has evolved considerably since initially reported in the early osteopathic literature. This has been acknowledged by chiropractic investigators [2,34]. Older papers describe or imply the rendition of mostly a single MUA procedure dose by osteopathic/medical physicians with an involved patient hospital stay [7,17,25,27,28]. Nowadays, MUA of the spine is usually administered in serial fashion [5,8,31], on an outpatient basis, with the principal provider type being chiropractors [39]. Paralyzing anesthetic drugs are no longer in use, while various types or combinations of hospital-based co-interventions are not part of the contemporary treatment regimen (i.e., shortwave diathermy [20], intramuscular medication [20], intramuscular vitamin E [20], muscle relaxants [17], vitamin B6 [17], various forms of traction [7,17,20,26-28,40] and fitted back brace [26]).

The contributing role of any or all of the early methods in the study outcomes previously reported is not known.

From an historical perspective, the eventual participation of chiropractors in spinal MUA occurred many years after orthopedic manipulation had fallen by the wayside and only after the larger osteopathic community hadn't taken acceptance to the MUA procedure [34]. One might deduce that an absence of perceived treatment efficacy for MUA was the principal causative factor for its generalized lack of popularity amongst allopathic physicians. As such, the contemporary chiropractic clinician should not rely upon decades old clinical papers, which cite a distinctly different MUA treatment regimen from that in use today, as an unconditional or rote support basis for MUA of the spine via conscious/deep sedation.

Proponents of the MUA procedure once categorized it as a last resort treatment option for those facing surgical intervention [38]. Nonetheless, under the domain of chiropractors MUA has arguably become a mode of care commonly administered under far less pressing clinical circumstances and with growing frequency. There is a general lack of published outcomes data in the peer reviewed medical literature to explain or support this element of the evolutionary process. Moreover, the manner in which the post-MUA therapy and rehabilitation component of care may contribute to the patient improvement claims frequently made by chiropractors is not known.

Review of the literature

Reviewing the medical literature on spinal manipulation under anesthesia presents a significant challenge on account of lack of a comparative nature of the procedure, and related components, over the course of many decades. Most published clinical studies on medicine assisted manipulation reflect largely positive outcomes. As such, some might consider MAM a universal treatment strategy for appropriately selected patients with spine-based musculoskeletal pain or disability. Nonetheless, by applying the levels of evidence schema introduced nearly a decade ago by Wright et al. [41] as a method to rate the more commonly cited or relied upon published clinical studies on MAM, the quality of research evidence can be gauged by way of a contemporary standard (Table 2). It is through this process that the lack of high quality supportive scientific evidence for spinal MUA is revealed.

Many of the MAM studies within the medical literature are of the case report or case series variety. Namely, each of numerous published reports spanning from 1949 to 2012 [3-6,8,10-12,16,18,19,21,22] accounts for only a select few patients undergoing MUA or MUJA/MUEA (ranging from 1 to 5 subjects). However, case reports or small case series are of limited value in that they are typically comprised of only successful cases, and are descriptive in nature as opposed to analytic/experimental [44,45]. The MUA case series by Morningstar and Strauchman cites inherent bias with a retrospective patient selection process [21]. Consequently, the case report/series study design lies relatively low in the hierarchy of medical evidence and specific cause and effect relationships cannot be determined [46].

The MUJA/MUEA treatment related case reports or case series offered by Aspegren, et al. [16], Ben-David and Raboy [11], Dougherty, et al. [9], Dreyfuss, et al. [18], Haldeman and Soto-Hall [1], Nelson, et al. [14] and Warr, et al. [30] all cite favorable results. It has been suggested or hypothesized that the efficacy of the MUJA procedure, or proposed manipulation following periarticular anesthetics, may be related to facilitation of the manipulative maneuver [47,48]. Specific to MUEA, it has been postulated that observed treatment efficacy for radiculopathic conditions of the cervical or lumbar regions is related to the combined effect of addressing both the inflammatory and mechanical components of pain [9].

In the management of chronic lumbosacral strain, the results of the studies conducted by Bremner [29] and Bremner and Simpson [49] were compared in determining patient response to two different treatment methods [49]. In the earlier study of 250 patients, manipulation of the lumbar spine under general anesthesia was performed, followed by physiotherapy for two weeks [29]. In the latter study involving 150 patients treated via physiotherapy three times per week for four weeks, treatment was comprised of deep massage to the lumbosacral spine, manipulation, strengthening exercises and, in some cases, short-wave diathermy [49]. The percentages of patients showing any improvement were 86.8% and 87.4%, respectively. Both treatment methods, either with or without MUA, were deemed to offer an equally beneficial immediate result.

Significantly positive outcomes for pain, patient work status and medication use were reported in the large MUA retrospective case series conducted by West, et al. [31]. However, those results are of uncertain value due to confounding factors with the study design. Namely, patient selection was not limited by diagnosis while patients were generically grouped by cervical or lumbar conditions despite the number of symptomatic anatomic regions. Furthermore, MUA was rendered on a multiregional basis for all patients rather than being directed at the region of primary diagnosis. Also, comparative post-MUA functional capacity outcomes data were generally collected six weeks after MUA, apparently only after the inception of an intensive post-MUA rehabilitation program. Last, and perhaps of greatest significance, this same study had been previously published, alternatively citing that 20 of the 177 patients in the treatment

Table 2 Synopsis of the routinely cited or reviewed published research papers on MAM of the spine

Author(s)	Publication year	No. of procedure doses	Study design	Level of research evidence[†]
		MUA or MAM*		
Kohlbeck FJ, et al. [13]	2005	1 to 3 (over consecutive weeks)	Cohort study (prospective)	II
Palmieri and Smoyak [15]	2002	1 to 4 (over the same number of days)	Cohort study (prospective)	II
Siehl D, et al. [23]	1971	1	Cohort study/RCT [#]	II
Morningstar and Strauchman [21]	2012	3 (over consecutive days)	Case series	IV
Morningstar and Strauchman [19]	2010	3 (over consecutive days)	Case report [+]	IV
Cremata E, et al. [5]	2005	3 (over consecutive days)	Case series	IV
Herzog J [4]	1999	3 (over consecutive days)	Case report	IV
West DT, et al. [31]	1999	3 (sequentially)	Case series	IV
West DT, et al. [42]	1998	3 (sequentially)	Case series	IV
Davis CG [3]	1996	At least 1 and up to 3 (consecutively or intermittently)	Case series	IV
Alexander GK [22]	1993	5 (serial)	Case report	IV
Davis CG, et al. [12]	1993	3 (over consecutive days)	Case reports	IV
Hughes BL [8]	1993	3 (daily basis)	Case report	IV
Greenman PE [6]	1992	1	Case report	IV
Chrisman OD, et al. [25]	1964	1	Case series	IV
Siehl, D [28]	1963	1 (91%), 2 or more (9%)	Case series	IV
Bremner, RA [29]	1958	1	Case series	IV
Mensor MC [26]	1955	1 (83%), 2 (17%)	Case series	IV
Soden CH [10]	1949	1	Case reports	IV
		MUEA/MUESI or MUJA[ℓ]		
Dougherty P, et al. [9]	2004	1 (67.5%), 2 (25%), 3 (6.25%), 4 (1.25%)	Case series	IV
Nelson L, et al. [14]	1997	1	Case series	IV
Aspegren DD, et al. [16]	1997	1	Case reports	IV
Dreyfuss P, et al. [18]	1995	1 or 2	Case reports	IV
Ben-David and Raboy [11]	1994	1	Case reports	IV
Warr AC, et al. [30]	1972	1	Case series	IV
Haldeman and Soto-Hall [1]	1938	1	Case series	IV

* With procedural application to one or more spinal regions via general anesthesia or conscious sedation.

[†] When applying the levels of evidence rating system for categorizing study quality, as put forth by Wright, et al. [41] and adopted by the *Journal of Bone & Joint Surgery* [41], *Spine, Clinical Orthopaedics and Related Research*, the North American Spine Society, the American Academy of Orthopaedic Surgeons, and the Pediatric Orthopaedic Society of North America [43].

[+] The case report study design has not been rated by Wright, et al. [41]. In terms of qualitative value it is likely most analogous to expert opinion (Level V evidence). However, in eliminating the appearance of bias toward underestimating its significance it has been coupled here with the case series study design and designated as Level IV evidence.

[#] Within the medical literature this study has been classified differently, as a Cohort study [13,34] and as an RCT [2]. As the final paper from Siehl, et al. [23] does not specifically cite the element of patient randomization, the Cohort study design classification appears to be correct. Nevertheless, the results reported [23] pertain to 47 of 147 patients (less than 80% follow-up). Therefore, even as an RCT, this study would qualify as Level II evidence under the rating system put forth by Wright, et al. [41].

[ℓ] With procedural application to specific spinal regions via MUEA/MUESI or MUJA (MAM agents applied locally).

Abbreviation key: *MAM*- medicine assisted manipulation, *MUA*- manipulation under anesthesia, *MUEA*- manipulation under epidural anesthesia, *MUESI*- manipulation under epidural steroid injection, *MUJA*- manipulation under joint anesthesia.

group were in receipt of "anesthetic/corticosteroid epidural injection" at the outset of MUA treatment for sequestered disc herniation [42]. The more recent West paper [31] offers no mention of this and does not address the potential therapeutic impact of the injection on the group of subjects that had received it relative to those who underwent MUA (conscious sedation) alone.

The prospective cohort studies undertaken by Kohlbeck, et al. [13] and Palmieri and Smoyak [15] refer to 42 and 38 subjects, respectively, in receipt of single or serial

MAM/MUA for chronic low back pain versus a control group. Between these two studies there are variations in technique application, the span of time between any serially administered procedure doses (consecutive days versus consecutive weeks), and the intravenous agents utilized. Although both clinical papers chronicle results that are encouraging (e.g., more improvement for the MAM/MUA treatment group in the patient-perceived outcome categories of pain and disability), neither study was conducted by way of a randomized trial. Both sets of authors acknowledge this fact and conclude that large-scale clinical studies (i.e., multi-site, randomized controlled trials) appear warranted in this area [13,15]. It should be noted that in the absence of randomization, it is significantly less likely that treatment and control groups will be balanced with regard to both the known and the unknown factors affecting outcome [46]. Therefore, while the results of each of these observational studies are both favorable and encouraging they are simply not conclusive enough to generalize that MAM or MUA via conscious sedation can be considered efficacious across the spectrum of chronic spine pain populations (low back or otherwise).

There is a general paucity of high quality clinical papers in the area of MUA management of intervertebral disc related conditions with a suspected neurological component of radiating pain into an extremity. In the presence of *EMG confirmed* lumbar nerve root compression, the study by Siehl, et al. [23] does not favor the use of MUA under that particular clinical circumstance. The authors of that paper opined that the trend of outcome deemed the procedure ineffective over the long term in the presence of positive EMG findings, with surgery likely required at some point. For lumbar disc herniation without EMG evidence of nerve root compression it was opined that MUA would probably offer lasting benefit [23]. Within the medical literature, this study has been alternately referred to as a Cohort study [13,34] and a randomized controlled trial [2]. Regardless of classification (both qualifying as Level II evidence), the findings of Siehl, et al. [23] were recently summarized in a literature synthesis put forth by the Scientific Commission of the Council on Chiropractic Guidelines and Practice Parameters [50]. Therefore, in the context of that seminal paper [23] it cannot be summarily assumed that absent electrodiagnostic testing, patient symptomatology of chronic lower back pain with a referred/radiating component into a lower extremity is necessarily indicative of a condition that may warrant or support consideration for MUA.

Commentary about the literature

MUA has been classified as both "surgical" [10,51] and "nonsurgical" [2]. Regardless of classification, recent multidisciplinary expert panel reviews of the interventions for neck and low back pain conditions do not include an analysis of any form of medicine assisted manipulation [52-55]. One might argue that the overall lack of high quality studies in this area, for specific clinical diagnoses, renders MUA of the spine controversial despite its seeming widespread use and strong theoretical basis. In contrast, the utilization of MUA to treat certain extremity conditions (i.e., frozen articulations of the shoulder or knee) has likely earned a greater degree of acceptance amongst practitioners and third party payers alike due to a gradually mounting body of supportive medical evidence [56-61]. So, despite the presence of MAM in the medical literature for many decades, questions remain as to whether MUA via conscious/deep sedation can be considered a clinically authenticated treatment option for acute or chronic neck and low back pain conditions across varying etiologies.

More than a decade ago an opinion paper cited that more than 20,000 patients in the US and the UK had received MUA since the late 1930's [32]. Since the publishing of that paper, certainly the number of chiropractors in the United States attaining MUA certification has grown. Considering this, as well as increasing popularity and a greater degree of MUA utilization within the chiropractic profession over that period, the relative paucity of published studies in the peer reviewed medical literature represents a glaring void. To date, as part of the natural progression of clinical research [62], the MUA protocols routinely used by chiropractors have not been subjected to a single large-scale randomized controlled trial for any spinal condition or diagnosis so as to reveal the evidence of efficacy or in serving to support serial MUA over a single procedure dose.

Advocates of spinal MUA may find themselves in a compromised position when they ignore the void of scientific evidence for this procedure. For the treatment of spine-based musculoskeletal pain/dysfunction most major third party payers in the United States have designated MUA "experimental/investigational". The sole basis for this unfavorable designation is the current lack of high quality evidence for MUA. However, these same payers take a favorable position with the allopathic version of MUA of the spine, when it involves the reduction of vertebral or pelvic fracture/dislocation [63-65]. The role of MUA in evaluating pelvic fracture stability following trauma has most recently been investigated [66].

The best evidence for MAM or MUA of the spine relates to the management of chronic low back pain (Level II evidence), as put forth in the controlled prospective cohort studies undertaken by Kohlbeck, et al. [13] and Palmieri and Smoyak [15]. However, these authors acknowledge the need for additional large scale studies in attaining more definitive data on treatment efficacy [13,15]. Consequently, the results of these studies should not be extrapolated as evidence of efficacy for MUA in treating different spine pain populations or when different agents/techniques from those outlined are implemented in similar spine pain populations. In terms of the vague nature of the manifestation diagnosis of pain (i.e., chronic low back pain), perhaps additional investigation would be beneficial in identifying specific clinical diagnoses of the low back that may be amenable to MUA. With regard to the treatment of EMG confirmed lumbar intervertebral disc related nerve root compromise, the only study undertaken to date [23] resulted in an outcome trend suggesting that MUA was ineffective over the long term (Level II evidence). Those same authors also opined that lasting improvement will probably be experienced in those with negative EMG-related low back pain with radiation to one or both legs.

There are no randomized controlled trials or published cohort studies on MUA management of specific diagnoses of the cervical or thoracic regions. As such, the efficacy of such treatment has yet to be adequately explored. As per the work of Krumhansl and Nowacek [38], despite a high percentage of favorable results attained for the 171 subjects treated by way of MUA for conditions of the lumbar and/or cervical regions, *not a single patient* received an extension of that care to the conjoining thoracic spine. Also, it was reported that relatively few (11%) of those same patients were in receipt of a second procedure dose. None required a third. In the large case series undertaken by Siehl, manipulation of the dorsal (thoracic) spine under general anesthesia was rendered "occasionally", while 9% of patients required more than one procedure dose [28]. Thus, in order to determine the efficacy of MUA for primary conditions of the cervical and thoracic regions, and in clarifying the dosing thresholds necessary for best patient outcomes, diagnosis specific comparative studies are needed.

There is no published medical evidence to support the common approach of universal MUA treatment of the entire axial spine in the management of an isolated regional condition (i.e., recalcitrant lumbar pain, with disabling range-of-motion loss). This remains true even in the presence of secondary and relatively innocuous complaints/physical findings of vertebral joint pain/dysfunction of other spinal regions. In fact, as reported by Krumhansl and Nowacek, following a single MUA procedure to the lumbar region, corrective mobilization of the upper thoracic and cervical regions is usually attained with a rigorous three day manual therapy regimen [38]. Also, relative to an initial MUA procedure dose to the lumbar region, subsequent application of MUA to treat cervical spine injuries is required infrequently (with about 5% of cases). Reportedly, this holds true even for injuries associated with rear-end vehicular collisions (with 20% of those cases selected for MUA) [38].

The clinical value of the distinct application of MUA to the shoulder and/or hip articulations, as a natural extension of MUA treatment of approximating vertebral/pelvic joints, has yet to be determined through scientific investigation. It is recognized that some of the commonly applied spine-related MUA maneuvers/techniques rely on the upper or lower extremity as a long lever. This serves to stretch the musculature from origin to insertion as it traverses both the targeted vertebral/pelvic motion units under care and the conjoining extremity. However, technique application does not signify that any incidental or intentionally induced joint cavitation from the glenohumeral or femoroacetabular articulations is an integral component of care such that it provides additional therapeutic benefit to the patient's treating spinal condition (whether or not there is an associated component of pain referral/radiation to the extremities). In fact, published MUA studies on the shoulder and hip joints are concerned solely with primary conditions of these articulations, such as adhesive capsulitis [57-59,67]. Consequently, any supportive medical evidence for the utilization of MUA to treat frozen shoulder or hip articulations does not serve as a clinical basis for the routine application of MUA to these extremity joints when rendered as an adjunctive form of care during the MUA management of a spine pain condition. This type of treatment approach has been criticized in the chiropractic literature [68].

There is a growing body of evidence on the use of MUA to treat frozen shoulder (adhesive capsulitis) [57-59] and post-operative fibroadhesions of the knee [60,61], when rendered as a single dose orthopedic procedure. However, a recent health technology assessment found limitations in the studies published on MUA management of frozen shoulder [69], with the only study deemed adequate revealing no evidence of better outcome with MUA over home exercise. For similar conditions of the hip joint (the femoroacetabular joint [67]), there is a general paucity of clinical papers in the peer reviewed medical literature.

Clinical considerations

Clinical issues of patient selection

Although manipulation of the spine under anesthesia is currently in general use by chiropractic professionals, it is an advanced form of treatment [35] not intended as a first-line therapy or routine service. For each of the varied forms of MAM, treatment is reserved for individuals who have already pursued traditional modes of care [3-5,7,9,11,12,14-16,18,25,31,33,36,38,47] (including, in part, spinal manipulation), but for whom the condition is recalcitrant [47]. Significant pain and dysfunction typically preclude a return to normal activities [5], whether personal, occupational or recreational. Acutely symptomatic conditions can be managed by MUA when immediate relief is desired but traditional modes of care including spinal manipulation are not tolerated [35] (i.e., with an acute idiopathic torticollis [36]). However, MUA is more commonly directed at the chronic and recalcitrant variety of musculoskeletal condition [32,38] which has not resolved as expected with conservative care or in accordance with the natural history of healing.

Descriptions of locked or immovable spinal joints have been offered as a primary patient qualifier for MUA [38,70,71]. This would suggest the presence of "a state of fixation" [71] by which the facet joint articulations of one or more vertebral motion units remain reflexogenically/biomechanically frozen or are bordering on pathological fusion. It is posited here that this level of vertebral joint "dysfunction" is seldom encountered in chiropractic practice.

It is well established that asymptomatic and/or atraumatic individuals can display positive findings upon magnetic resonance imaging of the cervical and lumbar regions [72-76], many of which are known phenomena of aging [77-79]. There is evidence that the anatomically mapped referral zones for neck and low back pain of sclerotomal and myotomal origin [80-85] can resemble or mimic patterns of radiating pain of dermatomal origin [86-90]. Both of these factors can confound the clinical picture when caring for patients with trauma induced spine pain conditions which include a referral/radiation component into an extremity. It's known that absent inflammation, spinal nerve root compression on its own does not cause pain, although physical signs of motor, deep tendon reflex and/or sensory deficits can occur [91,92]. Therefore, in the context of the findings of Siehl, et al. [23], each of these factors must be taken into consideration when patients exhibiting the aforesaid symptom complex are being evaluated for MUA.

The joint cavitation phenomenon

What makes chiropractic care unique in the realm of existing conservative management options for spine pain is the skilled manipulation component of that care. When spinal joints are manually manipulated they are moved passively to their physiological limit before receiving a dynamic thrust which separates the articular surfaces [93], resulting in joint cavitation (an audible crack) [93,94]. Joint cavitation is the consequence of an immediate reduction of intra-articular pressure and the liberation of gases from the synovial fluid, and results in a transitory period of joint surface separation due to the presence of a newly formed gas bubble [93,94]. The gapping of synovial joint surfaces, or the temporary induction of joint buoyancy, likely plays a role in the relief of joint pain and/or stiffness.

It was previously reported that a potential association between the therapeutic benefits attained with spinal manipulation and the joint cavitation phenomenon had yet to be fully investigated [95]. More recently, it has been revealed that a reduction in erector spinae muscle spindle stretch reflex activity occurs *only* when spinal manipulation is accompanied by an audible release [96]. Albeit preliminary, this might suggest a biological mechanism to the pain reducing effects of spinal manipulation. Joint cavitation may serve to interrupt muscle spindle stretch reflex excitability, part of the pain-spasm-pain cycle [96]. The analgesic/hypoalgesic effects of spinal manipulation have been discussed elsewhere [93,97-101], as have the mechanical/physiological benefits of increased joint range of motion [91,93,100] and a reduction of articular adhesions [93].

Clinical issues of manipulation technique

Thrust versus non-thrust techniques

Under the domain of chiropractic care lays numerous named spinal adjusting techniques [102-105], many of which are implemented with the intent of maneuvering synovial joints to the extent that cavitation is achieved. In theory, the audible release attained via different manipulation techniques could vary in terms of the side or vertebral level affected, with potential for better health outcomes upon modification of technique [106]. The Diversified technique is that which is most commonly utilized in chiropractic practice [107,108] and rendered with the clinical intent of eliciting joint cavitation. It is the only acceptable technique to utilize when delivering manipulations during the MUA procedure [35,109].

Two commonly utilized and well accepted chiropractic techniques that are applied without an explicit intent to elicit joint cavitation, on account of means of delivery, are the Activator Method and Cox Flexion Distraction. The former technique is administered by way of a handheld spring-loaded adjusting instrument that renders a low force impulse into spinal joints [110]. The latter technique is administered by way of a treatment table with breakaway sections that allow multi-planar distractive forces to be applied principally to intervertebral discs [111,112]. Although mechanically assisted manipulation with an impulse device such as the Activator adjusting instrument is categorized as a high velocity, low amplitude procedure [50], flexion distraction methods are considered within the realm of mobilization [50]. Hence, patients who have not received chiropractic treatment via manual manipulation techniques aimed at inducing joint cavitation have not undergone a trial of care akin to that which is utilized during the MUA procedure. Accordingly, it is with a patient's best interests in mind that adequate trials of in-office chiropractic manipulations should be comprised of one or another type of joint cavitation technique, assuming patient toleration, before the individual may be considered for potential placement into an MUA program.

Full spine versus regional manipulation

Many chiropractors adhere to a patient care ideology of treating the entire spine in achieving a state of structural and functional balance. However, for patients being managed by way of MUA, this philosophical precept is not supported by current medical evidence. As previously proffered by Krumhansl and Nowacek, corrective mobilization of the upper thoracic and cervical regions is usually attained with a rigorous three day manual therapy regimen following a single MUA procedure to the lumbar region [38]. Subsequent application of MUA to the cervical spine was reported to be infrequently required, even in cases of rear-end vehicular collisions [38]. As MUA is intended to be reserved for those exhibiting significant pain and dysfunction of a particular body region (which precludes normal activities [5]), the practice of full-spine application should not be routine but rather determined on a case-by-case basis with supportive clinical logic.

Treatment of a targeted spinal region via MUA necessitates the stretching of conjoining spinal regions incidental to the origin and insertion of the involved musculature. In and of itself, this does not constitute as MUA treatment of the secondary spinal region/s. Although conscious manipulation to a body region that conjoins another with pain or dysfunction can provide clinical benefit to the affected site [113-117], the evidence for this practice is limited and inconsistent [118]. That evidence should not be extrapolated to support the provision of multi-regional MUA care when treating a patient primarily for an isolated spinal condition. To the contrary, as reported by Krumhansl and Nowacek [38], evidence exists for the efficacy of short-term post-MUA office-based care in addressing secondary issues of spinal regions not treated via MUA.

MUA dosage

Divergent sets of protocols/indications for MUA exist [119,120] in part, with regard to the requisite conservative treatment timeframes associated with patient selection as well as procedure dose application. This raises questions as to what constitutes as the professional standard of care for MUA intervention and dosage. In the absence of a single and uniform process by which patients may qualify for and receive MUA it is easily inferred that the most fundamental decision points relied upon are lacking high quality supportive evidence. Instead, they rest upon consensus processes of different professional associations. Within the more recent chiropractic literature it has been said that the evidence to support the efficacy of MUA of the spine remains "largely anecdotal" [34], that various indications for MUA of the low back rest wholly upon the opinions and experiences of MUA practitioners [2] and that the types of spinal conditions most suitable for MUA are without clear-cut consensus [21].

The most recent review paper on MAM for chronic low back pain cites that there is "little evidence" to support the opinion that three MUA procedure doses, administered serially over the same number of days, are necessary to attain the best possible results [2]. This challenges the conventional chiropractic thinking and the more common practice of rendering MUA over three consecutive days. For what may be considered one of the seminal references on the subject of MUA, Krumhansl and Nowacek reported that over a 6 year period a total of 190 MUA procedures were performed on 171 subjects [38]. This would signify that an overwhelming percentage of those patients had received only a single procedure. Elsewhere, some of the chronic low back pain patients within the prospective cohort studies conducted by Kohlbeck, et al. [13] and Palmieri and Smoyak [15] were in receipt of only a single MUA or MAM procedure dose. Perhaps of greatest significance, a consensus document put forth by the American Academy of Osteopathy in 2005 qualifies that the MUA procedure is usually rendered as a single dose [119]. As such, chiropractors should be particularly attentive to individual patient needs rather than summarily presume that three MUA procedure doses would be appropriate or necessary for maximum therapeutic benefit. Also, broader consideration should be given to the potential for a perpetuation of favorable perceptions with treatment approaches that have yet to be substantiated by way of controlled clinical investigation [121].

Types of MUA treatment

MUJA has been said to be a clinical correlate of MUA [47]. However, it would be an oversimplification to compare MUJA or MUEA with the MUA procedure in general. Differences exist in the type, route and mode of action of the medication agents administered from one procedure to another. Therefore, as for the treatment of any particular clinical diagnosis, the existing base of literature on MUJA/MUEA should not be relied upon as evidence either for or against the efficacy of MUA of the spine via conscious sedation or deep sedation. Moreover, the emerging literature for use of MUA on frozen shoulders and post-operative knees is not generalizable to the spine.

Components of MUA treatment

Several clinical papers in the earlier MUA literature summarize the results for medium to large case series or offer a generic description about its utility as a successful means of managing patients with pain conditions of the spine [7,17,20,25-28]. For the most part, the principal context of the MUA care outlined in those papers is the provision of mostly a single procedure dose via osteopathic techniques with a hospital stay involving the concomitant administration of one or more types of co-interventions. Consequently, it would be unfitting to conclude that the findings of the studies or commentaries put forth by Clybourne [20], Chrisman, et al. [25], Mensor [26], Morey [7], Rumney [27], Siehl and Bradford [17] and Siehl [28] can be relied upon as evidence of efficacy with contemporary MUA protocols. Significant and numerous variations exist in the overall treatment approach cited in the past versus that of today.

Contemporary MUA protocols lack the support of high quality evidence. It would appear that the experience and observations of a limited number of individuals have shaped the consensus processes by which these protocols have been developed. Suffice it to say there is widespread acceptance of these protocols amongst chiropractors who either perform MUA or refer their patients for the like. Chiropractors have traditionally relied upon published protocols [120] for patient selection purposes as well as for guidance on the parameters for both MUA treatment and the post-MUA phase of care.

Post-MUA rehabilitation is proposed to be an integral and necessary component of MUA care if such treatment is to be of lasting benefit in the restoration of musculoskeletal function [21,35,122]. Following MUA, in order to deter the reformation of vertebral joint and/or myofascial adhesions during the course of healing, both spinal manipulation and a continuance of the stretching/traction type techniques utilized during MUA are to be employed, in part, at each post-MUA follow-up visit to the doctor's office [5]. With this approach, there would be no legitimate clinical purpose for the provision of MUA if, following its administration, a patient is simply discharged from chiropractic care. Furthermore, the purported benefits of the MUA procedure would theoretically be lost in the instance that a patient returns to office-based care absent the types of manipulation and soft tissue mobilization techniques/maneuvers that could be expected to stress the intersegmental elements to the degree necessary to prevent the reformation of adhesions and to maintain flexibility. Thus, for those who utilize this procedure, the pre-MUA, intra-MUA and post-MUA components of care be must be governed by clinical logical and decision making consistent with the fundamental adhesion-disruption theory upon which MUA has been built.

When chiropractic clinicians do not adhere to a patient-specific chiropractic care regimen leading up to, during, and following MUA of the spine, what develops over time is a patchwork of independent ideas, care methods and technique applications that collectively differ from how the procedure was ever intended to be rendered. This is not to suggest that manipulation of the spine under anesthesia be applied in cookbook fashion for all patients. However, without acknowledgement or consistency of the overall treatment regimen with supportive literature and its theoretical foundation to disrupt and then prevent the reformation of adhesions, the very premise of MUA becomes compromised. By lack of adherence to a more standardized means of selecting and applying all aspects of the procedure, chiropractors may place the future of MUA in jeopardy to the extent that patients who develop a need for the like may no longer have access.

Professional, ethical and legal considerations for the chiropractic clinician

Beyond the attainment of MUA certification chiropractors should strive to develop a good working knowledge of the substance of the related peer reviewed medical literature. The mere presence of clinical papers in the literature over an 80 year timespan does not summarily connote procedural efficacy. It is the responsibility of the MUA practitioner to understand the nature and scope of the evidence that pertains to the treatment of debilitating musculoskeletal conditions of different body regions. In accordance with the evidence, critical thinking skills and self-governance are necessary to the appropriate utilization and ethical application of the MUA service for each uniquely presenting patient. Nevertheless, it is recognized that lack of protocol/evidence awareness, financial enticement, entrepreneurial motivations and/or clinician assuredness for MUA can contribute to decision making that fails to best meet the needs of individual patients. A case can be made that the potential for indiscriminate use [34] has become a burgeoning issue in need of redress by the chiropractic profession, albeit in all likelihood few advocates of this procedure would be willing to acknowledge this.

Above all, chiropractic must serve the public interest [123]. This requires no explanation. Nevertheless, in its more recent history, it would appear that professionalism in chiropractic has been usurped by commercialism [123]. With broader regard to professional ethics, it has been said that, "*Despite the fact that a chiropractic practice is typically a commercial, for-profit enterprise, the chiropractor is not governed by the dictates of mercantilism but rather by professionalism... Thus, chiropractors, as health professionals, are expected to make recommendations that are in the best interest of the patient, superseding the doctor's pecuniary interests*" [124].

In order that chiropractors may better serve the public, a series of strategic steps were recently proposed for professional renewal in numerous areas including that of ethics [125]. Arguably, this matter has particular relevance to the chiropractic utilization of MUA within the personal injury arena. While purportedly providing an invaluable chiropractic service to those who are experiencing recalcitrant musculoskeletal conditions from an acceleration/deceleration trauma event, there is a seeming emergence of disregard by some in fulfilling basic patient selection criteria for a procedure that is seldom indicated. Accordingly, one might argue that MUA has more recently evolved into a one-size-fits-all treatment approach used in any capacity deemed appropriate by individual clinicians, at times without genuine regard for patient need [68], patient safety [126] or informed consent. This is unacceptable, and should no longer be tolerated by a profession that has yet to overcome negative public perception with regard to honesty/ethics [127] while still lacking cultural authority [123,128,129].

When provider activity surrounding patient selection for MUA lacks clarity, with potential for an ever growing percentage of patients being directed for the like, what might that imply about the efficacy of traditional in-office chiropractic treatment? For more than a century chiropractors have utilized conscious manipulation, adjunctive physiotherapeutic modalities and other conservative care measures to treat spine-based musculoskeletal conditions of varying etiologies. Principally, such treatment is aimed at correcting underlying mechanical dysfunctions or restrictions of spinal/extraspinal articulations and conjoining soft tissues. Care is also rendered for the purpose of accelerating the natural history of healing. Nonetheless, with increased utilization of MUA, particularly when this service is applied in comprehensive fashion after just a few short weeks of office-based care, some chiropractors are exhibiting a behavior that could easily be interpreted by others as an abandonment of routine treatment approaches. Thus, the trend of increasing MUA utilization and/or its metamorphosis into something different from that chronicled throughout the medical literature creates the appearance of a loss of confidence in the efficacy of traditional office-based chiropractic care methods. This is not beneficial for the profession, and could theoretically jeopardize future patient access to the services that are integral to present day office-based chiropractic care.

It is recognized that a lack of evidence of efficacy is not necessarily synonymous with lack of efficacy. Withholding any form of treatment due to the absence of supportive data from randomized controlled trials would be unnecessarily restrictive [130] and likely lead to a state of "therapeutic paralysis" [124]. Moreover, it is acknowledged that scores of testimonials from both doctors and patients have routinely cited the effectiveness of MUA in the treatment of chronic spine pain conditions. Nonetheless, as health care professionals charged with the public trust, chiropractors who perform spinal manipulation under anesthesia, or make referrals for the like, should know and rely upon existing published medical evidence when making clinical decisions for individual patients. Once the influences of anything other than the findings of bona fide clinical investigation or best practice consensus statements enter the patient-care decision making process, particularly with regard to a procedure that has had a history of being controversial [32,35,38,47], the integrity of the doctor patient relationship may become compromised. When educated health care professionals allow their views on patient care approaches to be shaped by testimonials (anecdotal evidence), as if such declarations are somehow akin to research evidence, a doctor's decision making abilities become compromised and, in essence, are relegated to the level of the laity. This can lead to a breach in the doctor's fiduciary duties and, in its broadest context, create and then perpetuate an artificial standard of care. This does not serve the public interest.

In contemporary times, pertinent to the rendition of MUA of the spine to individual patients, it is of utmost importance that chiropractors seek to understand the definition of evidence based clinical practice [56]. A patient that has reached clinical endpoint following sufficient trials of in-office manipulation and other modes of conservative care yet is still experiencing significant pain and disability, as measured by way of pain diagrams and disability measurement instruments [5], would be considered a complicated case that may justify consultation for MUA. Considering the deficiencies and differences noted across the existing literature and protocols, it is incumbent upon the MUA provider to substantiate a patient specific clinical rationale concerning the overall breadth of the MUA procedure to be rendered [37]. This pertains to the dysfunctional body region/s qualifying for such treatment and then, perhaps in accordance with the eighty percent threshold improvement criterion [120], the number of procedure doses that follow (whether applied serially [120] or intermittently [119]), if any. Nevertheless, the newly established American Association of Manipulation Under Anesthesia Providers (AAMUAP) alternatively recommends an approach for determining single versus serial MUA on a pre-MUA basis [131].

While the potential for patient complication with MUA exists regardless of the body region under treatment, the relative paucity of reported incidents or published case reports in this area [38,132] appears to indicate that the risk for complication is considerably low with properly selected patients. This matter has been discussed elsewhere [32,34]. Beyond the need for basic medical evidence awareness, chiropractors who regularly utilize MUA in their practices may soon find themselves giving consideration to looming issues of legality and a need to determine treatment alternatives to MUA in managing chronic spine pain patients. This follows a recent Texas court of appeals ruling which classifies MUA in that state as *"a surgical procedure excluded from the statutory scope of chiropractic practice"* [51].

Conclusion

In the MUA literature there is a long reported history of mostly favorable outcomes. Despite this, the evidence of treatment efficacy remains limited [119], with published studies that are generally weak in their methodological quality [2] and consistently varied across multiple domains which do not permit comparative analysis toward generalization [15]. An earlier chiropractic consensus process resulted in an assigned equivocal rating for MUA (approved for use in clinical practice but requiring further exploration) [133]. Similarly, a more recent evaluation of the clinical utility of MUA in the management of chronic low back pain resulted in no specific recommendations due to a lack of sufficient evidence [2].

In serving the public, chiropractors have a professional obligation to render care in accordance with the best available evidence. In view of the nature and scope of existing research and the outcomes of published professional assessments, the practitioner who is giving consideration to this treatment approach for individual patients should apply caution and tact before proceeding. If MUA is to remain a treatment option for chronic spine pain, it must be reserved for the most stubborn cases and/or under extenuating clinical circumstances. In addition, when appropriate, treatment should be applied to a targeted spinal region as a final resort to attempts at standard conservative treatment measures to alleviate pain and restore function. There is a void of high quality published medical evidence to support the practice of universal MUA treatment of the entire axial spine in the management of a sole regional condition, when there are concomitant but comparatively innocuous complaints/physical findings of vertebral joint pain/dysfunction of other spinal regions.

The three studies which likely represent the current best evidence for MUA via conscious/deep sedation pertain solely to the low back [13,15,23] (Level II evidence). Amongst these studies there are variations in the treating condition reported, the type of intravenous agents used, technique application employed and the number of procedures rendered. These variables pose a clinical challenge for the chiropractor who may be considering this mode of care. In determining the specific components of care to employ, breadth of treatment application and procedure dose, the clinician must rely upon this limited yet diverse evidence in the context of consensus based protocols that have been derived from the experiences and observations of a limited number of individuals. In the near future, chiropractors who perform manipulation under anesthesia may also find themselves confronted with challenges in the scope of practice domain, should the recent judicial battle of Texas [51] widen to other states.

Further research efforts by way of prospective, randomized trials are greatly needed in elevating the quality of research evidence either for or against spinal MUA via conscious/deep sedation and in better defining its role, if any, in the management of explicit spine-based neuromusculoskeletal conditions. Moreover, clinical trials are necessary in qualifying the indications and appropriate parameters of such treatment, including criteria for patient candidacy and optimal procedure dose application. Lastly, comparative studies are needed in clarifying if and under what circumstances MUA may be more efficacious over the long term versus a continuance of traditional office-based chiropractic management procedures or more invasive interventions that lie beyond the scope of chiropractic care. Without these research efforts, the efficacy of MUA relative to other interventions available for chronic spine pain will remain in question.

Abbreviations

MUA: Manipulation under anesthesia; MAM: Medicine assisted manipulation; MUJA: Manipulation under joint anesthesia; MUEA: Manipulation under epidural anesthesia; MUESI: Manipulation under epidural steroid injection.

Competing interests

The author declares that he has no conflicts of interest.

References

1. Haldeman KO, Soto-Hall R: **The Diagnosis and Treatment of Sacro-Iliac Conditions by the Injection of Procaine (Novocain).** *J Bone Joint Surg Am* 1938, **20**:675–685.
2. Dagenais S, Mayer J, Wooley JR, Haldeman S: **Evidence-informed management of chronic low back pain with medicine-assisted manipulation.** *Spine J* 2008, **8**(1):142–9.
3. Davis CG: **Chronic cervical spine pain treated with manipulation under anesthesia.** *Journal of the Neuromusculoskeletal System* 1996, **4**(3):102–15.
4. Herzog J: **Use of cervical spine manipulation under anesthesia for management of cervical disk herniation, cervical radiculopathy, and associated cervicogenic headache syndrome.** *J Manipulative Physiol Ther* 1999, **22**(3):166–70.
5. Cremata E, Collins S, Clauson W, Solinger AB, Roberts ES: **Manipulation under anesthesia: a report of four cases.** *J Manipulative Physiol Ther* 2005, **28**(7):526–533.
6. Greenman PE: **Manipulation with the patient under anesthesia.** *J Am Osteopath Assoc* 1992, **92**(9):1159–60, 1167–70.
7. Morey LW Jr: **Osteopathic manipulation under general anesthesia.** *J Am Osteopath Assoc* 1973, **73**(2):116–27.
8. Hughes BL: **Management of cervical disk syndrome utilizing manipulation under anesthesia.** *J Manipulative Physiol Ther* 1993, **16**(3):174–81.
9. Dougherty P, Bajwa S, Burke J, Dishman JD: **Spinal manipulation postepidural injection for lumbar and cervical radiculopathy: a retrospective case series.** *J Manipulative Physiol Ther* 2004, **27**(7):449–56.
10. Soden CH: **Osteopathic Manipulative Surgery Under General Anesthesia.** In *Yearbook- Academy of Applied Osteopathy.* Ann Arbor, MI: Edwards Brothers; 1949:188–95.
11. Ben-David B, Raboy M: **Manipulation under anesthesia combined with epidural steroid injection.** *J Manipulative Physiol Ther* 1994, **17**(9):605–9.
12. Davis CG, Fernando CA, Da Motta MA: **Manipulation of the low back under general anesthesia: case studies and discussion.** *Journal of the Neuromusculoskeletal System* 1993, **1**(3):126–134.

13. Kohlbeck FJ, Haldeman S, Hurwitz EL, Dagenais S: **Supplemental care with medication-assisted manipulation versus spinal manipulation therapy alone for patients with chronic low back pain.** *J Manipulative Physiol Ther* 2005, **28**(4):245–52.
14. Nelson L, Aspegren D, Bova C: **The use of epidural steroid injection and manipulation on patients with chronic low back pain.** *J Manipulative Physiol Ther* 1997, **20**(4):263–6.
15. Palmieri NF, Smoyak S: **Chronic low back pain: a study of the effects of manipulation under anesthesia.** *J Manipulative Physiol Ther* 2002, **25**(8):E8–E17.
16. Aspegren DD, Wright RE, Hemler DE: **Manipulation under epidural anesthesia with corticosteroid injection: two case reports.** *J Manipulative Physiol Ther* 1997, **20**(9):618–21.
17. Siehl D, Bradford WG: **Manipulation of the low back under general anesthesia.** *J Am Osteopath Assoc* 1952, **52**(4):239–42.
18. Dreyfuss P, Michaelsen M, Horne M: **MUJA: manipulation under joint anesthesia/analgesia: a treatment approach for recalcitrant low back pain of synovial joint origin.** *J Manipulative Physiol Ther* 1995, **18**(8):537–46.
19. Morningstar MW, Strauchman MN: **Management of a 59-year-old female patient with adult degenerative scoliosis using manipulation under anesthesia.** *J Chiropr Med* 2010, **9**(2):77–83.
20. Clybourne HE: **Manipulation of the low back region under anesthesia.** *J Am Osteopath Assoc* 1948, **48**(1):10–11.
21. Morningstar MW, Strauchman MN: **Manipulation under anesthesia for patients with failed back surgery: retrospective report of 3 cases with 1-year follow-up.** *J Chiropr Med* 2012, **11**(1):30–5.
22. Alexander GK: **Manipulation under anesthesia of lumbar post-laminectomy syndrome patients with epidural fibrosis and recurrent HNP.** *J Am Chiro Assoc* 1993, **30**(6):79–81.
23. Siehl D, Olson DR, Ross HE, Rockwood EE: **Manipulation of the lumbar spine with the patient under general anesthesia: evaluation by electromyography and clinical-neurologic examination of its use for lumbar nerve root compression syndrome.** *J Am Osteopath Assoc* 1971, **70:**433–40.
24. Ross HE, Siehl D: **Evaluation of manipulation of the lumbar spine under general anesthesia for lumbar nerve root compression syndrome, utilizing electromyographic and clinical neurologic examinations.** *J Am Osteopath Assoc* 1968, **67**(9):1027.
25. Chrisman OD, Mittnacht A, Snook GA: **A study of the results following rotatory manipulation in the lumbar intervertebral-disc syndrome.** *J Bone Joint Surg Am* 1964, **46:**517–24.
26. Mensor MC: **Non-operative treatment, including manipulation, for lumbar intervertebral disc syndrome.** *J Bone J Surg* 1955, **37A:**925–936.
27. Rumney IC: **Manipulation of the spine and appendages under anesthesia: an evaluation.** *J Am Osteopath Assoc* 1968, **68**(3):235–45.
28. Siehl D: **Manipulation of the spine under general anesthesia.** *J Am Osteopath Assoc* 1963, **62:**881–7.
29. Bremner RA: **Manipulation in the management of chronic low backache due to lumbosacral strain.** *Lancet* 1958, **4;1**(7010):20–1.
30. Warr AC, Wilkinson JA, Burn JM, Langdon L: **Chronic lumbosciatic syndrome treated by epidural injection and manipulation.** *Practitioner* 1972, **209**(249):53–9.
31. West DT, Mathews RS, Miller MR, Kent GM: **Effective management of spinal pain in one hundred seventy-seven patients evaluated for manipulation under anesthesia.** *J Manipulative Physiol Ther* 1999, **22**(5):299–308.
32. Gordon RC: **An evaluation of the experimental and investigational status and clinical validity of manipulation of patients under anesthesia: a contemporary opinion.** *J Manipulative Physiol Ther* 2001, **24**(9):603–11.
33. Francis R: **Spinal manipulation under general anesthesia: a chiropractic approach in a hospital setting.** *J Am Chiro Assoc* 1989, **26**(12):39–41.
34. Kohlbeck FJ, Haldeman S: **Medication-assisted spinal manipulation.** *Spine J* 2002, **2**(4):288–302.
35. Gordon RC (Ed): *Manipulation Under Anesthesia: Concepts in Theory and Application.* Boca Raton, FL: CRC Press Taylor & Francis Group; 2005.
36. Beckett RH, Francis R: **Spinal Manipulation Under Anesthesia.** In *Advances in chiropractic*, Volume 1. St. Louis: Mosby; 1994:325–340.
37. Williams HA: **Part II. manipulation under anesthesia: key aspects.** *Journal of the American Chiropractic Association* 1998, **35**(1):44. 46-9.
38. Krumhansl BR, Nowacek CJ: **Manipulation Under Anesthesia.** In *Modern manual therapy of the vertebral column.* Edited by Grieve GP. Edinburgh: Churchill Livingstone; 1986:777–786.
39. International MUA Academy of Physicians: Francis RS: *Manipulation Under Anesthesia: Historical Considerations.* Taylor & Francis Group; 2005 [http://muaphysicians.com/historical.html].
40. Mensor MC: **Non-operative treatment, including manipulation, for lumbar intervertebral-disc syndrome.** *J Bone Joint Surg Am* 1965, **47-A:**1073–4.
41. Wright JG, Swiontkowski MF, Heckman JD: **Introducing levels of evidence to the journal.** *J Bone Joint Surg Am* 2003, **85**(1):1–3 [http://jbjs.org/data/journalclub/1_85-1-1.pdf].
42. West DT, Mathews RS, Miller MR, Kent GM: **Effective management of spinal pain in 200 patients evaluated for manipulation under anesthesia.** *J Neurol Orthop Med Surg* 1998, **18:**31–42.
43. *Levels of Evidence For Primary Research Question.* http://www.spine.org/Documents/LevelsofEvidenceFinal.pdf.
44. Gehlbach SH: *Interpreting the Medical Literature.* 5th edition. New York: McGraw-Hill; 2006:13–30.
45. Brighton B, Bhandari M, Tornetta P 3rd, Felson DT: **Hierarchy of evidence: from case reports to randomized controlled trials.** *Clin Orthop Relat Res* 2003, **413:**19–24.
46. Guyatt G, Rennie D, Guyatt G, Rennie D: *User's Guide to the Medical Literature- Essentials of Evidence-Based Clinical Practice.* Chicago, IL: AMA Press; 2005:88–136.
47. Michaelsen MR: **Manipulation under joint anesthesia/analgesia: a proposed interdisciplinary treatment approach for recalcitrant spinal axis pain of synovial joint origin.** *J Manipulative Physiol Ther* 2000, **23**(2):127–9.
48. Wood L: **Acute locked facet syndrome and its treatment by manipulation under local periarticular anesthesia–Part I: Clinical perspective and pilot study proposal.** *J Manipulative Physiol Ther* 1984, **7**(4):211–7.
49. Bremner RA, Simpson M: **Management of chronic lumbosacral strain.** *Lancet* 1959, **28;2**(7109):949–50.
50. Lawrence DJ, Meeker W, Branson R, Bronfort G, Cates JR, Haas M, Haneline M, Micozzi M, Updyke W, Mootz R, Triano JJ, Hawk C: **Chiropractic management of low back pain and low back-related leg complaints: a literature synthesis.** *J Manipulative Physiol Ther* 2008, **31**(9):659–74.
51. TEXAS BOARD OF CHIROPRACTIC EXAMINERS v. TEXAS MEDICAL ASSOCIATION. TEXAS BOARD OF CHIROPRACTIC EXAMINERS: *Glenn Parker, Executive Director, and Texas Chiropractic Association, Appellants v. TEXAS MEDICAL ASSOCIATION, Texas Medical Board, and the State of Texas, Appellees. No. 03–10–00673–CV*; 2012. [http://caselaw.findlaw.com/tx-court-of-appeals/1605690.html].
52. Chou R, Qaseem A, Snow V, Casey D, Cross JT Jr, Shekelle P, Owens DK: **Diagnosis and treatment of low back pain: a joint clinical practice guideline from the American College of Physicians and the American Pain Society.** *Ann Intern Med* 2007, **147:**478–491.
53. Chou R, Loeser JD, Owens DK, Rosenquist RW, Atlas SJ, Baisden J, Carragee EJ, Grabois M, Murphy DR, Resnick DK, Stanos SP, Shaffer WO, Wall EM: **American Pain Society Low Back Pain Guideline Panel. Interventional therapies, surgery, and interdisciplinary rehabilitation for low back pain: an evidence-based clinical practice guideline from the American Pain Society.** *Spine* 2009, **34**(10):1066–77.
54. Hurwitz EL, Carragee EJ, van der Velde G, Carroll LJ, Nordin M, Guzman J, Peloso PM, Holm LW, Côté P, Hogg-Johnson S, Cassidy JD, Haldeman S: **Bone and Joint Decade 2000–2010 Task Force on Neck Pain and Its Associated Disorders. Treatment of neck pain: noninvasive interventions: results of the Bone and Joint Decade 2000–2010 Task Force on Neck Pain and Its Associated Disorders.** *Spine* 2008, **33**(4):123–52.
55. Carragee EJ, Hurwitz EL, Cheng I, Carroll LJ, Nordin M, Guzman J, Peloso P, Holm LW, Côté P, Hogg-Johnson S, van der Velde G, Cassidy JD, Haldeman S: **Bone and Joint Decade 2000–2010 Task Force on Neck Pain and Its Associated Disorders. Treatment of neck pain: injections and surgical interventions: results of the Bone and Joint Decade 2000–2010 Task Force on Neck Pain and Its Associated Disorders.** *Spine* 2008, **33**(4):153–69.
56. Lehman JJ, Jones RC: **The value of evidence-based practice.** *ACA News* 2012, **8**(7):16–21.
57. Sun J, Zhang L, Liu JS, Ma J, Li ZY: **Treatment of primary frozen shoulder with manipulation under anesthesia combined with arthroscopy [abstract].** *Zhongguo Gu Shang* 2011, **24**(6):490–2.
58. Khan JA, Devkota P, Acharya BM, Pradhan NM, Shreshtha SK, Singh M, Mainali L: **Manipulation under local anesthesia in idiopathic frozen shoulder–a new effective and simple technique.** *Nep Med Coll J* 2009, **11**(4):247–53.
59. Vastamäki H, Vastamäki M: **Motion and Pain Relief Remain 23 Years After Manipulation Under Anesthesia for Frozen Shoulder.** *Clin Orthop Relat Res 2013*, **471**(4):1245–50.

60. Ipach I, Mittag F, Lahrmann J, Kunze B, Kluba T: **Arthrofibrosis after TKA - Influence factors on the absolute flexion and gain in flexion after manipulation under anaesthesia.** *BMC Musculoskelet Disord* 2011, **12**(1):184.
61. Yeoh D, Nicolaou N, Goddard R, Willmott H, Miles K, East D, Hinves B, Shepperd J, Butler-Manuel A: **Manipulation under anaesthesia post total knee replacement: Long term follow up.** *Knee* 2012, **19**(4):329–31.
62. Haneline MT: *Evidence-Based Chiropractic Practice.* Sudbury, MA: Jones and Bartlett Publishers; 2007:24–27.
63. CIGNA Medical Coverage Policy: *Manipulation Under Anesthesia. Coverage Policy Number: 0276.* [http://www.cigna.com/customer_care/healthcare_professional/coverage_positions/medical/mm_0276_coveragepositioncriteria_spinal_manipulation_under_anesthesia.pdf].
64. UnitedHealthcare Medical Policy: *Manipulation Under Anesthesia. Policy Number 2013T0515G.* [https://www.unitedhealthcareonline.com/ccmcontent/ProviderII/UHC/en-US/Assets/ProviderStaticFiles/ProviderStaticFilesPdf/Tools%20and%20Resources/Policies%20and%20Protocols/Medical%20Policies/Medical%20Policies/Manipulation_Under_Anesthesia.pdf].
65. Empire Blue Cross Blue Shield Medical Policy: *Manipulation Under Anesthesia of the Spine and Joints other than the Knee. Policy Number: MED.00079.* [http://www.empireblue.com/medicalpolicies/policies/mp_pw_a050518.htm].
66. Tosounidis T, Kanakaris N, Nikolaou V, Tan B, Giannoudis PV: **Assessment of lateral compression type 1 pelvic ring injuries by intraoperative manipulation: which fracture pattern is unstable?** *Int Orthop* 2012, **36**(12):2553–8.
67. Luukkainen R, Sipola E, Varjo P: **Successful treatment of frozen hip with manipulation and pressure dilatation.** *Open Rheumatol J* 2008, **2**:31–2.
68. Cerf J: **Advances in Hospital Chiropractic.** *Dynamic Chiropractic* 2006, **24**(26). [http://www.dynamicchiropractic.com/mpacms/dc/article.php?id=51482].
69. Maund E, Craig D, Suekarran S, Neilson A, Wright K, Brealey S, Dennis L, Goodchild L, Hanchard N, Rangan A, Richardson G, Robertson J, McDaid C: **Management of frozen shoulder: a systematic review and cost-effectiveness analysis.** *Health Technol Assess* 2012, **16**(11):1–264.
70. International MUA Academy of Physicians: *How do you know if you need M.U.A.?.* [http://muaphysicians.com/what_is_mua.html].
71. Fisher G: *The New Millennium Chiropractic Survival Manual.* Montoursville, PA: Progressive Seminars; 2001:211–218.
72. Matsumoto M, Fujimura Y, Suzuki N, Nishi Y, Nakamura M, Yabe Y, Shiga H: **MRI of cervical intervertebral discs in asymptomatic subjects.** *J Bone Joint Surg Br* 1998, **80**(1):19–24.
73. Boden SD, McCowin PR, Davis DO, Dina TS, Mark AS, Wiesel S: **Abnormal magnetic resonance scans of the cervical spine in asymptomatic subjects. A prospective investigation.** *J Bone Joint Surg Am* 1990, **72**(8):1178–84.
74. Boden SD, Davis DO, Dina TS, Patronas NJ, Wiesel SW: **Abnormal magnetic resonance scans of the lumbar spine in asymptomatic subjects, a prospective investigation.** *J Bone Joint Surg Am* 1990, **72**(3):403–8.
75. Jensen MC, Brant-Zawadzki MN, Obuchowski N, Modic MT, Malkasian D, Ross JS: **Magnetic Resonance Imaging of the Lumbar Spine in People Without Back Pain.** *N Eng J Med* 1994, **331**:69–73.
76. Siivola SM, Levoska S, Tervonen O, Ilkko E, Vanharanta H, Keinänen-Kiukaanniemi S: **MRI changes of cervical spine in asymptomatic and symptomatic young adults.** *Eur Spine J* 2002, **11**(4):358–63.
77. Lehto IJ, Tertti MO, Komu ME, Paajanen HE, Tuominen J, Kormano MJ: **Age-related MRI changes at 0.1 T in cervical discs in asymptomatic subjects.** *Neuroradiology* 1994, **36**(1):49–53.
78. Guzman J, Haldeman S, Carroll LJ, Carragee EJ, Hurwitz EL, Peloso P, Nordin M, Cassidy JD, Holm LW, Côté P, van der Velde G, Hogg-Johnson S: **Clinical practice implications of the Bone and Joint Decade 2000–2010 Task Force on Neck Pain and Its Associated Disorders: from concepts and findings to recommendations.** *Spine* 2008, **33**(4):199–213.
79. Cheung KM, Karppinen J, Chan D, Ho DW, Song YQ, Sham P, Cheah KS, Leong JC, Luk KD: **Prevalence and pattern of lumbar magnetic resonance imaging changes in a population study of one thousand forty-three individuals.** *Spine* 2009, **34**(9):934–40.
80. Dwyer A, Aprill C, Bogduk N: **Cervical zygapophyseal joint pain patterns. I: a study in normal volunteers.** *Spine* 1990, **15**(6):453–7.
81. Aprill C, Dwyer A, Bogduk N: **Cervical zygapophyseal joint pain patterns. II: A clinical evaluation.** *Spine* 1990, **15**(6):458–61.
82. Feinstein B, Langton JN, Jameson RM, Schiller F: **Experiments on pain referred from deep somatic tissues.** *J Bone Joint Surg Am* 1954, **36-A**(5):981–97.
83. Borenstein DG, Wiesel SW, Boden SD: *Low Back Pain: Medical Diagnosis and Comprehensive Management.* 2nd edition. Philadelphia, PA: WB Saunders Co; 1995:28–57.
84. Jung JH, Kim HI, Shin DA, Shin DG, Lee JO, Kim HJ, Chung JH: **Usefulness of pain distribution pattern assessment in decision-making for the patients with lumbar zygapophyseal and sacroiliac joint arthropathy.** *J Korean Med Sci* 2007, **22**(6):1048–54.
85. Slipman CW, Jackson HB, Lipetz JS, Chan KT, Lenrow D, Vresilovic EJ: **Sacroiliac joint pain referral zones.** *Arch Phys Med Rehabil* 2000, **81**(3):334–8.
86. American Chiropractic Association: **Is That Low Back Pain Sclerotomal or Dermatomal? And Does it Really Matter.** *Journ Amer Chiropr Assoc* 1998, **35**(5):58–63.
87. Simmons JW Jr, Ricketson R, McMillin JN: **Painful lumbosacral sensory distribution patterns: embryogenesis to adulthood.** *Orthop Rev* 1993, **22**(10):1110–8.
88. Bove GM, Zaheen A, Bajwa ZH: **Subjective nature of lower limb radicular pain.** *J Manipulative Physiol Ther* 2005, **28**(1):12–4.
89. Milette PC, Fontaine S, Lepanto L, Breton G: **Radiating pain to the lower extremities caused by lumbar disk rupture without spinal nerve root involvement.** *Am J Neuroradiol* 1995, **16**:1605–1613.
90. Karppinen J, Malmivaara A, Tervonen O, Pääkkö E, Kurunlahti M, Syrjälä P, Vasari P, Vanharanta H: **Severity of symptoms and signs in relation to magnetic resonance imaging findings among sciatic patients.** *Spine* 2001, **26**(7). E149-54.
91. Cassidy JD, Thiel HW, Kirkaldy-Willis WH: **Side posture manipulation for lumbar intervertebral disk herniation.** *J Manipulative Physiol Ther* 1993, **16**(2):96–103.
92. Garfin SR, Rydevik B, Lind B, Massie J, Garfin SR, Rydevik B, Lind B, Massie J: **Spinal nerve root compression.** *Spine* 1995, **20**(16):1810–20.
93. Cassidy JD, Kirkaldy-Willis WH, Thiel HW: **Manipulation.** In *Managing Low Back Pain.* 3rd edition. Edited by Kirkaldy-Willis WH, Burton CV. NY: Churchill Livingstone; 1992:283–296.
94. Unsworth A, Dowson D, Wright V: **Cracking joints'. A bioengineering study of cavitation in the metacarpophalangeal joint.** *Ann Rheum Dis* 1971, **30**(4):348–58.
95. Reggars JW: **The therapeutic benefit of the audible release associated with spinal manipulative therapy. A critical review of the literature.** *Australas Chiropr Osteopathy* 1998, **7**(2):80–5.
96. Clark BC, Goss DA Jr, Walkowski S, Hoffman RL, Ross A, Thomas JS: **Neurophysiologic effects of spinal manipulation in patients with chronic low back pain.** *BMC Musculoskelet Disord* 2011, **12**:170.
97. Pickar JG: **Neurophysiological effects of spinal manipulation.** *Spine J* 2002, **2**(5):357–71.
98. Wright A: **Hypoalgesia post-manipulative therapy: a review of a potential neurophysiological mechanism.** *Man Ther* 1995, **1**(1):11–6.
99. George SZ, Bishop MD, Bialosky JE, Zeppieri G Jr, Robinson ME: **Immediate effects of spinal manipulation on thermal pain sensitivity: an experimental study.** *BMC Musculoskelet Disord* 2006, **7**:68.
100. Evans DW: **Mechanisms and effects of spinal high-velocity, low-amplitude thrust manipulation: previous theories.** *J Manipulative Physiol Ther* 2002, **25**(4):251–62.
101. Bishop MD, Beneciuk JM, George SZ: **Immediate reduction in temporal sensory summation after thoracic spinal manipulation.** *Spine J* 2011, **11**(5):440–446.
102. Simolo CA: **Bibliography of chiropractic and other techniques.** *J Chiropr Humanit* 2001, **10**:1–8.
103. McCoy M: **The Adjustment.** *The American Chiropractor* 2001, **23**(3):26–34.
104. Creed A, *et al*: **A close look at the adjustment- 10 great techniques.** *The American Chiropractor* 2002, **24**(3):25–32.
105. Epstein D: **Chiropractic technique: finding the right fit.** *The American Chiropractor* 2003, **25**(3):18–26.
106. Reggars JW: **Multiple channel recording of the articular crack associated with manipulation of the metacarpophalangeal joint, An observational study.** *Australas Chiropr Osteopathy* 1999, **8**(1):16–20.
107. Christensen M, Kerkhoff D, Kollasch MW: **Job analysis of chiropractic: a project report, survey analysis and summary of the practice of chiropractic within the United States.** Greeley: National Board of Chiropractic Examiners; 2000:129.
108. National Board of Chiropractic Examiners: *Job Analysis of Chiropractic: a project report, survey analysis and summary of the practice of chiropractic within the United States.* Greeley, Colorado, USA: National Board of Chiropractic Examiners; 2005:135.

109. Grant R: Manipulation Under Anesthesia syllabus. Logan College Of Chiropractic; April 2000.
110. **The Activator Instrument.** [http://www.activatorinstrument.com/].
111. Cox JM, Feller J, Cox-Cid J: **Distraction chiropractic adjusting: clinical application and outcomes of 1,000 cases.** *Top Clin Chiro* 1996, **3**(3):45–59.
112. Manison AM: **Chiropractic management using Cox cervical flexion-distraction technique for a disk herniation with left foraminal narrowing in a 64-year-old man.** *J Chiropr Med* 2011, **10**(4):316–321.
113. González-Iglesias J, Fernández-de-las-Peñas C, Cleland JA, Gutiérrez-Vega Mdel R: **Thoracic spine manipulation for the management of patients with neck pain: a randomized clinical trial.** *J Orthop Sports Phys Ther* 2009, **39**(1):20–7.
114. Bergman GJ, Winters JC, Groenier KH, Pool JJ, Meyboom-de Jong B, Postema K, van der Heijden GJ: **Manipulative therapy in addition to usual medical care for patients with shoulder dysfunction and pain: a randomized, controlled trial.** *Ann Intern Med* 2004, **141**(6):432–9.
115. Strunce JB, Walker MJ, Boyles RE, Young BA: **The immediate effects of thoracic spine and rib manipulation on subjects with primary complaints of shoulder pain.** *J Man Manip Ther* 2009, **17**(4):230–6.
116. Fernández-De-Las-Peñas C, Cleland JA, Huijbregts P, Palomeque-Del-Cerro L, González-Iglesias J: **Repeated applications of thoracic spine thrust manipulation do not lead to tolerance in patients presenting with acute mechanical neck pain: a secondary analysis.** *J Man Manip Ther* 2009, **17**(3):154–62.
117. Cleland JA, Mintken PE, Carpenter K, Fritz JM, Glynn P, Whitman J, Childs JD: **Examination of a clinical prediction rule to identify patients with neck pain likely to benefit from thoracic spine thrust manipulation and a general cervical range of motion exercise: multi-center randomized clinical trial.** *Phys Ther* 2010, **90**(9):1239–50.
118. Sillevis R, Cleland J, Hellman M, Beekhuizen K: **Immediate effects of a thoracic spine thrust manipulation on the autonomic nervous system: a randomized clinical trial.** *J Man Manip Ther* 2010, **18**(4):181–90.
119. *The American Academy of Osteopathy Journal*: **American Academy of Osteopathy Consensus Statement for Osteopathic Manipulation of Somatic Dysfunction under Anesthesia and Conscious Sedation.** Indainaoplis, IN: American Academy of Osteopathy; 2005, **15**(2):26–27.
120. National Academy of MUA Physicians: *The National Academy of MUA Physicians Standards and Protocols.* Manchester, MO: NAMUAP; 2008.
121. Hartman SE: **Why do ineffective treatments seem helpful? A brief review.** *Chiropr Osteopat* 2009, **17**:10.
122. International MUA Academy of Physicians: *Post-procedure care*; 2006 [http://muaphysicians.com/what_is_mua.html].
123. Vincent RE: *A Chiropractic License is a Social Contract-- Are You Serving the Public Interest?.* Federation of Chiropractic Licensing Boards Keynote Address; 2005.
124. Nelson CF, Lawrence DJ, Triano JJ, Bronfort G, Perle SM, Metz RD, Hegetschweiler K, LaBrot T: **Chiropractic as spine care: a model for the profession.** *Chiropr Osteopat* 2005, **13**:9.
125. Triano JJ, Goertz C, Weeks J, Murphy DR, Kranz KC, McClelland GC, Kopansky-Giles D, Morgan W, Nelson CF: **Chiropractic in North America: toward a strategic plan for professional renewal–outcomes from the 2006 Chiropractic Strategic Planning Conference.** *J Manipulative Physiol Ther* 2010, **33**(5):395–405.
126. LaMendola B: ***Medical safety spotlight growing- Man unresponsive after 'manipulation under anesthesia'.*** *March 22, 2009. Sun Sentinel.* Columbia, MO: Tribune Publishing; 2009 [http://articles.sun-sentinel.com/2009-03-22/news/0903210114_1_mua-chiropractor-procedure].
127. *Gallup:* ***Honesty/Ethics in Professions***. Copyright 2012, Gallup, Inc. All rights reserved. Cited with permission. Gallup retains all rights of republication. http://www.gallup.com/poll/1654/Honesty-Ethics-Professionas.aspx].
128. Murphy DR, Schneider MJ, Seaman DR, Perle SM, Nelson CF: **How can chiropractic become a respected mainstream profession? The example of podiatry.** *Chiropr Osteopat* 2008, **16**:10.
129. Keating JC Jr, Charlton KH, Grod JP, Perle SM, Sikorski D, Winterstein JF: **Subluxation: dogma or science?** *Chiropr Osteopat* 2005, **13**:17.
130. Bolton JE: **The evidence in evidence-based practice: what counts and what doesn't count?** *J Manipulative Physiol Ther* 2001, **24**(5):362–6.
131. THE GORDON MUA TECHNIQUE: About MUA- Determining the Number of MUAs. [http://backpainaway.info/about-mua.html].
132. Sambaziotis C, Plymale M, Lovy A, O'Halloran K, McCulloch K, Geller DS: **Pseudoaneurysm of the Distal Thigh After Manipulation of a Total Knee Arthroplasty.** *J Arthroplasty* 2012, **27**(7):1414.e5-7.
133. Haldeman S, Chapman-Smith D, Petersen DM: **Guidelines for Chiropractic Quality Assurance and Practice Parameters.** In *Proceedings of the Mercy Center Consensus Conference.* Gaithersburg, MD: Aspen Publishers; 1993:112.

Permissions

All chapters in this book were first published in CMT, by BioMed Central; hereby published with permission under the Creative Commons Attribution License or equivalent. Every chapter published in this book has been scrutinized by our experts. Their significance has been extensively debated. The topics covered herein carry significant findings which will fuel the growth of the discipline. They may even be implemented as practical applications or may be referred to as a beginning point for another development.

The contributors of this book come from diverse backgrounds, making this book a truly international effort. This book will bring forth new frontiers with its revolutionizing research information and detailed analysis of the nascent developments around the world.

We would like to thank all the contributing authors for lending their expertise to make the book truly unique. They have played a crucial role in the development of this book. Without their invaluable contributions this book wouldn't have been possible. They have made vital efforts to compile up to date information on the varied aspects of this subject to make this book a valuable addition to the collection of many professionals and students.

This book was conceptualized with the vision of imparting up-to-date information and advanced data in this field. To ensure the same, a matchless editorial board was set up. Every individual on the board went through rigorous rounds of assessment to prove their worth. After which they invested a large part of their time researching and compiling the most relevant data for our readers.

The editorial board has been involved in producing this book since its inception. They have spent rigorous hours researching and exploring the diverse topics which have resulted in the successful publishing of this book. They have passed on their knowledge of decades through this book. To expedite this challenging task, the publisher supported the team at every step. A small team of assistant editors was also appointed to further simplify the editing procedure and attain best results for the readers.

Apart from the editorial board, the designing team has also invested a significant amount of their time in understanding the subject and creating the most relevant covers. They scrutinized every image to scout for the most suitable representation of the subject and create an appropriate cover for the book.

The publishing team has been an ardent support to the editorial, designing and production team. Their endless efforts to recruit the best for this project, has resulted in the accomplishment of this book. They are a veteran in the field of academics and their pool of knowledge is as vast as their experience in printing. Their expertise and guidance has proved useful at every step. Their uncompromising quality standards have made this book an exceptional effort. Their encouragement from time to time has been an inspiration for everyone.

The publisher and the editorial board hope that this book will prove to be a valuable piece of knowledge for researchers, students, practitioners and scholars across the globe.

List of Contributors

Howard Vernon
Canadian Memorial Chiropractic College 6100 Leslie St., Toronto, Ontario, M2H 3J1, Canada

Aaron Puhl
Canadian Memorial Chiropractic College 6100 Leslie St., Toronto, Ontario, M2H 3J1, Canada

Reinhart
Canadian Memorial Chiropractic College 6100 Leslie St., Toronto, Ontario, M2H 3J1, Canada

Mario Millan
EA 4532 CIAMS, UFR STAPS, Univ Paris-Sud, Orsay, France
The Research Department, The Spine Centre of Southern Denmark, Hospital Lillebælt, Odense, Denmark
Institut Franco-Européen de Chiropratique, Paris, France

Charlotte Leboeuf-Yde
EA 4532 CIAMS, UFR STAPS, Univ Paris-Sud, Orsay, France
The Research Department, The Spine Centre of Southern Denmark, Hospital Lillebælt, Odense, Denmark
Institut Franco-Européen de Chiropratique, Paris, France
Institute of Regional Health Services Research, Faculty of Health Sciences, University of Southern Denmark, Odense, Denmark

Brian Budgell
Canadian Memorial Chiropractic College, Toronto, ON, Canada

Martin Descarreaux
Département de Chiropratique, Université du Québec à Trois-Rivières, Trois-Rivières, QC, Canada

Michel-Ange Amorim
EA 4532 CIAMS, UFR STAPS, Univ Paris-Sud, Orsay, France
Institut Universitaire de France, Paris, France

Peter Tuchin
Macquarie University, Bld E5A Rm 355, Waterloo Rd, North Ryde, Sydney, NSW 2109, Australia

Dwain M Daniel
Texas Chiropractic College, Pasadena, TX, USA

Harrison Ndetan
Parker University, Dallas, TX, USA

Ronald L Rupert
Parker University, Dallas, TX, USA

Daniel Martinez
Parker University, Dallas, TX, USA

Lisa C Carlesso
Toronto Western Research Institute, University Health Network, 399 Bathurst Street - MP11-328, Toronto, Ontario M5T 2S8, Canada

Joy C MacDermid
School of Rehabilitation Sciences McMaster University, Hamilton, Ontario, Canada
Clinical Research Lab, Hand and Upper Limb Centre, St. Joseph's Health Centre, London, Ontario, Canada

Anita R Gross
School of Rehabilitation Sciences McMaster University, Hamilton, Ontario, Canada

David M Walton
School of Physical Therapy, Western University, London, Ontario, Canada

P Lina Santaguida
Department of Clinical Epidemiology and Biostatistics, Hamilton, Ontario, Canada

O'Dane Brady
World Spine Care, PO Box 49, Mahalapye, Botswana

Scott Haldeman
University of California, Irvine, USA
University of California, Los Angeles, USA

Gwendolijne GM Scholten-Peeters
University of Applied Sciences AVANS, Research Group Diagnostics, PO Box 90116, Breda, RA 4800, The Netherlands
Department of General Practice, Erasmus Medical Centre, University Medical Center, PO Box 2040, Rotterdam, CA 3000, The Netherlands

Erik Thoomes
University of Applied Sciences AVANS, Research Group Diagnostics, PO Box 90116, Breda, RA 4800, The Netherlands
Department of General Practice, Erasmus Medical Centre, University Medical Center, PO Box 2040, Rotterdam, CA 3000, The Netherlands

Sophie Konings
Rotterdam University of Applied Sciences, Rotterdam, Department physical therapy, Museumpark 40, Rotterdam, CX 3015, The Netherlands

Michelle Beijer
Rotterdam University of Applied Sciences, Rotterdam, Department physical therapy, Museumpark 40, Rotterdam, CX 3015, The Netherlands

Karin Verkerk
Department of General Practice, Erasmus Medical Centre, University Medical Center, PO Box 2040, Rotterdam, CA 3000, The Netherlands
Rotterdam University of Applied Sciences, Rotterdam, Department physical therapy, Museumpark 40, Rotterdam, CX 3015, The Netherlands

Bart W Koes
Department of General Practice, Erasmus Medical Centre, University Medical Center, PO Box 2040, Rotterdam, CA 3000, The Netherlands

Arianne P Verhagen
University of Applied Sciences AVANS, Research Group Diagnostics, PO Box 90116, Breda, RA 4800, The Netherlands
Department of General Practice, Erasmus Medical Centre, University Medical Center, PO Box 2040, Rotterdam, CA 3000, The Netherlands

Annabel Kier
Welsh Institute of Chiropractic, University of South Wales, Treforest, Pontypridd CF38 2TE, UK

Matthew George
Private Practice, Worthing BN11 1PS, UK

Peter W McCarthy
Welsh Institute of Chiropractic, University of South Wales, Treforest, Pontypridd CF38 2TE, UK

Michael Schneider
School of Health and Rehabilitation Sciences, Department of Physical Therapy, University of Pittsburgh, Pittsburgh, PA, USA

Carlo Ammendolia
Institute of Health Policy, Management and Evaluation, University of Toronto, Toronto, Ontario, Canada

Donald Murphy
Clinical Director, Rhode Island Spine Center, Providence, RI, USA
Department of Family Medicine, Alpert Medical School of Brown University, Providence, RI, USA

Ronald Glick
Departments of Physical Medicine, Family Medicine, and Psychiatry, University of Pittsburgh, Pittsburgh, PA, USA

Sara Piva
School of Health and Rehabilitation Sciences, Department of Physical Therapy, University of Pittsburgh, Pittsburgh, PA, USA

Elizabeth Hile
School of Health and Rehabilitation Sciences, Department of Physical Therapy, University of Pittsburgh, Pittsburgh, PA, USA

Dana Tudorascu
School of Medicine, Biostatistics, Clinical and Translational Science Institute, University of Pittsburgh, Pittsburgh, PA, USA

Sally C Morton
Department of Biostatistics, Graduate School of Public Health, University of Pittsburgh, Pittsburgh, PA, USA

Dave Newell
AECC-Anglo European College of Chiropracti, 14-15 Parkwood Road, BH5 2DF, UK

Jonathan Field
Private practice, Bournemouth, UK

Nita Visnes
AECC, Bournemouth, UK

Mario Millan
EA 4532 CIAMS, UFR STAPS, University Paris-Sud, Paris, France
The Research Department, The Spine Centre of Southern Denmark Hospital Lillebælt, Lillebælt, Denmark

Charlotte Leboeuf-Yde
The Research Department, The Spine Centre of Southern Denmark Hospital Lillebælt, Lillebælt, Denmark
Institut Franco-Européen de Chiropratique, Paris, France
Institute of Regional Health Services Research, Faculty of Health Sciences, University of Southern Denmark, Odense, Denmark

Brian Budgell
Canadian Memorial Chiropractic College, Toronto, ON, Canada

Michel-Ange Amorim
EA 4532 CIAMS, UFR STAPS, University Paris-Sud, Paris, France
Institut Universitaire de France, Paris, France

Paul E Dougherty
Canandaigua Veterans Affairs Medical Center, Canandaigua, NY, USA
New York Chiropractic College, Seneca Falls, NY, USA
University of Rochester School of Medicine and Dentistry, Rochester, NY, USA

Jurgis Karuza
New York Chiropractic College, Seneca Falls, NY, USA
University of Rochester, Rochester, NY, USA
State University of New York College at Buffalo, Buffalo, NY, USA

Dorian Savino
Canandaigua Veterans Affairs Medical Center, Canandaigua, NY, USA

Paul Katz
University of Toronto, Toronto, ON, Canada
Medical Affairs, Baycrest Geriatric Centre, Toronto, Canada

Emiel van Trijffel
Department of Clinical Epidemiology, Biostatistics & Bioinformatics, Academic Medical Centre, University of Amsterdam, Amsterdam, the Netherlands
Institute for Master Education in Musculoskeletal Therapy, Amersfoort, the Netherlands

Robert Lindeboom
Department of Clinical Epidemiology, Biostatistics & Bioinformatics, Academic Medical Centre, University of Amsterdam, Amsterdam, the Netherlands

Patrick MM Bossuyt
Department of Clinical Epidemiology, Biostatistics & Bioinformatics, Academic Medical Centre, University of Amsterdam, Amsterdam, the Netherlands

Maarten A Schmitt
Institute for Master Education in Musculoskeletal Therapy, Amersfoort, the Netherlands

Cees Lucas
Department of Clinical Epidemiology, Biostatistics & Bioinformatics, Academic Medical Centre, University of Amsterdam, Amsterdam, the Netherlands

Bart W Koes
Department of General Practice, Erasmus MC University Medical Centre, Rotterdam, the Netherlands

Rob AB Oostendorp
Scientific Institute for Quality of Healthcare, Radboud University Nijmegen Medical Centre, Nijmegen, the Netherlands

Department of Rehabilitation, Physiotherapy and Manual Therapy, Faculty of Medicine and Pharmacology, Free University of Brussels, Brussels, Belgium

Craig Schulz
Wolfe-Harris Center for Clinical Studies, Northwestern Health Sciences University, 2501 W 84th St, Bloomington, MN 55431, USA

Brent Leininger
Wolfe-Harris Center for Clinical Studies, Northwestern Health Sciences University, 2501 W 84th St, Bloomington, MN 55431, USA

Roni Evans
Wolfe-Harris Center for Clinical Studies, Northwestern Health Sciences University, 2501 W 84th St, Bloomington, MN 55431, USA

Darcy Vavrek
Center for Outcome Studies, University of Western States, 2900 NE 132nd Ave, Portland, OR 97230, USA

Dave Peterson
Division of Chiropractic Sciences, University of Western States, 2900 NE 132nd Ave, Portland, OR 97230, USA

Mitchell Haas
Center for Outcome Studies, University of Western States, 2900 NE 132nd Ave, Portland, OR 97230, USA

Gert Bronfort
Wolfe-Harris Center for Clinical Studies, Northwestern Health Sciences University, 2501 W 84th St, Bloomington, MN 55431, USA

Maruti Ram Gudavalli
Biomechanics Core, Palmer Center for Chiropractic Research, 741 Brady street, Davenport, IA 52803, USA

Robert M Rowell
Diagnosis and Radiology Department, Palmer College of Chiropractic, 1000 Brady street, Davenport, IA 52803, USA

Kent Jason Stuber
Division of Graduate Education and Research, Canadian Memorial Chiropractic College, 6100 Leslie Street, Toronto, ON M2H 3J1, Canada

Shari Wynd
Texas Chiropractic College, 5912 Spencer Highway, Pasadena, TX 77505- 1699, USA

Carol Ann Weis
Division of Graduate Education and Research, Canadian Memorial Chiropractic College, 6100 Leslie Street, Toronto, ON M2H 3J1, Canada

Michael J Schneider
Department of Physical Therapy, School of Health and Rehabilitation Sciences, Clinical and Translational Science Institute, University of Pittsburgh, Pittsburgh, PA, USA

Roni Evans
Center for Spirituality and Healing, Integrative Health and Wellbeing Research Program, University of Minnesota, Minneapolis, MN, USA

Mitchell Haas
University of Western States, Portland, OR, USA

Matthew Leach
School of Nursing and Midwifery, University of South Australia, Adelaide, SA, Australia

Cheryl Hawk
Logan College of Chiropractic, Chesterfield, MO, USA

Cynthia Long
Palmer Center for Chiropractic Research, Palmer College of Chiropractic, Davenport, IA, USA

Gregory D Cramer
National University of Health Sciences, Lombard, IL, USA

Oakland Walters
The Commonwealth Medical College, Scranton, PA, USA

Corrie Vihstadt
Center for Spirituality and Healing, Integrative Health and Wellbeing Research Program, University of Minnesota, Minneapolis, MN, USA

Lauren Terhorst
Department of Occupational Therapy, School of Health and Rehabilitation Sciences, University of Pittsburgh, Pittsburgh, PA, USA

Peter D Chapman
6 Claredon Court, Alexander Heights 6064, WA, Australia

J Stomski
School of Health Professions, Murdoch University, 90 South St, Murdoch 6150, WA, Australia

Barrett Losco
Discipline of Chiropractic, School of Health Professions, Murdoch University, 90 South St, Murdoch 6150, WA, Australia

Bruce F Walker
Discipline of Chiropractic, School of Health Professions, Murdoch University, 90 South St, Murdoch 6150, WA, Australia

Søren O'Neill
Spine Centre of Southern Denmark, Lillebælt Hospital, Østre Hougvej 55, 5500 Middelfart, DK, Denmark
Institute of Regional Health Research, University of Southern Denmark, Campusvej 55, 5230 Odense, DK, Denmark

Øystein Ødegaard-Olsen
Spine Centre of Southern Denmark, Lillebælt Hospital, Østre Hougvej 55, 5500 Middelfart, DK, Denmark

Beate Søvde
Stathelle Healthcentre, Brugata 10, 3960 Stathelle, Norway

Amir M Arab
Department of Physical Therapy, University of Social Welfare and Rehabilitation Sciences, Velenjak, Tehran, Iran

Ailin Talimkhani
University of Social Welfare and Rehabilitation Sciences, Velenjak, Tehran, Iran

Noureddin Karimi
University of Social Welfare and Rehabilitation Sciences, Velenjak, Tehran, Iran

Fetemeh Ehsani
University of Social Welfare and Rehabilitation Sciences, Velenjak, Tehran, Iran

Donald R Murphy
Clinical Director, Rhode Island Spine Center, 600 Pawtucket Avenue, Pawtucket, RI 02860 USA
Clinical Assistant Professor, Alpert Medical School of Brown University, Box G-A, Providence, RI 02912 USA

Brian D Justice
Private Practice of Chiropractic, Rochester Chiropractic Group, 1687 English RoadRochester, NY 14616 USA

Ian C Paskowski
Medical Director, Medical Back Pain Program at Jordan Hospital, 10 Cordage Park Circle, Suite 225, Plymouth, MA 02360 USA

Stephen M Perle
Professor of Clinical Sciences, University of Bridgeport, Bridgeport, CT 06604 USA

Michael J Schneider
Assistant Professor, School of Health and Rehabilitative Sciences, University of Pittsburgh, 4028 Forbes Tower, Pittsburgh, PA 15260 USA

Andreas Tunset
Department of Sports Science and Clinical Biomechanics, University of Southern Denmark, Campusvej 55, Odense M DK-5230, Denmark

Per Kjaer
Department of Sports Science and Clinical Biomechanics, University of Southern Denmark, Campusvej 55, Odense M DK-5230, Denmark
Research Department, Spine Centre of Southern Denmark, Lillebaelt Hospital, Oestre Hougvej 55, Middelfart DK-5500, Denmark

Shadi Samir Chreiteh
DELTA, Venlighedsvej 4, Hørsholm DK-2970, Denmark

Tue Secher Jensen
Research Department, Spine Centre of Southern Denmark, Lillebaelt Hospital, Oestre Hougvej 55, Middelfart DK-5500, Denmark

Søren O'Neill
SMI Laboratory for Human Experimental Pain Research, Center for Sensory- motor Interaction, Department of Health Science and Technology, University of Aalborg, Fredrik Bajers Vej 7, Bld. D3, 9220 Aalborg, Denmark
RCF Spine Center of Southern Denmark, Lillebælt Hospital, Østre Hougvej 55, 5500 Middelfart, Denmark
SDU Institute of Regional Health Research, University of Southern Denmark, Campusvej 55, 5230 Odense, Denmark

Thomas Graven-Nielsen
SMI Laboratory for Human Experimental Pain Research, Center for Sensory- motor Interaction, Department of Health Science and Technology, University of Aalborg, Fredrik Bajers Vej 7, Bld. D3, 9220 Aalborg, Denmark

Claus Manniche
RCF Spine Center of Southern Denmark, Lillebælt Hospital, Østre Hougvej 55, 5500 Middelfart, Denmark
SDU Institute of Regional Health Research, University of Southern Denmark, Campusvej 55, 5230 Odense, Denmark

Lars Arendt-Nielsen
SMI Laboratory for Human Experimental Pain Research, Center for Sensory- motor Interaction, Department of Health Science and Technology, University of Aalborg, Fredrik Bajers Vej 7, Bld. D3, 9220 Aalborg, Denmark

Hoda McClymont and Chad Perry
School of Management and Enterprise, University of Southern Queensland, 4350 Toowoomba, QLD, Australia

Jeff Gow
School of Commerce, University of Southern Queensland, Toowoomba, Australia
Research Associate, Health Economics and HIV/AIDS Research Division (HEARD), University of KwaZulu-Natal, Westville Campus, Durban, South Africa

Dennis DiGiorgi
DC, CHCQM, CCIC, Consultant Practice- Whitestone, New York, USA